ATLAS OF
CARDIOVASCULAR RISK FACTORS

Volume Editor
J. Michael Gaziano, MD, MPH
Associate Professor of Medicine

Harvard Medical School

Chief, Division of Aging

Brigham and Women's Hospital

Boston, Massachusetts

Director, Massachusetts Veterans Epidemiology Research and Information Center (MAVERIC)

Director, Boston Geriatric Research, Education and Clinical Center (GRECC)

VA Boston Healthcare System

Jamaica Plain, Massachusetts

Series Editor
Eugene Braunwald, MD, MD (Hon), ScD (Hon)
Distinguished Hersey Professor of Medicine

Harvard Medical School

Chairman, TIMI Study Group

Brigham and Women's Hospital

Boston, Massachusetts

With 41 contributors

Developed by Current Medicine LLC.

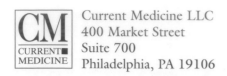

Current Medicine LLC
400 Market Street
Suite 700
Philadelphia, PA 19106

Developmental Editor: *Anthony Mirra*
Editorial Assistant: *Annmarie D'Ortona*
Cover Design: *William C. Whitman, Jr.*
Design and Layout: *Christine Keller-Quirk*
Illustrators: *Kim Broadbent, Theresa Englehart, Nicole Jones, Wieslawa Langenfeld, Maureen Looney, Deborah Lynam, John McCullough, Brian Mervine, Andrea Penka, and William C. Whitman, Jr.*
Assistant Production Manager: *Margaret La Mare*
Indexing: *Holly Lukens*

The photographs on the cover were provided by H. Thomas Aretz, MD, Michael B. Gravanis, MD, and F. John Service, MDCM, PhD.

Library of Congress Cataloging-in-Publication Data

Atlas of cardiovascular risk factors / volume editor, J. Michael Gaziano ; with 41 contributors.
    p. ; cm. - (Atlas of heart diseases)
  Includes bibliographical references and index.
  ISBN 1-57340-232-X
  1. Cardiovascular system--Diseases--Risk factors--Atlases. 2. Heart--Diseases--Risk factors--Atlases. I. Title: Cardiovascular risk factors. II. Gaziano, J. Michael (John Michael), 1961 - III. Atlas of heart disease (Unnumbered)
  [DNLM: 1. Heart Diseases--epidemiology--Atlases. 2. Risk Factors--Atlases. WG 17 A88156 2005]
  RA645.C34A89 2005
  614.5'91--dc22   2005049669

ISBN 1-57340-232-X

Printed in Hong Kong by Phoenix Color Asia

10 9 8 7 6 5 4 3 2 1

Preface

The world is in the midst of a two-century long transition from acute infectious illnesses and malnutrition to chronic illness dominated by cardiovascular disease as the major cause of death and disability. Coronary heart disease (CHD) is now the world's leading cause of death. This transition is occurring in every part of the globe among all races, ethnic groups, and cultures.

Once thought of as a natural consequence of aging, CHD is now understood to be very much a "man-made" disease, heavily influenced by the choices we make. The past 50 years have seen great progress in identifying a large number of lifestyle, as well as biochemical and even genetic, factors associated with heart disease. Our ever-increasing knowledge about the pathogenesis of atherosclerosis has enhanced our understanding of the substantial role these risk factors play in the development of CHD and have led to potential strategies to reduce the risk of developing or delaying its progression. Randomized trials demonstrated the benefits of various interventions for reducing the risk associated with some of the major risk factors.

Because many risk factors contribute to CHD risk, for most people, successful disease prevention or amelioration requires that we simultaneously address a spectrum of factors. Knowledge about risk factors can be used for two purposes. First, risk factor information can be used to assess the risk of a future event and to identify subgroups of individuals at very high risk. Second, many risk factors are potential targets for interventions to reduce risk. Some risk factors, such as age and gender, are useful only as predictors, whereas others, such as smoking and high blood pressure, serve as predictors and targets for intervention.

This Atlas provides a succinct overview and an update of current knowledge of the major causative factors for heart disease and other forms of cardiovascular disease and strategies to reduce the risk associated with those factors. It is intended to help physicians to understand how to use individual risk factor data to develop an integrated strategy that they believe will be the most successful for lowering risk in an individual patient. It begins with a discussion of the extent to which cardiovascular disease and it risk factors have grown over the past century around the word. The next three chapters introduce general concepts about risk factors, how to screen for them, and integrate the information into an assessment of overall risk. In subsequent chapters on each risk factor, we have provided detailed information on the strength of its association with the risk of CHD and the evidence of benefits of intervention strategies to reduce risk when available.

Later chapters discuss risk factors and prevention strategies in special populations including women, children, and the elderly. The final chapter outlines an integrated, logical strategy that physicians can easily implement to assess a patient's risk and then a systematic approach to developing a prescription for risk reduction. After determining the long-term risk, the clinician can implement the risk-reduction strategy that best suits a particular patient. I have prioritized these interventions into three categories based on the strength of the association of the risk factors with CHD and the evidence of benefit of the intervention.

Over the past 30 years, age-adjusted CHD mortality in the United States has dropped by more than 40%. However, there is concern that rates may once again be creeping up, fueled by an epidemic of obesity, diabetes, and physical inactivity—even among children—all major risk factors for heart disease. Given the abundance of information about how to prevent CHD, this is difficult to fathom. Similar trends are apparent in other developed countries. In much of the developing world, CHD rates are rising rapidly. The concepts presented in this volume provide a conceptual frame work to continue the favorable trends in the developed world and to slow the rise or even reverse these increasing trends in other parts of the globe.

J. Michael Gaziano, MD

Dedication

This book is dedicated to my parents who stimulated my love of the sciences early in life; to my many mentors and teachers who inspired me to learn, and to my wife, Anne, and children, Michaela, Dante and Liam, who give meaning to my every day.

J. Michael Gaziano, MD

Contributors

Robert Allan, PhD
Clinical Assistant Professor in Psychology
    and Psychiatry
Weill Medical College of Cornell University
Assistant Attending Psychologist
    in Psychiatry
New York Presbyterian Hospital
New York, New York

Ezra A. Amsterdam, MD
Professor
Department of Internal Medicine
University of California Davis School
    of Medicine
Associate Chief, Division of Cardiology
University of California Davis Medical Center
Sacramento, California

Shari S. Bassuk, ScD
Epidemiologist
Division of Preventive Medicine
Brigham and Women's Hospital
Boston, Massachusetts

Gerald S. Berenson, MD, MS
Professor
Departments of Epidemiology, Medicine,
    Cardiology, and Pediatric Cardiology
Tulane University Health Sciences Center
New Orleans, Louisiana

Thomas S. Bowman, MD, MPH
Instructor in Medicine
Harvard Medical School
Associate Physician
Department of Internal Medicine
Division of Aging
Brigham and Women's Hospital
VA Boston Healthcare System
Boston, Massachusetts

Edward Boyko, MD, MPH
Professor
Department of Medicine
University of Washington
Chief, General Internal Medicine
VA Puget Sound Health Care System
Seattle, Washington

Julie E. Buring, ScD
Professor of Medicine
Harvard Medical School
Brigham and Women's Hospital
Boston, Massachusetts

David Chiriboga, MD, MPH
Assistant Professor
Department of Family Medicine and
    Community Health
University of Massachusetts Medical School
Worcester, Massachusetts

S. Michael Clark, MD
Physician
Department of Internal and
    Preventive Medicine
Cooper Clinic
Dallas, Texas

Akshay S. Desai, MD, MPH
Fellow
Department of Cardiology and Medicine
Harvard Medical School
Fellow in Cardiology
Brigham and Women's Hospital
Boston, Massachusetts

Daniel E. Forman, MD
Assistant Professor of Medicine
Harvard Medical School
Director, Exercise Testing Laboratory
Brigham and Women's Hospital
Boston, Massachusetts
Clinical Scientist
Boston Geriatric Research, Education
    and Clinical Center (GRECC)
VA Boston Healthcare System
Jamaica Plain, Massachusetts

J. Michael Gaziano, MD, MPH
Associate Professor of Medicine
Harvard Medical School
Chief, Division of Aging
Brigham and Women's Hospital
Boston, Massachusetts
Director, Massachusetts Veterans
    Epidemiology Research and
    Information Center (MAVERIC)
Director, Boston Geriatric Research,
    Education and Clinical Center (GRECC)
VA Boston Healthcare System
Jamaica Plain, Massachusetts

Thomas A. Gaziano, MD, MSC
Instructor in Medicine
Department of Medicine
Harvard Medical School
Associate Physician of
    Cardiovascular Medicine
Brigham and Women's Hospital
Boston, Massachusetts

Larry W. Gibbons, MD, MPH
President
Cooper Clinic
Dallas, Texas

Heather L. Gornik, MD, MHS
Clinical Fellow
Department of Medicine
Harvard Medical School
Fellow in Cardiovascular Medicine
Brigham and Women's Hospital
Boston, Massachusetts

Francine Grodstein, ScD
Associate Professor
Department of Medicine
Harvard Medical School
Epidemiologist
Brigham and Women's Hospital
Boston, Massachusetts

Jiang He, MD, PhD
Professor and Chairman
Department of Epidemiology
Tulane University School of Public
    Health & Tropical Medicine
New Orleans, Louisiana

Paul A. Heidenreich, MD, MS
Assistant Professor
Department of Medicine
Stanford University
Stanford, California
Director of Echocardiography
VA Palo Alto Healthcare System
Palo Alto, California

Charles H. Hennekens, MD, DrPH
Professor of Medicine, Epidemiology
    and Public Health
University of Miami School of Medicine
Professor of Biomedical Science, Center
    of Excellence
Florida Atlantic University
Boca Raton, Florida

Frank B. Hu, MD, PhD
Associate Professor
Department of Nutrition
Harvard School of Public Health
Boston, Massachusetts

C. Tissa Kappagoda, MBBS, PhD
Professor
Department of Internal Medicine
University of California Davis School
   of Medicine
Director, Preventive Cardiology
University of California Davis
   Medical Center
Sacramento, California

Carlos S. Kase, MD
Professor and Chair
Department of Neurology
Boston University School of Medicine
Neurologist-in-Chief
Boston Medical Center
Boston, Massachusetts

Sekar Kathiresan, MD
Instructor
Department of Medicine
Harvard Medical School
Director, Cardiac Rehabilitation Program
Cardiology Division
Massachusetts General Hospital
Boston, Massachusetts

Arthur L. Klatsky, MD
Senior Consultant in Cardiology
Kaiser Permanente Medical Center
Oakland, California

Harlan M. Krumholz, MD, SM
Professor of Medicine, Epidemiology
   and Public Health
Department of Medicine
Division of Cardiovascular Medicine
Yale University School of Medicine
Director, Center for Outcomes Research
   and Evaluation
Yale-New Haven Hospital
New Haven, Connecticut

Tobias Kurth, MD, ScD
Instructor of Medicine
Division of Aging
Harvard Medical School
Associate Epidemiologist
Brigham and Women's Hospital
Boston, Massachusetts

JoAnn E. Manson, MD, DrPH
Professor of Medicine
Elizabeth F. Brigham Professor of
   Women's Health
Harvard Medical School
Chief, Division of Preventive Medicine
Brigham and Women's Hospital
Boston, Massachusetts

Daniel B. Mark, MD, MPH
Professor of Medicine
Department of Medicine
Duke Clinical Research Institute
Co-Director, Coronary Care Unit
Duke University Medical Center
Durham, North Carolina

Karin Nelson, MD, MSHS
Assistant Professor
Department of Medicine
University of Washington
Staff Physician
VA Puget Sound Health Care System
Seattle, Washington

Ira S. Ockene, MD, FACC
David and Barbara Milliken Professor
   of Preventive Cardiology
Director, Preventive Cardiology Program
Department of Medicine
University of Massachusetts Medical School
Worcester, Massachusetts

Christopher J. O'Donnell, MD, MPH
Assistant Professor
Department of Medicine
Massachusetts General Hospital
Harvard Medical School
Boston, Massachusetts
Associate Director
National Heart, Lung, and Blood Institute's
   Framingham Heart Study
Framingham, Massachusetts

Jorge Plutzky, MD
Assistant Professor of Medicine
Harvard Medical School
Director, The Vascular Disease
   Prevention Program
Brigham and Women's Hospital
Boston, Massachusetts

Gayle Reiber, PhD, MPH
Professor
Departments of Health Services
   and Epidemiology
University of Washington
Research Career Scientist
VA Puget Sound Health Care System
Seattle, Washington

Paul M Ridker, MD, MPH
Eugene Braunwald Professor of Medicine
Department of Medicine
Harvard Medical School
Director, Center for Cardiovascular
   Disease Prevention
Brigham and Women's Hospital
Boston, Massachusetts

Stephen Scheidt, MD
Professor of Clinical Medicine
Department of Cardiology
New York-Presbyterian Hospital
Weill Cornell Medical Center
New York, New York

Howard D. Sesso, ScD, MPH
Assistant Professor in Medicine
Department of Medicine
Harvard Medical School
Associate Epidemiologist
Brigham and Women's Hospital
Boston, Massachusetts

Peter H. Stone, MD
Associate Professor of Medicine
Department of Medicine
Cardiovascular Division
Harvard Medical School
Co-Director, Samuel A. Levine Cardiac Unit
Brigham and Women's Hospital
Boston, Massachusetts

Natalia Udaltsova, PhD
Data Consultant
Division of Research
Kaiser Permanente Medical Center
Oakland, California

Nanette K. Wenger, MD
Professor
Department of Medicine
Division of Cardiology
Emory University School of Medicine
Chief of Cardiology
Grady Memorial Hospital
Atlanta, Georgia

Paul K. Whelton, MD, MSc
Professor
Department of Epidemiology
Tulane University School of Public
   Health & Tropical Medicine
Department of Medicine
Tulane University School of Medicine
Senior Vice President for Health Sciences
Tulane University Health Sciences Center
New Orleans, Louisiana

Peter W. F. Wilson, MD
Professor
Department of Endocrinology, Diabetes
   and Medical Genetics
Medical University of South Carolina
Charleston, South Carolina

Contents

Historical Perspective on Heart Disease and Worldwide Trends

Thomas A. Gaziano and
J. Michael Gaziano

At the beginning of the 20th century, cardiovascular disease (CVD) was responsible for less than 10% of all deaths worldwide. Today, that figure is approximately 30%. In 2001, CVD became the number-one cause of death worldwide, and is now the leading cause of death in most developing regions with the exception of Sub-Saharan Africa [1–4].

Over the past two centuries, the Industrial and Technological Revolutions and the economic and social transformations associated with them have resulted in a dramatic shift in the causes of illness and death. Known as the *epidemiologic transition*, this shift is highly correlated with changes in personal and collective wealth (economic transition), social structure (social transition), and demographics (demographic transition). Omran [5] developed an excellent model of the epidemiologic transition, dividing the transition into three basic ages—Pestilence and Famine, Receding Pandemics, and Degenerative and Man-made Diseases (*see* Fig. 1-3). Olshansky and Ault [6] added a fourth stage—Delayed Degenerative Diseases—and troubling trends may foreshadow a fifth as-yet-unnamed stage of the epidemiologic transition. This stage is characterized by an epidemic of obesity and an increase in age-adjusted CVD mortality rates, which have been declining in developed countries.

Some parts of the developing world—for example, sub-Saharan Africa and parts of India—have yet to emerge from the Age of Pestilence and Famine, which is characterized by the predominance of malnutrition and infectious disease, and by the infrequency of CVD. The Age of Receding Pandemics is marked by increases in wealth that lead to improved nutrition because of better availability of food, improved sanitation, and access to vaccines and antibiotics. The Age of Degenerative Man-made Diseases includes dramatic lifestyle changes in diet, activity levels, and behaviors such as smoking that set the stage for the emergence of atherosclerosis. The average lifespan increases beyond 50 years of age and mortality, from CVD in particular and other noncommunicable diseases, exceeds mortality from malnutrition and infectious diseases. The predominant form of CVD is coronary heart disease, but ischemic stroke also emerges as a significant cause of mortality and morbidity. Cancer rates also rise rapidly. The emerging market economies of the former Soviet socialist states currently fall into this category. In the Age of Delayed Degenerative Diseases, CVD and cancer continue to be the major causes of morbidity and mortality. However, in industrialized nations, technologic advances such as bypass surgery are implemented, and because of widespread primary and secondary prevention efforts, deaths are prevented. Age-adjusted CVD mortality tends to decline.

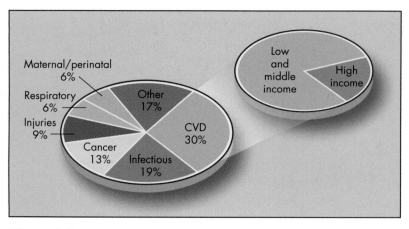

Figure 1-1.
Changing patterns of mortality (20th to 21st century). A century ago, cardiovascular disease (CVD) accounted for less than 10% of all deaths worldwide. Today, CVD is responsible for approximately 30% of all deaths [1]. This increase can be traced to a dramatic shift in the health status of people around the world during the 20th century and to a major change in the distribution of disease. Before 1900, infectious diseases and malnutrition were the most common causes of death; but, primarily because of improved nutrition and public health measures, they have gradually been supplanted by CVD and cancer in most countries. As these improvements continue to spread to developing countries, CVD mortality rates are also increasing. In fact, today, approximately 80% of the global burden of CVD death occurs in low- and middle-income countries.

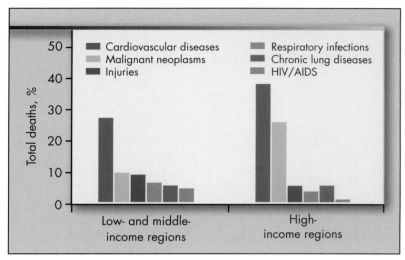

Figure 1-2.
Cardiovascular disease (CVD) is also now the leading cause of death in developing countries. In seminal work by Murray and Lopez [2] in the 1990s, CVD was predicted to be the number-one cause of death and disability worldwide by 2020 mainly because of an increase in low- and middle-income countries. In fact, by 2001, CVD became the leading cause of death in the developing world as it had been in the developed world since the middle of the 1900s [1,3,4]. Nearly half of all deaths in high-income (developed) countries and approximately 28% of deaths in low- and middle-income (developing) countries are the result of CVD [1]. Other causes of death, such as injuries, respiratory infections, nutritional deficiency, and HIV/AIDS, collectively still play a predominant role in certain regions, but it is clear now that, even in these areas, CVD is a significant cause of mortality.

Typical Stages of the Epidemiologic Transition

Stage	Description	Deaths related to CVD, %	Predominant CVD type
Pestilence and Famine	Predominance of malnutrition and infectious diseases as causes of death; high rates of infant and child mortality; low mean life expectancy	< 10	Rheumatic heart disease, cardiomyopathies caused by infection and malnutrition
Receding Pandemics	Improvements in nutrition and public health lead to decrease in rates of deaths related to malnutrition and infection; precipitous decline in infant and child mortality rates	10–35	Rheumatic valvular disease, hypertension, coronary heart disease, and stroke
Degenerative and Man-made Diseases	Increased fat and caloric intake and decrease in physical activity lead to emergence of hypertension and atherosclerosis; with increase in life expectancy, mortality from chronic, noncommunicable diseases exceeds mortality from malnutrition and infectious disease	35–65	Coronary heart disease and stroke
Delayed Degenerative Diseases	CVD and cancer are the major causes of morbidity and mortality; better treatment and prevention efforts help avoid deaths among those with disease and delay primary events; age-adjusted CVD morality declines; CVD affecting older and older individuals	40–50	Coronary heart disease, stroke, and congestive heart failure

Figure 1-3.
Four typical stages of the epidemiologic transition. The emergence of high cardiovascular disease (CVD) incidence in all regions of the world reflects changes that have occurred to varying degrees across the world. The Industrial and Technological Revolutions and their associated economic and social transformations have resulted in dramatic shifts in the diseases responsible for illness and death. Known as the *epidemiologic transition*, these changes in morbidity and mortality are linked to changes in personal and collective wealth (economic transition), social structure (social transition), and demo

graphics (demographic transition). Omran [5] developed an insightful model of the epidemiologic transition. He divided the transition into three basic ages—Pestilence and Famine, Receding Pandemics, and Degenerative Man-made Diseases. A fourth stage, Delayed Degenerative Diseases, was added by Olshansky and Ault [6]. However, countries tend to enter these stages at different times. The progression from one stage to the next usually proceeds in a predictable manner, with the rate and the nature of cardiovascular diseases changing over the course of the transition. (*Adapted from* Omran [5].)

Atlas of Cardiovascular Risk Factors

Age of Pestilence and Famine (1800s to 1900)	Age of Receding Pandemics (1900 to 1930)	Age of Degenerative and Man-made Diseases (1930 to 1965)	Age of Declining Degenerative Disease (1965 to 2000)	Age of ? (2000+)
Agrarian economy, rural lifestyles	Industrialization/urbanization	Increased urbanization and industrialization	Fully industrialized	Overweight and obesity increase at alarming pace
Tuberculosis, pneumonia, and diarrheal disease cause most deaths	Major change in diet and activity	Improved health care systems	Improved standard of care and prevention measures for those with, and at risk of, CVD	Diabetes and hypertension are increasing
CVD and cancer mortality < 10% of the total	Emergence of a public health infrastructure	Mortality rates related to malnutrition and infectious disease continue to decrease	Decreased smoking	Decline in smoking rates has leveled off
	Mortality rates related to malnutrition and infectious disease decline	Increased smoking and high-fat diet; lower activity levels	CVD and stroke rates decline	Only a minority of the population meets minimal physical activity recommendations
	CVD and cancer mortality rates increase	CHD, stoke, and cancer mortality rates continue to increase	Some cancer mortality rates fall while others increase	

Figure 1-4.
Timeline of epidemiologic transition in the United States. The United States, like other established market economies, has passed through the four stages of the epidemiologic transition. From its founding until approximately 1900, the United States was in the Age of Pestilence and Famine. Tuberculosis and other infectious diseases accounted for the majority of deaths; cardiovascular disease (CVD) accounted for less than 10% of all deaths. By the turn of the century, the society was still largely agrarian, but industrialization and urbanization were well under way. Per capita income and life expectancy were increasing— from approximately 35 years to 47.8 years for men and 50.7 years for women. Rapid social changes around this time signaled the beginning of the Age of Receding Pandemics. These changes included industrialization, the emergence of a public health structure and improvements in the water supply, with a decline in infectious disease deaths and an increase in CVD mortality. By the middle of the century, with an increase in smoking rates, a high-fat diet, and lower activity levels, the Age of Degenerative and Man-made Diseases reached its peak with coronary heart disease (CHD) and stroke as the leading causes of death. In the latter part of the 20th century, the United States entered the Age of Declining Degenerative diseases with improved techniques to treat and prevent CVD and a decline in smoking rates. The United States experienced a significant decline in CVD mortality rates as a result. Troubling trends may signal that the country is entering a fifth as-yet-unnamed phase of the epidemiologic transition, which may be characterized by an epidemic of obesity.

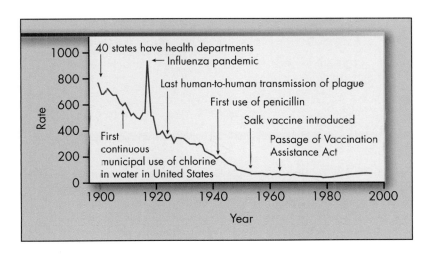

Figure 1-5.
Decline in mortality because of infectious disease in the United States (1900 to 1996). Early in the 20th century, the United States entered the Age of Receding Pandemics as the primarily rural, agricultural-based economy shifted to an urban, industrial-based economy. Food supplies became more abundant, but the consumption of fruits and vegetables declined as consumption of meats and grains increased. With the emergence of a public health infrastructure, municipal use of chlorine to disinfect water became widespread, and pasteurization and other improvements in food handling were introduced. Between 1900 and 1930, life expectancy increased by 10 years, and infectious disease mortality rates fell dramatically, largely because of rapidly declining infant, childhood, and adolescent mortality from malnutrition and infectious diseases. Age-adjusted CVD mortality, however, was on the rise. Around 1930, the Unites States entered the Age of Degenerative and Man-made Diseases.

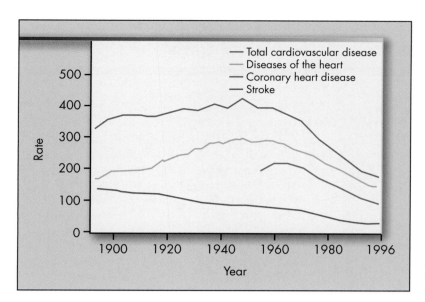

Figure 1-6.
Increase and decline in heart disease rates through the epidemiologic transition in the United States (1900 to 1996). In the 1930s and 1940s, smoking and fat consumption continued to rise, as did the prevalence of heart disease. The United States had entered the third phase of the epidemiologic transition, the Age of Degenerative and Man-made Diseases. By 1955, 55% of adult men were smoking, and fat consumption represented approximately 40% of total calories. Americans were also becoming more sedentary as a result of continued mechanization and urbanization and the rise of the suburbs after World War II; more people were driving instead of walking and bicycling. Another important development affecting the health of Americans post–World War II was the growth of the health care industry. By the late 1950s, more than two thirds of the working population had some form of private insurance [7]. As the 1960s progressed, age-adjusted cardiovascular disease mortality rates began to decline, marking the beginning of the fourth phase of the transition, the Age of Delayed Degenerative Diseases. Since then, there have been substantial reductions in rates of mortality from stroke and coronary heart disease. This decline can be attributed primarily to two main factors—therapeutic advances and prevention measures targeted at people with cardiovascular disease, as well as those potentially at risk for it [8–10]. Healthier lifestyles may have actually had an even greater impact on the decline in age-adjusted rates of death. For example, improvements in diet because of access to fresh fruits and vegetables year-round in developed countries may have contributed to declining cholesterol mean levels before effective drug therapy was widely available.

Economic, Demographic, and Social Transitions: Trends in the United States During the 20th Century

Trend	1900	1930	1970	2000
Population (in millions), *n*	76	123	203	281
Mean income	N/A	$15,050 (1947)	$26,333	$29,058
Age-adjusted CVD mortality (per 100,000)	325	390	699	341
Age-adjusted CHD mortality (per 100,000)	N/A	N/A	448	186
Age-adjusted smoke mortality (per 100,000)	140	100	148	57
Urbanization, %	39	56	74	76
Life expectancy	49.2	59.3	70.8	76.9
Smoking				
Cigarettes per capita, *n*	54	1185	3969	1977
Smokers, %	N/A	N/A	37.4	23.3
Total caloric intake, *kcal*	3500	3300	3200	3800
Fat intake (total calories), %	31.6	37.3	41.2	33
Cholesterol level, *mg/dL*	N/A	N/A	216	204
Overweight or obese individuals, %	N/A	N/A	47.7	64.5

Figure 1-7.
Economic, demographic, and social transitions: trends in the United States during the 20th century. Parallel transformations—economic, demographic, and social—accompanied the epidemiologic transition in the United States during the past century. Increasing per capita income marked the economic transition. Social transition was driven by industrialization that sparked a large number of changes, including urbanization. Sixty percent of the population lived in rural settings in 1900, compared with only 20% at the beginning of the 21st century. Changes in lifestyle associated with these economic and social transitions caused shifts in the profile of risk behaviors and risk factors for disease. These included decreased physical activity, increased smoking, and dramatic changes in diet, such as a higher percentage of meat and other foods high in fat. The result was an increase in coronary heart disease (CHD) and stroke mortality, indicators that a country is in the third phase of the epidemiologic transition, the Age of Degenerative and Man-made Diseases. Then, as the pendulum swung back, during the fourth phase of the transition (the Age of Declining Degenerative Diseases), smoking rates fell, and the diet became less fat laden. However, even within a given country, segments of the population may undergo the epidemiologic transition at varying rates. The transitions generally begin among those with higher socioeconomic status, and eventually spread to those with lower socioeconomic status. CVD—cardiovascular disease; N/A—not available. (*Data from* US Census Bureau and National Center for Health Statistics, Centers for Disease Control and Prevention.)

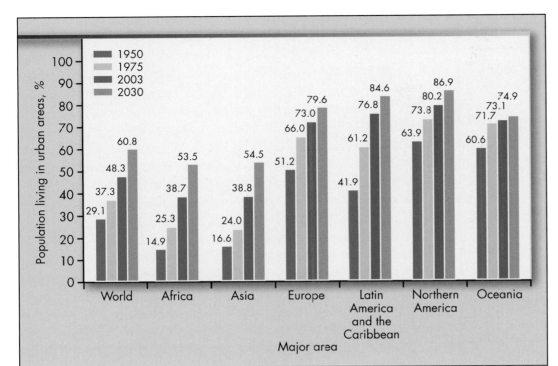

Figure 1-8.
Number of people living in urban areas. Several parallel transformations accompany the epidemiologic transition and include economic, demographic, and social transitions. The latter is driven by industrialization and is typically accompanied by urbanization. As a major social force, urbanization affects living standards and lifestyle and affords the opportunity to develop organized health care systems. Virtually every part of the world has seen a shift from rural to urban life. In the United States, for example, at the beginning of the 20th century, 60% of the population lived in rural settings compared with only 20% at the beginning of the 21st century. In Latin America, Asia, and Africa, a similar shift has occurred over the second half of the 20th century. However, the shift is relative. Latin America and the Caribbean have become highly urbanized, with more than 75% of residents living in urban areas in 2003, whereas Asia and Africa are still primarily rural [11].

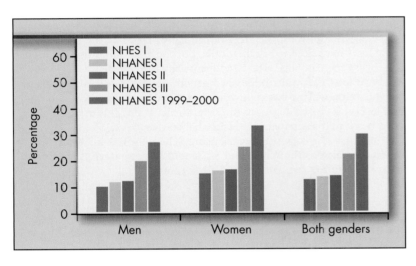

Figure 1-9.
Obesity emerging as a new health concern. Although rates of coronary heart disease and stroke fell 2% to 3% per year through the 1970s and 1980s, the rate of decline has slowed. In the United States, physical activity continues to decline as total caloric intake increases. Overweight and obesity are escalating at an alarming pace, while rates of type 2 diabetes, hypertension, and lipid abnormalities associated with obesity are on the rise. This trend is not unique to only developed countries, however. According to the World Health Organization, worldwide more than 1 billion adults are overweight and 300 million are clinically obese. Even more disturbing are increases in childhood obesity, leading to large increases in diabetes and hypertension. If these trends continue, age-adjusted cardiovascular disease mortality rates could increase in the United States and in other countries in the coming years. These changes suggest that the United States could be entering a fifth as-yet-unnamed phase of the epidemiologic transition, characterized by an epidemic of obesity. NHANES—National Health and Nutrition Examination Survey; NHES—National Health Examination Survey.

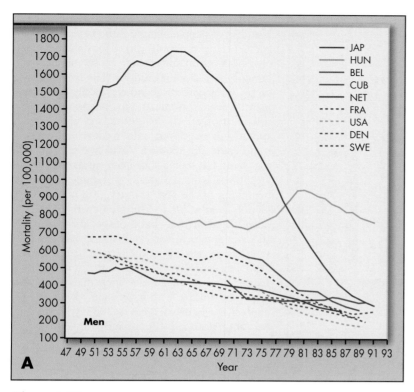
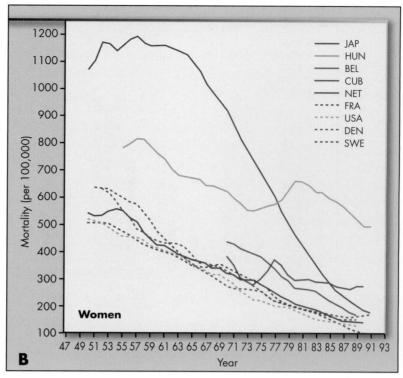

Figure 1-10.

Japan's epidemiologic transition compared with other high-income countries. **A,** Men. **B,** Women. Japan's epidemiologic transition is unique compared with other high-income countries. In many developed countries, the epidemiologic transition started approximately 100 to 150 years ago and followed a pattern similar to the United States. In Japan, the transition started later, but proceeded much more rapidly. Japan is unique among the established market economy countries. As the rate of communicable diseases fell in the early part of the 20th century, stroke rates increased dramatically, eventually becoming the highest in the world by the middle of the century. Coronary heart disease (CHD) rates, however, did not rise as sharplyas they did in other industrialized countries, and have remained lower. Since the 1970s, stroke rates have declined dramatically, but there are indications of a possible recent increase in CHD. The historically lower heart disease rates may be at least partly attributable to genetic factors, but it is more likely that the average plant-based, low-fat diet and the resultant low cholesterol levels have played a more important role. If CHD is increasing, it could be related to changes in dietary habits that Japan, like so many other countries, is currently experiencing. These include a 7.4-fold increase in dairy consumption and a 5.3-fold increase in consumption of fats and oils in the last half of the 20th century [12].

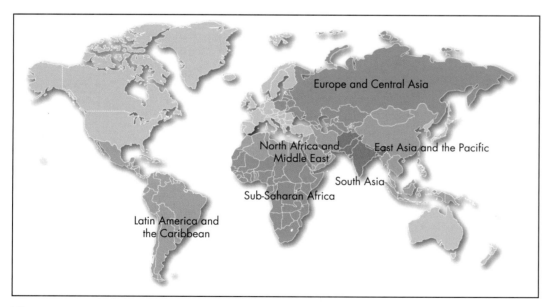

Figure 1-11.

Geographic and economic regions of the developing world. With the exception of Japan, most high-income countries followed the epidemiologic transition outlined by the United States example. The six developing regions are at various phases of the epidemiologic transition. Where development has occurred, it often has been at a more compressed rate than in the high-income countries. The World Bank treats all high-income countries as one region even though they are not geographically contiguous, and then divides the remaining low- and middle-income countries into six geographic regions. High-income countries (gross national income per capita > $9205) include the established market economies of North America, western Europe, Australia, New Zealand, and Japan. The six regions are East Asia and the Pacific (EAP) with China representing the bulk of its population, Europe and Central Asia (ECA), Latin America and the Caribbean (LAC), Middle East and North Africa (MNA), South Asia (SAR) with India as its largest member, and sub-Saharan Africa (SSA).

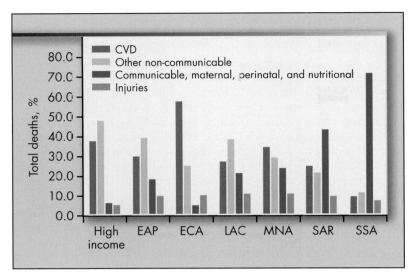

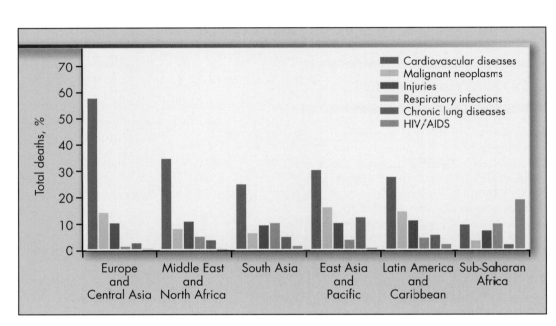

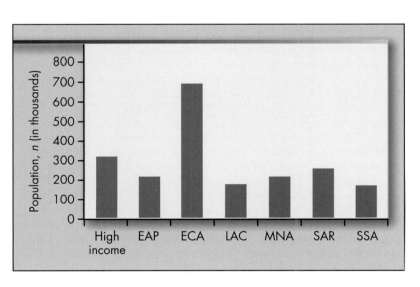

Figure 1-12.

Burden of disease for the economic regions of the world. National health and disease profiles vary widely by country and by region. These vast differences in burden of disease are readily apparent across the economic and geographic sectors of the world. For example, life expectancy in Japan (81.8 years) is more than twice that in Sierra Leone (34 years) [13]. The Europe and Central Asia (ECA) region consisting mostly of the emerging market economies of the former socialist states, is dominated by the highest rates of cardiovascular disease (CVD) mortality in the world. However, in the sub-Saharan Africa (SSA) region, over 60% of deaths are the result of so-called group I diseases (communicable, maternal and perinatal conditions, and nutritional deficiencies). In India, Bangladesh, and other countries that comprise the high-mortality developing countries of the South Asia Region (SAR), 40% of deaths are from group I diseases. In contrast, group I diseases account for just 6% of deaths in high-income countries. EAP—East Asia and the Pacific; LAC—Latin America and the Caribbean; MNA—Middle East and North Africa.

Figure 1-13.

Shifting worldwide burden of heart disease: top six causes of death in low- and middle-income countries. An epidemiologic transition much like the one that occurred in the United States over the past century is taking place throughout the world. As was the case in the United States during the first half of the 1900s, cardiovascular disease (CVD) rates have risen steadily across the globe. As a result of these trends, CVD is the leading cause of death in all World Bank regions with the exception of Saharan Africa, where HIV/AIDS has emerged as the leading cause of mortality [1]. At the close of the 20th century, 28% of all deaths worldwide were because of CVD, with the majority of deaths occurring in developing countries [2]. Between 1990 and 2020, ischemic heart disease alone is anticipated to increase by 120% for women and 137% for men in developing countries, compared with age-related increases of between 30% and 60% in developed countries [14].

Figure 1-14.

Cardiovascular disease (CVD) deaths per 100,000 population. Although 80% of CVD deaths come from the low- and middle-income regions, the death rates for most regions are still less than the rate of the high-income countries of 320 per 100,000 annually. The marked exception is the Europe and Central Asia regions, which have a rate of 690 CVD deaths per 100,000, more than double that of the high-income countries. ECA—Europe and Central Asia; EAP—East Asia and the Pacific; LAC—Latin America and the Caribbean; MNA—Middle East and North Africa; SAR—South Asia Region; SSA—sub-Saharan Africa.

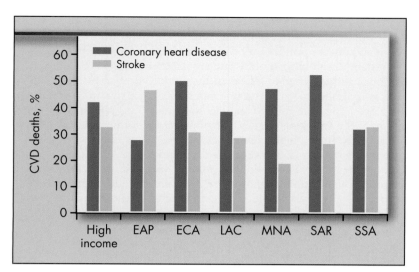

Figure 1-15.
The relative contribution of coronary heart disease and stroke to cardiovascular disease mortality across world regions. The consistent pattern for most high-income countries going through the epidemiologic transition has been high rates of stroke (mostly hemorrhagic). This is because hypertension appears to be the first risk factor to develop along the epidemiologic transition pathway. Only in the third phase, with increased diabetes, increased smoking rates, and adverse lipid profiles, do coronary heart disease (CHD) rates climb. This is also accompanied by better control of severe hypertension, reducing the rates of hemorrhagic stroke to be replaced by ischemic stroke. Most regions appear to follow this pattern and have a predominance of CHD. The two exceptions are sub-Saharan Africa (SSA) and the East Asia Pacific (EAP) region. SSA is in the earlier phase of the epidemiologic transition. The EAP region's pattern is dominated by China's population and appears to be a result of its stage in the transition, but perhaps it is also following a pattern similar to Japan's, which is dominated by more strokes and less CHD deaths. CVD—cardiovascular disease; ECA—Europe and Central Asia; LAC—Latin America and the Caribbean; MNA—Middle East and North Africa; SAR—South Asia Region.

Status of the Epidemiologic Transition in 2004

Transition stage	World's population, %	Regions
Pestilence and Famine	11	Sub-Saharan Africa; parts of all regions excluding high-income
Receding Pandemics	38	South Asia; parts of Latin America and the Caribbean and southern East Asia and the Pacific
Degenerative and Man-made Diseases	35	Europe and Central Asia, Latin America and the Caribbean, Middle East and North Africa, northern East Asia and the Pacific, and urban parts of most regions, especially India
Delayed Degenerative Diseases with increasing obesity	15	High-income countries, parts of Latin America and the Caribbean

Figure 1-16.

Status of the epidemiologic transition in 2004. With roughly 840 million people, the United States and the other established market economy countries (Canada, Australia, New Zealand, western Europe, and Japan), currently comprise a little more than 15% of the world's population. Rapid declines in coronary heart disease (CHD) and stroke rates since the early 1970s indicate that these countries are in the fourth phase of the epidemiologic transition, the Age of Delayed Degenerative Diseases. In these countries, CHD rates tend to be two- to fivefold higher than stroke rates. Although it is unclear why, in Portugal and Japan the opposite is true, with stroke rates higher than CHD rates. Despite large regional variations, HIV/AIDS-plagued sub-Saharan Africa remains largely in the first phase of the epidemiologic transition, which is marked by communicable disease rates that far exceed those of chronic diseases. Heterogeneity is also apparent throughout the rest of the developing world—even within countries. Some regions of India,

for example, appear to be in the first phase of the transition, whereas others are in the second or even the third phase. China looks to be straddling the second and third phases with apparent regional differences in cardiovascular disease (CVD) rates. A north-south gradient has emerged, with higher CVD rates in northern China than in southern China. Within the Middle East and North Africa region, the majority of the Middle Eastern Crescent appears to be entering the third phase of the epidemiologic transition; increasing economic wealth has been accompanied by a rapid increase in CVD. As a whole, Latin America seems to be in the third phase also, but this region, as defined by the World Bank, includes all of South America, where residents of some countries are still at risk of contracting malaria and dengue fever, and those portions are still in the first transitional phase. The Europe and Central Asia regions are firmly in the peak of the third phase of the transition, with CVD representing 60% of all deaths.

Double Burden of Disease in Low-income Countries (Deaths by Cause)

Region	Communicable diseases*	Noncommunicable conditions
Africa	7779	2252
The Americas	875	4543
Eastern Mediterranean	1746	2030
Europe	567	8112
Southeast Asia	5730	7423
Western Pacific	1701	9000

*Includes maternal and perinatal conditions and nutritional deficiencies.

Figure 1-17.

Double burden of disease in low-income countries. Most developing countries now face the "double burden" presented by communicable and noncommunicable disease. Limited resources are stretched thin as they struggle to address an epidemic of heart disease while continuing to battle HIV/AIDS, tuberculosis, and other infectious diseases. In so-called "young" developing countries, with a high proportion of citizens under 65, the onset of CVD will occur among ever-younger people, posing a threat to economic and social development [15]. The level of death and disability attributable to cardiovascular disease in the labor force will be much greater than in Western nations, now or even in the past. If this tide is to be reversed, the next 20 years will be important, as the prevalence of risk factors for chronic disease, driven by urbanization and globalization, increases in many of these countries. (*Adapted from* Reddy and Yusuf [15].)

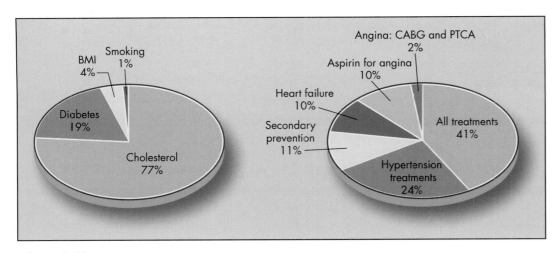

Figure 1-18.

The epidemiologic tranisition in the East Asia Pacific region (Beijing, 1984–1999; additional deaths attributable to risk factor changes [*left panel*]; deaths prevented or postponed by treatments [*right panel*]). The diversity of economic circumstances in these countries is reflected in the status and character of the epidemiologic transition across the region. Average life expectancy in South Korea (mean annual per capital gross national product [GNP] of $9700 and a high-income country according to the World Bank) is 75 years, compared with 57 years in Cambodia (per capita GNP of $240). The rapid economic expansion in several of these countries has been accompanied by the expected shift to urbanization and associated lifestyle changes. In the most industrialized countries, such as Singapore, cardiovascular disease (CVD) rates mirror those in the established market and emerging market economies, with CVD predominating as a major cause of death, and CHD mortality rates twice as high as stroke mortality rates. Since the 1950s, life expectancy in China has nearly doubled from 37 years to 71 years [13]. Approximately 60% of its inhabitants still live outside urban centers, and, as is the case in most developing countries, there is an urban/regional gradient for CHD, stroke, and hypertension, with higher rates in urban centers (although they are not as great as those seen in India and sub-Saharan Africa). In general, China appears to be straddling the second and third stages of a Japanese-style epidemiologic transition, with CVD rates higher than 35% (although dominated by stroke, not CHD), because they are in the established market economies and the emerging market economies. In urban China, the death rate from coronary disease rose by 53% from 1988 to 1996. Major features of the transition there are very high smoking rates—approximately 60% in men—and hypertension, much of which remains untreated. Changes in diet are also apparent. In Beijing, between 1982 and 1992, the intake of food from animal sources increased by 6%, animal sources of protein increased 18%, and fat intake increased from 21.6% of total energy to 30.6% [16]. BMI—body mass index; CABG—coronary artery bypass surgery; PTCA—percutaneous transluminal coronary angioplasty.

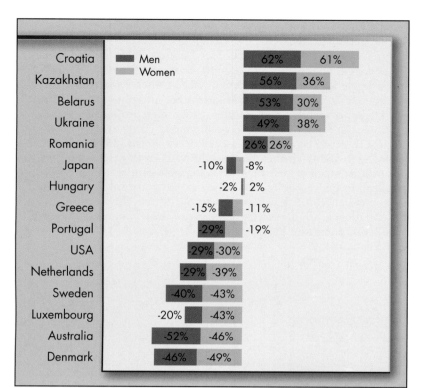

Figure 1-19.
Percentage change in coronary heart disease death rates in people aged 35 to 74 years (1988–1998). The emerging market economies, which consist of the former socialist states of Europe, are largely in the third phase of the epidemiologic transition. As a group, they have the highest rates of cardiovascular disease (CVD) mortality in the world, similar to those seen in the United States in the 1960s when CVD was at its peak. Croatia, Kazakhstan, Belarus, Ukraine, and Romania have significant increases in the coronary heart disease death rates. In Russia, life expectancy for men has dropped precipitously since 1986, from 71.6 to approximately 59 years today, shorter than that of men in three fourths of the world's countries. Russia's overall death rate jumped by nearly a third during the 1990s, primarily because of heart disease and violent deaths. Nearly two thirds of Russian men smoke. The economic, political, and social instability appear to have taken their toll, with widespread alcohol abuse reported. CVD rates have been stable in Bulgaria, Romania, Hungary, and Poland; in the Czech Republic and Slovenia, age-adjusted CVD rates have been declining. Even so, CVD rates remain generally higher than in western Europe. (*Adapted from* Mathers [1].)

A. Latin American and Caribbean Trends in the Percentage of Total Protein from Vegetables and Animals (1964 to 1996)

	Southern Cone	Brazil	Andean Region	Mexico	Central America	Latin Caribbean
Vegetable protein, %						
1964–1966	47.7	68.5	62.1	73.6	68.2	58.2
1974–1976	48.0	63.6	60.2	67.4	63.1	59.1
1984–1986	47.9	59.8	58.7	62.9	64.7	57.4
1994–1996	41.7	51.4	57.3	60.7	64.9	56.3
Animal protein, %						
1964–1966	52.3	31.5	37.9	26.4	33.2	41.8
1974–1976	52.0	36.4	39.8	32.6	36.8	40.9
1984–1986	52.1	40.2	41.3	37.1	35.3	42.6
1994–1996	58.3	48.6	42.7	39.3	35.1	43.7

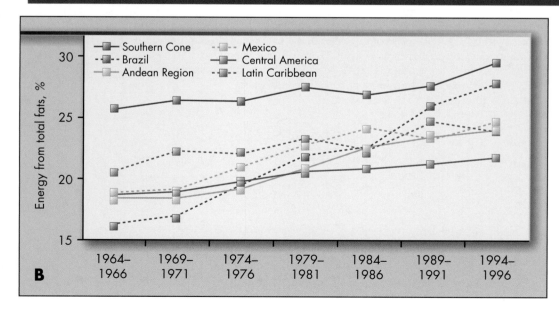

Figure 1-20.
A–C, The epidemiologic transition in Latin America and the Caribbean. In recent decades, average life expectancy in this part of the world has risen by 20 years to 71 years of age, and the quality of nutrition has steadily improved. Over a similar time period, the region has seen a switch to animal from vegetable as a source of protein and an increase in fat intake as a percentage of energy. As a whole, Latin America appears to be in the third phase of the epidemiologic transition, although there are vast regional differences. Approximately one quarter of the citizens live in poverty, and many are still at risk of contacting malaria or dengue. In addition, Chagas disease continues to be a major problem, with as much as 30% of the population infected

(*continued on next page*)

C. Latin American and Caribbean Trends in Energy Available from Fruits, Vegetables, and Starchy Roots

	Southern Cone	Brazil	Andean Region	Mexico	Central America	Latin Caribbean
Fruits, % energy						
1964–1966	0.3	4.3	10.4	3.3	4.1	11.6
1974–1976	0.3	4.2	9.0	3.1	5.0	9.3
1984–1986	0.3	4.0	7.2	3.5	3.6	8.2
1994–1996	0.3	2.5	2.4	1.9	1.8	2.8
Change	None	-1.8	-7.9	-1.4	-2.3	-8.9
Vegetables, % energy						
1964–1966	1.8	0.7	1.8	0.6	1.7	0.9
1974–1976	1.8	0.7	1.5	0.7	0.7	1.1
1984–1986	1.8	0.8	1.2	1.0	1.1	1.0
1994–1996	2.5	0.9	1.2	0.9	0.7	0.8
Change	0.7	0.2	-0.6	0.3	-1.0	-0.1
Starchy roots, % energy						
1964–1966	8.5	11.2	10.9	0.9	1.4	8.0
1974–1976	7.9	8.6	9.8	0.8	1.3	5.3
1984–1986	7.5	6.3	7.7	0.8	1.3	3.2
1994–1996	6.5	4.9	6.4	0.8	1.3	3.8
Change	-2.0	-6.3	-4.4	-0.1	-0.1	-4.1

A. Arab Middle Eastern Trends in Daily Dietary Energy and Fat Supplies

	Calories, kcal			Fat, g		
Country	1971	1997	Increase, %	1971	1997	Increase, %
Egypt	2351	3287	39.8	47.1	57.6	22.3
Iraq	2258	2619	16	42.5	77.2	81.6
Jordan	2436	3014	23.7	58.5	86.2	47.4
Kuwait	2637	3096	17.4	71.4	94.7	32.6
Lebanon	2356	3277	39.1	62.9	107.8	71.4
Libya	2457	3289	33.9	74.1	106.1	43.2
Saudi Arabia	1876	2783	48.3	32.3	78.6	143.3
Sudan	2180	2395	10	66.3	75.3	13.6
Syria	2342	3351	43	61.9	92.9	50.1
Tunisia	2279	3283	44	56.8	92.9	63.6
Yemen	1779	2051	15.3	30.2	36.5	20.8
United Arab Emirates	3093	3390	9.6	85.6	109	27.3

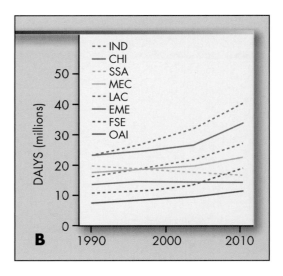

Figure 1-20. **continued** with the parasite that causes it. Today, cardiovascular disease (CVD) accounts for approximately 31% of all deaths, but that figure is expected to rise to 38% by 2020 [2]. Although coronary heart disease rates are higher than stroke rates (although not to the degree seen in the established market economies), the combination of these two accounts for more than 75% of CVD in this region. CVD rates are beginning to decline in some countries. However, those countries with the lowest CVD rates are facing the steepest increases in CVD mortality. (*Adapted from* Bermudez and Tucker [17].)

Figure 1-21.
The epidemiologic transition in the Middle East and North Africa. In this region, increasing economic wealth has been characteristically accompanied by urbanization, but uncharacteristically accompanied by increasing fertility rates as infant and childhood mortality rates declined. The result has been a young mean age of the population (*ie*, 44% younger than 15 years of age). The rate of cardiovascular disease (CVD) has been increasing rapidly, and CVD is now the leading cause of death, accounting for 25% to 45% of total deaths. The traditional high-fiber diet, low in fat and cholesterol, has rapidly changed to a Western diet. Over the past few decades, daily per capita fat consumption (**A**) has increased in most of these countries, ranging from a 13.6% increase in Sudan to a 143.3% increase in Saudi Arabia [18]. According to a review of three national surveys, in Iran, the prevalence of overweight and obesity was as high as 50% among men and 66% among women in the 40–69 age group [19]. As in the established market economies (**B**), coronary heart disease is the predominant cause of CVD, with approximately three CHD deaths for every stroke death. Rheumatic heart disease remains a major cause of morbidity and mortality, but the number of hospitalizations for rheumatic heart disease is rapidly declining. This region is entering the third phase of the epidemiologic transition. CHI—China; DALYs—disability-adjusted life-years; EME—emerging market economies; FSE—former Socialist economies; IND—India; LAC—Latin America and the Caribbean; MEC—Middle Eastern countries; OAI—other Asian islands; SSA—sub-Saharan Africa. (*Panel A Adapted from* Musaiger [18]; *panel B data from* the World Health Organization.)

Diabetes in South Asia: Estimated Prevalence 2000 and 2025

Country	Percentage (people, *n*) 2000	Percentage (people, *n*) 2025
Bangladesh	2.2 (1564)	3.1 (4032)
Bhutan	2.1 (19)	2.3 (39)
India	4.0 (22,878)	6.0 (57,243)
Maldives	2.5 (3.2)	3.0 (9.2)
Nepal	2.2 (263)	2.6 (638)
Pakistan	7.1 (5310)	8.7 (14,523)
Sri Lanka	2.6 (318)	3.5 (617)

Estimated Number of Rheumatic Heart Disease Cases in Children (5- to 14-year-olds)

Region	Cases, *n*
Sub-Saharan Africa	1,008,207
China	176,576
South-Central Asia	734,786
Asia (other)	101,822
Latin America	136,971
Eastern Mediterranean and North Africa	153,679
Eastern Europe	40,366
Pacific	7744
Developed countries	33,330

Figure 1-22.
Diabetes in the South Asia region: India. With more than one billion people, India has about one sixth of the world's population, and the vast majority still reside in rural settings. Nonetheless, India is experiencing an alarming increase in heart disease, which appears to be linked to changes in lifestyle and diet, rapid urbanization, and possibly an underlying genetic component. Diabetes also is a major health issue; India has 31.6 million diabetic individuals, more than any other country. This number is expected to reach 57.2 million by 2025 [20]. The World Health Organization estimates that 60% of the world's cardiac patients will be Indian by 2010. Concern has been expressed that rising rates of death and disability because of cardiovascular disease (CVD) among relatively young residents will seriously affect productivity and impose economic burdens on the country. Today, approximately 50% of CVD-related deaths occur below the age of 70, compared with approximately 22% in the West. Between 2000 and 2030, approximately 35% of all CVD deaths in India will occur in the 35–64 age group, compared with only 12% in the United States and 22% in China. (*Adapted from* Ghaffar *et al.* [20].)

Figure 1-23.
Rheumatic heart disease in sub-Saharan Africa. Almost 75% of the 40 million adults and children living with HIV/AIDS reside in sub-Saharan Africa, an epidemic that will definitely influence the natural history of cardiovascular disease (CVD) [21]. Cardiac involvement is a common sequela of infection with HIV. Accurate countywide data are not generally available, and most data come from urban centers and sampling in rural areas. Overall, CVD is responsible for approximately 10% of all deaths in sub-Saharan Africa. In keeping with patterns characteristic of the earlier phases of the epidemiologic transition, stroke is the dominant form. With increasing urbanization, average daily physical activity among urban dwellers is falling, and smoking rates are increasing. Hypertension has emerged as a major public health concern and hypertensive disease accounts for the dominance of stroke [22]. Rheumatic heart disease and cardiomyopathies, the latter mostly caused by malnutrition, various viral illnesses, and parasitic organisms, are also important causes of CVD mortality and morbidity. (*Data from* the World Health Organization.)

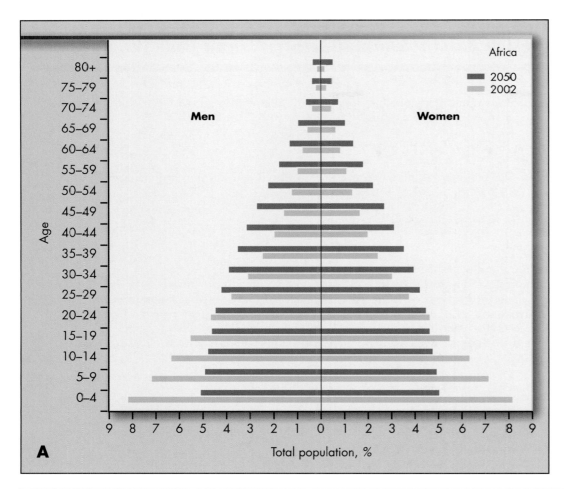

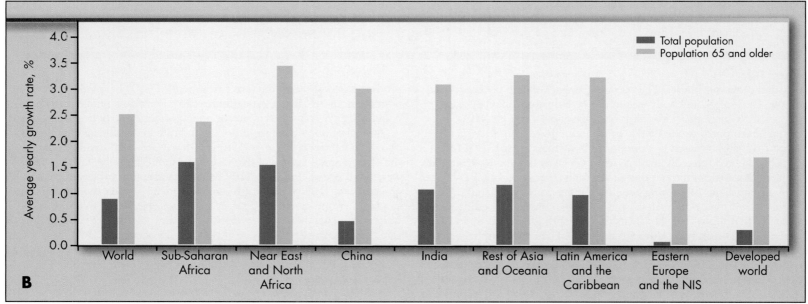

Figure 1-24.
A and **B**, The world's aging population. A demographic profile of the world over the next 25 years shows that the segment of the population aged 65 and older is projected to grow faster than any other segment in all world regions [23]. In 2002, approximately 7% of the world's population had reached retirement age, a number that is predicted to double by 2020 and more than triple by 2050. By 2040, more than 20% of United States citizens will be 65 or older. In China and Russia, that number will be around 20%, while in Brazil and India—so-called "young countries"—approximately 8% to 14% of residents will have reached 65 years of age. Because cardiovascular disease mortality increases as population longevity increases, there will be economic implications as the disease becomes clinically manifest and more people require treatment. NIS—newly independent states of the former Soviet Union.

Social and Economic Impact of High Blood Pressure, Cholesterol, and Body Weight Issues

Global cost of smoking

Health care costs associated with smoke-related illnesses result in a global net loss of $200 billion per year, with one third of these losses occurring in developing countries

Global cost of diabetes

Between 4% and 5% of health budgets are spent on diabetes-related illnesses

Latin America and the Caribbean

Permanent disabilities resulting from diabetes cost $50 billion in 2000, whereas costs associated with insulin, hospitalization, consultations, and care totaled $10.6 billion

United States, Australia and Europe

Reports from 2002 indicate that up to 10% of health budgets are spent on diabetes-related illnesses

Global cost of heart disease and obesity

United States

The direct costs of physical inactivity accounted for an estimated $24 billion in health care costs (1995)

Health problems related to obesity, such as heart disease and type-2 diabetes, cost the United States approximately $177 billion per year

Cholesterol-reducing medications were the top-selling medications of 2003, generating approximately $13.9 billion in sales

The American Heart Association estimates that stroke will cost a total of $53.6 billion in 2004; direct costs for medical care and therapy will average $33 billion and indirect costs from lost productivity will be approximately $20.6 billion

In 2001, the National Stroke Association estimated that the average cost per patient for the first 90 days after stroke was $15,000, although 10% of cases cost more than $35,000

United Kingdom

More than 4% of the National Health Services spending was on stroke-related service in 2000

Netherlands

Stroke was estimated to be responsible for 3% of total health care costs in the Netherlands in 1994; 7% of the costs were for the population aged 75 and older. Stroke was second on the list of most costly disease for the elderly, after dementia, and these costs are expected to increase by 40% by 2015

Singapore

Average hospital costs for stroke were reported at $5000 per patient in 2000.

Global costs of heart disease medication

The number of individuals who die or are disabled by coronary heart disease and stroke could be cut in half with wider use of a combination of drugs that costs just $14 per year

Figure 1-25.
Social and economic impact. The economic impact of high levels of blood pressure, cholesterol, and body weight can be estimated indirectly using data that show more than two thirds of cardiovascular disease (CVD) burden can be attributed to these risks. In addition, more than three quarters of type 2 diabetes is caused by nonoptimal body mass levels [3]. A recent report highlighted the economic impact of CVDs in developing economies, stemming largely from the fact that such a high proportion of CVD burden occurs among adults of working age [14]. In five countries surveyed (Brazil, India, China, South Africa, and Mexico), conservative estimates indicated that at least 21 million years of future productive life are lost because of CVD each year. Although no detailed data exist on the direct economic burden of the individual risk factors, the costs of CVD treatment in developing countries is significant and appears similar to that in developed countries. In South Africa, for example, 2% to 3% of gross domestic product was devoted to the direct treatment of CVD or roughly 25% of the South African health care expenditures [24]. For many middle-income countries, high body mass is already an important cause of health inequities.

An indication of possible future expenditure in developing countries is also provided by current expenditure in developed countries. For example, the United States estimated that direct and indirect costs of CVD in 2003 were $350 billion. In 1998, $109 billion was spent on hypertension, or approximately 13% of the health care budget [25]. Studies are limited, but suggest that obesity-related diseases are responsible for 2% to 8% of all health care expenditures in developed countries. In 1991, 2.5% of health care costs in New Zealand were attributable to obesity. In 1996, $22 billion was attributed to obesity-related CVD in the United States, which amounts to 17% of CVD-related health expenditures [26]. (*Data from* the World Health Organization.)

A. Estimated Disability-adjusted Life Years: 2010–2030

DALYs	By 2010	By 2020	By 2030
CVD DALYs: average number of DALYs	15.3 million	169 million	187 million
Burden of CVD: percentage of all DALYs	10.4%	11.0%	11.6%
CVD rankings globally	Coronary heart disease: 3rd; stroke: 5th	Coronary heart disease: 3rd; stroke: 4th	Coronary heart disease: 3rd; stroke 4th
CVD rankings in developing countries	Coronary heart disease: 4th; stroke: 8th	Coronary heart disease: 3rd; stroke: 6th	Coronary heart disease: 3rd; stroke: 5th

Figure 1-26. (*continued on next page*)

B. *Estimated Morbidity Related to Heart Disease: 2010–2030*

Deaths	By 2010	By 2020	By 2030
CVD deaths: annual number of all deaths	18.1 million	20.5 million	24.2 million
CVD deaths: percentage of all deaths	30.8%	31.5%	32.5
CHD deaths: percentage of all male deaths	13.1%	14.3%	14.9
CHD deaths: percentage of all female deaths	13.6%	13.0%	13.1
Stroke deaths: percentage of all male deaths	5.2%	9.8%	10.4
Stroke deaths: percentage of all female deaths	11.5%	11.5%	11.8
CVD deaths from cigarette smoking: annual number of deaths	1.9 million	2.6 million	

Figure 1-26. *continued*

The future: estimated disability-adjusted life-years (DALYs) (**A**) and heart-disease–related morbidity (**B**). A global cardiovascular disease (CVD) epidemic is rapidly evolving, with the burden of disease shifting. Twice as many deaths from CVD now occur in developing countries as developed countries [13]. The vast majority of CVD can be attributed to conventional risk factors, such as smoking and obesity. Even in sub-Saharan Africa, a developing region with high mortality, high blood pressure, high cholesterol, tobacco, and alcohol use, as well as low vegetable and fruit consumption, are already among the top risk factors for disease [27]. Because of the lag time associated with CVD risk factors,

especially in children, the full effect of exposure to these factors will only be seen in the future. Information from more than 100 countries shows that more 13- to 15-year-old children smoke than ever before, and studies show that obesity levels in children are increasing markedly in countries as diverse as Brazil, China, India, and almost all island states [14]. Population-wide efforts to reduce risk factors through multiple economic and educational policies and programs will reap savings later in medical and other direct costs as well as indirectly in improved quality of life and economic productivity. CHD—coronary heart disease. (*Data from* the World Health Organization.)

References

1. Mathers CD: *Deaths and Disease Burden by Cause: Global Burden of Disease Estimates for 2001 by World Bank Country Groups.* Disease Control Priorities Project Working Paper 18. Available at http://www.fic.nih.gov/dcpp/wps.html.

2. Murray CJL, Lopez AD: *The Global Burden of Disease.* Cambridge: Harvard School Of Public Health; 1996.

3. Rodgers A, Vaughn P: *World Health Report 2002: Reducing Risks, Promoting Healthy Life.* Edited by Murray C, Lopez A. Geneva: World Health Organization; 2002.

4. The World Health Organization web site. Available at http://www.who.int/ncd/cvd.

5. Omran AR: The epidemiologic transition: a theory of the epidemiology of population change. *Milbank Mem Fund Q* 1971, 49:509.

6. Olshansky SJ, Ault AB: The fourth stage of the epidemiologic transition: the age of delayed degenerative diseases. *Milbank Mem Fund Q* 1986, 64:355.

7. Starr P: *The Social Transformation of American Medicine.* New York: Basic Books; 1982.

8. Goldman L, Cook EF: The decline in ischemic heart disease mortality rates: an analysis of the comparative effects of medical interventions and changes in lifestyle. *Ann Intern Med* 1984, 101:825.

9. Hunink MG, Goldman L, Toteson AN, *et al.*: The recent decline in mortality from coronary heart disease, 1980–1990: the effect of secular trends in risk factors and treatment. *JAMA* 1997, 277:535.

10. Cooper R, Cutler J, Desvigne-Nickens P, *et al.*: Trends and disparities in coronary heart disease, stroke, and other cardiovascular diseases in the United States: findings of the national conference on cardiovascular disease prevention. *Circulation* 2000, 102:3137.

11. United Nations Department of Economic and Social Affairs/Population Division: *World Urbanization Prospects: The 2003 Revision.* New York: United Nations Population Division; 2004.

12. Drewnowski A, Popkin BM: The nutrition transition: new trends in the global diet. *Nutr Rev* 1997, 55:31.

13. Beaglehole R, Irwin A, Prentice T: *World Health Report 2003: Shaping the Future.* Edited by Evans T, Beaglehole R. Geneva: World Health Organization; 2003.

14. Leeder S, Raymond S, Greenberg H: *A Race Against Time: The Challenge of Cardiovascular Disease in Developing Countries.* New York: Trustees of Columbia University; 2004.

15. Reddy KS, Yusuf S: Emerging epidemic of cardiovascular disease in developing countries. *Circulation* 1998, 97:596–601.

16. Yusuf S, Reddy S, Ounpuu S, Anand S: Global burden of cardiovascular diseases part I: general considerations, the epidemiologic transition, risk factors, and impact of urbanization. *Circulation* 2001, 104:2746–2753.

17. Bermudez OI, Tucker KL: Trends in dietary patterns of Latin American populations. *Cad Saude Publica* 2003, 19(suppl):S87–S99.

18. Musaiger AO: Diet and prevention of coronary heart disease in the Arab Middle East countries. *Med Princ Pract* 2002, 11(suppl):9–16.

19. Sheikholeslam R, Mohamad A, Mohammad K, Vaseghi S: Non communicable disease risk factors in Iran. *Asia Pac J Clin Nutr* 2004, 13(suppl):S100.

20. Ghaffar A, Reddy KS, Singhi M: Burden of non-communicable diseases in South Asia. *BMJ* 2004, 328:807–810.

21. *Report on the Global HIV/AIDS Epidemic.* Geneva: United Nations Programme on HIV/AIDS; 2002.

22. Bertrand E: Cardiovascular disease in developing countries. In *Cardiology.* Edited by Dalla Volta S. New York: McGraw-Hill; 1999:825–834.

23. *US Census Bureau Global Population Profile: 2002.* Washington, DC: US Government Printing Office; 2004.

24. Pestana J, Steyn K, Leiman A, Hartzenberg GM: The direct and indirect costs of cardiovascular disease in South Africa in 1991. *S Afr Med J* 1996, 86:679–684.

25. Hodgson TA, Cai L: Medical care expenditures for hypertension, its complications, and its comorbidities. *Med Care* 2001, 39:599–615.

26. Wang G, Zheng ZJ, Heath G, *et al.*: Economic burden of cardiovascular disease associated with excess body weight in U.S. adults. *Am J Prev Med* 2002, 23:1–6.

27. World Health Organization: *Atlas of Heart Disease and Stroke.* Geneva: World Health Organization; 2004.

About Risk Factors

J. Michael Gaziano

Once thought of as a natural consequence of aging, cardiovascular disease (CVD) is now understood to be predominately a "man-made" disease, heavily influenced by the choices we make. The past 50 years have seen great progress in identifying a large number of these lifestyle risk factors, as well as biochemical and genetic factors, associated with CVD. In addition, basic research and clinical studies have significantly expanded our knowledge of the pathophysiology of atherosclerosis, thereby shedding light on the impact risk factors can have on the disease process [1].

In the 1950s and 1960s, several kinds of epidemiologic studies helped establish a definitive cause and effect between certain "risk factors" and CVD. For example, the Seven Countries Study [2], a large cross-cultural study, proved that CVD rates varied around the world, implicating environmental factors. Migration studies comparing CVD prevalence among those of the same ethnic background living in geographically diverse locations lent further credence to the theory that environmental factors played a key role in the development of CVD [3]. In fact, migration studies described differences in the prevalence of various environmental factors such as cigarette smoking that may have contributed to the differences in the rates of disease. By 1961, published data from the landmark Framingham Heart Study [4] showed that hypertension, high cholesterol, and smoking all increased the risk of heart disease. It was here that it appears the term *risk factor* was coined.

Evidence about risk factors has come from a variety of sources. Autopsy studies have shown that atherosclerosis can begin at an early age if risk factors—the same risk factors that lead to CVD in adults—are present [5,6]. Basic research and physiologic studies provide insight into the mechanisms underlying atherogenesis and help elucidate the biologic plausibility of potential interventions to modify these effects. Human observational studies, such as case-control studies and prospective cohorts, are extremely useful in establishing risk attributable to a single factor. Randomized trials are helpful in confirming causation and are essential in establishing interventions to modify the risk.

Risk factors can be divided into two groups: those that predict risk and those that are targets for intervention [7]. Some risk factors, such as an unhealthy diet, fall into both categories. The protective effect of prophylactic aspirin, for example, for the primary and secondary prevention of CVD is an example of an intervention for which there is not an easily measurable corresponding risk factor [8]. This simple measure is an inexpensive way to cut individual risk, as well as population risk. Data from the World Health Organization prove that CVD, which was once considered a "rich country" disease, and the risk factors associated with it, are now taking their toll in low- and middle-income countries [9]. One way that these countries can address this increasing burden is to promote taking an aspirin per day. Because CVD is now the leading cause of death worldwide, widespread deployment of affordable preventive strategies should have high priority in developed and developing countries.

The ideal risk factor is one that is common and for which the published data consistently demonstrate a strong and independent association with CVD. The added knowledge should enhance our ability to predict disease. The assessment of that risk factor should be easy, low-risk, reliable, and low in cost. Ideally, the factor would be modifiable and effective interventions would be established through trials.

This chapter reviews the development of the concept of a risk factor in the prediction of risk as well as interventions for reducing risk. Risk factors can come from predisposing factors such as gender or age, from behaviors such as smoking, from physiologic measures such as blood pressure, from blood markers, or markers of quiescent disease [10,11]. The presence of known CVD is even a risk factor for future events. In subsequent chapters, other authors will summarize the totality of evidence on the various risk factors. In the final chapter of this book, recommendations for the use of the major risk factors in everyday practice will be summarized.

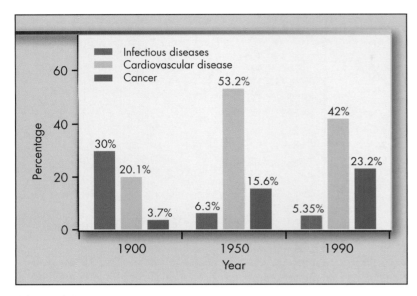

Figure 2-1.
Changes in leading causes of death. As nutrition and living conditions improved and medical technology advanced, deaths from infectious diseases steadily declined during the 20th century, while morbidity from chronic conditions increased. Cardiovascular disease (CVD) in general and coronary heart disease (CHD) in particular became the leading cause of morbidity and mortality in the developed world in the 20th century.

Cardiovascular disease recently became the number one cause of death in the developing world. This dramatic rise and then modest decline underscores the importance of prevention in dealing with CVD. The hospital-based health care system first responded by introducing therapies to address the acute manifestations of this chronic disease. In the latter half of the 20th century, much attention was focused on strategies for preventing the development of CVD (primary prevention) and preventing secondary events in those with existing disease (secondary prevention). These efforts resulted in the decline in age-adjusted rates of CVD evident here in the later part of the 20th century. Similar trends are occurring around the world.

Types of Studies Used in Establishing Preventive Strategies

Basic research
  In vitro studies
  Animal studies
Physiologic studies
Epidemiologic studies
  Descriptive studies
    Case reports
    Cross-sectional surveys
    Cross-cultural comparison studies
    Temporal trend studies
  Analytic studies
    Observational
      Case-control studies
      Cohort studies
  Intervention (randomized trials)
Cost-efficacy studies
Meta-analyses

Steps in Disease Prevention

Measure the burden of disease in the population
Understand disease mechanisms
Identify risk factors
Establish intervention strategies
Risk and cost/benefit analyses
Establish guidelines
Implement guidelines

Figure 2-2.
Steps in disease prevention. There are several steps in disease prevention, but we do not necessarily proceed through these steps in a purely sequential fashion. Progress in disease prevention can occur in each of these areas simultaneously. To effectively prevent disease, we must first measure the burden of disease in the population. It is useful to develop an understanding of the underlying disease mechanisms that will point to better ways to detect the disease, determine factors that will predict disease, and identify potential targets for intervention to reduce the chance of developing a disease. The next step is to develop and test interventions, usually in large-scale randomized trials. This testing will permit health economists to determine if these interventions are worthwhile in terms of their risks and costs. The last step in prevention is to establish and then implement guidelines to lower the chance that an individual will develop this disease, and, at a population level, reduce the burden of the disease.

Prevention strategies can be directed to the individual patient or to the population as a whole. In individuals, the focus is on preventing or delaying the onset of disease, or minimizing its consequences in those who have it. From a population standpoint, prevention refers to reducing the overall burden of the disease in the population and its consequences. Both strategies play an important role.

Figure 2-3.
Establishing preventive strategies. The first step in determining whether a risk factor is a potential marker of and target for intervention is establishing definitive cause and effect. Data from several types of research are needed to establish a causal relationship between exposure and disease. Basic research and physiologic studies, for example, have provided insight into the mechanisms underlying atherogenesis and helped elucidate the biologic plausibility of potential interventions to modify these effects. The development of preventive strategies also depends heavily on complementary methods of population research, including descriptive studies (cross-sectional surveys and cross-cultural analyses), analytic studies (case-control and prospective cohort studies), and intervention studies (randomized trials). Each kind of study has strengths and weaknesses. For example, observational studies are extremely useful in establishing risk attributable to a single factor, particularly when the effect of a given factor is large, as is the case for smoking and lung cancer. However, when searching for small-to-moderate effects, the level of uncontrolled confounding in observational studies may be as large as the probable risk reduction itself. In such cases, randomized trials are essential for confirming causation. Once established, interventions to modify the risk must be developed and tested to ensure that the magnitude of the associated risk is on par with the benefit derived from the intervention; randomized trials generally provide the best data on this.

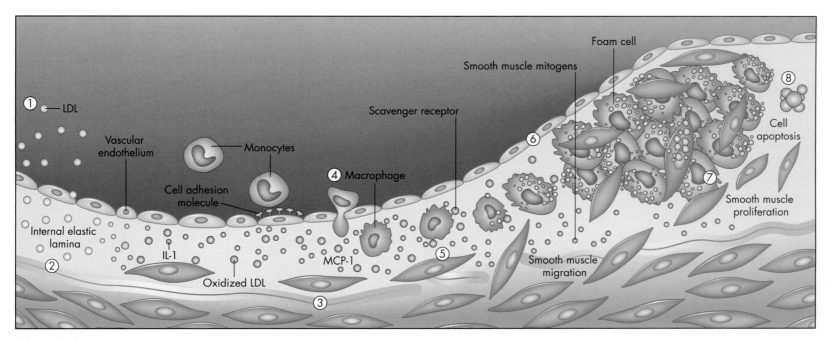

Figure 2-4.

Schematic of the evolution of atherosclerotic plaque. Over the past several decades, basic research and clinical studies have led to an in-depth understanding of the atherosclerotic process. This image schematically presents the development of atherosclerotic plaque [1]. Lipoprotein particles first accumulate in the artery wall. These particles become damaged and induce local cytokine, adhesion molecule, and chemoattractant production. What results is the migration of monocytes into the artery wall. These monocytes are transformed into resident macrophages. Smooth muscle cells divide and accumulate in the growing plaque. The plaque then becomes more fibrotic and later calcified. Improved understanding of the pathology of the atherosclerotic process has helped in identifying risk factors that are causally linked to the disease by providing a biologically plausible explanation. IL-1—interleukin-1; LDL—low-density lipoprotein; MCP—monocyte chemoattractant protein. (*Adapted from* Libby [1].)

Figure 2-5.

Mechanisms underlying the formation of a coronary thrombus [10]. Plaque that accumulates in the coronary arteries is vulnerable to fissuring. Mild-to-moderate stenoses that undergo lesser degrees of fissuring usually lead to incomplete occlusion of the vessel. However, with deeper plaque fissures or more severe stenoses, plaques can rupture, leading to the formation of a thrombus. A better understanding of the pathophysiologic mechanisms of atherosclerosis has contributed to the understanding of how various risk factors cause cardiovascular disease.

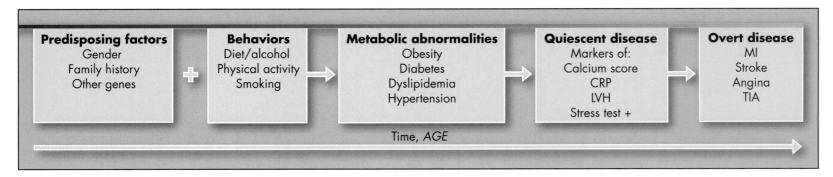

Figure 2-6.

Progression of atherosclerosis. Our knowledge of the biologic process of atherosclerosis has led to a working model for the progression of this disease. Heart disease is caused by a number of factors coming together. Most people with cardiovascular disease have small, concurrent adverse

(*continued on next page*)

Figure 2-6. continued

changes in multiple risk factors rather than extreme deviations in any single risk factor. Left unchecked, atherosclerosis will proceed along a continuum. Predisposing factors such as genes interact with behavioral factors, *eg*, the type of diet an individual follows, whether he or she drinks alcohol, and the amount of exercise one gets on a regular basis. This combination of predisposing factors and behaviors can lead to metabolic abnormalities, such as dyslipidemia, hypertension, obesity, and diabetes, which may eventually result in quiescent disease. One can obtain clues to this underlying disease and quiescent disease by using various diagnostic tests. An exercise stress test or a calcium score, or possibly a C-reactive protein (CRP)

measurement can be used as an assessment of underlying disease. Eventually this quiescent disease may become overt in the form of a transient ischemic attack (TIA), a myocardial infarction (MI), or another cardiovascular event. Factors that are useful in predicting who is at risk can come from any stage in this process. For example, a family history of heart disease or a behavior such as smoking is a risk factor. A metabolic factor like high cholesterol is also a risk factor. A measure of underlying disease such as a calcium score or left ventricular hypertrophy (LVH) on an echocardiogram can be used to predict future events. Finally, the existence of disease, as evidenced by having an MI, also predicts future events.

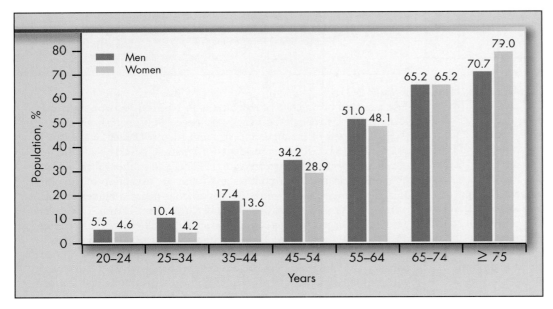

Figure 2-7.
Data from many different types of epidemiologic studies have advanced our knowledge of cardiovascular disease (CVD) risk. Descriptive studies, which include cross-sectional surveys, cross-cultural analyses, and studies of population-based temporal trends, contributed significantly to our understanding of risk factors associated with CVD. What was probably the first well-established risk factor for heart disease came from the observation that the prevalence of this disease increases with age and male gender [12]. In addition, male gender emerged early on as being clearly associated with coronary heart disease. (*Data from* American Heart Association; *adapted from* Penckhofer [12].)

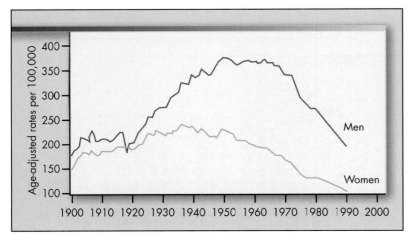

Figure 2-8.
Analysis of temporal trends in disease rates over time has suggested that environmental factors that also changed, such as diet and activity level, may have a major impact on cardiovascular disease (CVD) risk. In the United States during the 1800s, CVD was a relatively rare cause of morbidity and mortality, whereas infectious disease and malnutrition were prevalent. Then, over the course of the 20th century, heart disease rates trended upward, a change that was obvious to health care providers. As mean life expectancy increased, some felt that the increase in heart disease was merely a consequence of aging. However, in the latter half of the century, the decline in age-adjusted CVD rates clearly showed that this was not the case. (*Adapted from* Feinleib [13].)

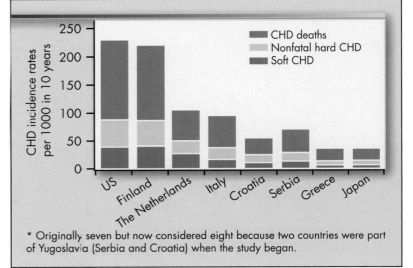

* Originally seven but now considered eight because two countries were part of Yugoslavia (Serbia and Croatia) when the study began.

Figure 2-9.
Differences in rates of cardiovascular disease (CVD) around the world were also a clue that environmental factors played a major role in coronary heart disease (CHD). The first and probably most famous cross-cultural study to examine CVD risk is the Seven Countries Study, which started collecting baseline data in 1958 in 16 cohorts on three continents, North America, Europe, and Japan. It was the first to quantify true differences in prevalence, incidence, and mortality for CHD among populations with various geographic, ethnic, and cultural characteristics [2]. The 10-year follow-up data showed high incidence rates in North America and northern Europe, whereas rates were low in southern Europe and Japan. Fivefold or greater differences existed in the 10-year hard CHD (CHD deaths plus hard nonfatal CHD, including myocardial infarction) rates between the countries with the highest and lowest rates. This study also suggested that CVD was likely multifactorial. (*Adapted from* Kfomhut *et al.* [2].)

About Risk Factors

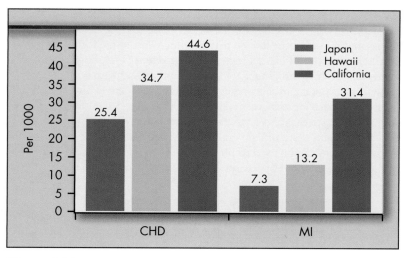

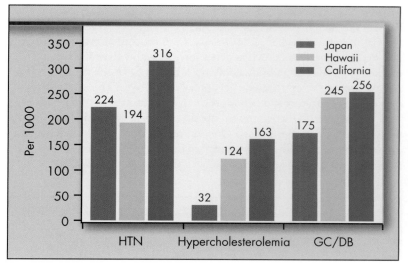

Figure 2-10.

Age-adjusted prevalence of coronary heart disease (CHD): graph from Ni-Hon-San study. Migration studies provided further evidence that the environment played an important role in cardiovascular disease (CVD). One of the best-known migration studies examining risk factors and heart disease patterns was the Ni-Hon-San Study, which began in 1965 and compared CVD risk factors and deaths from ischemic heart disease among Japanese men living in Japan, Hawaii, and San Francisco. Comparing men of the same ethnic background eliminated the potential confounding effect of genetic factors. Disease rates were highest in California, lowest in Japan, and intermediate in Hawaii, indicating that some change in environmental or living habits has altered susceptibility to CVD. CHD is defined by major and minor Q/QS abnormalities: Minnesota codes 1-1-1 through 1-3-6. MI—myocardial infarction. (*Adapted from* Marmot *et al.* [3].)

Figure 2-11.

Age-adjusted prevalence of risk factors in Ni-Hon-San cohorts. The Ni-Hon-San study reported on the prevalence of coronary heart disease (CHD) in men of Japanese ancestry and the prevalence of associated risk factors [3]. California residents of Japanese descent had a higher prevalence of definite hypertension (HTN) and higher mean blood pressures than the other cohorts and, with the exception of the oldest and the youngest age groups, the Japan cohort had a higher prevalence of hypertension than was seen in Hawaii. A Japan-Hawaii-California gradient emerged for increasing prevalence of elevated serum cholesterol (> 260 mg/100 mL). The frequency of hyperglycemia/diabetes was approximately equal in Hawaii and California, but in both of these cohorts, the frequency was greater than in Japan. Overall, compared with the Japanese cohort, the study found that the American cohorts had a greater prevalence of CHD risk factors and CHD. GC/DB—hyperglycemia or history of diabetes. (*Adapted from* Marmot *et al.* [3].)

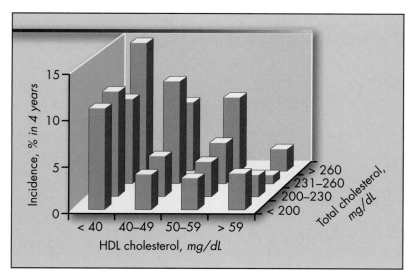

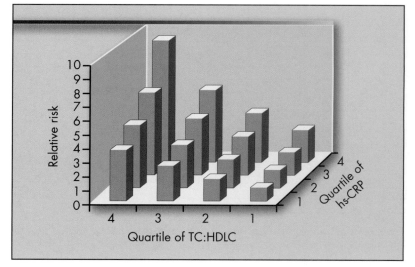

Figure 2-12.

High-density lipoprotein (HDL) predictive value: men and women without coronary heart disease (CHD) history. The Framingham Heart Study and other cohort studies identified a number of risk factors for CHD. In the 1960s and 1970s, smoking and high blood pressure were clearly established as risk factors for CHD. In addition, blood-based markers appeared as important predictors of disease, with the emergence of cholesterol levels as clear risk factors. This image illustrates the independent relationship of total cholesterol and HDL cholesterol with incident CHD in men and women [14]. In addition to the Framingham Heart Study, a number of other large-scale cohort studies, as well as smaller case-control studies, have clearly established factors, such as smoking, high blood pressure, and lipids, as causative agents in the development of CHD. (*Adapted from* Castelli *et al.* [14].)

Figure 2-13.

High-sensitivity C-reactive protein (hs-CRP), lipids, and risk of future coronary events: the Women's Health Study. Predictive value of inflammatory markers. Since the establishment of cholesterol as a biomarker predicting coronary heart disease (CHD), newer biomarkers have emerged as important predictors of disease. hs-CRP appears to be one of the strongest, as evidenced by a nested, case-control study among 28,263 apparently healthy postmenopausal women [15]. Of 12 biomarkers evaluated in this study, hs-CRP was the most significant predictor of the risk of cardiovascular events. The addition of this measurement increased the predictive value of models using only standard lipid screening, particularly when regression analyses were based on cut-off points for quartiles (rather than cut-off points for the division of the study group into thirds) and analysis of the ratio of total cholesterol to high-density lipoprotein cholesterol (TC:HDLC) as opposed to total cholesterol alone. (*Adapted from* Ridker *et al.* [15].)

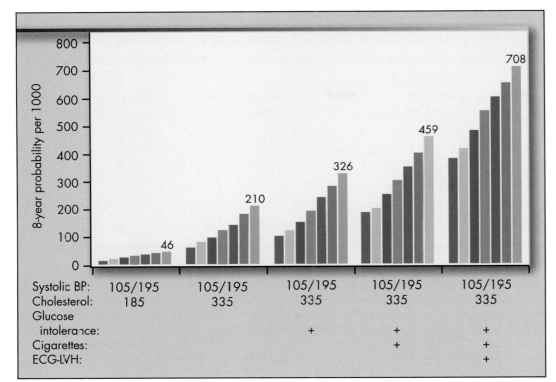

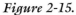

Systolic BP:	105/195	105/195	105/195	105/195	105/195
Cholesterol:	185	335	335	335	335
Glucose intolerance:			+	+	+
Cigarettes:				+	+
ECG-LVH:					+

Figure 2-14.

Risk of cardiovascular disease in men age 40 according to systolic blood pressure (SBP) and risk profile. Risk factors can work together to increase risk. This image from the Framingham Heart Study shows that having multiple risk factors can dramatically increase the 8-year probability of developing coronary heart disease [16]. The authors of this 1976 paper wrote, "Coronary disease does not really begin with crushing chest pain, pulmonary edema, shock, angina or ventricular fibrillation, but rather with more subtle signs like a poor coronary risk profile." And they conclude, "Most cases of angina pectoris or myocardial infarction represent medical failures; the conditions should have been detected years earlier for preventive management." ECG-LVH—electrocardiographic left ventricular hypertrophy. (*Adapted from* Kannel [16].)

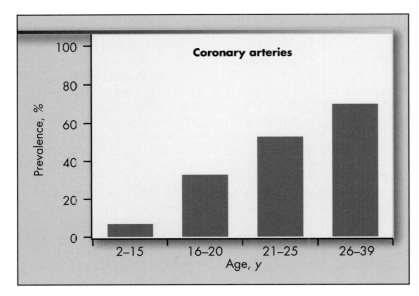

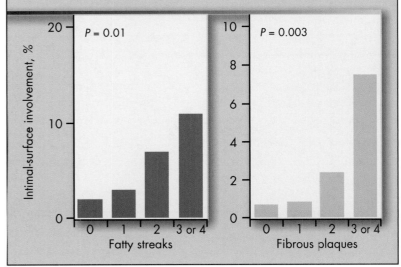

Figure 2-15.

Bogalusa Heart Study graph of prevalence in coronary arteries. The Bogalusa Heart Study contributed important evidence that, even in childhood and early adulthood, the traditional risk factors that predict cardiovascular events among middle-aged and older adults are largely the same as those that predict atherosclerotic lesions in children and young adults [5]. The study demonstrated that the prevalence of fatty streaks and raised fibrous-plaque lesions (shown here) in the coronary arteries of young people who died of noncardiac causes increased with age; the prevalence of fibrous plaques reached 69% in those 26 to 39 years old. It also showed that elevations in body mass index, systolic blood pressure, and other risk factors are significantly related to the extent of atherosclerotic lesions. Body mass index, systolic blood pressure, low-density lipoprotein cholesterol levels, triglyceride levels, and cigarette smoking were highly correlated with the number of lesions in the aorta and the coronary arteries. (*Adapted from* Berenson *et al.* [5].)

Figure 2-16.

Effect of multiple risk factors on the extent of atherosclerosis in the coronary arteries in children and young adults. The Bogalusa Heart Study found that as the number of traditional risk factors (including high values for body mass index, systolic blood pressure, and low-density lipoprotein cholesterol) increases, so does the severity of asymptomatic coronary and aortic atherosclerosis in young people [5]. In individuals with 0, one, two, and three or four risk factors, 1.3%, 2.5%, 7.9%, and 11.0%, respectively, of the intimal surface of the coronary arteries was covered with fibrous plaques. The extent of fatty-streak lesions in the coronary artery was 8.5 times as great in persons with three or four risk factors as in those with none, and the extent of fibrous plaque lesions in the coronary arteries was 12 times as great. Because behavioral and lifestyle patterns learned in childhood tend to continue into adulthood, it seems reasonable to assume that the presence of these traditional risk factors in children is likely to lead to cardiovascular events later in life. (*Adapted from* Berenson *et al.* [5].)

About Risk Factors

	Low-risk	No risk factors high but 1 or more unfavorable	One only risk factor high	Two or more risk factors high
Women, *n*	1469	1558	3217	1058
Person-years of follow-up	43,168	43,036	94,115	30,803
Deaths, *n*	2	3	23	19
Rate per 1000 person-years	0.7	0.7	2.4	5.4
Hazard ratio (95% CI)				
Age-adjusted	0.10 (0.02–0.45)	0.12 (0.04–0.42)	0.47 (0.26–0.87)	1.00
Multivariate-adjusted	0.12 (0.03–0.50)	0.13 (0.04–0.45)	0.49 (0.26–0.90)	1.00

Figure 2-17.

Chicago Heart Association mortality rates. Is there empiric evidence that reducing risk factors really reduces the risk of developing cardiovascular disease? A long-running study, the Chicago Heart Association Detection Project in Industry, assessed the relationship of cardiovascular risk factors measured in young women on subsequent mortality [17]. Five major risk factors (blood pressure, cholesterol level, body mass index, presence of diabetes, and smoking status) were measured at baseline in more than 7000 women between the ages of 18 and 39 without prior evidence of coronary heart disease (CHD). Participants were divided into four groups: low-risk; 0 risk factors high but one or more unfavorable; one only risk factor high; and two or more risk factors high. The study showed that among women who initially had favorable levels of all five major risk factors, CHD and cardiovascular disease were rare, and that long-term and all-cause mortality were much lower after 31 years compared with the other participants. The presence of high levels of major risk factors at baseline was associated with much higher mortality risk. The mortality rate among those with no risk factors was only 12% of those with two or more risk factors. (*Adapted from* Daviglus *et al.* [17].)

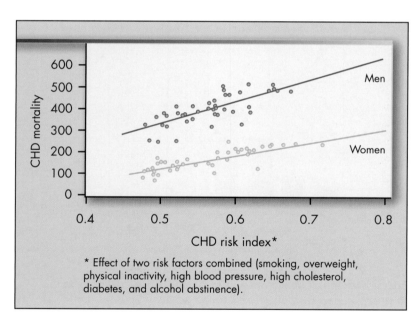

* Effect of two risk factors combined (smoking, overweight, physical inactivity, high blood pressure, high cholesterol, diabetes, and alcohol abstinence).

Figure 2-18.

The relationship between coronary heart disease (CHD) mortality (mortality from CHD among people age 45–74) and CHD risk factors in 49 states: 1991; risk at the population level. The effect that was apparent among individuals in Figure 2-19 can be seen at a population level. The data plotted illustrates the association between a composite of risk (coronary heart disease risk index) that is based on each state's level of risk factors and the risk of coronary heart disease in that state demonstrating a clear association [13].

It is important that society gauge individual and population risk by determining incidence, prevalence, and population-attributable risk. *Incidence* reflects the frequency of new cases of disease or a risk factor during a certain period; *prevalence* reflects the proportion of individuals with a given condition or factor at a single point in time. Population-attributable risk, or how much of the population's risk of disease is attributable to a given factor, is driven by the proportion of the public with a given risk factor and the magnitude of the associated risk. It is an important concept for determining resource allocation between various preventive interventions [18].

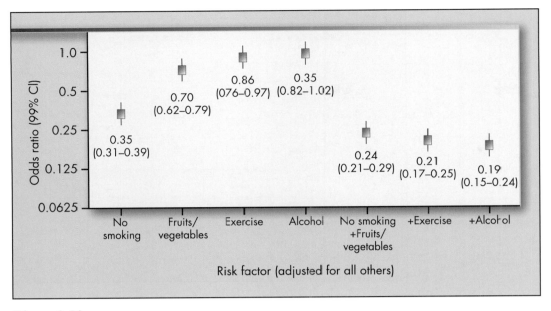

Figure 2-19.

The INTERHEART study. This concept discussed previously can be further extended cross-culturally. Current knowledge about potentially modifiable cardiac risk factors is primarily derived from developed countries. To expand this database, INTERHEART, a recent case-control study, investigated the strength of the association between acute myocardial infarction (MI) and nine risk factors in participants recruited from 52 countries [19]. Researchers used structured questionnaires, physical examinations, and blood samples from 15,152 cases and 14,820 control subjects to assess risk. Odds ratios and the population-attributable risk were evaluated for risk factors and their combinations in the overall population and in different age groups and geographic regions. The study found that abnormal lipids, smoking, hypertension,

diabetes, abdominal obesity, psychosocial factors, low consumption of fruits and vegetables, no alcohol intake, and irregular physical activity account for most of the risk of MI worldwide in both genders and at all ages in all regions. Conversely, a healthy lifestyle that includes daily consumption of fruits and vegetables and regular exercise was shown to reduce the risk of acute myocardial infarction, conferring an odds ratio of 0.60. The risk was further reduced (odds ratio of 0.21) if in addition to eating a healthy diet and exercising, an individual also avoided smoking. Although the relative importance of every risk factor varied, raised lipids, smoking, and psychosocial factors were the most important risk factors in all regions of the world. (*Adapted from* Yusuf *et al.* [19].)

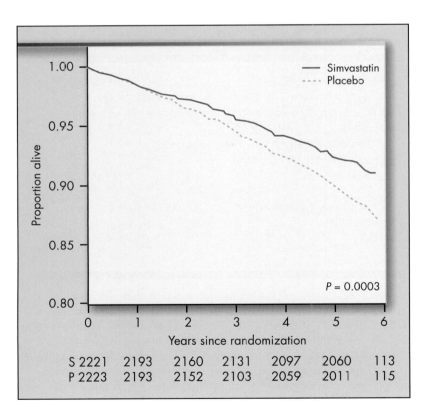

Figure 2-20.

Randomized trials: Kaplan-Meier curves for all-cause mortality. The discussion so far has focused on the ability of risk factors to predict who at an individual level will likely develop cardiovascular disease in the future or predict rates of disease at a population level. The next step is to develop interventions that can reduce the risk of developing disease or delay its onset or progression.

Randomized trials also have played a critical role in firmly establishing cause and effect and clearly demonstrating that an intervention can reduce the risk of coronary heart disease (CHD). The randomized trial provides not only confirmation of cause and effect but also permits quantification of the benefits of a given intervention. Effective treatments for hypertension and dyslipidemia have been tested in large-scale trials. The Scandinavian Simvastatin Survival Study Group (4S) [20] trial is one such large-scale trial that clearly demonstrated reduced risk of CHD among those with known CHD who were given a statin. (*Adapted from* Scandinavian Simvastatin Survival Study Group (4S) [20].)

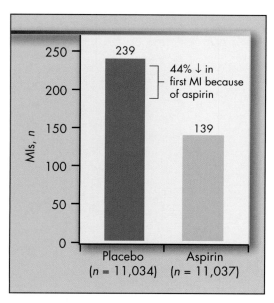

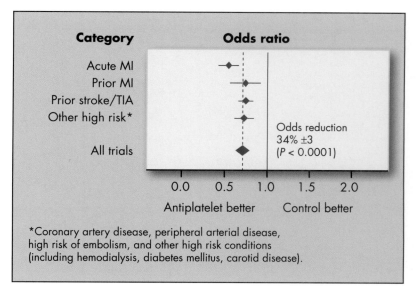

Figure 2-21.

Myocardial infarction (MI) in the Physicians' Health Study. In addition to identifying risk factors, randomized trials established new interventions that could prevent events. A good example of this is the use of aspirin in primary and secondary prevention of coronary heart disease (CHD). Aspirin was shown to reduce CHD events among those having an acute MI and among those with existing cardiovascular disease. The Physicians' Health Study was the first large-scale primary prevention trial to demonstrate the protective effects of aspirin in healthy men [21]. This study introduced a new concept of a prophylactic agent that could lower future risk.

Figure 2-22.

Antithrombotic Trialists' Collaboration: reduction in risk of nonfatal myocardial infarction (MI). Trials are clearly useful in establishing the benefits and understanding the risks of any given intervention. Meta-analyses play an important role in summarizing data from many trials to provide the best quantitative estimate of the effect of an intervention. One of the best examples is the Antithrombotic Trialists' Collaboration [8] on the effects of aspirin in secondary prevention of MI. (*Adapted from* Antithrombotic Trialists' Collaboration [8].)

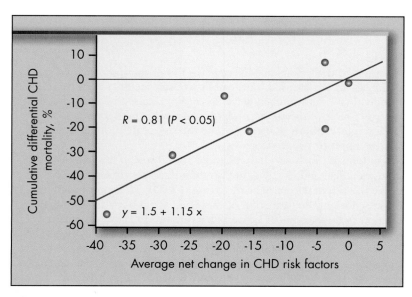

Figure 2-23.

Although most prevention studies focus on changing a single risk factor, several have attempted to measure the impact of simultaneously changing multiple risk factors. The results have been mixed. These multifactorial trials have generally demonstrated a change in risk factor levels or composite scores among those receiving intervention. However, this change has not always translated into lower event rates. Explanations for this inconsistency include the possibility that the magnitude of intervention was too small or that control patients may also have improved their health habits over time. One thing that is clear from these trials is that multiple simultaneous interventions can reduce risk when the planned interventions are large enough and are adequately implemented. In an analysis of seven multiple intervention trials, Kornitzer [22] plotted change in the multiple logistic function of risk against the reduction in risk of coronary heart disease (CHD). The strong linear relationship suggests that as long as risk factors are truly modified, event rates will also be reduced. (*Adapted from* Kornitzer [22].)

Prevalence of Coronary Risk Factors in the United States

Risk factor	Prevalence, %
Total cholesterol of 200 mg/dL or greater	50.7
LDL cholesterol of 130 mg/dL or greater	45.8
HDL cholesterol < 40 mg/dL	26.4
Blood pressure 140/90 mm Hg or greater	32.8
Current cigarette smoker	28
Diabetes mellitus	5.5 (physician diagnosed)
Overweight and obese adults	64.5
Obese adults	30.5
Inactive	31–55 (depending on race)

Figure 2-24.

Prevalence of coronary risk factors in the United States. Despite some declines in several risk factors, there remain many targets for intervention [23]. Overweight and obesity top the list, followed closely by the lack of physical activity. Globally, more than one billion adults are overweight— at least 300 million of whom are obese—the result of changes in diet and exercise brought about by industrialization, urbanization, and economic development. Recognizing this, in 2004 the World Health Assembly endorsed the World Health Organization Global Strategy on Diet, Physical Activity, and Health, a broad-ranging approach to improving all aspects of nutrition that recommended at least 30 minutes of regular, moderate-intensity physical activity on most days. (*Adapted from* American Heart Association [23].)

Risk Factors for Coronary Heart Disease, Cardiovascular Disease, and Stroke

High-mortality developing countries

Risk factor	Prevalence, %pp
High blood pressure*	2.5
Tobacco use*	2.0
High cholesterol*	1.9
Underweight	14.9
Unsafe sex	10.2
Unsafe water, sanitation, and hygiene	5.5
Indoor smoke from solid fuels	3.7
Zinc deficiency	3.2
Iron deficiency	3.1
Vitamin A deficiency	3.0

Low-mortality developing countries

Risk factor	Prevalence, %
High blood pressure*	5.0
Tobacco use*	4.0
High cholesterol*	2.1
Alcohol*	6.2
Obesity*	2.7
Low fruit and vegetable intake	1.9
Underweight	3.1
Indoor smoke from solid fuels	1.9
Iron deficiency	1.8
Unsafe water, sanitation, and hygiene	1.7

Developed countries

Risk factors	Prevalence, %
High blood pressure*	10.9
Tobacco use*	12.2
High cholesterol*	7.6
Alcohol*	9.2
Obesity*	7.4
Low fruit and vegetable intake*	3.9
Physical inactivity*	3.3
Illicit drug use	1.8
Unsafe sex	0.8
Iron deficiency	0.7

*Major cardiovascular disease risk factors.

Figure 2-25.
Risk factors for heart disease. Once thought of as a "rich country" disease, cardiovascular disease and the risk factors associated with it are now taking their toll in low- and middle-income countries. In its 2002 World Health Report, the World Health Organization (WHO) found that even in the poorest regions of the world, common risk factors such as high blood pressure, high cholesterol, and obesity are contributing to a rising burden of serious disease and untimely death. In 2003, the WHO launched the SuRF (Surveillance of Risk Factors) Report 1, which captured for the first time chronic disease risk factor profiles from more than 170 member states [9]. SuRF 1 is the first step in a major ongoing initiative to collect data helpful in predicting the future burden of cardiovascular disease and other chronic diseases to identify potential interventions and health policies to reduce risk, especially in developing countries. (*Adapted from* Mackay and Mensah [9].)

Evaluating Risk Factors

High prevalence of the risk factors
Consistency of prospective data
Strength and independence of association
Improve predictive value
Biologic plausibility
Standardized measure
Low cost
Potentially modifiable
Risk reduction in randomized trials
Interventions are worth the risks and costs

Figure 2-26.
Evaluating risk factors. Over the past few decades, basic research and human physiologic studies have provided researchers with a basic understanding of the pathophysiology of atherosclerosis. Human observational studies have identified risk factors that clearly predict future risk and serve as potential targets for interventions to lower risk. Randomized trials have in some cases demonstrated the utility of practical preventive interventions.

The ideal risk factor is one that is common and for which the published data consistently demonstrate a strong and independent association with CVD. The added knowledge should enhance researchers' ability to predict disease. The assessment of that risk factor should be easy, low risk, reliable, and low cost. Ideally, the risk factor would be modifiable, and effective interventions would be established through trials.

References

1. Libby P: The vascular biology of atherosclerosis. In *Braunwald's Heart Disease: A Textbook of Cardiovascular Medicine*, edn 7. Philadelphia: Elsevier Saunders; 2005:921–937.

2. Kfomhut D, Menotti M, Blackburn H: *Prevention of Coronary Disease, Diet, Lifestyle, and Risk Factors in the Seven Countries Study.* Norwell, MA: Kluwer Academic Publishers; 2002.

3. Marmot MG, Syme LS, Kagan A, *et al.*: Epidemiologic studies of coronary heart disease and stroke in Japanese men living in Japan, Hawaii and California: prevalence of coronary and hypertensive heart disease and associated risk factors. *Am J Epidemiol* 1975, 102:514–525.

4. Kannel WB, Dawber TR, Kagan A, *et al.*: Factors of risk in the development of coronary heart disease: six-year follow-up experience. The Framingham Study. *Ann Intern Med* 1961, 55:33–50.

5. Berenson GS, Srinivasan SR, Bao W, *et al.*: Association between multiple cardiovascular risk factors and atherosclerosis in children and young adults. The Bogalusa Heart Study. *N Engl J Med* 1998, 338:1650–1656.

6. Relationship of atherosclerosis in young men to serum lipoprotein cholesterol concentrations and smoking: a preliminary report from the Pathobiological Determinants of Atherosclerosis in Youth (PDAY) Research Group. *JAMA* 1990, 264:3018–3024.

7. Gaziano JM: Primary and secondary prevention of coronary heart disease. In *Braunwald's Heart Disease: A Textbook of Cardiovascular Medicine*, edn 7. Philadelphia: Elsevier Saunders; 2005:921–937.

8. Antithrombotic Trialists' Collaboration: Collaborative meta-analysis of randomized trials of antiplatelet therapy for prevention of death, myocardial infarction, and stroke in high risk patients. *BMJ* 2002, 324:71–86.

9. Mackay J, Mensah GA: *The Atlas of Heart Disease and Stroke.* Spring Lake, MI: World Health Organization; 2004.

10. Fuster V, Badimon JJ: The pathogenesis of coronary artery disease and the acute coronary syndrome. *N Engl J Med* 1992, 326:242–250.

11. Newman WP III, Freedman DS, Voors AW, *et al.*: Relation of serum lipoprotein levels and systolic blood pressure to early atherosclerosis: the Bogalusa Heart Study. *N Engl J Med* 1986, 314:138–144.

12. Penckhofer S: Cardiovascular risk factors in women. *J Myo Isch* 1992, 4:25–46.

13. Feinleib M: Trends in heart disease in the United States. *Am J Med Sci* 1995, 310:s8–s14.

14. Castelli WP, Garrison RJ, Wilson PW: Incidence of coronary heart disease and lipoprotein cholesterol levels. The Framingham Study. *JAMA* 1986, 256:2835–2838.

15. Ridker P, Hennekens C, Buring J, *et al.*: C-reactive protein and other markers of inflammation in the prediction of cardiovascular disease in women. *N Engl J Med* 2000, 342:836–843.

16. Kannel WB: Some lessons in cardiovascular epidemiology from Framingham. *Am J Cardiol* 1976, 37:269–282.

17. Daviglus ML, Stamler J, Pirzada A, *et al.*: Favorable cardiovascular risk profile in young women and long-term risk of cardiovascular and all-cause mortality. *JAMA* 2004, 292:1588–1592.

18. The Burden of Chronic Disease and the Future of Public Health. National Center for Chronic Disease Prevention and Health Promotion, US Centers for Disease Control and Prevention. Available at http://www.cdc.gov/nccdphp/burden_pres/bcd_09.htm.

19. Yusuf S, Hawken S, Ounpuu S, *et al.*: Effect of potentially modifiable risk factors associated with myocardial infarction in 52 countries (the INTERHEART study): case-control study. *Lancet* 2004, 364:937–952.

20. Scandinavian Simvastatin Survival Study Group (4S): Randomized trial of cholesterol lowering in 4444 patients with coronary heart disease: the Scandinavian Simvastatin Survival Study (4S). *Lancet* 1994, 344:1383–1389.

21. Steering Committee of the Physicians' Health Study Research Group: Final report on the aspirin component of the ongoing Physicians' Health Study. *N Engl J Med* 1989, 321:129–135.

22. Kornitzer M: Changing individual behavior. In *Coronary Heart Disease Epidemiology: From Aetiology to Public Health.* Edited by Marmot M, Elliott P. Oxford, UK: Oxford University Press; 1992:492.

23. American Heart Association: *2004 Heart Disease and Stroke Statistical Update.* Dallas: American Heart Association; 2004.

Coronary Heart Disease Risk: Origins, Factors, and Utility

Peter W. F. Wilson

Coronary heart disease (CHD) is largely attributable to arteriosclerosis, a disease process that develops in adolescence. The term *risk factor* was first used in publications from the Framingham Heart Study in the late 1950s and early 1960s [1]. Analyses described higher levels of cholesterol, blood pressure, and cigarette smoking that together augmented the chances of developing CHD over 6 years of follow-up; single factors were generally not responsible for the development of clinical vascular events. Since that time, a variety of advances have led to the development of key factors that are easy to assess and are consistently related to greater risk of initial CHD events, including age, gender, blood pressure, lipids, smoking, and diabetes mellitus.

The type of clinical CHD event that occurs first varies by age and gender. For example, angina pectoris is the most common first CHD event in women, followed by myocardial infarction, and CHD death; sudden cardiac death is extremely uncommon in women. However, among men a myocardial infarction is the most common first CHD event, followed by angina pectoris and coronary death [2]. CHD in women tends to occur after menopause, and rates are significantly higher than for other common diseases of aging, including fractures, cerebrovascular disease, breast cancer, and uterine cancer.

Higher levels of cholesterol have been consistently related to a greater risk for CHD, and high-density lipoprotein (HDL) cholesterol is a major fraction of cholesterol in the plasma. HDL cholesterol levels are an important determinant of risk for CHD and myocardial infarction even when the total cholesterol level is known. The 12-year incidence of myocardial infarction was positively related to cholesterol level and inversely to HDL cholesterol level in Framingham women (*see* Fig. 3-2) [3]. At a total cholesterol level less than 211 mg/dL, the HDL cholesterol levels were inversely related to risk of developing myocardial infarction in women. Similar results were obtained for men and other studies, helping to provide the rationale for cholesterol and HDL cholesterol screening to assess cardiovascular disease (CVD) risk.

Effective lipid therapies over the past two decades have shown that improving total, low-density lipoproteins (LDL) and HDL cholesterol levels, with the emphasis on the LDL fraction, leads to lower risk of initial and recurrent CHD events. In general, more cholesterol lowering has led to a greater reduction in risk of initial and recurrent CHD in these studies. The effectiveness of therapy in these trials has largely been premised on the intention to treat, not on the degree of cholesterol lowering achieved or the ability to reach predefined target levels of cholesterol or LDL cholesterol.

Blood pressure levels that do not meet the criteria for hypertension increase the risk for a first major vascular event, and long-term comparisons have shown that the risk of CVD is increased in persons with high normal blood pressure (systolic pressure 130–139 mm Hg with diastolic 85–89 mm Hg). As high normal pressure level is a common condition, this level of blood pressure accounts for a sizable fraction of CVD events and on a population basis is nearly as important as hypertension itself [4].

The prevalence of cigarette smoking has declined in the United States since the 1960s, and this habit generally doubles the risk of vascular outcomes. Regular and filter cigarettes have similar adverse effects on CHD risk [5]. Low-tar and low-nicotine cigarettes have shown no reduction in CVD risk in comparisons with products that are higher in tar and nicotine [6]. Cessation of cigarette smoking was associated with half the risk for CVD death 1 to 2 years after quitting in men screened as part of the Multiple Risk Factor Intervention Trial study [7].

Risk of CHD is generally increased twofold among younger men and threefold among younger women with type-2 diabetes mellitus [8]. Data from Finland have suggested that the risk for a heart attack in persons with diabetes is very similar to the risk for persons who have had a heart attack, and are at risk for subsequent heart attack. This result led to the concept of type 2 diabetes mellitus as a CHD risk equivalent, and emphasizes the need for aggressive treatment of risk factors in persons with type 2 diabetes mellitus to prevent CVD events [9].

Risk for CVD events can be estimated with multivariable prediction equations that use a score sheet, pocket calculator, or computer. The variables age, systolic blood pressure, smoking, cholesterol, HDL cholesterol, and diabetes mellitus are commonly used to estimate risk for initial CHD events, using separate equations for men and women; risk varies according to the combinations of risk factors [10]. This approach has been validated in the United States across

several observational studies. A variety of population research techniques are used in this setting, including testing the ability of the variables to discriminate new cases from noncases and calibrating equations for use in other locales [11]. Estimation of CHD risk is generally valid for middle-class, white populations in North America and Europe where risk factors and heart disease rates approximate the experience of studies such as Framingham that provided the estimates. Overestimates of CHD risk may be obtained in other locales, such as in China or Hawaii [11,12].

Using a slightly different set of variables, equations that estimate CHD risk have been developed in Germany to predict initial CHD events in men [13]. European investigators from several countries have also developed algorithms to estimate risk of CHD disease mortality [14].

Estimating CHD risk can help clinicians to match the estimated risk of CHD with aggressiveness of risk factor management. Using a multivariable equation approach is a dynamic process, and new information is constantly being evaluated as it may change the approach. It is important to assess whether new information improves the overall prediction of CHD within a population. Accuracy and precision of the new measurement, standardization of the technique, low correlation with existing predictive variables, validation in other observational studies, and biologic relevance are examples of features that need to be considered prior to the inclusion of newer variables into risk-estimating approaches [15,16].

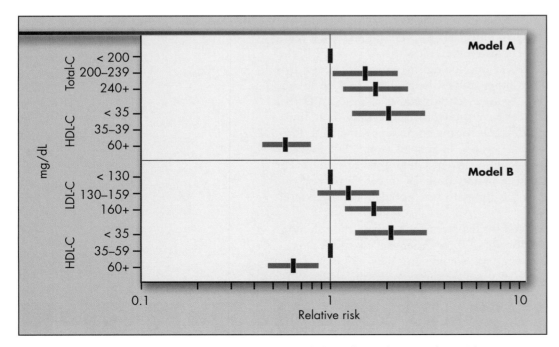

Figure 3-1.
Twelve-year incidence of myocardial infarction from the Framingham cohort for women. Total cholesterol and high-density lipoprotein cholesterol (HDL-C) are critical risk factors for the development of initial coronary heart disease (CHD) events. This figure shows the Framingham evidence for risk of total CHD incidence (myocardial infarction, angina pectoris, coronary heart disease death) for men according to quartile of total cholesterol and quartile of HDL-C. The general trends for total cholesterol and for HDL-C are statistically related to CHD risk. Within the lowest quartile of cholesterol the HDL-C levels were related to CHD risk, which led to the inclusion of HDL-C as part of initial screening to assess CHD risk. Similar data were obtained for women. (*Adapted from* Abbott *et al.* [3].)

Figure 3-2.
Twelve-year coronary heart disease incidence according to lipid categories in women. Data are shown for Framingham women at risk for initial coronary heart disease events in statistical models that included 1) age, cholesterol category, and high-density lipoprotein (HDL-C) category in the *top panel* (Model A) or age, low-density lipoprotein cholesterol (LDL-C) category, and HDL-C category in the *bottom panel* (Model B). The results showed that there was little advantage to include LDL-C in the initial screening for coronary heart disease risk, and total cholesterol assessment provided reliable estimates of risk. Similar data were obtained for men. (*Adapted from* Wilson *et al.* [10].)

Atlas of Cardiovascular Risk Factors

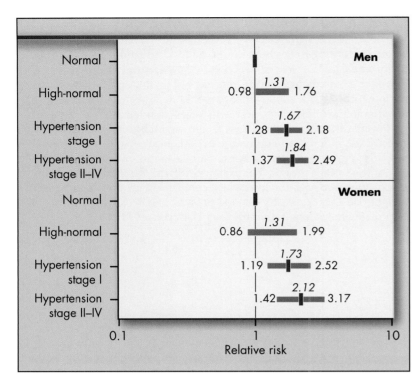

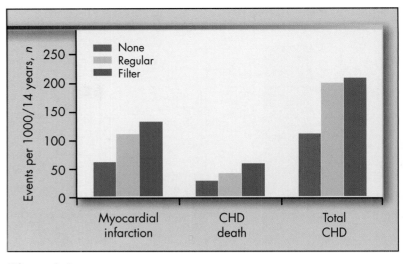

Figure 3-3.
Twelve-year coronary heart disease incidence according to blood pressure category. The incidence of coronary heart disease events was related to category of blood pressure in Framingham men and women over 12 years of follow-up. Successively higher blood pressure categories imparted greater risk for events and these effects were evident within the range typically considered to be normal blood pressure. (*Adapted from* Wilson *et al.* [10].)

Figure 3-4.
Fourteen-year incidence in men: cigarette smoking and coronary heart disease (CHD) Framingham Heart Study. Filter and regular (nonfilter) cigarette smoking was related to greater risk of CHD events (myocardial infarction, CHD death, and total CHD) in Framingham participants. (*Adapted from* Castelli *et al.* [5].)

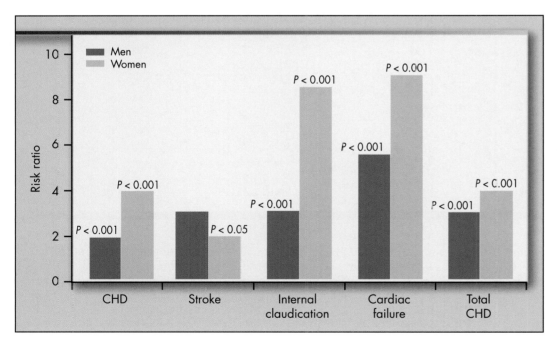

Figure 3-5.
Diabetes and cardiovascular disease risk in the Framingham cohort aged 35 to 64 years: 30-year follow-up. Diabetes mellitus generally led to an increased risk of cardiovascular events in Framingham Heart Study participants. Typically a doubling of risk for events was evident for men and often a tripling of risk was found for women in the age group 35 to 64 years at baseline. Actual risks varied according to the cardiovascular disease outcome being studied. CHD—coronary heart disease. (*Adapted from* Wilson [8].)

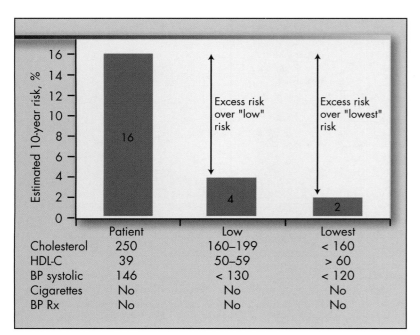

	Patient	Low	Lowest
Cholesterol	250	160–199	< 160
HDL-C	39	50–59	> 60
BP systolic	146	< 130	< 120
Cigarettes	No	No	No
BP Rx	No	No	No

Figure 3-6.

Estimated 10-year hard coronary heart disease (CHD) risk in a 55-year-old man according to levels of various factors. Equations that estimated risk for initial CHD events allowed individual calculations of risk as shown for a hypothetical person represented by the vertical bar on the left, in which the risk factors present would be expected to lead to a 16% risk of an initial CHD event over a 10-year follow-up interval. Low-risk and lowest-risk comparison groups are provided. Excess risk can be estimated as the difference between the hypothetical person's estimate and comparison groups. Relative risk estimates also can be estimated as the ratio of the various groups. For example, the risk for the hypothetical person compared with the lowest risk comparison group would be 16/2, an eightfold greater risk. BP—blood pressure; HDL-C—high-density lipoprotein cholesterol. (*Adapted from* Wilson *et al.* [10].)

Coronary Heart Disease Prediction with Risk Factor Algorithms

Risk factor	Wilson *et al.* [10]	Adult Treatment Panel III (2001 National Institutes of Health)	D'Agostino *et al.* [11]	Assmann *et al.* [13]	Euro-SCOR
Source	Framingham	Framingham	Framingham	Prospective Cardiovascular Münster study (PROCAM)	Europe
Age interval	5 years	5 years	5 years	5 years	5 years
Gender	Yes	Yes	Yes	Men	Yes
BP levels	JNC-VI	BP systolic	BP systolic	BP systolic	BP systolic
BP Rx	No	Yes	No	No	No
Cholesterol	Yes	Yes	Yes	No	Yes
HDL-C	Yes	Yes	Yes	Yes	No
LDL-C	Optional	No	No	Yes	No
Cigarettes	Yes	Yes	Yes	Yes	Yes
Diabetes	Yes	No	Yes	Yes	Yes
ECG-LVH	No	No	No	MI history	No
Event	Total CHD	Hard CHD	Hard CHD	Hard CHD	CHD death

Figure 3-7.

Coronary heart disease (CHD) with risk factor algorithms. A variety of CHD risk-estimating equations have been developed by Framingham and European investigators. Many of the variables used to estimate risk are similar and the overall effects are to rank individuals and provide estimates of absolute risk for disease.

BP—blood pressure; ECG-LVH—echocardiography left ventricular hypertrophy; HDL-C—high-density lipoprotein cholesterol; LDL-C—low-density lipoprotein cholesterol. (*Adapted from* Wilson *et al.* [10], D'Agostino *et al.* [11], Assmann *et al.* [13], and Conroy *et al.* [14].)

Performance Measures for Risk Estimation

Discrimination
  Ability of the model to distinguish events from nonevents
      (C-statistic used as measure)
Calibration
  Closeness of predicted probability to observed (adjusted
      Hosmer-Lemeshow chi-square < 20 and calibration bar
      plot as measures)

Figure 3-8.

Performance measures for risk estimation. Risk estimation can be characterized by the ability to provide good discrimination and calibration. The specialized definitions are provided in this table. Discrimination is the ability of the model to distinguish events from nonevents, using the C-statistic as a performance measure. However, calibration may often be needed to provide accurate estimates of absolute risk in other settings, and it is defined as the closeness of predicted probability to observed, in which adjusted Hosmer-Lemeshow chi-square statistics and calibration bar plots are used as measures. (*Adapted from* D'Agostino *et al.* [11].)

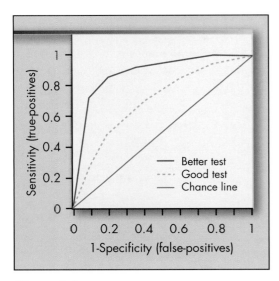

Figure 3-9.
Receiver operative characteristic (ROC) curves and disease prediction. ROC curves are used to describe the relationship between a diagnostic test (or estimating equation) and disease outcome. The abscissa is the false-positive rate and the ordinate is the true-positive rate. The chance line is the *diagonal line* and has an area under the ROC of 0.50. Higher area under the ROC denotes better risk estimation. The typical ROC for CHD risk estimation using traditional variables is in the 0.75–0.80 range. (*Adapted from* D'Agostino *et al.* [11].)

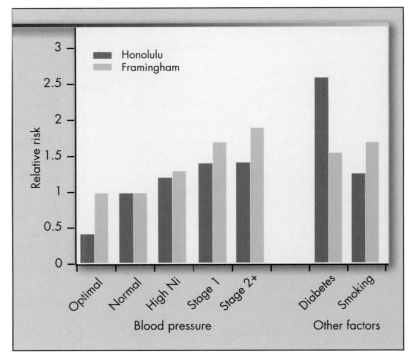

Figure 3-10.
Relative risk for coronary heart disease in men from the Honolulu Heart Study and the Framingham Heart Study: 10-year follow-up. Relative risk estimates for coronary heart disease outcomes are shown for Honolulu men and Framingham men according to two blood pressure categories: diabetes mellitus and smoking history. Relative risk estimates were generally similar in each of these population settings, with the exception of diabetes mellitus, which was associated with a greater relative risk for events in the Honolulu men than in Framingham men. Ni—nickel. (*Adapted from* D'Agostino *et al.* [11].)

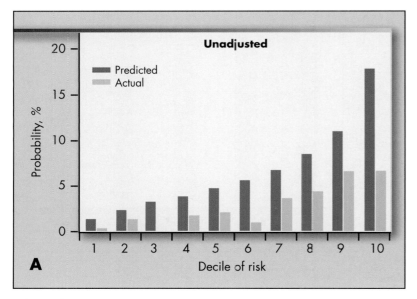

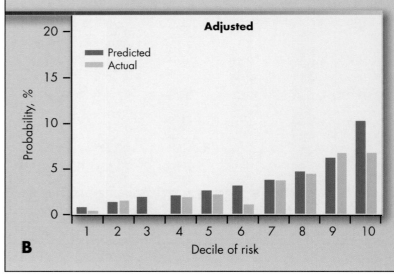

Figure 3-11.
Honolulu Heart Study hard coronary heart disease (CHD) prediction with Framingham equations. Prediction of hard CHD events (myocardial infarction and CHD death) in Honolulu men was undertaken with Framingham CHD risk-estimating equations. The deciles of risk are shown for the Honolulu men and the estimated risks are typically double that of the actual experience when no adjustments were used for the estimating equations (**A**). However, when the Framingham risk equations were adjusted according to the event experience and the mean risk factor levels of the Honolulu participants, the estimates were fairly close to what was actually observed (**B**). (*Adapted from* D'Agostino *et al.* [11].)

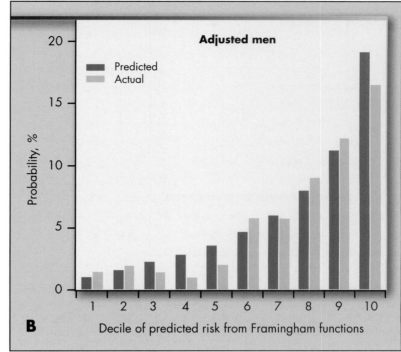

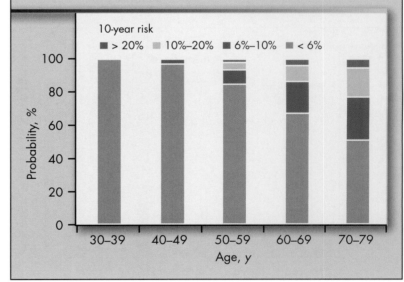

Figure 3-12.
Estimation of 10-year hard coronary heart disease (CHD) risk in Chinese men using Framingham Heart Study CHD functions. Prediction of hard CHD events (myocardial infarction and CHD death) in Chinese men was undertaken with Framingham CHD risk-estimating equations. The deciles of risk are shown for the Chinese men and the estimated risks are typically four times that of the actual experience

when no adjustments were used for the estimating equations (**A**). However, when the Framingham risk equations were adjusted according to the event experience and the mean risk factor levels of the Chinese participants, the estimates were fairly close to what was actually observed (**B**). (*Adapted from* Liu *et al.* [12].)

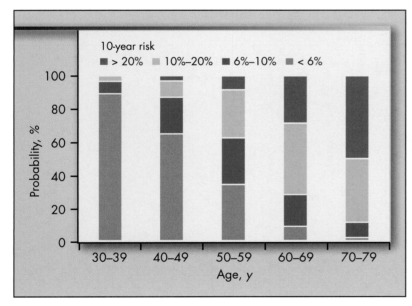

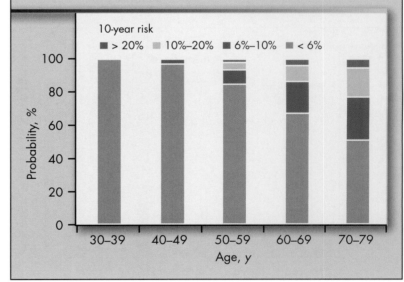

Figure 3-13.
Estimated 10-year hard coronary heart disease (CHD) risk: Framingham Heart Study offspring and cohort men. The risk of hard CHD (myocardial infarction, CHD death) according to age decile is shown for Framingham men according to several categories of CHD risk (< 6%, 6%–10%, 10%–20%, and > 20% over 10 years). Most men are at very low risk up to age 40 years. After age 50 years the majority of men are at intermediate risk, and high risk (> 20%/10 years) is an important contributor only after 60 years of age. (*Adapted from* Pasternak *et al.* [17].)

Figure 3-14.
Estimated 10-year hard coronary heart disease (CHD) risk: Framingham Heart Study offspring and cohort women. The risk of hard CHD (myocardial infarction, CHD death) according to age decile is shown for Framingham women according to several categories of CHD risk (< 6%, 6%–10%, 10%–20%, and > 20% over 10 years). Most women are at very low risk throughout adulthood. Only after age 60 years are many women at intermediate or high risk. (*Adapted from* Pasternak *et al.* [17].)

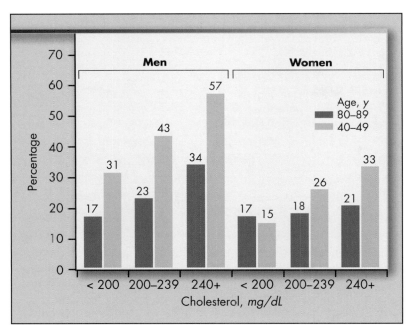

Figure 3-15.
The cumulative lifetime risk of coronary heart disease (CHD) for Framingham participants according to low, middle, and high cholesterol categories and baseline age of 40 to 49 and 80 to 89 years is shown for men and women. At younger and older ages the risk for men is higher. Even men and women who survive to age 80 years and have yet to experience CHD have significant risk for later CHD that varies with cholesterol level, ranging from 17% to 34% in men and 17% to 21% in women. (*Adapted from* Lloyd-Jones *et al.* [18].)

Factor	Prevalence	Relative odds	PAR, %
Familial hypercholesterolemia	0.002	35	6.4
Familial defective apolipoprotein B100	0.0014	40	0.4
Type III dyslipidemia	0.0025	40	1
MTHFR gene homozygote	0.10	1.16	2
ε-4 allele	0.25	1.53	11

Figure 3-16.
Risk factors and estimated coronary heart disease (CHD) risk. Risk for CHD according to a variety of genetic markers and lipid levels is estimated from Framingham offspring data. This table shows the prevalence of the factor, relative risk, and population attributable risk percent (PAR) related to the factor. The PAR represents the potential effect that eliminating the factor may have on the occurrence of the disease. For example, heterozygous familial hypercholesterolemia is found in approximately one in 500 persons, has a high relative risk for CHD, and is found in only 6% of persons with a myocardial infarction. The apolipoprotein ε4 allele is present in approximately 24% of the population, the relative risk for CHD, but the PAR is approximately 11%. (*Adapted from* Wilson *et al.* [19].)

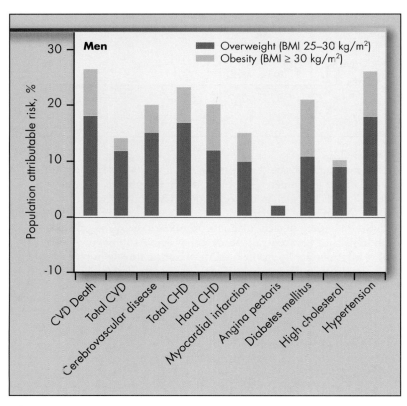

Figure 3-17.
The population attributable risk percent for overweight (body mass index [BMI] 25–30 kg/m²) and obesity (BMI > 30 kg/m²) in relation to a variety of cardiovascular disease (CVD) risk factors and CVD outcomes is shown for men. In general, approximately 25% of CVD outcomes can be attributed to excess adiposity and the effects of overweight are generally greater that what is observed for frank obesity. CHD—coronary heart disease. (*Adapted from* Wilson *et al.* [20].)

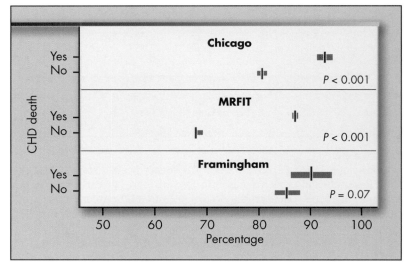

Figure 3-18.
The presence of major cardiovascular disease (CVD) risk factors (cholesterol level > 240 mg/dL, systolic pressure > 140 mm Hg), before the occurrence of coronary heart disease (CHD) death during follow-up, was investigated in men 40–59 years with diastolic pressure > 90 mm Hg, smoking, or diabetes mellitus at baseline. Individuals were screened from the Chicago Heart Study, Multiple Risk Factor Intervention Trial (MRFIT), and Framingham Heart Study. Most of the participants (> 90% in Chicago Heart Study, 85% in MRFIT, and 90% in Framingham) who experienced CHD death had at least one major risk factor. (*Adapted from* Greenland *et al.* [21].)

Criteria for Novel Risk Factors

Standardized measurements
Gradient of effects
Linear, extremes, logarithmic
Clinically important
Can generally intervene on factor
Usually low correlations with existing factors

Figure 3-19.
Criteria for novel risk factors. A variety of issues are important in the evaluation of risk factors that might help to improve coronary heart disease risk estimation, including whether the factors are standardized, the gradient of effects is linear, observed only at extremes, or logarithmic. Additional considerations are whether the factor is clinically important, it is possible to intervene on the factor, and there are usually low correlations between important new factors and traditionally accepted.

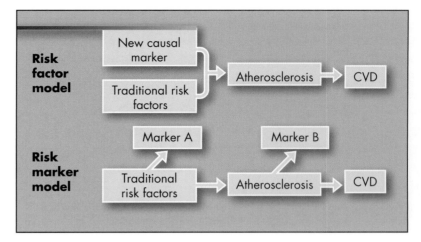

Figure 3-20.
Alternative models for role of risk factors and markers in cardiovascular disease (CVD). *Risk factor* is a term used to describe a mechanism that is along a causal pathway for the development of CVD; the term *risk marker* characterizes effects that are thought to result from a disease process and are not causal. (*Adapted from* Pearson *et al.* [22].)

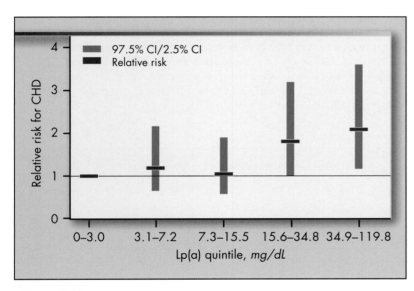

Figure 3-21.
Lipoprotein(a) [Lp(a)] level and risk for coronary heart disease (CHD) in Lipid Research Clinics men aged 35 to 59 with 7 to 10 years of follow-up. Lp(a) has been related to the occurrence of CHD outcomes in a variety of studies with varying results, partly because the particles vary in composition from person to person and make standardization difficult. In addition, as shown in this figure, it appears that the relation between CHD risk and Lp(a) level is not linear, as shown for participants from the Lipid Research Clinics Program, in which an increased risk for CHD was only observed for men at the fourth and fifth quintile of Lp(a). (*Adapted from* Schaefer *et al.* [23].)

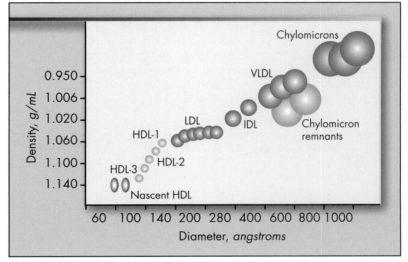

Figure 3-22.
Serum lipoprotein size and density. Serum lipoproteins in the plasma vary according to diameter and buoyancy in the plasma, with triglyceride-rich particles, such as chylomicrons, having the greatest buoyancy and size. A variety of subparticles have been characterized, and several methods, including nuclear magnetic resonance, gradient gel electrophoresis, and ultracentrifugation, are available to quantify them. HDL—high-density lipoprotein; IDL—intermediate-density lipoprotein; LDL—low-density lipoprotein; VLDL—very low-density lipoprotein.

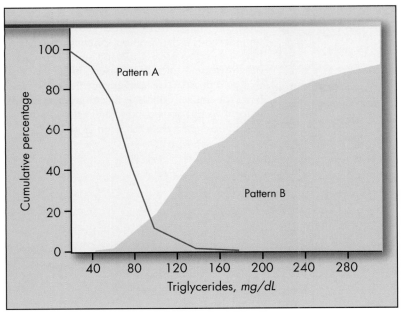

Figure 3-23.
Cumulative distribution of adjusted triglyceride levels by low-density lipoprotein subtype. The cumulative distribution of small, dense low-density lipoprotein particles (*pattern B*) is proportional to the concentration of triglycerides in the plasma. The opposite effect (*pattern A*), in which the low-density lipoprotein particles are larger and more buoyant, is more likely to be observed at low concentrations of triglycerides in the plasma. (*Adapted from* Austin *et al*. [24].)

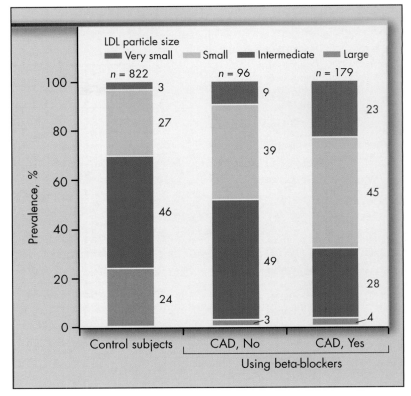

Figure 3-24.
Prevalence of coronary artery disease (CAD) and low-density lipoprotein (LDL) particle size in men. The proportion of Framingham participants with small, dense LDL particles was related to the prevalence of CAD and use of beta-blockers in the population. Although reports have generally shown that persons with coronary heart disease are more likely to have small, dense LDL particles, they have not consistently shown that LDL particle size estimation helps to improve coronary heart disease risk assessment. (*Adapted from* Campos *et al*. [25].)

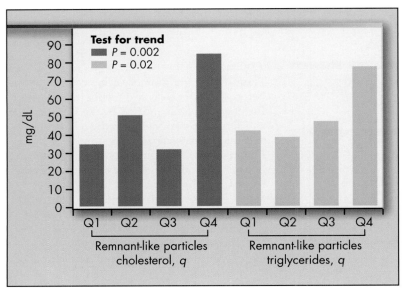

Figure 3-25.
Remnant lipoprotein particles and cardiovascular disease risk prevalence: Framingham Heart Study Offspring Women Examination 4. Concentration of remnant lipoprotein particles assessed by an immunoassay were related to the prevalence of cardiovascular disease in Framingham Offspring Women, using assays that evaluated the triglyceride or the cholesterol concentration of the particles. (*Adapted from* McNamara *et al*. [26].)

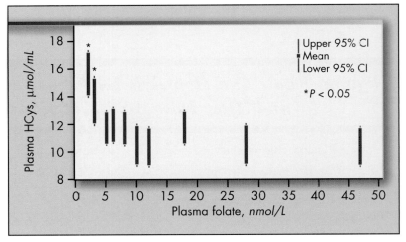

Figure 3-26.
Mean homocysteine (HCys) plasma level by decile of plasma folate: Framingham Heart Study cohort. Higher HCys levels have been found for persons with lower intakes and blood concentrations of B vitamins such as folate, B6, and B12. This figure shows that the two bottom deciles of plasma folate in the original Framingham cohort were likely to have higher HCys than others in the population sample. (*Adapted from* Selhub *et al*. [27].)

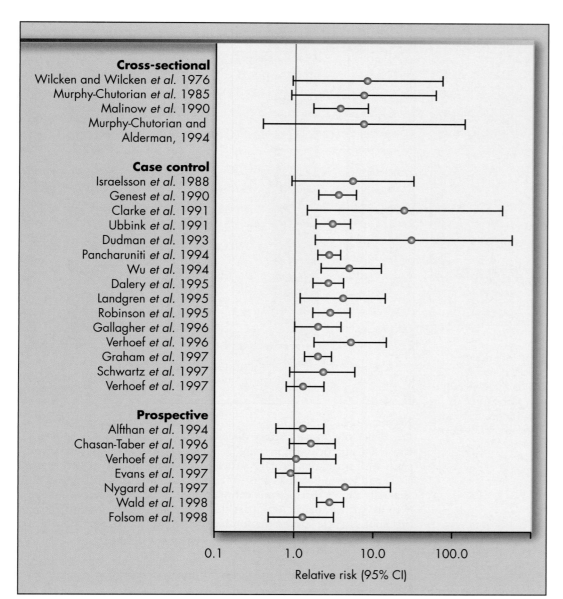

Figure 3-27.
Coronary heart disease and elevated homocysteine levels. Higher homocysteine levels have been related to greater risk for initial coronary heart disease events in cross-sectional, case control, and prospective studies, but the trend has been for smaller effects in recent years, especially for investigations conducted in the United States. (*Adapted from* Christen *et al.* [28].)

Plasma Folate and Homocysteine Concentrations Before and After Folic Acid Fortification

Plasma characteristic	Before	After
Mean folate, *ng/mL*	4.6	10
Folate < 3 ng/mL	22%	1.7%
Mean total homocysteine, *μmol/L*	10.1	9.4
Total homocysteine > 13 μmol/L	18.7%	9.8%

Figure 3-28.
Plasma folate and homocysteine concentrations before and after folic acid fortification. Folate fortification was mandated by the US Food and Drug Administration in the late 1990s, and the effects were studied in the Framingham Offspring before and after the policy went into effect. The prevalence of low folate in the blood declined greatly from approximately 22% to 2%, and the frequency of an elevated homocysteine greater than 13 umol/L was much less (19% before and 10% after). (*Adapted from* Jacques *et al.* [29].)

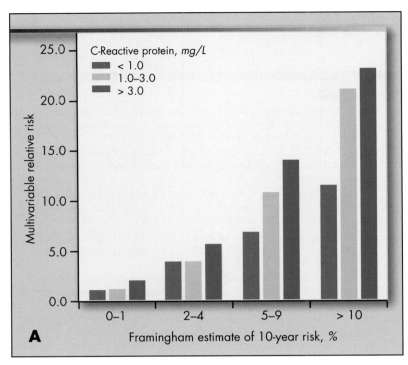

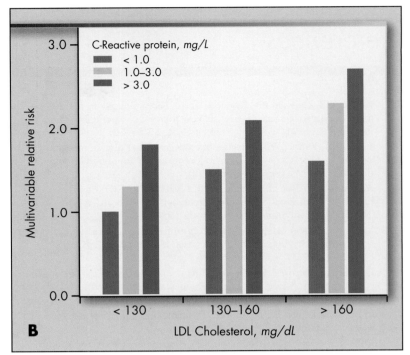

Figure 3-29.

Relative risk for cardiovascular disease according to C-reactive protein and Framingham risk score and low-density lipoprotein cholesterol. Inflammatory markers, especially high-sensitivity C-reactive protein, have been investigated in several studies for a relation with risk for cardiovascular disease outcomes. In multivariable risk assessment of health professionals, the high-sensitivity C-reactive protein levels were shown to help improve the assignment of risk category (**A**) and the effects were generally observed at the three LDL cholesterol levels (**B**) that were studied. (*Adapted from* Ridker *et al.* [30].)

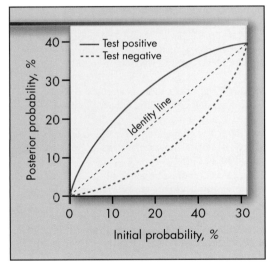

Figure 3-30.

Incorporating decision analysis: serial testing and risk of coronary heart disease. Serial testing is being evaluated as part of the role of new cardiovascular disease risk factors. If a test is repeated and the identical result is obtained, the prior and posterior probability of developing (or having) disease will not change. This application of Bayes' Theorem was used to assess the utility of exercise treadmill testing for cardiovascular disease in the 1980s and is now being used for CHD risk assessment. (*Adapted from* Wilson *et al.* [31].)

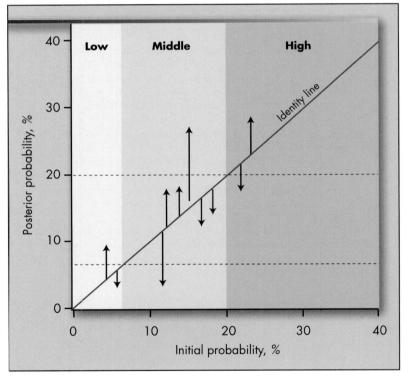

Figure 3-31.

Serial testing and risk of disease. The prior and posterior probabilities of disease are hypothetically illustrated for low-, middle-, and high-risk for CHD, taking the suggested cutoff values (< 6% low-risk, 6%–20% intermediate-risk, > 20% high-risk over 10 years) recommended by experts. The utility of an additional novel test, over and above traditional testing, can be considered as the difference in risk between the *identity line* and the tip of the *arrow*. In some cases the additional test will lead to a lower risk estimation, and in some cases, the opposite will be observed. It has been suggested that the greatest utility will arise when additional testing leads to a reassignment outside the 6% to 20% square that is in the center of the figure. (*Adapted from* Wilson *et al.* [31].)

Coronary Heart Disease Risk: Origins, Factors, and Utility

1. Kannel WB, Dawber TR, Kagan A, *et al.*: Factors of risk in the development of coronary heart disease: six year follow-up experience. The Framingham Study. *Ann Intern Med* 1961, 55:33–50.

2. Lerner DJ, Kannel WB: Patterns of coronary heart disease morbidity and mortality in the sexes: a 26-year follow-up of the Framingham population. *Am Heart J* 1986, 111:383–390.

3. Abbott RD, Wilson PW, Kannel WB, Castelli WP: High density lipoprotein cholesterol, total cholesterol screening, and myocardial infarction. The Framingham Study. *Arteriosclerosis* 1988, 8:207–211.

4. Vasan RS, Larson MG, Leip EP, *et al.*: Impact of high-normal blood pressure on the risk of cardiovascular disease. *N Engl J Med* 2001, 345:1291–1297.

5. Castelli WP, Garrison RJ, Dawber TR, *et al.*: The filter cigarette and coronary heart disease: the Framingham Study. *Lancet* 1981, 2:109–113.

6. Palmer JR, Rosenberg L, Shapiro S: "Low yield" cigarettes and the risk of nonfatal myocardial infarction in women. *N Engl J Med* 1989, 320:1569–1573.

7. Ockene JK, Kuller LH, Svendsen KH, Meilahn E: The relationship of smoking cessation to coronary heart disease and lung cancer in the Multiple Risk Factor Intervention Trial (MRFIT). *Am J Public Health* 1990, 80:954–958.

8. Wilson PW: Diabetes mellitus and coronary heart disease. *Am J Kidney Dis* 1998, 32(suppl):S89–S100.

9. Haffner SM, Lehto S, Ronnemaa T, *et al.*: Mortality from coronary heart disease in subjects with type 2 diabetes and in nondiabetic subjects with and without prior myocardial infarction. *N Engl J Med* 1998, 339:229–234.

10. Wilson PW, D'Agostino RB, Levy D, *et al.*: Prediction of coronary heart disease using risk factor categories. *Circulation* 1998, 97:1837–1847.

11. D'Agostino RB, Grundy S, Sullivan LM, Wilson P: Validation of the Framingham coronary heart disease prediction scores: results of a multiple ethnic groups investigation. *JAMA* 2001, 286:180–187.

12. Liu J, Hong Y, D'Agostino RB, *et al.*: Predictive value for the Chinese population of the Framingham CHD risk assessment tool compared with the Chinese Multi-Provincial Cohort Study. *JAMA* 2004, 291:2591–2599.

13. Assmann G, Cullen P, Schulte H: Simple scoring scheme for calculating the risk of acute coronary events based on the 10-year follow-up of the prospective cardiovascular Munster (PROCAM) study. *Circulation* 2002, 105:310–315.

14. Conroy RM, Pyorala K, Fitzgerald AP, *et al.*: Estimation of ten-year risk of fatal cardiovascular disease in Europe: the SCORE project. *Eur Heart J* 2003; 24:987–1003.

15. Wilson PW: Metabolic risk factors for coronary heart disease: current and future prospects. *Curr Opin Cardiol* 1999, 14:176–185.

16. Mosca L: C-reactive protein: to screen or not to screen? *N Engl J Med* 2002, 347:1615–1617.

17. Pasternak RC, Abrams J, Greenland P, *et al.*: 34th Bethesda Conference: task force #1. Identification of coronary heart disease risk: is there a detection gap? *J Am Coll Cardiol* 2003, 41:1863–1874.

18. Lloyd-Jones DM, Wilson PW, Larson MG, *et al.*: Lifetime risk of coronary heart disease by cholesterol levels at selected ages. *Arch Intern Med* 2003, 163:1966–1972.

19. Wilson PW, Myers RH, Larson MG, *et al.*: Apolipoprotein E alleles, dyslipidemia, and coronary heart disease. The Framingham Offspring Study. *JAMA* 1994, 272:1666–1671.

20. Wilson PW, D'Agostino RB, Sullivan L, *et al.*: Overweight and obesity as determinants of cardiovascular risk: the Framingham experience. *Arch Intern Med* 2002, 162:1867–1872.

21. Greenland P, Knoll MD, Stamler J, *et al.*: Major risk factors as antecedents of fatal and nonfatal coronary heart disease events. *JAMA* 2003, 290:891–897.

22. Pearson TA, Mensah GA, Alexander RW, *et al.*: Markers of inflammation and cardiovascular disease: application to clinical and public health practice: a statement for healthcare professionals from the Centers for Disease Control and Prevention and the American Heart Association. *Circulation* 2003, 107:499–511.

23. Schaefer EJ, Lamon-Fava S, Jenner JL, *et al.*: Lipoprotein(a) levels and risk of coronary heart disease in men: the Lipid Research Clinics Coronary Primary Prevention Trial. *JAMA* 1994, 271:999–1003.

24. Austin MA, King MC, Vranizan KM, Krauss RM: Atherogenic lipoprotein phenotype: a proposed genetic marker for coronary heart disease risk. *Circulation* 1990, 82:495–506.

25. Campos H, Genest JJ Jr, Blijlevens E, *et al.*: Low density lipoprotein particle size and coronary artery disease. *Arterioscler Thromb* 1992, 12:187–195.

26. McNamara JR, Shah PK, Nakajima K, *et al.*: Remnant-like particle (RLP) cholesterol is an independent cardiovascular disease risk factor in women: results from the Framingham Heart Study. *Atherosclerosis* 2001, 154:229–236.

27. Selhub J, Jacques PF, Wilson PWF, *et al.*: Vitamin status and intake as primary determinants of homocysteinemia in the elderly. *JAMA* 1993, 270:2693–2698.

28. Christen WG, Ajani UA, Glynn RJ, Hennekens CH: Blood levels of homocysteine and increased risks of cardiovascular disease: causal or casual? *Arch Intern Med* 2000, 160:422–434.

29. Jacques PF, Selhub J, Bostom AG, *et al.*: The effect of folic acid fortification on plasma folate and total homocysteine concentrations. *N Engl J Med* 1999, 340:1449–1454.

30. Ridker PM, Rifai N, Rose L, *et al.*: Comparison of C-reactive protein and low-density lipoprotein cholesterol levels in the prediction of first cardiovascular events. *N Engl J Med* 2002, 347:1557–1565.

31. Wilson PW, Smith SC Jr, Blumenthal RS, *et al.*: 34th Bethesda Conference: task force #4. How do we select patients for atherosclerosis imaging? *J Am Coll Cardiol* 2003, 41:1898–1906.

Screening Tests

Daniel B. Mark

Some may argue that performing life-saving procedures and administering powerful medicines are the principal tasks of the doctor. This chapter argues rather that the principal tool of the physician is information and that the principal tasks are risk stratification and decision-making. Without the proper data, each patient remains a closed book and decision-making is no more than a game of darts. Risk stratification is the process that ties information about the patient to a decision about how to manage the patient's illness. Thus, it becomes a critical undertaking for medical practitioners to understand the properties of the tests they use and the principles required to turn test results into risk information that can guide management.

This chapter focuses on use of screening tests for cardiovascular diseases. Screening is often understood to refer to the search for occult disease among the apparently healthy. Much of this chapter will consider screening tests in this context. However, screening tests can also be used to stratify risk among those with known disease. Thus, we will also consider several examples of this type of screening. The chapter is organized into four main sections: 1) key concepts related to screening and risk stratification, 2) basics of screening for primary prevention, 3) specific screening test use for primary prevention, and 4) screening for secondary prevention: selected examples. Although the focus of the chapter is on atherosclerotic coronary artery disease, many of the principles developed here apply as well to other forms of cardiovascular disease.

Key Concepts

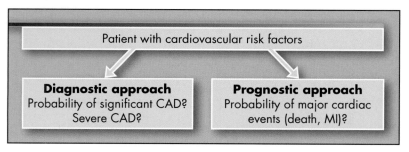

Patient with cardiovascular risk factors

Diagnostic approach
Probability of significant CAD?
Severe CAD?

Prognostic approach
Probability of major cardiac
events (death, MI)?

Figure 4-1.
Diagnosis versus prognosis. There are two general approaches to risk
stratification that focus on diagnosis and prognosis, respectively.
Diagnostic risk stratification seeks to answer the question, how likely is
it that my patient has significant coronary artery disease (CAD)?
Prognostic risk stratification, however, seeks the answer to the question:
how likely is it that my patient will die or experience major cardiac morbidity, especially in the near future? Although this may seem a semantic
distinction, it is actually quite important. From an anatomic vantage,
three-vessel CAD is the most severe form of the disease. However, it is
possible to demonstrate that some groups of three-vessel CAD have an
excellent prognosis, equal to that of patients with much less severe
CAD. MI—myocardial infarction.

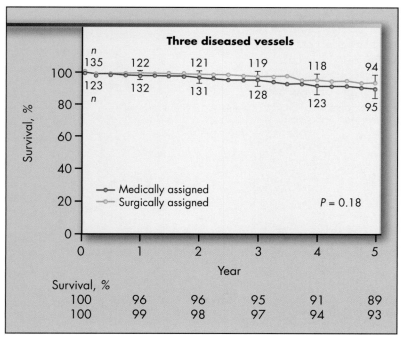

Survival, %
100	96	96	95	91	89
100	99	98	97	94	93

Figure 4-3.
Diagnostic predictions: major outcomes. Much of the literature on cardiovascular testing focuses on diagnostic endpoint. The most common of these
are "significant coronary artery disease," defined as ≥ 75% diameter stenosis
in one or more major coronary arteries, and "severe coronary artery disease," defined as three-vessel or left main disease. Although these outcomes
have persuaded many that the goal of testing is to find anatomic disease, it
is worth reporting that, in many research studies, these endpoints have
been selected because of relative convenience; they are easier to assess than
prognosis, which can take years and substantial additional expense to evaluate. However, there are some subsets of three-vessel disease that are quite
low risk and some subsets of less anatomically severe coronary artery disease
that are high risk. This point is well illustrated by the excellent survival in
the three-vessel disease subgroup of the medical arm of the randomized
portion of the Coronary Artery Surgery Study, shown in this figure.

Incremental Value of Test Information: Definition

Given what is already known about the patient's risk level
What new risk information does the test provide?

Figure 4-2.
Incremental value of test information. A test should always be interpreted in
light of information already known. There are several reasons for this. First, it
is inefficient to ignore simple readily available clinical information in favor of
more expensive additional testing. Second, ignoring the relationship between
what is already known and the apparently new information collected from a
test may result in biased estimates of outcomes, as will be discussed later in
relationship to Bayes' theorem. Two examples of incremental information can
be offered to illustrate this point. First, a patient who is predicted to be moderate risk based on clinical data and is predicted to be high risk after a test
demonstrates that a test with incremental value alters (correctly) the risk
assessment, which (presumably) leads to a change in management.
Alternatively, a low-risk patient based on clinical data who is still low risk after
the test does not gain anything in terms of risk stratification from the test.

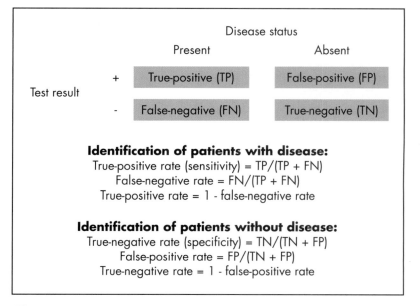

Disease status

		Present	Absent
Test result	+	True-positive (TP)	False-positive (FP)
	−	False-negative (FN)	True-negative (TN)

Identification of patients with disease:
True-positive rate (sensitivity) = TP/(TP + FN)
False-negative rate = FN/(TP + FN)
True-positive rate = 1 - false-negative rate

Identification of patients without disease:
True-negative rate (specificity) = TN/(TN + FP)
False-positive rate = FP/(TN + FP)
True-negative rate = 1 - false-positive rate

Figure 4-4
Measures of diagnostic test accuracy. We can conceptualize a test as any
measurement or assessment made on a patient, including asking history
questions and doing an examination. Conventionally, however, most
physicians think of a test as a technology-based examination that follows the initial assessment. For simplicity, test results are often
dichotomized into "positive" or high-risk and "negative" or low-risk,
and the accuracy of the test can then be defined in terms of how well it
identifies patients with disease or at high risk (ideally, all such patients
should have a positive test) and how well it identifies patients without
disease or at low risk (ideally, all these patients should have a negative
test). Test sensitivity and its converse, the false-negative rate, reflect
accuracy in identifying patients with disease. Test specificity and its converse, the false-positive rate, reflect test accuracy in correctly identifying
patients without disease.

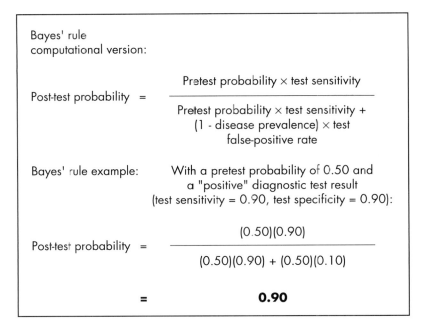

Bayes' rule
computational version:

$$\text{Post-test probability} = \frac{\text{Pretest probability} \times \text{test sensitivity}}{\text{Pretest probability} \times \text{test sensitivity} + (1 - \text{disease prevalence}) \times \text{test false-positive rate}}$$

Bayes' rule example: With a pretest probability of 0.50 and a "positive" diagnostic test result (test sensitivity = 0.90, test specificity = 0.90):

$$\text{Post-test probability} = \frac{(0.50)(0.90)}{(0.50)(0.90) + (0.50)(0.10)}$$

$$= \mathbf{0.90}$$

Figure 4-5.
Bayes' rule and measures of disease probability. The relationship between what we believe about a patient's diagnosis or prognosis before we do a test (the pretest probability of disease or an adverse outcome) and our corresponding assessment after we get the test results (the post-test probability of disease or an adverse outcome) is given by Bayes' rule. Conceptually, Bayes' rule states that the post-test probability of the outcome of interest is a function of the pretest probability of that outcome and the accuracy of the test (as reflected by sensitivity and specificity). There are several computational forms of Bayes' rule. This figure shows the conceptual form and an example of the calculations involved. (*Adapted from* Mark [1].)

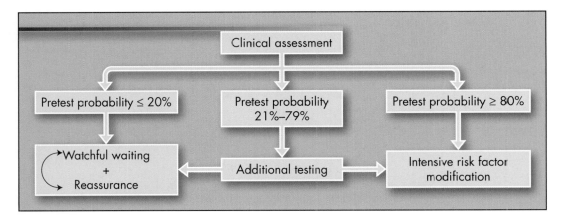

Figure 4-6.
Decision thresholds. Even the most accurate predictions of risk are not useful until they are combined with some decision rules. In general, we wish to take aggressive diagnostic and therapeutic steps with high-risk patients and use conservative management for low-risk subjects. In order to do this, we need to define what high and low risk mean operationally. For example, in the diagnosis of significant coronary artery disease, a probability of coronary artery disease exceeding 80% could be considered a "high-risk" threshold. If the probability of coronary artery disease before testing is 50% (essentially a coin toss) and the diagnostic test performed raises that probability greater than 80%, the doctor becomes certain enough of his diagnosis to make a management decision. Complete certainty (*ie*, a probability of 100%) cannot be achieved. Thus, even when the diagnosis seems beyond doubt, there is always a small probability of error. The "quest for certainty" may lead to use of additional testing with very low yield (*eg*, increase probability of disease from 90% to 95% without changing management). This figure illustrates the concept of a diagnostic threshold in terms of diagnostic probabilities, but the concept is just as easily expressed in terms of prognosis (*see* Fig. 4-15).

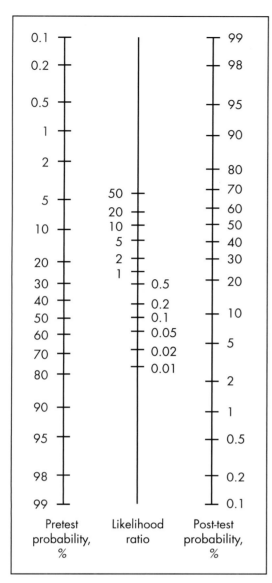

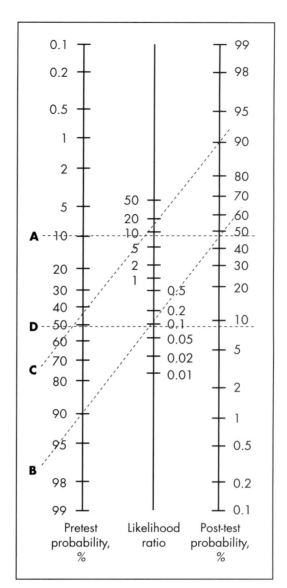

Figure 4-7.

Bayes' rule likelihood ratio form. Nomogram for converting pretest probabilities to post-test probabilities for a diagnostic test result with a given likelihood ratio. This figure shows a nomogram of Bayes' rule that allows calculation of the post-test probability of disease from the pretest probability and the likelihood ratio. The likelihood ratio for a positive test is calculated as sensitivity/(1-specificity), the probability of a positive test in a patient with disease over the probability of a positive test in a patient without disease. The likelihood ratio for a negative test is calculated as (1-sensitivity)/specificity or the probability of a false-positive test over the probability of a true negative test. A hypothetic very accurate test, say one with 99% sensitivity and 99% specificity, would have a likelihood ratio for a positive test of 99 (0.99/0.01 = 99) and a likelihood ratio for a negative test of 0.01 (0.01/0.99 = 0.01). In practice, any test with a likelihood ratio for a positive test 9 or over and 0.11 or less for a negative test is considered to be quite accurate (*eg*, with a sensitivity of 0.90 and a specificity of 0.90, the likelihood ratio for a positive test would be 9). Obviously, a likelihood ratio of 1.0 does not change the pretest probability (*eg*, a sensitivity and specificity of 50% would yield a likelihood ratio of 1). A likelihood ratio greater than 1 will increase the post-test probability, whereas a likelihood ratio less than 1 will decrease it relative to the pretest probability. Tests with high sensitivity and low specificity have likelihood ratios for positive tests close to 1.0 (*eg*, 90% sensitivity and 60% specificity yields a likelihood ratio of 1.5), whereas tests with low sensitivity and high specificity and likelihood ratios less than 1.0 (*eg*, sensitivity 60% and specificity 90%, yields a likelihood ratio of 0.67). (*Adapted from* Centre for Evidence-based Medicine [2].)

Figure 4-8.

Key concept of Bayes' rule. Nomogram for converting pre-test probabilities to post-test probabilities for a diagnostic test result with a given likelihood ratio. Working some examples of Bayes' rule reveals a basic pattern of many different combinations of pretest probabilities and test results. If the pretest probability is low (*eg*, ≤ 10%), even a "positive" result from a very accurate test (*eg*, sensitivity and specificity ≥ 90%) will not raise the post-test probability to the high range (*eg*, ≥ 90%). Conversely, if the pretest probability is high, even a "negative" result of a very accurate test will not lower the post-test probability to a range in which disease can be excluded. The biggest impact of testing on decision making, therefore, comes in testing patients in the intermediate pretest probability range (*eg*, 30%–70%). This can be readily demonstrated by trying different scenarios of pretest probability and test accuracy using the likelihood ratio nomogram of Bayes' rule introduced in Figure 4-7. This figure considers a hypothetic positive test with sensitivity and specificity at 90%: likelihood ratio for a positive test = 9, likelihood ratio for a negative test = 0.11. With a pretest probability of 10%, a positive test raises the post-test probability to about 50% (case A). Similarly, with a pretest probability of 90%, a negative test lowers the post-test probability to approximately 50% (case B). In both cases, therefore, with fairly secure pretest probabilities, a contrary test result can do no more than to move the clinician from a fairly secure diagnosis to complete uncertainty (50:50 chance of being correct). Contrast this with the positive (case C) and negative (case D) results from the same test used on a patient with a pretest probability of disease of 50%. In both of these latter cases, the test result moves the clinician from uncertainty to a secure diagnostic region. (*Adapted from* Centre for Evidence-based Medicine [2].)

Multivariable Alternatives to Bayes' Rule

Logistic regression
   Prediction of binary event (disease/no disease; dead/alive)
Cox regression
   Time to an event (*eg*, survival time; event-free survival time)

Figure 4-9.

Multivariable alternatives to Bayes' rule. Bayes' rule, as outlined here-with, works best for diagnostic problems involving simple tests whose results can be summarized as "positive" or "negative." Diagnostic tests with more complex results and prognostic tests are more difficult to adapt to this simple model. For these situations, multivariable statistical models have been used with great success. The major drawback of such methods is their computational complexity, which makes it impossible for clinicians to generate estimates in their heads. Although adaptation to handheld computers and similar devices is possible for these models, few clinicians are willing to take the time to do this. A few exceptions will be discussed later in the chapter, including the Framingham risk score and the Thrombolysis in Myocardial Infarction risk scores. Nomograms offer an alternative form of the models that may be more accessible for practicing clinicians.

One of the most commonly used regression models to evaluate diagnostic problems is logistic regression. Logistic regression models predict the probability of an event on a 0 to 1 scale. In addition, they can simultaneously account for multiple pretest patient characteristics and multiple data items from the diagnostic test. Thus, they provide a much more powerful platform than Bayes' rule for developing risk stratification scores.

Logistic regression is useful in prognostic predictions in which the interest is in the risk of an event within a specific time interval and the exact time when the event occurs in that interval does not matter. A model to predict death in the next year, for example, would treat a death at 1 day and at 1 year as being equivalent. Cox regression models are useful in dealing with prognostic predictions when the time until an event does matter. A Cox model would be able to account for enhanced survival time over an interval of follow-up instead of at one specific point.

Cost effectiveness: general concepts

- Cost effectiveness (CE) = cost to produce one extra unit of health benefit (*eg*, life year)
- Ratio of incremental costs to incremental benefits

$$CE \ Ratio = \frac{C_{New} - C_{Usual \ care}}{HB_{New} - HB_{Usual \ care}}$$

- Economically attractive therapies have CE ratio ≤ $50,000/life-year saved

Figure 4-10.

Cost effectiveness: general concepts. Cost effectiveness is a type of analysis that attempts to compare the yield of different investments in the health care system [3]. The cost effectiveness ratio, the primary measure of such analyses, expresses the relationship between extra or incremental benefits provided and the associated incremental costs. To permit comparisons across different types of health care, many analyses express cost effectiveness as the cost to add one additional life year or one additional quality-adjusted life year with the new therapy or management strategy in question relative to "standard care." One common reference standard is hemodialysis for chronic renal failure. It costs the US federal government approximately $50,000 to keep a chronic renal failure patient alive for a year on dialysis. Thus, any medical care with an incremental cost-effectiveness ratio of $50,000 per life year or less is considered "economically attractive." By contrast, medical care with a ratio over $100,000 per added life year is considered "economically unattractive." The middle range is the economic grey zone. C—costs; HB—health benefits.

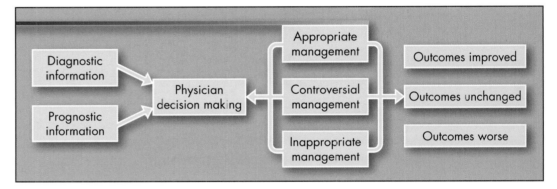

Figure 4-11.

Cost effectiveness of diagnostic tests. One of the challenges of examining the economics of screening tests is that, unlike therapies, screening tests do not usually alter health directly. Rather, the information provided by the test must be used judiciously by the physician to alter management and thereby improve outcome. Although it is possible to calculate cost effectiveness ratios in terms of cost to reach a "correct diagnosis" or cost per positive test result, there is little evidence that such intermediate endpoints clearly translate into better patient outcomes. Because doctors do not always use test information to alter management appropriately, the connection between different testing strategies and better outcomes can be difficult to draw. Most of the work in this area has used decision models to connect ideal physician behavior to expected changes in outcome and thereby estimate possible cost effectiveness of testing.

A. Step 1

Age, y	Points
30–34	-1
35–39	0
40–44	1
45–49	2
50–54	3
55–59	4
60–64	5
65–69	6
70–74	7

B. Step 2

LDL cholesterol

mg/dL	mmol/L	Points
< 100	2.59 or less	-3
100–129	2.60–3.36	0
130–159	3.37–4.14	0
160–189	4.15–4.91	1
190 or greater	4.92 or greater	2

C. Step 3

HDL cholesterol

mg/dL	mmol/L	Points
< 35	0.90 or less	2
35–44	0.91–1.16	1
45–49	1.17–1.29	0
50–59	1.30–1.55	0
60 or greater	1.56 or greater	-1

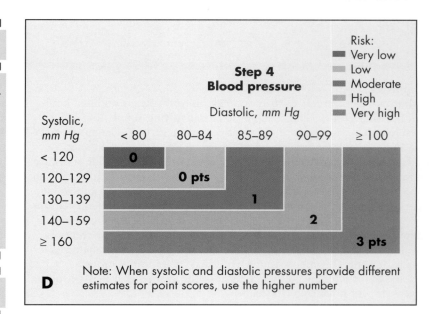

Step 4 Blood pressure

Risk:
- Very low
- Low
- Moderate
- High
- Very high

Systolic, mm Hg	Diastolic, mm Hg < 80	80–84	85–89	90–99	≥ 100
< 120	0				
120–129		0 pts			
130–139			1		
140–159				2	
≥ 160					3 pts

Note: When systolic and diastolic pressures provide different estimates for point scores, use the higher number

D

E. Step 5

Diabetes	Points
No	0
Yes	2

F. Step 6

Smoker	Points
No	0
Yes	2

G. Step 7 (Sum of Steps 1–6)

Risk factor	Points
Age	—
LDL cholesterol	—
HDL cholesterol	—
Blood pressure	—
Diabetes	—
Smoking status	—
Point total	—

Figure 4-12.

A–I, Framingham Risk Score: coronary disease risk prediction score sheet for men based on low-density lipoprotein (LDL) cholesterol level. Primary prevention seeks to abort the disease processes before they manifest as irreversible morbidity or mortality. Before one can prevent, one must be able to identify susceptible candidates, *ie*, those at increased risk. For apparently healthy subjects, the first and still most widely used tool for this purpose is the Framingham Coronary Disease Risk Score [4]. The key concept behind this prediction tool is that patient-level risk is a function of multiple individual risk factors, which operate to increase or reduce the global risk level. This approach further implies that preventive treatment should be applied according to global risk rather than the level of one individual risk factor. The major components of the Framingham Risk Score are weighted as illustrated in this figure, with the weights being derived from regression models. The model predicts total coronary heart disease risk: angina pectoris, myocardial infarction, or coronary disease death. CHD—coronary heart disease; HDL—high-density lipoprotein. (*Adapted from* Anderson *et al.* [4].)

(*continued on next page*)

H. Step 8
(Determine CHD Risk from Point Total)

Point total	10-year CHD risk, %
-3 or less	1
-2	2
-1	2
0	3
1	4
2	4
3	6
4	7
5	9
6	11
7	14
8	18
9	22
10	27
11	33
12	40
13	47
14 or greater	56 or greater

I. Step 9
(Compared with Men of the Same Age)

Age, y	Average 10-year CHD risk, %	Low* 10-year CHD risk, %
30–34	3	2
35–39	5	3
40–44	7	4
45–49	11	4
50–54	14	6
55–59	16	7
60–64	21	9
65–69	25	11
70–74	30	14

*Low risk was calculated for a man the same age, normal blood pressure, LDL cholesterol 100–129 mg/dL, HDL cholesterol 45 mg/dL, nonsmoker, and no diabetes.

Figure 4-12. continued

A. Step 1

Age	Points
30–34	-9
35–39	-4
40–44	0
45–49	3
50–54	6
55–59	7
60–64	8
65–69	8
70–74	8

B. Step 2

LDL Cholesterol mg/dL	mmol/L	Points
< 100	2.59 or less	-2
100–129	2.60–3.36	0
130–159	3.37–4.14	0
160–489	4.15–4.91	2
190 or greater	4.92 or greater	2

Figure 4-13.

A–I, Framingham Risk Score: coronary disease risk prediction score sheet for women based on low-density lipoprotein (LDL) cholesterol level. Primary prevention seeks to abort the disease processes before they manifest as irreversible morbidity or mortality. Before one can prevent, one must be able to identify susceptible candidates, *ie*, those at increased risk. For apparently healthy subjects, the first and still most widely used tool for this purpose is the Framingham Coronary Disease Risk Score [4]. The key concept behind this prediction tool is that patient-level risk is a function of multiple individual risk factors, which operate to increase or reduce the global risk level. This approach further implies that preventive treatment should be applied according to global risk rather than the level of one individual risk factor. The major components of the Framingham Risk Score are weighted as illustrated in this figure, with the weights being derived from regression models.

The model predicts total coronary heart disease risk: angina pectoris, myocardial infarction, or coronary disease death. CHD—coronary heart disease; HDL—high-density lipoprotein. (*Adapted from* Anderson *et al.* [4].)

(*continued on next page*)

C. Step 3

HDL Cholesterol

mg/dL	mmol/L	Points
< 35	0.90 or less	5
35–44	0.91–1.16	2
45–49	1.17–1.29	1
50–59	1.30–1.55	0
60 or greater	1.56 or greater	-2

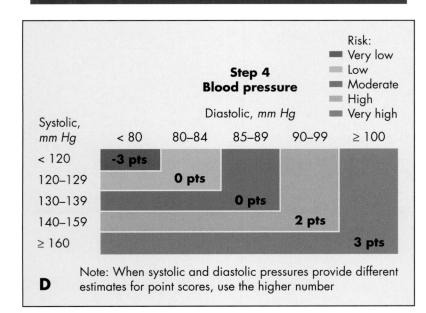

Step 4
Blood pressure

Note: When systolic and diastolic pressures provide different estimates for point scores, use the higher number

E. Step 5

Diabetes	Points
No	0
Yes	4

F. Step 6

Smoker	Points
No	0
Yes	2

G. Step 7 (Sum of Steps 1–6)

Risk factor	Points
Age	—
LDL Cholesterol	—
HDL Cholesterol	—
Blood pressure	—
Diabetes	—
Smoking status	—
Point total	—

H. Step 8
(Determine CHD Risk from Point Total)

Point total	10-year CHD risk, %
-2 or less	1
-1	2
0	2
1	2
2	3
3	3
4	4
5	5
6	6
7	7
8	8
9	9
10	11
11	13
12	15
13	17
14	20
15	24
16	27
17 or greater	32 or greater

I. Step 9
(Compared with Women of the Same Age)

Age, y	Average 10-year CHD risk, %	Low* 10-year CHD risk, %
30–34	< 1	< 1
35–39	1	< 1
40–44	2	2
45–49	5	3
50–54	8	5
55–59	12	7
60–64	12	8
65–69	13	8
70–74	14	8

*Low risk was calculated for a woman the same age, normal blood pressure, LDL cholesterol 100–129 mg/dL, HDL cholesterol 55 mg/dL, nonsmoker, and no diabetes.

Figure 4-13. continued

Definitions of Risk Levels and Link with Management

Risk level	Management		
Step 1	Initial office-based assessment in all asymptomatic adults using multiple coronary disease risk factors/global risk assessment		
	Low risk (approximately 35% of patients)	**Intermediate risk (approximately 40% of patients)**	**High risk (approximately 25% of patients)**
Step 2	Low-risk patients have a low-risk Framingham risk score and no major coronary heart disease risk factors	Intermediate-risk patients have at least one major risk factor outside the desirable range or a positive family history of coronary heart disease; global risk estimate is 0.6%–2.0% per year	High-risk patients are those with established coronary heart disease; other forms of atherosclerotic disease including peripheral arterial disease, abdominal aortic aneurysm, carotid artery transient ischemic attack or stroke; and middle-aged or older patients with type 2 diabetes or multiple other risk factors (hard coronary heart disease risk > 20% in 10 years)
Step 3	Based on low-risk status, provide reassurance and retest in approximately 5 years	Intermediate-risk patients may benefit from noninvasive testing for further risk assessment	High-risk patients are candidates for intensive risk factor intervention; noninvasive testing of asymptomatic patients is not required to determine treatment goals

Figure 4-14.
Definitions of risk levels and link with management. The use of a global risk assessment tool, such as the Framingham Risk Score, yields a prediction of the risk of future clinical coronary disease over 10 years. To assist in interpretation of the resulting prediction, comparison is often made with average age and gender comparable subjects

(*see* step 9 of Figs. 4-12 and 4-13). Alternatively, one may define an arbitrary threshold risk level for intermediate- and high-risk categories, as shown in this figure [4]. Subjects at high risk are judged suitable for intensive risk factor modification and in some cases additional noninvasive testing. (*Adapted from* Greenland *et al.* [5].)

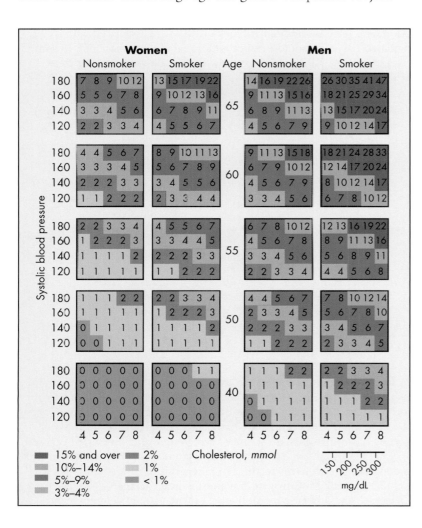

Figure 4-15.
Alternatives to Framingham. There are at least 10 published risk model alternatives to the Framingham Risk Score, although none has achieved the same level of clinical use and acceptance. The Framingham model's generalizability is limited in part by the relatively homogenous population used to develop it. One of the most widely used alternatives is the risk score for fatal cardiovascular disease developed by the Systematic Coronary Risk Evaluation (SCORE) project using data from 12 European cohort studies involving 205,178 persons [6]. As shown in this figure, the SCORE nomogram calculates 10-year risk of cardiovascular death based on age, gender, systolic blood pressure, and total cholesterol. Alternative forms are available using the high-density lipoprotein–total cholesterol ratio and for subjects at low risk of cardiovascular disease. One weakness of the SCORE model is the absence of diabetes as a risk factor. Diabetes was excluded because it was not reliably measured in the cohorts used to develop the scores. (*Adapted from* Conroy *et al.* [6].)

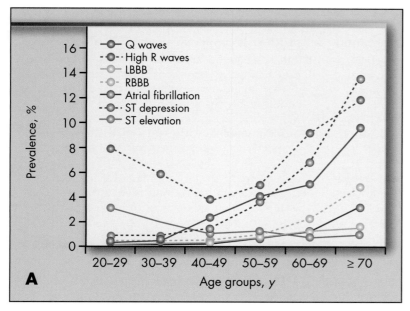

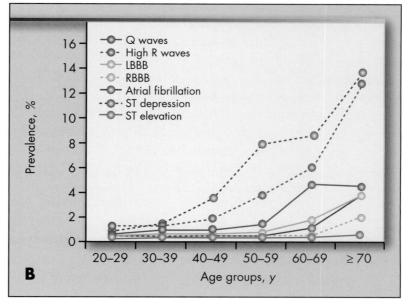

Figure 4-16.

Twelve-lead ECG. The resting 12-lead ECG is the most frequently performed diagnostic test in cardiovascular medicine, with an estimated 75 million tests performed each year in the United States. Recently, Ashley *et al.* [7] reviewed 22 studies (1966–1999) that used the ECG as a screening test. This figure shows the summary prevalence of ECG abnormalities by type of abnormality in men (**A**) and women (**B**). For all of these findings, the sensitivity was too low to make the ECG a

practical screening test in the asymptomatic population, although some findings, such as Q-wave myocardial infarction ([MI] "silent MI"), left ventricular hypertension (LVH) with strain, ST depression, atrial fibrillation, and left-bundle branch block (LBBB) are associated with a clear increased risk and should prompt additional investigation and, in some cases, therapies. RBBB—right bundle branch block. (*Adapted from* Ashley *et al.* [7].)

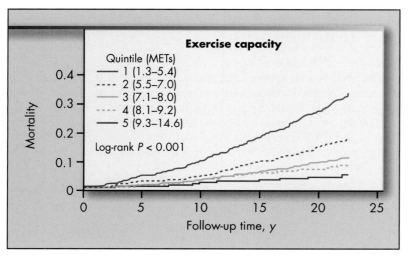

Figure 4-17.

Exercise ECG. No study has examined the effect of screening with the exercise ECG test on patient outcomes. A number of cohort studies have examined the predictive value of exercise test parameters in asymptomatic subjects. In a cohort study from Olmstead County, exercise capacity was an independent predictor of all-cause mortality in men and women [8]. In a recent report on the 20-year follow-up of women in the Lipid Research Clinics Prevalence Study, low exercise capacity was an independent predictor of mortality in 2994 initially asymptomatic women [9]. As shown in this figure, separating patients into quintiles of risk based on exercise metabolic equivalent (MET) level achieved provides powerful risk stratification.

The proportion of subjects in exercise ECG screening studies found to have coronary disease severe enough to potentially benefit from coronary bypass surgery was less than 3% [10]. The American College of Cardiology/American Heart Association Guideline on Exercise Testing has not endorsed the use of screening exercise testing because of concerns about low accuracy in the asymptomatic population, as well as concerns about harms relating to false-positive results [11]. These include unneeded invasive studies and medical therapies as well as the adverse effects of a false medical label on the patient's employment, insurance, and general well-being. (*Adapted from* Mora *et al.* [9].)

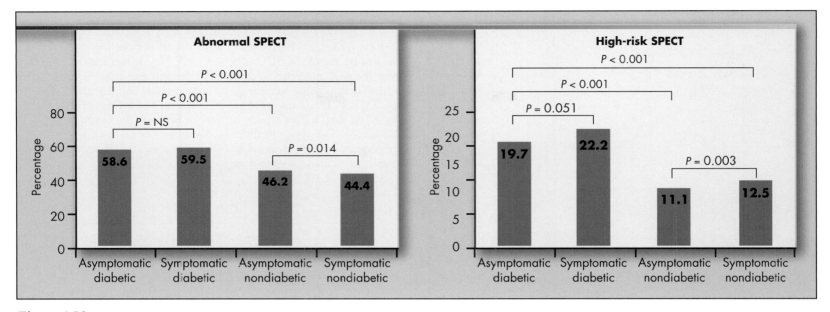

Figure 4-18.
Exercise/stress imaging. Exercise or stress perfusion imaging and echocardiography have not been as well studied in the asymptomatic population as has exercise ECG testing. As written earlier, most studies of diagnostic testing do not directly evaluate the effects of testing on patient outcomes. Rather, they record how many "cases" are discovered, assuming that finding a subject with putative disease will ultimately lead to patient benefit. Given the very low prevalence of significant coronary artery disease in the unselected asymptomatic population, recent studies have concentrated on diabetics, because this is a group known to be particularly at risk. One representative study compared asymptomatic and symptomatic diabetics referred to the Mayo Clinic for stress single-photon emission computed tomography (SPECT) studies [12]. As shown in this figure, the prevalence of abnormal and high-risk scans was about the same in asymptomatic and symptomatic groups. In the ongoing Detection of Ischemia in Asymptomatic

Diabetics (DIAD) study, 1123 type 2 diabetes patients aged 50 to 75 without known coronary artery disease are being randomized to adenosine sestamibi stress testing or clinical follow-up only [13]. In the stress testing arm, 22% of subjects had evidence of ischemia. Results of the planned 5-year follow-up for difference in clinical outcomes are expected in 2007. In an earlier study of 407 asymptomatic volunteers aged 40 to 76 in the Baltimore Longitudinal Study on Aging, the combination of abnormal exercise ST depression and a perfusion defect on thallium scintigraphy was associated with a 48% cardiac event rate (death, myocardial infarction, or new angina) over 4.6 years of follow-up [14]. If only one test was positive, the risk of events was the same (8%) as when both tests were negative (7%). The probability of this concordant test result was a direct function of age, with up to 15% of patients in their 80s having such a result. (*Adapted from* Miller *et al.* [12].)

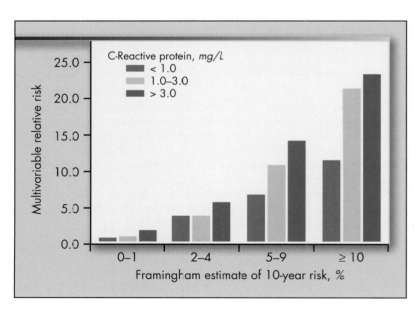

Figure 4-19.
High sensitivity C-reactive protein (CRP). CRP is an inflammatory marker that rises in response to a variety of types of tissue injury, including inflammatory diseases, trauma, infections, and malignancies. Recent work has shown that CRP is also a marker of atherothrombotic disease and possibly a mediator of that disease, as well. There are over a dozen prospective studies in subjects without clinically manifest disease showing that CRP is a strong predictor of future cardiovascular events [15]. There are also some data showing that the predictive value of CRP in this population is independent of global risk scores, such as the Framingham Risk Score [16]. What remains controversial is whether CRP provides clinically useful information beyond such global scores and what the therapeutic implications of an elevated CRP are. In 27,939 apparently healthy women in the Nurses' Health Study, CRP level stratified risk beyond the risk information in the Framingham Risk Score, as shown here. This analysis, however, lacks information about absolute risk levels, which is the primary concern in clinical management. (*Adapted from* Ridker *et al.* [16].)

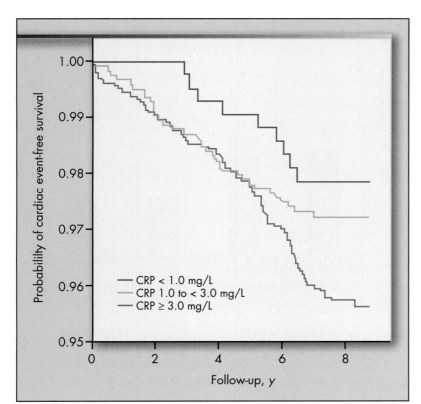

Figure 4-20.

C-Reactive protein (CRP) and absolute risk. When CRP levels are displayed on a Kaplan-Meier survival plot, the corresponding absolute risk levels can be seen [15]. As can be seen, CRP levels less than 1.0 mg/L confer the best prognosis in this cohort. At approximately 5 years, there is a further distinction between level between 1.0 and 2.9 mg/L and levels 3.0 mg/L and over. However, at the end of 8 years of follow-up, there is less than a 3% absolute difference between the best and worst CRP groups. The apparent difference is magnified by the choice of scale displayed on the y-axis. On a 0 to 100 scale, the difference would be barely evident. (*Adapted from* Ridker [15].)

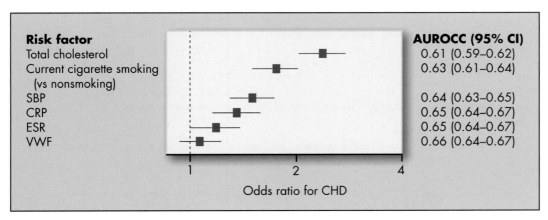

Figure 4-21.

C-Reactive protein (CRP) and prediction of coronary heart disease (CHD). In a case-control study derived from a large prospective cohort, 2459 patients who had had a nonfatal myocardial infarction or died from CHD were compared with 3969 controls without CHD [17]. Dividing the combined population into tertiles based on CRP level and adjusting for established risk factors yielded an odds ratio of 1.45 for (CHD with high versus low CRP level. This was similar to but not quite as large as the odds ratio for established risk factors, such as smoking and elevated cholesterol. Calculation of the area under the receiver operating characteristic curve (AUROCC) for each risk factor

starting with the strongest (total cholesterol) and adding each one to the model showed that none of these risk factors alone is very powerful in identifying subjects at risk for major cardiac events. Further, the incremental value of CRP in this context is quite modest. Perhaps the main message from these data on CRP is that this new test is not the panacea for screening patients for risk of CHD. Whether it should be routinely used for this purpose continues to be debated. ESR—erythrocyte sedimentation rate; SBP—systolic blood pressure; VWF—von Willebrand factor. (*Adapted from* Danesh *et al.* [17].)

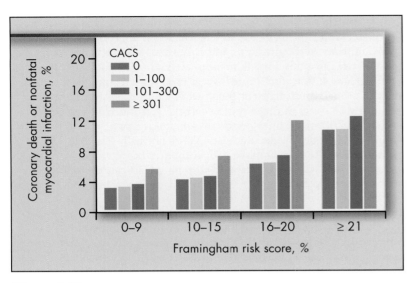

Figure 4-22.

Testing for coronary calcium. Predicted 7-year event rates from COX regression model for coronary heart disease death or nonfatal myocardial infarction for categories of Framingham Risk Score or coronary artery calcium score (CACS). The imperfect performance of clinical data, serologic tests, and exercise testing as methods to identify early preclinical atherosclerosis has led to the investigation of a variety of imaging techniques as a means to find early evidence of disease. One of the most widely studied such markers is coronary calcium. The prevalence of any detectable coronary calcium increases with age and for any age is less common in women than men. Coronary calcium indicates atherosclerosis but not all coronary atherosclerosis exhibits calcification. The amount of calcium present is correlated roughly with the extent of coronary plaque but reveals nothing about the severity of the stenosis or the likelihood of a future plaque event. There are now two main CT-based techniques that are used for screening for coronary calcium. Electron beam computer tomography (EBCT) is the more commonly used method and uses a fixed radiograph source to make serial slices of the whole heart during a single breath-hold acquisition period. Multidetector CT scanners mechanically rotate the radiographic source around the patient and therefore are slower than EBCT. The spiral scan mode moves the gantry around the patient, acquiring data continuously while the table carrying the patient is advanced at a constant speed. Both methods are sensitive to small amounts of coronary calcium and may detect incidental noncoronary abnormalities in the field of view. Several scoring methods have been developed to reflect a semiquantitative assessment of amount of calcium present. A variety of studies have reported that higher calcium scores equate with higher risk of future cardiac events. Whether this risk is independent of clinical and laboratory risk factors remains less well defined. In one prospective population-based study of 1416 asymptomatic adults, CACS added statistically significant prognostic information to the Framingham Risk Score for higher risk but not lower risk subjects [18]. These results are shown in this figure for four levels of the Framingham Risk Score and four levels of CACS. What is unclear from these data is how the modest incremental information from the coronary calcium test would alter management. In fact, the proper management of a "positive" calcium scan has yet to be clearly defined. In addition, the value of serial testing has not yet been settled. (*Adapted from* Greenland *et al.* [18].)

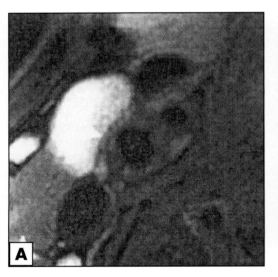
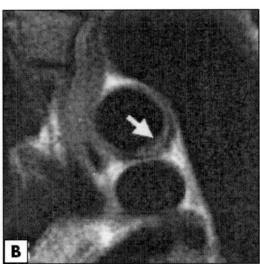
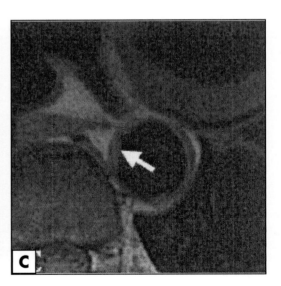

Figure 4-23.

Complex carotid and aortic plaques detected in a 71-year-old woman by use of high-resolution in vivo MRI. **A,** Left carotid artery plaque. **B,** Aortic arch plaque (*arrow*). **C,** Descending aortic plaque (*arrow*). Some early studies have shown that cardiac magnetic resonance can visualize atherosclerotic lesions in the aorta, including discerning the composition of the plaques. Some preliminary work has also shown that these images can be observed serially to evaluate the effects of cholesterol-lowering therapy on plaque composition. Magnetic resonance has been used to demonstrate atherosclerotic plaque in the thoracic and abdominal aorta and the carotid arteries, as shown in this figure from the Mount Sinai group [19]. At present, use of magnetic resonance to examine the coronary tree noninvasively is still a research activity. (*From* Fayad *et al.* [19]; with permission.)

Screening Tests

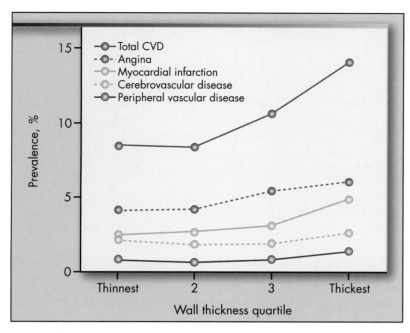

Figure 4-24.
Carotid ultrasound. Although originally a diagnostic test for subjects with suspected cerebrovascular disease, carotid ultrasound also has been used in epidemiologic studies to identify occult atherosclerotic disease. The underlying concept is that atherosclerosis is a diffuse disease involving many of the medium- and large-sized arteries of the body and that the carotid is a medium-sized artery that is readily examined with high-resolution ultrasound. When used for screening in this manner, the primary measurement obtained is the thickness of the intima-media (IMT) layers of the common carotid. Carotid IMT can be assessed with B-mode ultrasound (two-dimensional) or two-dimensional guided M-mode images. Because IMT is normally less than 1 mm, measurements are usually made with computer-based calipers. Besides measuring IMT, carotid ultrasound screening tests can identify focal nonobstructive plaques.

Epidemiologic studies have found a linear relationship with increasing carotid IMT and increasing risk from future cardiovascular disease (CVD). Increasing carotid IMT values over time identified higher risk subjects. In addition to atherosclerosis, increasing age and hypertension increase carotid IMT, making identification of an abnormal cutoff value problematic. Thus, several groups have proposed use of an age-adjusted nomogram to identify abnormal values. To date, carotid IMT assessment remains primarily a research tool. In the Atherosclerosis Risk in Communities (ARIC) Study, B-mode ultrasound measurements of carotid IMT were made on 13,870 middle-aged subjects [20]. As shown in this figure, the prevalence of CVD increased as a function of carotid IMT, with the highest prevalence in the 25% of subjects with the thickest carotid walls. (*Adapted from* Burke *et al.* [20].)

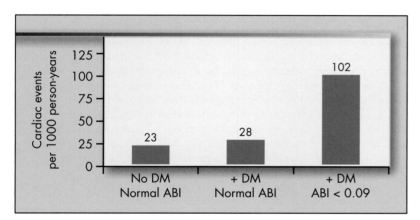

Figure 4-25.
Ankle brachial index (ABI). The ABI is the ratio of systolic blood pressures at the ankle and the brachial artery. The underlying concept is that atherosclerotic disease more often affects the vascular supply to the legs than to the arms, and subjects with peripheral vascular disease also have coronary artery disease. However, it is important to check blood pressure in both arms to avoid overlooking possible subclavian stenosis. If the two blood pressures are significantly different, the higher one should be used in calculating the ABI. Both legs are evaluated and an ABI for each is calculated. The ABI is considered abnormal if it is ≤ 0.90. Because it implies significant vascular obstruction to blood flow, the ABI detects disease at a later stage than the carotid intima-media or brachial artery reactivity testing.

In a population-based cohort of male subjects from Malmo, Sweden, the presence of asymptomatic diabetes (DM) with a normal ABI increased cardiac events modestly over a 14-year follow-up [21]. However, when DM was coupled with an abnormal ABI, as shown in this figure, the cardiac event rate was significantly ($P < 0.001$) increased.

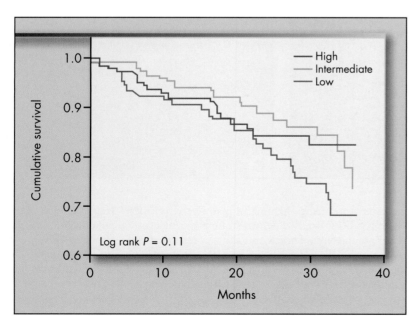

Figure 4-26.
Brachial artery reactivity. Brachial artery reactivity testing is a research technique that tests for endothelial dysfunction, an early sign of atherosclerotic disease. Under normal circumstances, the vascular endothelium produces nitric oxide, a potent vasodilator, in response to local factors affecting blood flow. When shear stress increases on the vascular endothelium because of, for example, increased blood flow, the endothelial cells synthesize and release more nitric oxide to dilate the artery in question. This response is the basis for brachial artery reactivity testing [22]. A high-resolution ultrasound scan is taken of the brachial artery to measure diameter at baseline. A blood pressure cuff is then used to occlude the artery for a period of approximately 5 minutes to create downstream ischemia and consequent hyperemia (with vasodilatation). When the cuff is released, the flow down the brachial artery is significantly increased for the next several minutes. During this period, a second set of images of the brachial artery are obtained and the ratio of post- to pre-occlusion/release diameters is calculated. Normal individuals are expected to increase diameter by approximately 10%, but older individuals may have an attenuated response.

Although brachial artery reactivity has some appeal as a research tool, it has so far not proved practical as a clinical screening test, in part because of substantial variability of the test results over time independent of clinical reasons for change. (*Adapted from* Fathi *et al.* [23].)

Atlas of Cardiovascular Risk Factors

Thus far in this chapter, we have considered the use of screening tests to search for evidence of disease in asymptomatic subjects not known to have coronary artery disease. The test data build on clinical data to generate an increasingly refined (and hopefully more accurate) risk assessment, which can be used to guide therapy. In this section, we will examine a few examples of the use of tests in subjects with symptoms possibly caused by coronary artery disease.

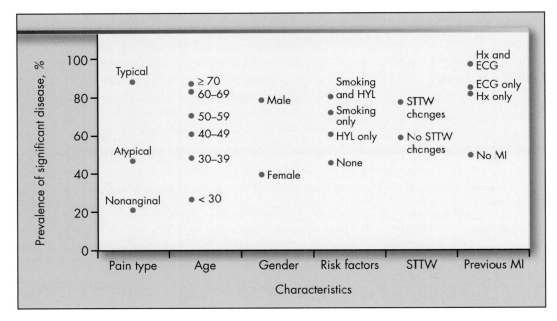

Figure 4-27.
Risk prediction with symptoms suspected to be coronary artery disease (CAD). In the diagnostic evaluation of chest pain symptoms, a few simple clinical assessments provide substantial predictive information. In particular, the clinician's judgment about the extent to which the patients' symptoms are typical for angina pectoris is a very important part of the pretest risk assessment [24]. Age and gender are also important as is evidence of a prior myocardial infarction (MI) on ECG. Hx—history; HYL—hyperlipidemia. (*Adapted from* Pryor *et al.* [24].)

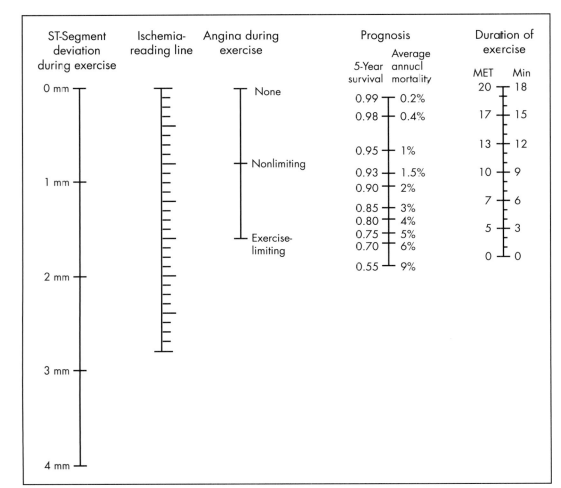

Figure 4-28.
Risk stratification using treadmill exercise testing. As reported earlier, prognostic risk algorithms tend to be more complex than diagnostic ones and the challenge for developers of these tools has been to balance accuracy with user-friendliness. One attempt to achieve this balance is represented by the Duke Treadmill Score [25]. This figure shows the reduction of the original Cox model–based score to a nomogram that is fairly simple to use. The Duke Treadmill Score contains only three variables and by design does not include clinical variables. Attempts to develop composite clinical-exercise test scores have been hampered by the added complexity associated with the addition of five or more clinical factors in addition to the exercise test result variables. (*Adapted from* Mark *et al.* [25].)

A. Risk Prediction with Acute Coronary Syndromes: TIMI ST Increased MI Risk Score

Points	Risk factor
2	Age 65–75
3	Age 75 or older
3	SBP < 100
2	Heart rate > 100
2	Killip class II or greater
1	Anterior ST increased or LBBB
1	Diabetes, history of HBP, history of angina
1	Weight < 67 kg
1	Time to treatment > 4 hours
Total possible 0–14	

B. Risk Predictions with Acute Coronary Syndromes: TIMI Non-ST Increased Acute Coronary Syndrome Risk Score

Points	Risk factor
1	Age 65 years or older
1	Three or more risk factors for CAD
1	Prior CAD 50% or greater stenosis
1	ST deviation on presenting ECG
1	Two or more anginal events in past 24 hours
1	Use of aspirin in previous 7 days
1	Increased serum cardiac markers

Figure 4-29.

Risk prediction with acute coronary syndromes. Probably the best known risk model used in the care of acute coronary syndrome patients is the Thrombolysis in Myocardial Infarction (TIMI) risk score. Two TIMI risk scores have been developed: one for ST elevation myocardial infarction (MI) [26] and one for unstable angina and non-ST elevation MI [27]. **A,** The score for ST elevation is relatively complex, with some factors receiving more weight than others. **B,** By contrast, the non-ST elevation acute coronary syndrome (ACS) score has fewer factors and equal weighting, making it more likely that clinicians can remember it and will therefore use it. CAD—coronary artery disease; HBP—high blood pressure; LBBB—left-bundle branch block; SBP—systolic blood pressure.

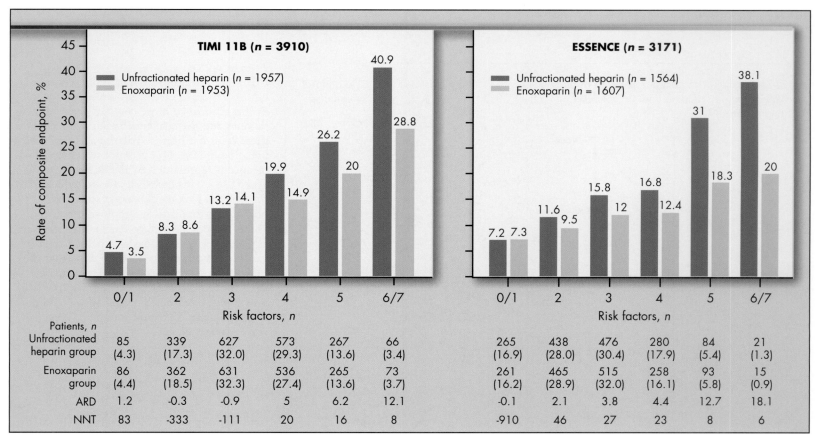

Figure 4-30.

One critical aspect of risk score development is validation. Many risk scores can be developed with statistical regression software, and in the population used to derive the score, performance may appear pretty good. However, the value of the score relates to its performance in new populations. Thus, a score should be considered for clinical practice only after it has undergone robust validation, preferably in a population separate from the derivation subjects. In the case of the Thrombolysis in Myocardial Infarction (TIMI) non-ST elevation acute coronary syndrome risk score, several independent populations have been used to demonstrate the robust nature of the prognostic stratification provided. In this figure, two separate clinical trial populations testing enoxaparin versus unfractionated heparin were used to show that the TIMI score stratified risk well [27]. ARD—absolute risk difference; ESSENCE—Efficacy and Safety of Subcutaneous Enoxaparin in non–Q-wave coronary events; NNT—number needed to treat. (*Adapted from* Antman *et al.* [27].)

References

1. Mark DB: Economic issues in clinical medicine. In *Harrison's Principles of Internal Medicine*. Edited by Braunwald E. Philadelphia: McGraw-Hill; 2001.

2. Centre for Evidence-based Medicine: Likelihood ratios. Available at http://www.cebm.net/likelihood_ratios.asp.

3. Mark DB, Hlatky MA: Medical economics and the assessment of value in cardiovascular medicine: part I. *Circulation* 2002,106:516–520.

4. Anderson KM, Wilson PW, Odell PM, Kannel WB: An updated coronary risk profile: a statement for health professionals. *Circulation* 1991, 83:356–362.

5. Greenland P. Smith SC Jr, Grundy SM: Improving coronary heart disease risk assessment in asymptomatic people: role of traditional risk factors and noninvasive cardiovascular tests. *Circulation* 2001, 104:1863–1867.

6. Conroy RM, Pyorala K, Fitzgerald AP, *et al.*: Estimation of ten-year risk of fatal cardiovascular disease in Europe: the SCORE project. *Eur Heart J* 2003, 24:987–1003.

7. Ashley EA, Raxwal V, Froelicher V: An evidence-based review of the resting electrocardiogram as a screening technique for heart disease. *Prog Cardiovasc Dis* 2001, 44:55–67.

8. Roger VL, Jacobsen SJ, Pellikka PA, *et al.*:. Prognostic value of treadmill exercise testing: a population-based study in Olmsted County, Minnesota. *Circulation* 1998, 98:2836–2841.

9. Mora S, Redberg RF, Cui Y, *et al.*: Ability of exercise testing to predict cardiovascular and all-cause death in asymptomatic women: a 20-year follow-up of the lipid research clinics prevalence study. *JAMA* 2003, 290:1600–1607.

10. Fowler-Brown A, Pignone M, Pletcher M, *et al.*: Exercise tolerance testing to screen for coronary heart disease: a systematic review for the technical support for the U.S. Preventive Services Task Force. *Ann Intern Med* 2004, 140:W9–W24.

11. Gibbons RJ, Balady GJ, Bricker JT, *et al.*: ACC/AHA 2002 guideline update for exercise testing: summary article: a report of the American College of Cardiology/American Heart Association Task Force on Practice Guidelines (Committee to Update the 1997 Exercise Testing Guidelines). *Circulation* 2002, 106:1883–1892.

12. Miller TD, Rajagopalan N, Hodge DO, *et al.*: Yield of stress single-photon emission computed tomography in asymptomatic patients with diabetes. *Am Heart J* 2004, 147:890–896.

13. Wackers FJ, Young LH, Inzucchi SE, *et al.*: Detection of silent myocardial ischemia in asymptomatic diabetic subjects: the DIAD study. *Diabetes Care* 2004, 27:1954–1961.

14. Fleg JL, Gerstenblith G, Zonderman AB, *et al.*: Prevalence and prognostic significance of exercise-induced silent myocardial ischemia detected by thallium scintigraphy and electrocardiography in asymptomatic volunteers. *Circulation* 1990, 81:428–436.

15. Ridker PM: Clinical application of C-reactive protein for cardiovascular disease detection and prevention. *Circulation* 2003, 107:363–369.

16. Ridker PM, Koenig W, Fuster V: C-reactive protein and coronary heart disease. *N Engl J Med* 2004, 351:295–298.

17. Danesh J, Wheeler JG, Hirschfield GM, *et al.*: C-reactive protein and other circulating markers of inflammation in the prediction of coronary heart disease. *N Engl J Med* 2004, 350:1387–1397.

18. Greenland P, LaBree L, Azen SP, *et al.*: Coronary artery calcium score combined with Framingham score for risk prediction in asymptomatic individuals. *JAMA* 2004, 291:210–215.

19. Fayad ZA, Fuster V, Nikolaou K, Becker C: Computed tomography and magnetic resonance imaging for noninvasive coronary angiography and plaque imaging: current and potential future concepts. *Circulation* 2002, 106:2026–2034.

20. Burke GL, Evans GW, Riley WA, *et al.*: Arterial wall thickness is associated with prevalent cardiovascular disease in middle-aged adults. The Atherosclerosis Risk in Communities (ARIC) Study. *Stroke* 1995, 26:386–391.

21. Ogren M, Hedblad B, Engstrom G, Janzon L: Prevalence and prognostic significance of asymptomatic peripheral arterial disease in 68-year-old men with diabetes: results from the population study 'men born in 1914' from Malmo, Sweden. *Eur J Vasc Endovasc Surg* 2005, 29:182–189.

22. Fathi R, Marwick TH: Noninvasive tests of vascular function and structure: why and how to perform them. *Am Heart J* 2001, 141:694–703.

23. Fathi R, Haluska B, Isbel N, *et al.*: The relative importance of vascular structure and function in predicting cardiovascular events. *J Am Coll Cardiol* 2004, 43:616–623.

24. Pryor D3, Harrell FE Jr, Lee KL, *et al.*: Estimating the likelihood of significant coronary artery disease. *Am J Med* 1983, 75:771–780.

25. Mark DB, Shaw L, Harrell FE Jr, *et al.*: Prognostic value of a treadmill exercise score in outpatients with suspected coronary artery disease. *N Engl J Med* 1991, 325:849–853.

26. Morrow DA, Antman EM, Charlesworth A, *et al.*: TIMI risk score for ST-elevation myocardial infarction: A convenient, bedside, clinical score for risk assessment at presentation: an intravenous nPA for treatment of infarcting myocardium early II trial substudy. *Circulation* 2000, 102:2031–2037.

27. Antman EM, Cohen M, Bernink PJ, *et al.*: The TIMI risk score for unstable angina/non-ST elevation MI: A method for prognostication and therapeutic decision making. *JAMA* 2000, 284:835–842.

5

Nonmodifiable Risk Factors: Gender, Race, and Family History

Howard D. Sesso

With the large number of modifiable risk factors for cardiovascular disease (CVD) that have been identified over the past few decades, considerable progress has been made in the primary prevention of CVD. Behavioral and pharmacologic interventions have targeted these modifiable risk factors and helped influence dramatic reductions in mortality from CVD. Yet despite these tremendous steps forward, the incidence of CVD remains alarmingly high. Besides the plethora of modifiable risk factors for CVD, however, three key nonmodifiable risk factors—gender, race, and family history—remain critically important when considering a patient for their risk of developing CVD. These three risk factors represent a combination of genotypic, phenotypic, and cultural characteristics that contribute to the etiology of CVD. Gender, race, and family history provide valuable risk factor information that can be obtained easily and cheaply in a doctor's office. An improved understanding of what these nonmodifiable risk factors represent will improve risk prediction, an important first step in prevention.

Gender not only represents a set of unique physiologic differences that may impact the risk of CVD, but also a risk factor in and of itself. Gender is often viewed as a proxy, which can be described by differences in blood pressure, lipids, and other clinical and behavioral characteristics. The prevalence and incidence of CVD are markedly different comparing men and women over the course of the past few decades in the United States. These differences are a function of biology and behavior, the relative contributions of which are difficult to quantify. Patterns in smoking rates, obesity, physical activity, hypertension, and cholesterol levels tend to differ in men and women. More knowledge is clearly needed on how the unique aspects of being male and female promote the development of CVD, based on known and still unidentified biologic mechanisms.

Race shares many parallels with gender in the sense that biology and behavior contribute to its importance as a risk factor for CVD. Although considerable progress has been made in lowering cardiovascular death rates in the United States, the lowering of death rates has been proportionally greater in white men and women than minorities. This observation reflects not only biology and behavior, but also access to treatment and care. Many conventional cardiovascular risk factors illustrate differences among the major racial groups. In particular, rates of physical inactivity and obesity differ widely in whites, blacks, and other racial groups. The common clinical manifestations of being inactive and overweight—diabetes mellitus, hypertension, and dyslipidemia—also explain in part the differences in the incidence and mortality rates of different racial groups. Although it remains unclear what role race in and of itself may play in the development of CVD, an improved knowledge of how race impacts various risk factors, treatment, and diagnosis has the potential to reduce some of the observed differences in CVD among various racial groups.

The final nonmodifiable risk factor for CVD in this chapter, family history, represents an individual's genetic makeup, but also may include acquired behavioral factors. Individuals with a positive family history of CVD typically have a wide range of genetic and phenotypic components whereby that person may be predisposed to be at a higher risk of CVD. Most major cardiovascular risk factors often cluster within families. However, few data are available on the entire range of genetic and phenotypic factors necessary to examine the extent to which each contribute to the risk associated with family history of CVD. A patient's family history of CVD can be measured in a multitude of ways; conventional definitions tend to focus on parental history with an early, "premature" onset of CVD. However, family history of CVD is propagated through parents and influenced by siblings, grandparents, cousins, and other family members. Studies suggest that as more information on family history is known, its ability to predict future CVD risk improves. In this regard, family history of CVD is a noninvasive risk factor that can be easily obtained in regular physician visits, the knowledge of which can guide primary prevention efforts.

Gender

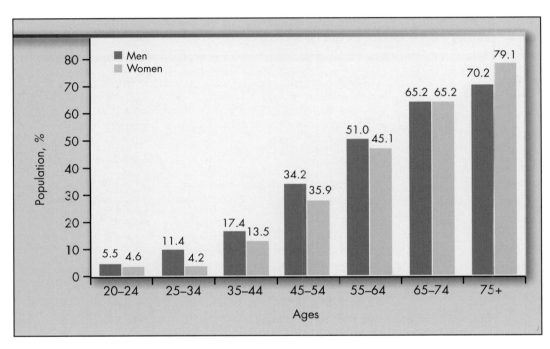

Figure 5-1.
Prevalence of cardiovascular disease in American adults aged 20 years and older. Cardiovascular disease is more prevalent in men than in women through early and middle adulthood (younger than 65 years). However, the prevalence of cardiovascular disease is roughly equal by age 65, and elderly women are more likely to have cardiovascular disease. Traditional views on these prevalence patterns in men and women suggested that menopause and its associated hormonal changes, as well as its subsequent impact on other cardiovascular risk factors in women, was largely responsible for the catch-up in rates by women during middle adulthood [1]. However, several other differences in cardiovascular risk factors may be responsible, but it remains unclear why there is such a wide discrepancy in the prevalence of cardiovascular disease at younger ages. (*Adapted from* the American Heart Association [2].)

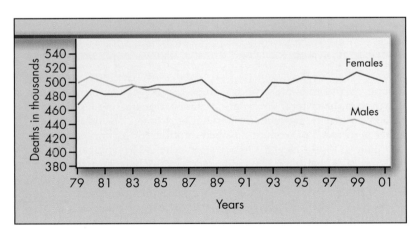

Figure 5-2.
Age-adjusted trends in the number of deaths related to cardiovascular disease in men and women in the United States from 1979 through 2001. The death rates have steadily decreased in men and have increased slightly in women. Changes in smoking status are commonly alluded to as a major reason for the discrepant trends; whereas smoking rates in men began to decrease considerably after the initial epidemiologic studies on smoking and health in the 1950s, which was followed by the Surgeon General's report on smoking. Smoking rates in women did not drop as dramatically, resulting in a relatively steady rate of cardiovascular disease mortality over time. The absolute number of deaths from cardiovascular disease in the United States is higher in women than men due to demographic shift. The prevalence of cardiovascular disease is higher in women than in men among those aged 65 years or older. In addition, more women are alive at older ages than men. In the United States during 2002, there were 137 million men and 143.3 million women, of whom 10.8% of men and 14.3% of women are aged 65 years or older [3]. These and other factors contribute to the difference in the absolute number of cardiovascular deaths. (*Adapted from* the American Heart Association [4].)

Unique Differences Between Men and Women

Genetic (*eg*, Y chromosome in men)
Hormonal (*eg*, higher levels of testosterone in men vs higher levels of estradiol in women)
Reproductive (*eg*, differences in organ systems)
Behavioral (*eg*, use of oral contraceptives in women)

Figure 5-3.
Potential biologic differences in men versus women as a guide to understanding potential differences in the impact of cardiovascular disease. Although gender is a nonmodifiable risk factor for cardiovascular disease, we can begin to identify potential risk factors specific to men and women that may help to explain the differences in cardiovascular disease risk. These include a broad spectrum of genetic, hormonal, reproductive, and behavioral factors. The role of hormones in cardiovascular disease prevention remains controversial [1]. Observational studies suggested that hormone replacement therapy, by which estrogen levels were maintained after menopause and positively impacted risk factors like high-density lipoprotein cholesterol, reduced the risk of cardiovascular disease. However, clinical trial evidence has proven the contrary, with the results from the Women's Health Initiative demonstrating that hormone replacement therapy did not reduce the risk of cardiovascular disease [5].

Comparison of Adult Men Versus Women for the Prevalence of Various Cardiovascular Risk Factors

Diseases and cardiovascular risk factors	Men	Women
High blood pressure		
Prevalence, %	33.1	32.1
Mortality	18,900	27,900
Tobacco use		
Prevalence, %	25.2	20.7
Blood cholesterol		
Total cholesterol 200 mg/dL or greater, %	50.4	50.9
Total cholesterol 240 mg/dL or greater, %	17.2	19.1
LDL cholesterol 130 mg.dL or greater, %	48.5	43.3
HDL cholesterol < 40 mg/dL, %	39.0	14.9
Physical inactivity		
Prevalence, %	32.5 (whites only)	36.2 (whites only)
Overweight and obesity		
Overweight: 25 kg/m^2 or greater, %	67.2	61.9
Obese: 30 kg/m^2 or greater, %	27.5	33.4
Diabetes mellitus		
Physician-diagnosed, %	5.5	5.5
Undiagnosed, %	3.3	2.5
Pre-diabetes, %	9.3	5.3

Figure 5-4.
Comparison of adult men versus women for the prevalence of various cardiovascular risk factors. When traditional cardiovascular risk factors, including high blood pressure, tobacco use, blood cholesterol, physical inactivity, overweight and obesity, and diabetes mellitus are compared by gender, we can begin to understand differences in rates of cardiovascular disease. For example, low high-density lipoprotein (HDL) cholesterol (less than 40 mg/dL) is much more prevalent in men than in women, reflecting in part the hormonal differences in men versus women. Because HDL cholesterol has been shown to be a powerful predictor of cardiovascular disease, it may be postulated that low HDL cholesterol is a more common pathway through which cardiovascular disease may develop in men than in women. Women tend to be less physically active than men. With women less likely to exercise frequently than men, behavioral interventions aimed at increasing levels of physical activity may be more important among women. In addition, the higher percentage of women classified as obese (30 kg/m^2 or greater) according to World Health Organization criteria [6], compared with men, indicates that body mass index and obesity have greater roles in women for the development of cardiovascular disease. Such comparisons of risk factors, although cross-sectional in nature, offer important insight into which cardiovascular risk factors may be more or less amenable to intervention in men and women, helping to shape primary prevention recommendations and guidelines. (*Adapted from* the American Heart Association [4,7].)

National Health and Nutrition Examination Survey: Prevalence of Obesity

Study	20–29 Years	30–39 Years	40–49 Years	50–59 Years	60–69 Years	70–79 Years*	80 + Years†	Total prevalence (≥ 20 years)	Age-adjusted total prevalence (20–74 years)
Men									
NHES I	9.0	10.4	11.9	13.4	7.7	8.6	—	10.5	10.4
NHANES I	8.0	13.3	14.2	15.3	10.3	11.1	—	12.0	11.8
NHANES II	8.1	12.1	16.4	14.3	13.5	13.6	—	12.3	12.3
NHANES III	12.5	17.2	23.1	28.9	24.8	20.0	8.0	19.5	19.9
Women									
NHES I	6.1	12.1	17.1	20.4	27.2	21.9	—	16.2	15.1
NHANES I	8.2	15.1	17.6	22.0	24.0	21.9	—	16.7	16.1
NHANES II	9.0	16.8	18.1	22.6	22.0	19.4	—	16.8	16.5
NHANES III	14.6	25.8	26.9	35.6	29.8	25.0	15.1	25.0	24.9
Total									
NHES I	7.5	11.3	14.6	17.0	18.0	15.7	—	13.4	12.8
NHANES I	8.1	14.2	15.9	18.7	17.9	17.3	—	14.4	14.1
NHANES II	8.6	14.5	17.3	18.7	18.1	16.9	—	14.7	14.5
NHANES III	13.5	21.5	25.0	32.3	27.5	22.9	12.6	22.3	22.5

*For NHANES I and II, the upper age in the survey was only 74 years; therefore, estimates in this category only include patients aged 70–74 years.
†Data from this group are only available from NHANES III.

Figure 5-5.
Prevalence of obesity (defined according to World Health Organization criteria as a body mass index of 30 kg/m² or greater) by age, gender, and survey, which covers changes over approximately four decades starting in the 1970s. For the National Health and Nutrition Examination Survey (NHANES) I and NHANES II, the estimates in the 70–79 year category are for those aged 70–74 years only because the upper age limit for the survey was 74 years. The largest increases in the prevalence of obesity occurred from NHANES II to NHANES III, with obesity increasing by approximately 50% in men and women. The expected spikes in the rates of cardiovascular disease have not been realized yet, although other clinical manifestations have already become apparent; the rates of diabetes and hypertension are increasing. NHES—National Health Examination Survey. (*Adapted from* the Centers for Disease Control [8].)

Cardiovascular Risk Factors for Men and Women

Risk factor	Men	Women
Total cholesterol	VS	VS
LDL	VS	VS
HDL	S	VS
Triglycerides	M	S
Apo A-I	VS	VS
Apo-B	VS	VS
Apo(a)	S	M to S
Smoking	S	S to VS
Diabetes	S	VS
Physical inactivity	S	S
Family history of cardiovascular disease	S	S
Alcohol consumption	M	M
BMI	S	S
WHR	VS	VS
Hypertension	S	S
Family history	S	S to VS
Hormones	M	VS
Homocysteine	M	M
Fibrinogen	S	S
Inflammation (*eg*, CRP)	M	S
Infection (*eg*, ChP, HP)	P	P
Psychosocial factors	M	M

Figure 5-6.
A sampling of cardiovascular risk factors and possible differences by gender in the magnitude of risk associated with the risk of cardiovascular disease. When considering how gender may serve as a nonmodifiable risk factor for cardiovascular disease, the prevalence of various risk factors, as well as the magnitude of risk, is important (*see* Fig. 5-5). The attributable risk takes into account the prevalence of the risk factor in question as well as the magnitude of cardiovascular risk associated with that risk factor. There is considerable subjectivity in determining the risk factors that may be of greater or lesser magnitude in men and women. By and large, for most conventional risk factors that are common in men and women, the magnitude of risk is typically observed to be roughly equivalent. Because the rates of cardiovascular disease tend to be higher in elderly men than in women at younger ages, many prospective epidemiologic studies will report greater magnitudes of relative risks of cardiovascular disease in women. However, the absolute risk of cardiovascular disease may remain higher for men. Apo—apolipoprotein; BMI—body mass index; ChP—*Chlamydia pneumoniae*; CRP—C-reactive protein; HDL—high-density lipoprotein; HP—*Helicobacter pylori*; LDL—low-density lipoprotein; M—modest risk factor; P—protective factor; S—strong risk factor; VS—very strong risk factor; WHR—waist-hip ratio. (*Adapted from* Roeters van Lennep *et al.* [9].)

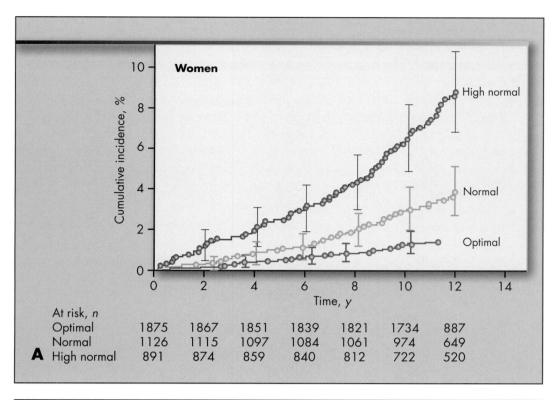

At risk, n							
Optimal	1875	1867	1851	1839	1821	1734	887
Normal	1126	1115	1097	1084	1061	974	649
A High normal	891	874	859	840	812	722	520

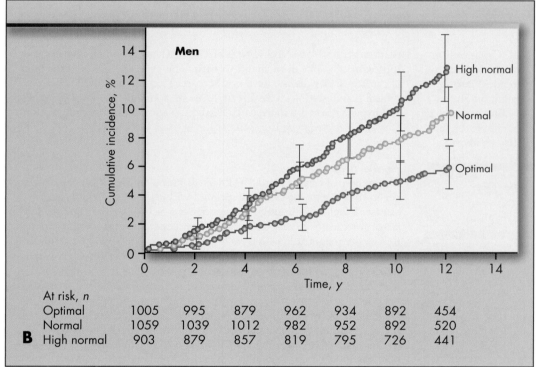

At risk, n							
Optimal	1005	995	879	962	934	892	454
Normal	1059	1039	1012	982	952	892	520
B High normal	903	879	857	819	795	726	441

Figure 5-7.
Blood pressure category and incidence of cardiovascular disease in men (**A**) and women (**B**). The impact of blood pressure on the risk of cardiovascular disease represents an excellent example of differences in the absolute and relative risks of cardiovascular disease, using data from the Framingham Heart Study [10]. These data were from 6859 men and women who were initially free from hypertension (systolic blood pressure [SBP] < 140 mm Hg and diastolic blood pressure [DBP] < 90 mm Hg) and cardiovascular disease. The 10-year cumulative incidence of cardiovascular disease was calculated among subjects aged 35–64 years for optimal (SBP < 120 mm Hg and DBP < 80 mm Hg), normal (SBP 120–129 mm Hg or DBP 80–84 mm Hg), or high-normal ([now classified as prehypertension according to JNC 7] SBP 130–139 mm Hg or DBP 85–89 mm Hg) in men and women.

Compared with those with optimal blood pressure levels, the multivariate-adjusted relative risks of cardiovascular disease for high-normal blood pressure was 2.5 (95% CI, 1.6–4.1) in women and 1.6 (1.1–2.2) in men. Blood pressure, even within the normal range, could be considered an important risk factor for cardiovascular disease in men and women, this figure indicates additional information beyond the magnitude of the relative risks. Women appear to have a more deleterious impact from elevations in blood pressure, with a greater relative risk. Even in the range of nonhypertensive blood pressure levels among middle-aged and older adults, blood pressure was a strong risk factor in the development of cardiovascular disease. (*Adapted from* Vasan *et al.* [10].)

Race

Projected Changes in the United States Population According to Race and Hispanic Origin: 2020–2050

	2020		2030		2040		2050	
	Population (in millions)	Total, %	Population (in millions)	Total, %	Population (in millions)	Total, %	Population (in millions)	Total, %
Total (aged 65 or older)	335.8 (54.6)	100 (16.3)	363.6 (71.4)	100 (19.6)	391.0 (80.0)	100 (20.4)	419.8 (86.7)	100 (20.6)
White*	250.6	77.6	275.7	75.8	280.7	78.9	302.6	72.1
Black*	45.4	13.5	50.4	13.9	68.9	14.3	61.4	14.6
Asian*	18.0	5.4	22.6	6.2	28.0	7.1	33.4	8.0
All other races	11.8	3.5	14.8	4.1	18.4	4.7	22.4	5.3
Hispanic (of any race)	(50.8)	(17.8)	(79.0)	(20.1)	(87.6)	(22.3)	(102.6)	(24.4)
Non-Hispanic white	(205.9)	(61.3)	(209.2)	(57.5)	(210.3)	(53.7)	(210.3)	(50.1)

*No other race, includes Hispanics.

Figure 5-8.
Projected changes in the United States population from 2020 through 2050 according to race and Hispanic origin. Over the next several decades, there will continue to be dramatic increases in the number of minorities in the United States, with the greatest percentage gains among Asians and Hispanics. There will be implications of these projected increases in various racial groups on the national rates of cardiovascular disease. Broad-based and individual primary prevention strategies will need to become more sensitive to the similarities and differences that each of the groups demonstrates for various cardiovascular risk factors. (*Adapted from* the US Bureau of the Census [3].)

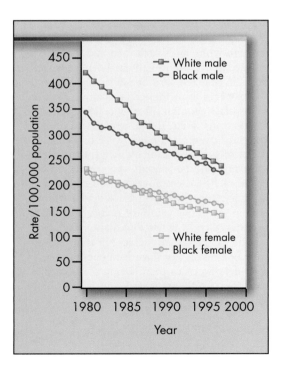

Figure 5-9.
Temporal trends from 1980 through 1997 in death rates for coronary heart disease that are adjusted for the 2000 standard for age, according to gender and race. Although there has been considerable progress in the lowering of death rates from coronary heart disease across all groups, the lowering of death rates has been proportionally greater in white men and women. As a result, death rates for coronary heart disease have become roughly equal in white and black men, whereas white women now have lower rates than black women. One oft-cited explanation for the slower reductions in coronary heart disease death rates is not risk factors per se, but rather the quality of care after an incident event. Better access to treatment, intervention, and follow-up care by whites compared with blacks has been demonstrated in numerous studies [11], which in turn would lead to lower rates of subsequent coronary heart disease death. (*Adapted from* Cooper *et al.* [12].)

Average Annual Percentage Change for Age-adjusted Total and Cause-specific Death: 1999–2002

Cause of death	White men	White women	Black men	Black women
All causes	-1.3	-1.1	-1.8	-2.3
CVD*	-3.2	-3.4	-2.3	-3.4
Heart disease	-3.3	-3.7	-2.6	-3.7
CHD	-4.0	-4.9	-3.0	-4.6
CHF	-0.6	-1.0	-1.1	-1.6
Stroke	-3.3	-3.3	-2.4	-3.3
Non-CVD	-0.1	0.4	-1.5	-1.5

*Does not include congenital malformations of the circulatory system.

Figure 5-10.
More recent data on the average annual percent change from 1999 through 2002 for age-adjusted total and cause-specific death according to gender and race. The declines in cardiovascular disease (CVD) and coronary heart disease (CHD) mortality have continued from the prior two decades in all subgroups, although the declines in cardiovascular disease mortality continue at a steeper slope for white versus black men. Among women, declines in mortality appear to have become relatively similar in whites and blacks. CHF—congestive heart failure. (*Adapted from* the National Heart, Lung, and Blood Institute [13].)

Temporal Changes in the Age-standardized Incidence Rates of Cardiovascular Disease

Outcome	1971–1982 Cohort Incidence per 10,000 person-years	1982–1992 Cohort Incidence per 10,000 person-years
White men		
Cardiovascular disease	342.6	264.2
Coronary heart disease	177.0	151.2
Acute myocardial infarction	79.6	73.4
Stroke	57.0	42.1
White women		
Cardiovascular disease	246.8	190.8
Coronary heart disease	101.7	90.1
Acute myocardial infarction	30.0	36.3
Stroke	39.2	31.2
Black men		
Cardiovascular disease	368.6	291.1
Coronary heart disease	162.7	132.6
Acute myocardial infarction	62.4	61.6
Stroke	75.6	75.7
Black women		
Cardiovascular disease	303.1	262.1
Coronary heart disease	122.7	118.0
Acute myocardial infarction	33.1	37.4
Stroke	69.5	50.9

Figure 5-11.
Temporal changes in the age-standardized incidence rates of cardiovascular disease. Using data from the first National Health and Nutrition Examination Survey Epidemiologic Follow-up Study, two cohorts (10,869 subjects in the 1971–1982 cohort and 9774 in the 1982–1992 cohort) of participants aged 35 to 74 years were created to generate age-standardized incidence rates of cardiovascular disease according to gender and race. Despite the enormous public health implications of cardiovascular disease, there are few published data on its incidence and its temporal patterns in nationally representative samples, according to gender and race. These data reinforce the observation that the declines in cardiovascular mortality are not just a function of improvements in secondary prevention, reflecting treatment of existing cardiovascular disease. The reductions in cardiovascular disease incidence in white and black men and women indicate that there must have been improvements in selected cardiovascular risk factors. The patterns in incidence rates among white versus black women offer several interesting observations. First, the absolute rates of incident cardiovascular disease were higher in blacks versus whites for men and women at both time points. Second, the relative difference in incident cardiovascular disease was much greater comparing black versus white women. Moreover, rates of myocardial infarction increased in white *and* black women, possibly reflecting an increase in their prevalence of smoking or improvements in the identification of women having a myocardial infarction. (*Adapted from* Ergin *et al.* [14].)

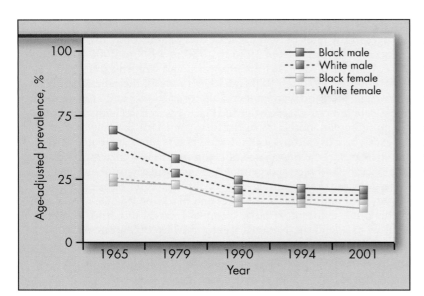

Figure 5-12.
Among adults from the United States aged 18 years and older, differences in age-adjusted smoking rates by race and gender, comparing white with blacks also by gender from 1965 through 2001. These changes in smoking status over time represent one possible environmental difference that may account for the excess risk of cardiovascular disease associated with black individuals. Smoking rates have systematically decreased in whites and blacks, as well as in men and women. In particular, the smoking rates for white and black men in 2001 are less than half the rates from 1965. Smoking rates in white and black women, which were initially less than men in 1965, have not decreased as much proportionally. The lower rates over the past few decades are not exclusive to whites and blacks; other racial groups also have experienced declines in smoking. Based on 2001 rates of smoking, there are modest differences with blacks smoking less than whites. Given the greater incidence rates of cardiovascular disease in blacks than in whites, smoking does not appear to clearly explain such differences, although the duration and amount that individuals smoked may also be informative. (*Adapted from* the National Heart, Lung, and Blood Institute [13].)

Prevalence of Cardiovascular Risk Factors Among White, Black, and Mexican-American Men and Women

Cardiovascular risk factors	White men	Black men	Mexican-American men	White women	Black women	Mexican-American women
High blood pressure						
Prevalence, %	32.2	41.6	34.5	29.5	44.7	29.9
Mortality	53,400	7900	NA	21,400	5900	NA
Tobacco use						
Prevalence, %	25.1	27.6	NA	21.7	18.0	NA
Blood cholesterol						
Total cholesterol 200 mg/dL or greater, %	51.0	37.3	54.3	53.6	46.4	44.7
Total cholesterol 240 mg/dL or greater, %	17.8	10.6	17.8	19.9	17.7	13.9
LDL cholesterol 130 mg/dL or greater, %	49.6	46.3	43.6	43.7	41.6	41.6
HDL cholesterol < 40 mg/dL, %	40.5	24.3	40.1	14.5	13.0	18.4
Physical inactivity						
Prevalence, %	32.5	44.1	NA	36.2	55.2	NA
Overweight and obesity						
Overweight: 25 kg/m^2 or greater, %	67.4	60.7	74.7	57.3	77.3	71.9
Obese: 30 kg/m^2 or greater, %	27.3	28.1	28.9	30.1	49.7	39.7
Diabetes mellitus						
Physician-diagnosed, %	5.4	7.6	8.1	4.7	9.5	11.4
Undiagnosed, %	3.0	2.8	5.8	2.1	4.7	3.9
Pre-diabetes, %	9.4	8.0	12.1	4.8	6.8	6.7

Figure 5-13.
Comparison of white, black, and Mexican-American men and women for the prevalence of various cardiovascular risk factors. These data provide insights into some of the relevant differences in cardiovascular risk factors among white, black, and Mexican-American men and women that may help explain ethnicity and race as a cardiovascular risk factor. The prevalence of high blood pressure is of particular concern among black men and women, and is a major reason why stroke rates in blacks tend to be higher than in whites and other racial groups. Total and low-density lipoprotein (LDL) cholesterol, along with low high-density lipoprotein (HDL) cholesterol, are roughly equivalent in white and Mexican-American men, whereas black men had lower rates of adverse lipid levels. White women had the highest prevalence of elevated total cholesterol and LDL cholesterol. Of particular concern is the high prevalence of physical inactivity among blacks, coupled with the high rates of obesity, especially among black women. This combination of inactivity and excess body weight is of major concern among blacks and Mexican-Americans, and particularly among women, and represents a major pathway through which race serves as a risk factor for the development of cardiovascular disease. One manifestation of physical inactivity and excess body weight—diabetes—is considerably higher in black women and Mexican-American men and women compared with whites. This rise in diabetes prevalence may be a harbinger of future increases in cardiovascular morbidity and mortality in blacks and Mexican-Americans, possibly making race and ethnicity an even greater discriminator for cardiovascular disease risk. NA—no data available. (*Adapted from* the American Heart Association [15–17].)

Nonmodifiable Risk Factors: Gender, Race, and Family History

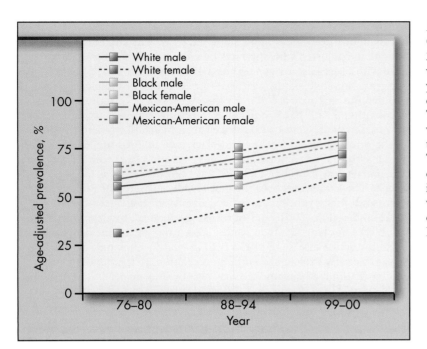

Figure 5-14.
Changes in the rates of being at least overweight (body mass index of 25 kg/m² or greater) from 1976 to 1980 to 1999 to 2000 comparing white, black, and Mexican-American men and women aged 20 to 74 years. Between 1976 to 1980 and 1999 to 2000, the prevalence of overweight men and women increased for each race and ethnic group. These data indicate that longitudinal changes in risk factors like body weight represent another cardiovascular risk factor that may account for the excess risk of cardiovascular disease that is often attributed to race. The increases in the prevalence of being overweight increased systematically regardless of race and gender. One particularly troublesome trend is that Mexican-Americans have especially high rates of being overweight, although the rates in whites and blacks on average appear to be catching up. (*Adapted from* the National Heart, Lung, and Blood Institute [13] and the National Center for Health Statistics [18].)

Prevalence of Overweight and Obesity According to Age, Gender, and Survey Type: 1988–1994

| | Age group, y | | | | | | | Total | | |
| | | | | | | | | | Age-adjusted | |
Group	20–29	30–39	40–49	50–59	60–69	70–79	80+	Crude	Age 20+	Age 20–74
Body mass index 25.0 kg/m² or greater										
Men										
Non-Hispanic white	41.7%	58.7%	67.0%	72.9%	72.2%	64.8%	51.9%	60.6%	59.5%	59.6%
Non-Hispanic black	50.1%	54.0%	63.9%	65.5%	62.2%	53.7%	48.5%	56.7%	56.9%	57.5%
Mexican-American	49.9%	68.2%	78.5%	80.6%	71.8%	65.4%	60.5%	63.9%	66.7%	67.1%
Women										
Non-Hispanic white	27.7%	41.1%	48.3%	62.8%	61.9%	55.9%	49.5%	47.4%	45.8%	45.5%
Non-Hispanic black	50.0%	63.0%	75.0%	78.1%	79.5%	76.4%	54.2%	66.0%	66.4%	66.5%
Mexican-American	52.7%	66.7%	77.5%	76.9%	78.5%	61.0%	50.9%	65.9%	66.6%	67.6%
Body mass index 30.0 kg/m² or greater										
Men										
Non-Hispanic white	12.0%	17.1%	22.7%	30.6%	25.3%	20.4%	7.7%	19.9%	19.5%	20.0%
Non-Hispanic black	19.1%	20.3%	22.3%	21.5%	25.6%	19.5%	11.1%	20.7%	20.7%	21.3%
Mexican-American	13.3%	17.9%	32.9%	37.1%	26.6%	18.5%	4.4%	20.6%	22.5%	23.1%
Women										
Non-Hispanic white	13.1%	22.4%	22.6%	33.5%	28.3%	23.7%	14.3%	22.7%	22.2%	22.4%
Non-Hispanic black	23.4%	35.5%	44.6%	50.1%	45.4%	38.3%	20.5%	36.7%	36.8%	37.4%
Mexican-American	22.4%	34.7%	44.7%	43.0%	39.1%	24.3%	19.1%	33.3%	33.4%	34.2%

Figure 5-15.
Prevalence of being overweight (body mass index 25 kg/m² or greater) or obese (body mass index 30 kg/m² or greater) according to age, gender, and survey from 1988 through 1994. Differences in the data sources and data analyses account for some of the discrepancies comparing this figure with Figure 5-14. Being overweight or obese begins at an alarmingly early age, particularly among non-Hispanic blacks and Mexican-Americans. Approximately half of non-Hispanic black and Mexican-American men and women aged 20 to 29 years were already overweight. Furthermore, nearly half of those women were already obese, translating to nearly one quarter of all non-Hispanic black and Mexican-American women aged 20 to 29 years. This suggests that race may be an important risk factor for cardiovascular disease that begins at

an early age for body mass index. Interventions to reduce and maintain healthy body weights in non-Hispanic and Mexican-American men and women must begin as early as possible, and cover the wide range of dietary, environmental, and cultural determinants of health to aim to reduce the prevalence of being overweight or obese. Another interesting observation in these data is that the prevalence of being overweight plateaus from 50 to 69 years then goes down at older age, reflecting the fact that subjects with a lower body mass index are more likely to survive to that age. For obesity, the prevalence generally peaks at an earlier age, at 50 to 59 years, followed by a parallel decline in prevalence with age. (*Adapted from* the Centers for Disease Control [19].)

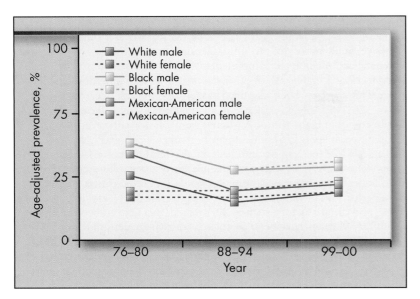

Figure 5-16.
Differences in the age-adjusted prevalence of hypertension (defined as a systolic blood pressure 140 mm Hg or greater, diastolic blood pressure 90 mm Hg or greater, or antihypertensive treatment) by race and gender, comparing white, black, and Mexican-American individuals aged 20 to 74 years. These data represent an important environmental difference that may account for the excess risk of cardiovascular disease and those changes in risk over time. The initial reductions in the prevalence of hypertension from 1976–1980 to 1988–1994 in whites and blacks, but not Mexican-Americans, reflected improvements in body weight in conjunction with other coronary risk factors such as increased physical activity and heart-healthy diets. However, with the recent surge in body weight, the data from 1999 to 2000 may have caused an increase in the prevalence in hypertension in white, black, and Mexican-American men and women that offers no immediate hope of abating. The overall rates of hypertension at present are comparable for whites and Mexican-Americans despite the higher rates of obesity in Mexican-Americans. Black men and women continue to have a considerably higher prevalence of hypertension that may be related to genetic and cultural differences that have yet to be fully explained. (*Adapted from* the National Heart, Lung, and Blood Institute [13,20].)

Family History

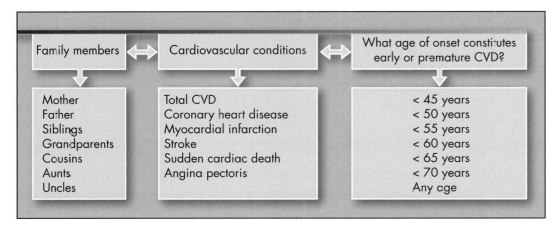

Figure 5-17.
What constitutes a family history of cardiovascular disease (CVD)? Three components may need to be considered, including which biologic family members are affected, what are the cardiovascular conditions, and what is the age of onset. An individual's genetic makeup is directly impacted by their mother and father, who are typically the focus of determining a patient's family history of CVD. However, clues to genetic traits can be observed in siblings, cousins, and other family members. Moreover, various definitions of parental history of CVD in the existing literature neglect the separate effects of paternal and maternal history [21]. Second, the conventional definition of family history of CVD is often limited to family history of myocardial infarction, without regard to other CVD outcomes. Granted, myocardial infarction represents some of the most

severe manifestation of CVD along with stroke, but other cardiovascular outcomes are typically not included in the definition of family history. Finally, family history is ordinarily classified as premature or early, but the age cut-off for that designation is arbitrary [22]. Most often, CVD in a biologic parent before age 55 for the father and before age 65 for the mother is considered a positive family history of CVD, according to the clinical guidelines from the National Cholesterol Education Program Third Adult Treatment Panel [23] and Seventh Joint National Committee on Prevention, Detection, Evaluation, and Treatment of High Blood Pressure [24]. However, given the low incidence rates of CVD and myocardial infarction in women before age 65 [2], this definition may overemphasize paternal history of CVD.

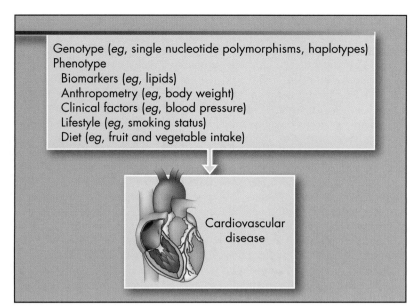

Genotype (*eg*, single nucleotide polymorphisms, haplotypes)
Phenotype
  Biomarkers (*eg*, lipids)
  Anthropometry (*eg*, body weight)
  Clinical factors (*eg*, blood pressure)
  Lifestyle (*eg*, smoking status)
  Diet (*eg*, fruit and vegetable intake)

Cardiovascular disease

Figure 5-18.

Manifestations of a family history of cardiovascular disease. Individuals with a positive family history of cardiovascular disease typically have a wide range of genetic and phenotypic components whereby that person may be predisposed to be at a higher risk of cardiovascular disease. Numerous genetic markers have already been identified as elevating the risk of cardiovascular disease [25]. Phenotypic evidence of a family history of cardiovascular disease comes in many forms. A positive family history of cardiovascular disease impacts lipids [26], inflammatory markers [27], and hemostatic markers [28]. Hypertension and diabetes also tend to have a familial component that is represented by a family history of cardiovascular disease. In addition, most major cardiovascular risk factors often cluster within families. Lifestyle and dietary factors, such as physical activity, smoking, alcohol intake, and dietary factors, such as fiber intake, also tend to be similar within families. Mothers have been postulated to have greater influences on their children's dietary and behavioral patterns retained later in life [21]. No single study has yet to incorporate the entire array of genetic and phenotypic factors to examine the extent to which the independent effect of family history of cardiovascular disease may be mediated by these factors.

A. Impact of Premature Paternal Cardiovascular Disease Risk Factors on Offspring

Model adjustment	Risk for offspring CVD, odds ratio (95% CI)			
	None	Paternal CVD	Maternal CVD	Paternal and maternal
Offspring men				
Unadjusted	1.0	3.0 (1.7–5.0)	3.4 (2.1–5.6)	3.3 (1.2–9.0)
Age-adjusted	1.0	2.7 (1.6–4.7)	2.4 (1.5–4.0)	3.1 (1.1–8.3)
Multivariable-adjusted*	1.0	2.2 (1.2–3.9)	1.7 (1.0–2.9)	2.4 (0.9–6.8)
Offspring women				
Unadjusted	1.0	2.7 (1.3–5.8)	3.2 (1.7–6.0)	4.3 (1.2–15)
Age-adjusted	1.0	2.8 (1.3–6.1)	2.3 (1.2–4.5)	4.1 (1.1–15)
Multivariable-adjusted*	1.0	1.7 (0.7–3.9)	1.7 (0.8–3.4)	2.8 (0.7–11)

B. Impact of Nonpremature Paternal Cardiovascular Disease Risk Factors on Offspring

Model adjustment	Risk for offspring CVD, odds ratio (95% CI)			
	None	Paternal CVD	Maternal CVD	Paternal and maternal
Offspring men				
Unadjusted	1.0	3.0 (1.9–4.6)	4.1 (2.4–6.8)	5.2 (2.8–9.8)
Age-adjusted	1.0	2.0 (1.2–3.1)	1.8 (1.0–3.2)	2.4 (1.2–4.8)
Multivariable-adjusted*	1.0	1.6 (1.0–2.5)	1.3 (0.7–2.4)	1.8 (0.9–3.7)
Offspring women				
Unadjusted	1.0	2.6 (1.5–4.6)	3.5 (1.7–6.9)	3.9 (1.7–9.0)
Age-adjusted	1.0	1.6 (0.9–3.0)	1.7 (0.8–3.7)	1.7 (0.7–4.1)
Multivariable-adjusted*	1.0	1.1 (0.6–2.1)	1.2 (0.5–2.9)	1.0 (0.4–2.7)

*Adjusted for age, total/high-density lipoprotein cholesterol ratio, systolic blood pressure, antihypertensive therapy, diabetes, body mass index, and current smoking status.

Figure 5-19.

A and **B**, Impact of parental history of cardiovascular disease (CVD) on the risk of CVD. Using data from the Framingham Offspring Study, a United States population-based epidemiologic cohort established in 1971, 2302 men and women aged 30 years or older with parents in the original Framingham Heart Study were examined for their risk of developing CVD according to the presence of premature (onset age < 55 years in father, < 65 years in mother) CVD [29]. The definition of CVD included confirmed reports of coronary death, myocardial infarction, coronary insufficiency, angina pectoris, atherothrombotic stroke, intermittent claudication, and cardiovascular death. It appears that a premature paternal history of CVD is at least as important as a premature maternal history for men and women. When both parents have a premature history of CVD, women in particular have a considerably higher risk of developing CVD, with 2.8 times the risk compared with women lacking any premature parental history. When the presence of nonpremature (onset age 55 years or older in father, 65 years or older in mother) CVD was considered, the relative risks were greatly reduced and not significant. These data suggest that only an early or premature parental history of CVD may be clinically relevant in patients when considering the long-term risk of developing cardiovascular disease. (*Adapted from* Lloyd-Jones *et al.* [29].)

Impact of Age of Maternal History of Myocardial Infarction on the Risk of Cardiovascular Disease

	Age of maternal myocardial infarction					
	None	< 50 years	50–59 years	60–69 years	70–79 years	80 years or older
Men (CVD cases)	17,984 (2178)	38 (4)	215 (40)	514 (107)	606 (127)	326 (66)
Age-adjusted relative risk	1.00 (referent)	1.05 (0.40–2.81)	1.94 (1.42–2.65)	1.89 (1.56–2.29)	1.69 (1.42–2.03)	1.18 (0.92–1.51)
Multivariate-adjusted relative risk*	1.00 (referent)	1.00 (0.38–2.68)	1.88 (1.37–2.58)	1.88 (1.55–2.29)	1.67 (1.39–2.00)	1.17 (0.91–1.50)
Women (CVD cases)	33,304 (451)	433 (14)	884 (17)		3175 (73)	
Age-adjusted relative risk	1.00 (referent)	2.59 (1.52–4.41)	1.50 (0.93–2.44)		1.55 (1.21–1.99)	
Multivariate-adjusted relative risk*	1.00 (referent)	2.57 (1.51–4.37)	1.33 (0.80–2.23)		1.52 (1.18–1.96)	

*Adjusted for age, body mass index, smoking status, exercise, and alcohol consumption. Addition covariates for men include aspirin and beta-carotene treatment; for women, aspirin and vitamin E treatment, postmenopausal status, and postmenopausal hormone use.

Figure 5-20.

Impact of age of maternal history of myocardial infarction (MI) on the risk of cardiovascular disease (CVD). In another investigation, 22,071 men from the Physicians' Health Study and 39,876 women from the Women's Health Study with data on parental history and age of MI were prospectively observed for the risk of CVD [21]. Rather than focus on the presence or absence of premature CVD, focus on the effect of various categories of maternal and paternal age of MI. A total of 9.6% of women reported a maternal history with a maternal age of less than 50 years compared with only 2.2% of men. In men, even a maternal age of MI of 70 to 79 years was significantly associated with a 67% increased risk of CVD. Women with a maternal age of MI of 60 years or older also had a significant 52% increased risk of CVD, suggesting that history of maternal MI may be important regardless of maternal age. (*Adapted from* Sesso *et al.* [21].)

Impact of Age of Paternal History of Myocardial Infarction and Relative Risk of Cardiovascular Disease

	Age of paternal myocardial infarction					
	None	< 50 years	50–59 years	60–69 years	70–79 years	80 years or older
Men (CVD cases)	15,510 (1713)	499 (91)	125 (198)	1717 (260)	1273 (191)	440 (69)
Age-adjusted relative risk	1.00 (referent)	2.22 (1.80–2.75)	1.66 (1.43–1.93)	1.39 (1.22–1.59)	1.19 (1.02–1.38)	0.94 (0.74–1.20)
Multivariate-adjusted relative risk*	1.00 (referent)	2.19 (1.77–2.72)	1.64 (1.42–1.91)	1.42 (1.24–1.62)	1.16 (1.00–1.36)	0.92 (0.72–1.18)
Women (CVD cases)	28,025 (401)	1587 (31)	2600 (42)		5480 (83)	
Age-adjusted relative risk	1.00 (referent)	1.76 (1.22–2.55)	1.30 (0.94–1.80)		1.09 (0.84–1.36)	
Multivariate-adjusted relative risk*	1.00 (referent)	1.63 (1.12–2.39)	1.33 (0.96–1.84)		1.13 (0.89–1.43)	

*Adjusted for age, body mass index, smoking status, and alcohol intake. Additional covariates for men included aspirin and beta-carotene treatment; for women, aspirin and vitamin E treatment, postmenopausal status, and postmenopausal hormone use.

Figure 5-21.

Impact of age of paternal history of myocardial infarction (MI) on the risk of cardiovascular disease (CVD). Again, considering 22,071 men from the Physicians' Health Study and 39,876 women from the Women's Health Study with data on parental history and age of MI, we prospectively observed these subjects for the risk of CVD. We next considered the effect of paternal age of MI on cardiovascular risk. A greater proportion of women (16.4%) with a paternal history of MI reported an earlier paternal age (< 50 years) versus men (9.6%). Compared with men having no paternal history of MI, earlier paternal ages of MI had greater magnitudes of cardiovascular risk that decreased as the paternal age increased. However, a paternal age of 70 to 79 years remained significantly associated with an increased risk of CVD in men. In contrast, women with a paternal age of MI of 60 years or older had no increased risk of CVD. (*Adapted from* Sesso *et al.* [21].)

Nonmodifiable Risk Factors: Gender, Race, and Family History

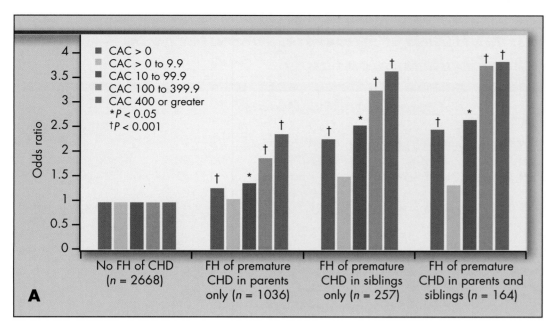

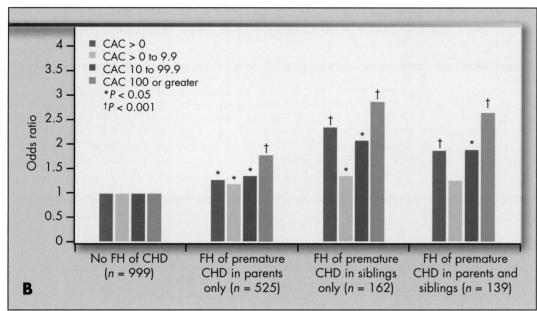

Figure 5-22.
A and **B**, Sibling history may be more important than parental history of premature coronary heart disease (CHD) for the development of coronary artery calcification (CAC). Sibling history of cardiovascular disease may be problematic to ascertain depending on whether a patient even has any siblings or knowledge of their health conditions, as well as whether siblings may be of an age for cardiovascular disease. In a large study of 8549 asymptomatic men and women, the association of a family history of premature (< 55 years of age in men and women) CHD with CAC determined from electron beam tomography scanning [30]. Odds ratios compare sequentially higher scores of CAC for individuals with a premature parental history of CHD only, a premature sibling history of CHD only, and a premature history of CHD in parents and siblings. Notably, in men *and* women, there was a highly and more strongly significant association between premature sibling history of CHD as compared with premature parental history. These findings suggest that siblings also contribute important information on family history of cardiovascular disease, perhaps more strongly than parental history. In addition, primary prevention strategies may need to expand the definition of family history to include parental and sibling history of premature cardiovascular disease. This is especially relevant when parents or siblings may have died at a relatively younger age by which time cardiovascular disease had not had an ample opportunity to develop. FH—family history. (*Adapted from* Nasir *et al.* [30].)

Utah Family Tree Study: Results from Families at Risk of Coronary Heart Disease and Stroke: 1983–1996

CHD and stroke FRS	Families, n (%)	Relatives with CHD and stroke at an early age, n (%)	Relatives with CHD and stroke at any age, n (%)	Concentration factor		Type of family history
				Early	Any age	
CHD						
2.0 or greater	1227 (1.0)	2797 (16.8)	3418 (6.6)	16.8	6.3	Very strong positive
1.0 or greater	3917 (3.2)	5756 (34.7)	9556 (17.6)	10.8	5.5	Strong positive
0.5 or greater	17,064 (14.0)	11,968 (72.1)	26,222 (48.4)	5.2	3.5	Positive
< 0.5	105,091 (86.0)	4634 (27.9)	27,960 (51.6)	0.3	0.6	Average
Total	122,155	16,602	54,182	1.0	1.0	
Stroke						
2.0 or greater	1246 (1.0)	860 (18.7)	2661 (11.9)	18.7	11.9	Very strong positive
1.0 or greater	1727 (1.4)	1004 (21.8)	3645 (16.2)	15.6	11.1	Strong positive
0.5 or greater	13,106 (10.7)	3937 (85.6)	15,171 (67.6)	8.0	6.3	Positive
< 0.5	109,049 (89.3)	663 (14.4)	7254 (32.3)	0.2	0.4	Average
Total	122,155	4600	22,425	1.0	1.0	

Figure 5-23.

Detailed information on family history of cardiovascular disease provides clinically relevant and targeted primary prevention efforts. Through the use of a standardized quantitative family risk score, derived from data on cardiovascular disease and risk factor information on a subject's first-degree relatives, including siblings, parents, and children [31], a potentially more thorough perspective of family history of cardiovascular disease can be obtained. In this study, data were obtained from 122,155 Utah families as part of the large, population-based Health Family Tree Study [32]. Only 14% of 122,155 Utah families (all races combined) had a positive family history defined as a family risk score of 0.5 or greater, and yet these families accounted for more than 72% of all persons with early coronary heart disease (CHD). However, a very strong family history of CHD occurred in only 1% of the population, but these families included nearly 17% of the early cases of CHD. For stroke, 10.7% of families had a positive family history and accounted for 86% of

early strokes and even 68% of strokes regardless of age. Among the 1% of families with a very strong positive family history of stroke, 18.7% of the early cases of stroke were included. The concentrating factor, defined as the percentage of events divided by the percentage of families for each family history classification, increases with greater strength of the positive family history definition. For CHD and stroke, having any family history increases the likelihood of having that cardiovascular end-point. In addition, as there is a greater concentration of family history of CHD and stroke within a specific family, the likelihood of having a cardiovascular event continues to rise dramatically. These data indicate that the risk associated with a positive family history of cardiovascular disease is greater when accounting for a greater number of primary at-risk relatives. In this regard, limiting family history to parental history may be insufficient in the primary prevention of cardiovascular disease. FRS—Family Risk Score. (*Adapted from* Williams *et al.* [32].)

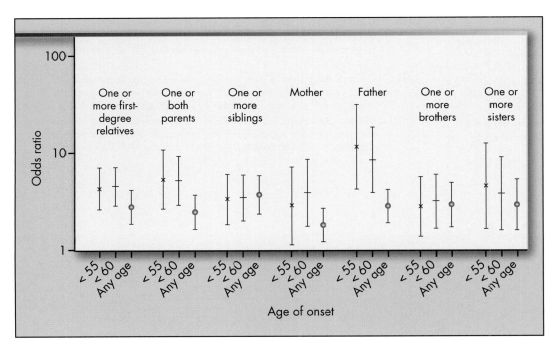

Figure 5-24.

Possible combinations of family members that may comprise a family history of cardiovascular disease and risk of coronary heart disease. In an Australian study of 403 cases of coronary heart disease and 236 controls, various definitions of family history of coronary heart disease were considered attempted to estimate the additional information provided by more complex or comprehensive family history definitions [22]. This figure compares the odds ratios of coronary heart disease for different family history definitions, as well as considering premature history (< 55 men or < 60 women) or any history at all. All definitions were predictive of coronary heart disease, and with premature family history having a slightly stronger magnitude of risk. Models were then fit to quantitate the improvement in the prediction of coronary heart disease with more this more detailed information compared with a "simple" definition of one or more first-degree family member with coronary heart disease at any age. (*Adapted from* Silberberg *et al.* [22].)

References

1. Rossouw JE: Hormones, genetic factors, and gender differences in cardiovascular disease. *Cardiovasc Res* 2002, 53:550–557.

2. American Heart Association: *Heart Disease and Stroke Statistics: 2004 Update.* Dallas: American Heart Association; 2003.

3. US Bureau of the Census: National Population Projections. Available at http://www.census.gov/population/www/projections/natsum.html.

4. American Heart Association: *Men and Cardiovascular Diseases: Heart Disease and Stroke Statistics—2004 Update.* Dallas: American Heart Association; 2003.

5. Rossouw JE, Anderson GL, Prentice RL, *et al.*: Risks and benefits of estrogen plus progestin in healthy postmenopausal women: principal results from the Women's Health Initiative randomized controlled trial. *JAMA* 2002, 288:321–333.

6. World Health Organization: *Physical Status: The Use and Interpretation of Anthropometry.* Geneva, Switzerland: World Health Organization; 1995.

7. American Heart Association: *Women and Cardiovascular Diseases: Heart Disease and Stroke Statistics—2004 Update.* Dallas: American Heart Association; 2003.

8. Centers for Disease Control: National Center for Health Statistics unpublished tabulations. Available at http://www.cdc.gov/nchs/data/nhanes/overweight.pdf.

9. Roeters van Lennep JE, Westerveld HT, Erkelens DW, van der Wall EE: Risk factors for coronary heart disease: implications of gender. *Cardiovasc Res* 2002, 53:538–549.

10. Vasan RS, Larson MG, Leip EP, *et al.*: Impact of high-normal blood pressure on the risk of cardiovascular disease. *N Engl J Med* 2001, 345:1291–1297.

11. Lillie-Blanton M, Maddox TM, Rushing O, Mensah GA: Disparities in cardiac care: rising to the challenge of Healthy People 2010. *J Am Coll Cardiol* 2004, 44:503–508.

12. Cooper R, Cutler J, Desvigne-Nickens P, *et al.*: Trends and disparities in coronary heart disease, stroke, and other cardiovascular diseases in the United States: findings of the national conference on cardiovascular disease prevention. *Circulation* 2000, 102:3137–3147.

13. National Heart, Lung, and Blood Institute: *Morbidity and Mortality: 2004 Chart Book on Cardiovascular, Lung, and Blood Diseases.* Available at http://www.nhlbi.nih.gov/resources/docs/04_chtbk.pdf.

14. Ergin A, Muntner P, Sherwin R, He J: Secular trends in cardiovascular disease mortality, incidence, and case fatality rates in adults in the United States. *Am J Med* 2004, 117:219–227.

15. American Heart Association: *African-Americans and Cardiovascular Diseases: Heart Disease and Stroke Statistics—2004 Update.* Dallas: American Heart Association; 2003.

16. American Heart Association: *Whites and Cardiovascular Diseases: Heart Disease and Stroke Statistics—2004 Update.* Dallas: American Heart Association; 2003.

17. American Heart Association: *Hispanics/Latinos and Cardiovascular Diseases: Heart Disease and Stroke Statistics—2004 Update.* Dallas: American Heart Association; 2003.

18. National Center for Health Statistics: *Health, United States, 2004.* Available at http://www.cdc.gov/nchs/hus.htm.

19. Centers for Disease Control: National Center for Health Statistics unpublished tabulations. Available at http://www.cdc.gov/nchs/data/nhanes/overweight.pdf.

20. National Heart, Lung, and Blood Institute: Unpublished tabulation from the public use data tapes, National Health and Nutrition Examination Survey, 1971–1975, 1976–1980, 1988–1994, 1999–2000. Bethesda, Maryland: National Center for Health Statistics; 1999.

21. Sesso HD, Lee IM, Gaziano JM, *et al.*: Maternal and paternal history of myocardial infarction and risk of cardiovascular disease in men and women. *Circulation* 2001, 104:393–398.

22. Silberberg JS, Wlodarczyk J, Fryer J, *et al.*: Risk associated with various definitions of family history of coronary heart disease. The Newcastle Family History Study II. *Am J Epidemiol* 1998, 147:1133–1139.

23. Executive Summary of the Third Report of the National Cholesterol Education Program (NCEP) Expert Panel on Detection, Evaluation, and Treatment of High Blood Cholesterol in Adults (Adult Treatment Panel III). *JAMA* 2001, 285:2486–2497.

24. Chobanian AV, Bakris GL, Black HR, *et al.*: The seventh report of the Joint National Committee on Prevention, Detection, Evaluation, and Treatment of High Blood Pressure: The JNC 7 Report. *JAMA* 2003, 289:2560–2571.

25. Gibbons GH, Liew CC, Goodarzi MO, *et al.*: Genetic markers: progress and potential for cardiovascular disease. *Circulation* 2004, 109:IV47–IV58.

26. Hippe M, Vestbo J, Bjerg AM, *et al.*: Cardiovascular risk factor profile in subjects with familial predisposition to myocardial infarction in Denmark. *J Epidemiol Community Health* 1997, 51:266–271.

27. Margaglione M, Cappucci G, Colaizzo D, *et al.*: C-reactive protein in offspring is associated with the occurrence of myocardial infarction in first-degree relatives. *Arterioscler Thromb Vasc Biol* 2000, 20:198–203.

28. Pankow JS, Folsom AR, Cushman M, *et al.*: Familial and genetic determinants of systemic markers of inflammation: the NHLBI family heart study. *Atherosclerosis* 2001, 154:681–689.

29. Lloyd-Jones DM, Nam BH, D'Agostino RB Sr., *et al.*: Parental cardiovascular disease as a risk factor for cardiovascular disease in middle-aged adults: a prospective study of parents and offspring. *JAMA* 2004, 291:2204–2211.

30. Nasir K, Michos ED, Rumberger JA, *et al.*: Coronary artery calcification and family history of premature coronary heart disease: sibling history is more strongly associated than parental history. *Circulation* 2004, 110:2150–2156.

31. Williams RR, Hunt SC, Barlow GK, *et al.*: Health family trees: a tool for finding and helping young family members of coronary and cancer prone pedigrees in Texas and Utah. *Am J Public Health* 1988, 78:1283–1286.

32. Williams RR, Hunt SC, Heiss G, *et al.*: Usefulness of cardiovascular family history data for population-based preventive medicine and medical research (the Health Family Tree Study and the NHLBI Family Heart Study). *Am J Cardiol* 2001, 87:129–135.

Cigarette Smoking/Cessation

Thomas S. Bowman and
Charles H. Hennekens

There were 1.2 billion smokers worldwide during the year 2000, with a projected increase to 1.6 billion by 2030 [1]. During this time period, deaths related to tobacco use are projected to increase from 4.9 million to 10 million annually. For cardiovascular disease, the hazards of smoking relate to the amount currently smoked, whereas for cancer they relate to duration; thus the effects of smoking occur decades after the exposure. In developed countries, cigarette smoking increased during the first half of the 20th century, and cancer-related deaths have occurred in the last half of the century. Because smoking prevention is likely to affect adolescents or young adults, the only hope of substantially reducing tobacco-related deaths in the first half of the 21st century is for current smokers to stop. Even into middle age, smoking cessation is remarkably effective and removes all cardiovascular risk within a few years and, even after 5 to 10 years, a substantial amount of the cancer risk associated with tobacco use [2].

In the United States, there were 45.8 million (22.5%) current smokers in 2002, with a large variation by gender, age, geography, race, income, and education [3,4]. Men (25.2%) are more likely to smoke than women (20.0%), but rates among men have declined more than among women [4]. Among all high school students, the time at which almost all tobacco use starts [5], smoking rates in 1997 were 36.4% and by 2003 had declined substantially to 21.9% [6]. At the beginning of high school, 9th graders already smoke at a high rate (17.4%), which increases steadily into 12th grade (26.2%) [6], and peaks among 18 to 24 year olds (28.5%). Smoking rates then decline with age and with selective early morality among smokers, with a rate of 9.3% among those aged 65 years or older [4].

Among the 50 US states, there are significant variations in smoking rates, with the highest prevalence in Kentucky (30.8%) and the lowest in Utah (12.0%) [4]. Among ethnic groups, Native Americans have a high rate of smoking (40.8%), whereas whites (23.6%) and blacks (22.4%) have similar rates, and Hispanics (16.7%) and Asians (13.3%) have rates lower than the national average [4]. Adults living below the poverty level are more likely to smoke (32.9%) than those living at or above the poverty level (22.2%). Over the past 20 years, college graduates have decreased their rates from 22% to 12.1%, which is far lower than that among those without a high school diploma (27.6%) [4].

In the United States, tobacco use was responsible for 435,000 deaths in the year 2000 [8]. Patients with diabetes [9], on dialysis [10], and women who take oral contraceptives who also smoke [11] have increased risks of cardiovascular disease. The economic toll, including loss of productivity and medical-related costs, was estimated at $157 billion annually from 1995 to 1999 [12].

Four stages of the global tobacco epidemic have been described, beginning with rapidly increasing tobacco use currently occurring in sub-Saharan Africa [13]. The second stage is characterized by increasing tobacco use and an increasing number of tobacco-related deaths, which is occurring in China, Japan, and Latin America [14]. Eastern Europe is in the third stage in which tobacco use peaks and then slowly declines while mortality from smoking continues to increase. The United States, Canada, and western Europe are in a fourth stage in which tobacco use declines, but tobacco-related deaths remain high.

The benefits of stopping smoking have been clearly demonstrated in many case-control and prospective cohort studies [15]. The British Doctor's Study, with 50 years of follow-up, has the longest duration and has demonstrated the increased mortality associated with smoking as well as the health benefits of quitting [2]. In another prospective cohort study of women who stopped smoking, the risk of cardiovascular disease was reduced by one third within 2 years of cessation, with a further decline within 10 to 14 years to the baseline risk of those who never smoked [16]. For older individuals (aged > 65 years) without cardiovascular disease, current smoking doubled the risk of cardiovascular death, whereas former smokers had a risk similar to those who never smoke [17]. Among women with diabetes, smoking cessation decreased the risk of coronary heart disease [9], and for those who have already had a myocardial infarction, smoking cessation also decreases mortality, regardless of gender, length of follow-up, location, or time period [18].

Although quitting is clearly beneficial and many smokers would like to quit, tobacco smoking has addictive components [19]. In this regard, counseling and pharmacotherapy are effective at increasing cessation rates [20]. The "five As" (Ask, Advise, Assess, Assist, and Arrange) are commonly used for those who wish to quit, whereas the "five Rs" (Relevance, Risks, Rewards, Roadblocks, and Repetition) are used to motivate smokers to quit. Nicotine replacement relieves withdrawal symptoms and is available over the counter [21], and bupropion is a prescription medication that increases smoking cessation rates [22] and prevents relapses in those who have quit [23].

The US Surgeon General has released 28 reports about tobacco, beginning with the landmark 1964 document that widely publicized smoking as a major cause of lung cancer and led to a decrease in cigarette consumption [24]. The 2004 report from the US Surgeon

General reviewed the causal relationship between smoking and damage to almost every organ in the human body, while emphasizing that quitting has immediate as well as long-term health benefits [25].

Several strategies on a national, state, and local level have been used to reduce tobacco use. Taxation of cigarettes reduces demand, but tax rates vary across states. The lowest rates are in areas with local tobacco growers and higher rates of smoking. Legislation has been used to ban smoking in public places and provide clean indoor air [26]. Litigation against tobacco manufacturers led to the landmark 1998 Master Settlement Agreement between 46 states and the four major US tobacco companies; however, the public health impact remains unclear [27].

In the United States, tobacco cessation efforts have included education and legislative strategies, including taxation and establishing smoke-free workplaces. In California, a tobacco control program started in 1989 has helped create smoke-free environments and clean indoor air, with subsequent decreases in cigarette consumption and heart disease mortality [26]. A national goal of Healthy People 2010 is to reduce the prevalence of cigarette smoking to less than 12%, with a rate of less than 16% among adolescents [28]. The World Health Organization is working to standardize global tobacco control measures through the Framework Convention on Tobacco Control, the world's first public health treaty [29]. The Framework Convention on Tobacco Control is an international agreement to address the global tobacco epidemic, with provisions to reduce demand for tobacco and strategies to limit supply. The United States signed the treaty in 2004 and in early 2005 the document awaited US Senate ratification, a process that would make it legally binding [30]. To achieve the important goal of reducing tobacco use, comprehensive programs for cessation and prevention will be necessary among all socioeconomic groups and ethnicities [25]. Tobacco consumption is the leading cause of premature death in the United States and is rapidly becoming a worldwide problem. Sustained efforts will be essential to reduce smoking rates in the United States and across the globe.

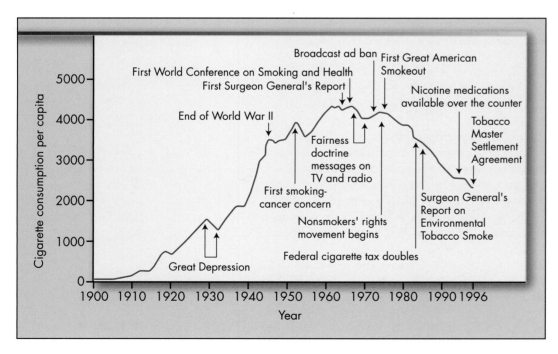

Figure 6-1.
Yearly adult cigarette consumption per capita and major smoking and health events in the United States. In the 20th century, rates of cigarette smoking have increased, with few pauses, until the 1960s when health warnings were first issued by the US Surgeon General and anti-tobacco efforts began. Many factors have contributed to the steady decline in consumption over the past four decades, including education about health risks, improved therapies for cessation, taxes on tobacco, litigation, and legislation to create smoke-free public places. (*Data from* US Department of Agriculture, 1986 Surgeon General's Report.)

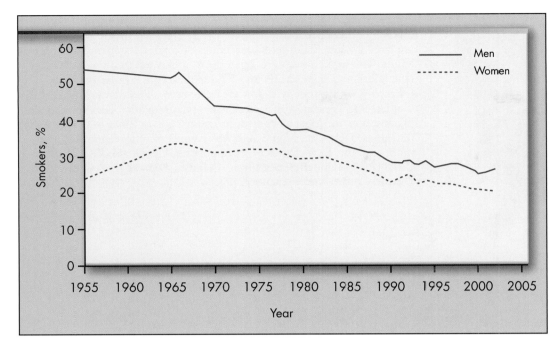

Figure 6-2.
Cigarette smoking trends among men and women older than 18 years: 1955 to 1997. Since the 1960s, smoking rates have continued to decline, and by 2002 there were more former smokers than current smokers in the United States. There have been persistent gender differences in smoking rates with a gap that has narrowed over time. In 2002, the rate among men (25.2%) remained higher than that among women (20.0%). (*Adapted from* Schoenborn *et al.* [3] and Centers for Disease Control and Prevention [4].)

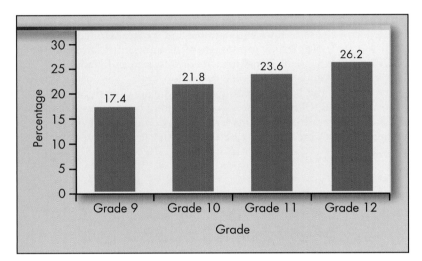

Figure 6-3.
Percentage of high school students who smoked cigarettes on one or more of the 30 days preceding the survey, United States, 2003. Most tobacco use begins at an early age. In 2003, students in the first year of high school already smoked at a rate of 17.4%, and smoking rates steadily increased through high school. Overall rates among high school students have recently decreased, with 12th graders smoking at a rate of 42.8% in 1999 and 26.2% in 2003. Because smoking rates are associated with failing or dropping out of high school earlier, school-based antismoking efforts are being targeted to younger students before they leave school. (*Adapted from* Centers for Disease Control and Prevention [6].)

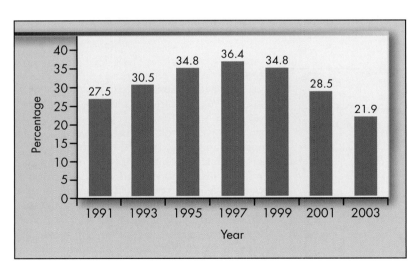

Figure 6-4.
Percentage of high school students who reported current cigarette smoking (one or more of the 30 days preceding the survey): 1991 to 2003. Current smoking rates among all high school students peaked in 1997, and then there has been a dramatic decline toward the national Healthy People 2010 goal of 16%. In this age group, rates are similar among males and females. Because nearly all smoking begins early in life, the decrease among high school students may lead to a lower national smoking rate later in the 21st century. (*Adapted from* Centers for Disease Control and Prevention [6].)

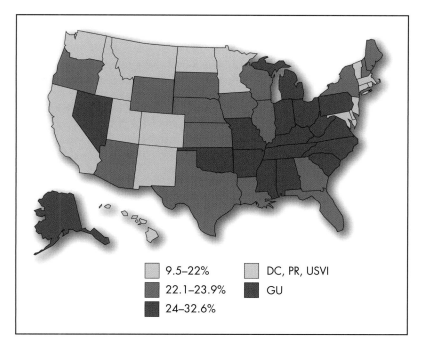

Figure 6-5.
Smoking prevalence in the United States, 2002. In the 50 states, there are large geographic differences in rates of cigarette smoking among adults. The highest rates are generally found in tobacco-growing states (the South and upper Midwest). The highest rate is in Kentucky, a tobacco-growing state with low cigarette taxes. The Centers for Disease Control and Prevention has established recommended per capita spending amounts for tobacco control programs, and in 2004 only four states (Arkansas, Delaware, Maine, and Mississippi) were investing this minimum amount. DC—District of Columbia; GU—Guam; PR—Puerto Rico; USVI—United States Virgin Islands. (*Adapted from* Centers for Disease Control and Prevention [7].)

9.5–22%   DC, PR, USVI
22.1–23.9%   GU
24–32.6%

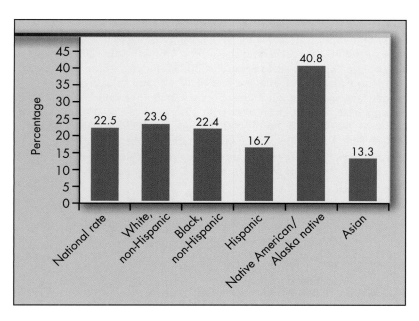

Figure 6-6.
Prevalence of cigarette smoking: national and by race, United States, 2002. Among racial/ethnic groups, there are substantial differences in tobacco use, with Asians smoking at the lowest rate and Native Americans smoking at nearly twice the national rate. National health objectives (Healthy People 2010) include reducing disparities in population subgroups. Closing these gaps will require comprehensive, sustained tobacco-control programs targeted to populations at risk. (*Adapted from* Centers for Disease Control and Prevention [4].)

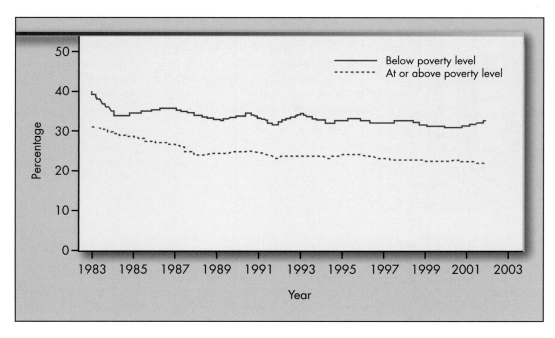

Figure 6-7.
Current cigarette smoking trends among adults 18 years of age and older by poverty level: 1983 to 2002. Income level is highly correlated with smoking. Although overall smoking rates have declined over the past 20 years, declines among those below the poverty level have plateaued and differences based on income may be increasing. Low-income smokers often lack health insurance to pay for cessation aids, and those in low-wage jobs frequently lack social support to quit. Several national programs are targeted at low-income populations, including telephone quit lines and media campaigns. (*Adapted from* Centers for Disease Control and Prevention [4].)

Atlas of Cardiovascular Risk Factors

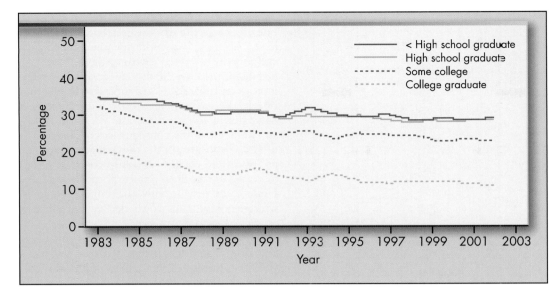

Figure 6-8.
Current cigarette smoking trends among adults 18 years of age and older by education level: 1983 to 2002. More education is correlated with a lower rate of smoking. Among college graduates, declines in smoking have been substantial and continuous. In contrast, those with a high school or less than a high school education continue to have a much higher smoking rate. National efforts to substantially reduce rates of smoking may need to be targeted toward smokers with lower levels of education. (*Adapted from* Centers for Disease Control and Prevention [4].)

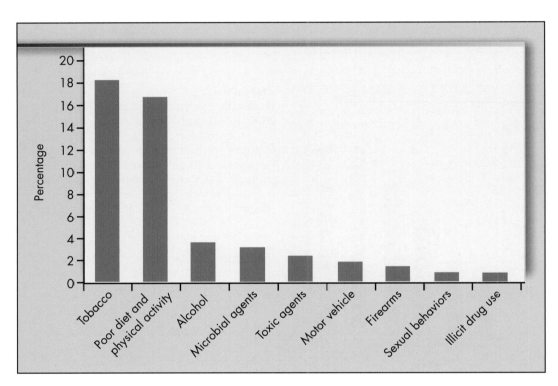

Figure 6-9.
Actual causes of death in the United States: 2000. Despite the declines in tobacco use, the leading cause of death in the United States remains tobacco use. The effects of tobacco use can be felt for years later on, and the health effects of prior smoking will lead to increased mortality rates for decades. Because it is possible to completely stop tobacco exposure, reducing this preventable cause of death would lead to significant health benefits across the entire population. (*Adapted from* Mokdad *et al.* [8].)

Smoking-attributable Mortality in the United States: 1999

Disease	Total	Predominant disease, *n*
Malignant neoplasms	154,180	With trachea, lung, bronchus neoplasm, 123,186
Cardiovascular disease	145,441	With ischemic heart disease, 88,409
Respiratory disease	105,129	With chronic obstructive pulmonary disease, 77,818

Figure 6-10.
Smoking-attributable mortality in the United States: 1999. The chronic effects of tobacco exposure lead to many diseases, including malignancies, cardiovascular disease, and respiratory disease. The Surgeon General has found a causal link between tobacco and a substantial number of diseases and concluded that smoking generally diminishes the health of all smokers. Cessation of smoking can improve many of these consequences and reduce the increased mortality rate found among smokers. (*Adapted from* Centers for Disease Control and Prevention [31].)

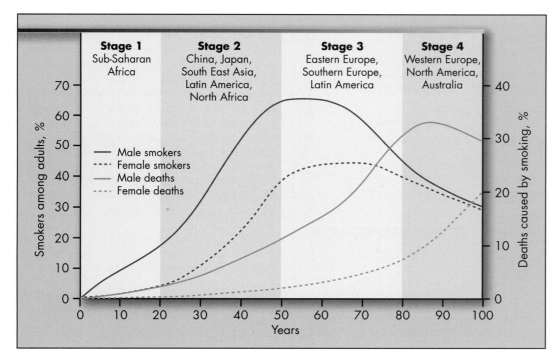

Figure 6-11.
Four stages of the worldwide tobacco epidemic. Tobacco use is a worldwide phenomenon, and four stages of the global epidemic have been described. In the first stage, smoking rates increase as tobacco-related mortality begins to rise. In the second stage, tobacco use climbs while deaths from tobacco also rise, leading to an awareness of the consequences of chronic tobacco exposure. In the third stage, tobacco use peaks and declines as deaths continue to increase (the result of prior exposure). The United States is currently in a fourth stage in which smoking rates slowly decline and tobacco-related mortality among men begins to decline while still increasing among women. Smoking-related effects tend to occur earlier and to a greater degree in men compared with women. (*Adapted from* Lopez *et al.* [13].)

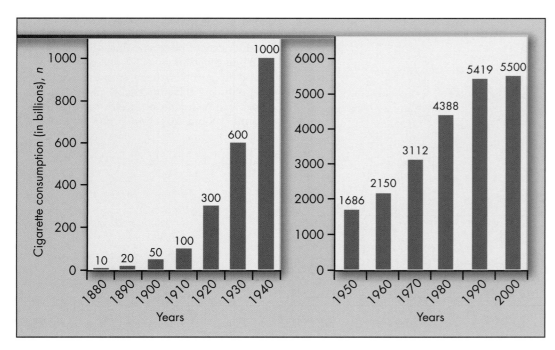

Figure 6-12.
Worldwide cigarette consumption: 1880 to 2000. Worldwide consumption of cigarettes has had exponential growth since 1880, but started to plateau by the late 20th century. International consumption patterns have changed as countries move through the four stages of the worldwide tobacco epidemic. (*Data from* the World Health Organization.)

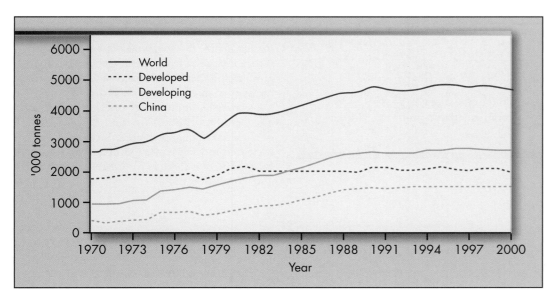

Figure 6-13.
Global cigarette consumption trends: 1970 to 2000. Global cigarette consumption increased steadily through 1990 and has since flattened. Developed nations have been steady consumers of cigarettes, while developing nations, particularly China, have been responsible for the global increases in consumption over the past 30 years. (*Data from* Food and Agriculture Organization of the United Nations, Rome, 2003.)

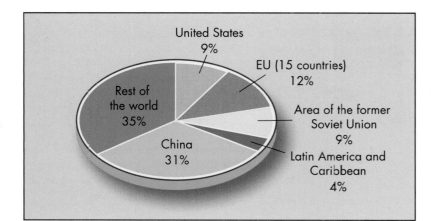

Figure 6-14.
Global cigarette consumption by world region: 1999. In 1999, the
United States consumed 9% of the world's production of cigarettes, and
the expanding market in China was consuming almost a third of all
cigarettes produced in the world. In China, over 60% of men aged 35
to 74 years smoke, whereas the reported rate among women is 7%,
indicating a gender imbalance and highlighting the urgent need for
international antismoking efforts. (*Data from* Food and Agriculture
Organization of the United Nations, Rome, 2003 and *adapted from*
Gu *et al.* [32].)

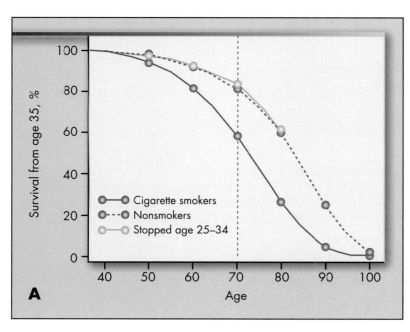

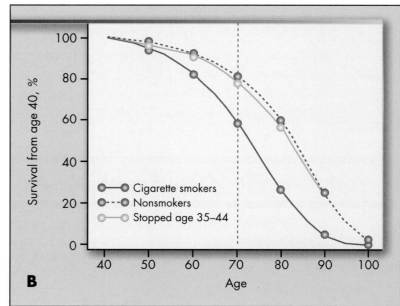

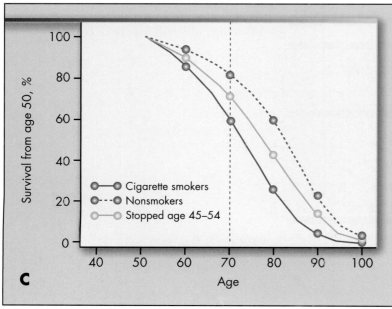

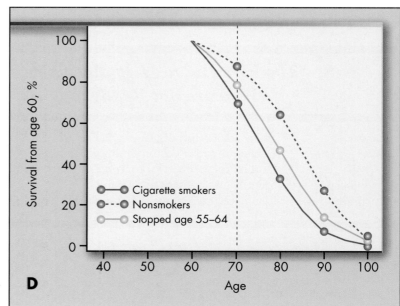

Figure 6-15.
A–D, The mortality benefit after smoking cessation at four age ranges.
These four figures show the effect on survival when current smokers in
this study stop smoking at age 25 to 34, age 35 to 44, age 45 to 54, or
age 55 to 64 years, and the mortality rate is compared with those who
never smoked. Smoking cessation has a mortality benefit at any age, and
quitting earlier has the most health benefit. **A,** Smokers who quit at age
30 have a survival curve that is similar to those who never smoked.

B, Smokers who quit at age 40 have a slightly increased mortality risk
compared with those who never smoked. **C,** Smokers who quit at age 50
have a mortality rate that is in between that of a current smoker and
those who never smoked. **D,** Smokers who quit at age 60 had a lower
mortality rate compared with those who continued to smoke. (*Adapted
from* Doll *et al.* [2].)

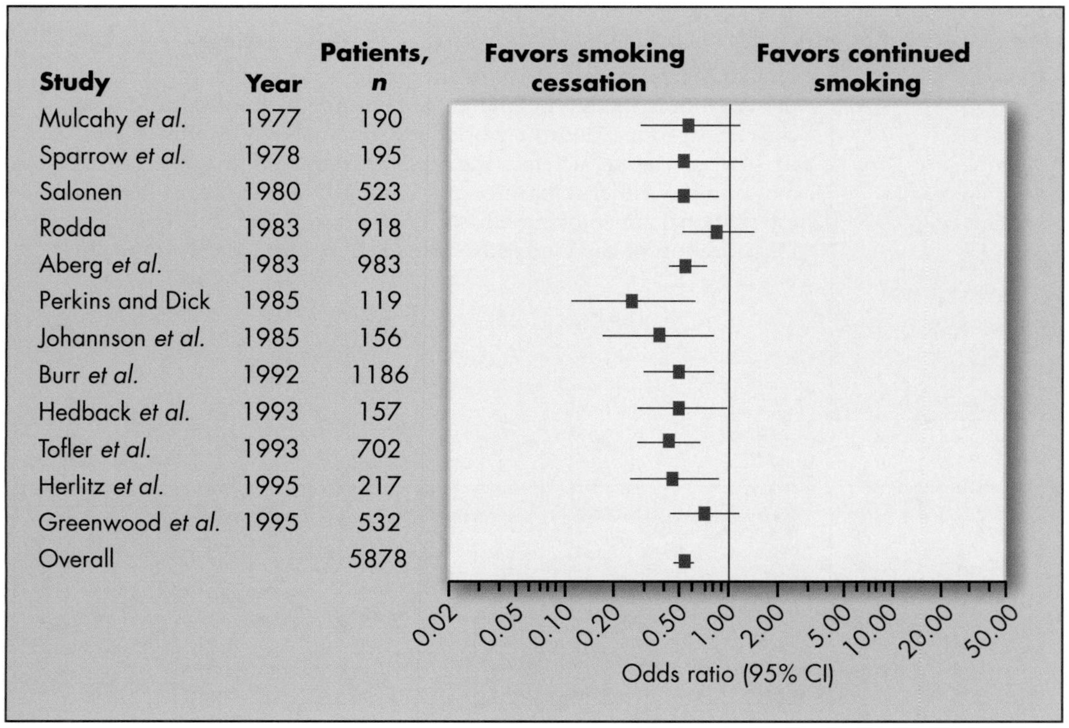

Study	Year	Patients, n	Favors smoking cessation ←	→ Favors continued smoking
Mulcahy et al.	1977	190		
Sparrow et al.	1978	195		
Salonen	1980	523		
Rodda	1983	918		
Aberg et al.	1983	983		
Perkins and Dick	1985	119		
Johannson et al.	1985	156		
Burr et al.	1992	1186		
Hedback et al.	1993	157		
Tofler et al.	1993	702		
Herlitz et al.	1995	217		
Greenwood et al.	1995	532		
Overall		5878		

Odds ratio (95% CI): 0.02 0.05 0.10 0.20 0.50 1.00 2.00 5.00 10.00 20.00 50.00

Figure 6-16.
Reduction in mortality with smoking cessation after myocardial infarction. In a meta-analysis, smoking cessation was associated with a lower mortality rate after a myocardial infarction in 12 cohorts over a mean of 4.8 years. Odds ratios ranged from 0.29 to 0.84, with a combined odds ratio of 0.54 (95% CI; 0.46–0.62), a magnitude comparable with other therapeutic interventions. A benefit to smoking cessation was observed in every group, with results consistent across study location, patient gender, year of study, and length of follow-up. (*Adapted from* Wilson *et al.* [18].)

A. "The Five As" to Assess Willingness to Quit

Ask	Identify and document tobacco use status for every patient at every visit
Advise	In a clear, strong, and personalized manner, urge every tobacco user to quit
Assess	Is the tobacco user willing to make a quit attempt this time?
Assist	For the patient willing to make a quit attempt, use counseling and pharmacotherapy
Arrange	Schedule follow-up contact, in person or by telephone, preferably < 1 week after quit date

B. "The Five Rs" to Help Motivated Patients Who are not Ready to Quit

Relevance	Tailor advice and discussion to each patient
Risks	Outline the risks of continuing to smoke
Rewards	Outline the benefits of quitting smoking
Roadblocks	Identify any barriers to quitting
Repetition	Reinforce the motivational message at every visit

Figure 6-17.
A and **B**, The five major steps to intervention: "The Five As" and "The Five Rs." The "five As" (*panel A*) are commonly used to identify those who smoke and assess willingness to quit. When a patient is ready, the health care provider can assist with counseling, pharmacotherapy, and arrange close follow-up. For patients who are not ready to quit smoking, the "five Rs" (*panel B*) can be used to reinforce the risks of smoking and highlight the benefits of cessation. If a patient can be motivated to quit, then the health care provider can assist with therapy and arrange follow-up. (*Adapted from* Fiore *et al.* [19].)

Pharmacotherapy for Smoking Cessation

First-line pharmacotherapy	Trials, *n*	Odds ratio for smoking abstinence (95% CI)
Nicotine replacement	103	1.77 (1.66–1.88)
Patch		1.81 (1.63–2.02)
Gum		1.66 (1.52–1.81)
Nasal spray		2.35 (1.63–3.38)
Inhaled nicotine		2.14 (1.44–3.18)
Sublingual tablet/lozenge		2.05 (1.62–2.59)
Bupropion	19	2.06 (1.77–2.40)
Second-line pharmacotherapy		
Nortriptyline	4	2.79 (1.70–4.59)
Clonidine	6	1.89 (1.30–2.74)

Figure 6-18.
Pharmacotherapy for smoking cessation. There have been many trials of pharmacotherapy for smoking cessation. The nicotine patch, gum, and lozenge are available over the counter. The second-line agents are not approved by the US Food and Drug Administration for smoking cessation and may have significant side effects. Combination therapy with more than one nicotine replacement therapy agent is not approved by the US Food and Drug Administration. Combining bupropion and nicotine replacement does not increase quit rates more than using only bupropion. (*Adapted from* The Cochrane Library [33].)

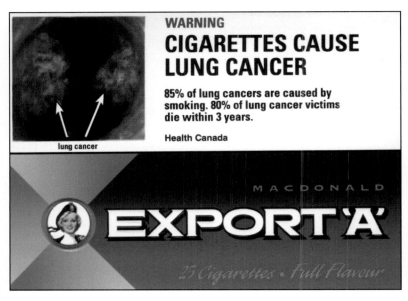

Figure 6-19.
Sample health warning. Since the year 2000, cigarettes for sale in Canada are required to have one of 16 health warnings printed on each package. Inside each pack is a five paragraph warning that provides more detailed health information. Designed to be noticeable, informative, and provide a magnitude of the risk associated with smoking, these types of warnings have been adopted by many other countries. Recent proposals for new labels will be directed to smokers with low literacy skills. The Framework Convention on Tobacco Control (FCTC), sponsored by the World Health Organization, is an international anti tobacco treaty that was signed and ratified by Canada in 2004. The United States became the 108th nation to sign the treaty in mid-2004, and as of early 2005, the treaty awaits ratification in the US Senate. (*From* Health Canada.)

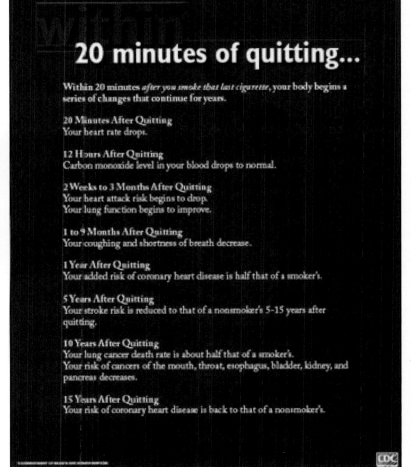

Figure 6-20.
Sample informational poster. In the United States, the Centers for Disease Control and Prevention provides resources for quitting, including informational posters that inform smokers of the benefits of quitting smoking. Within the Centers for Disease Control and Prevention is the Office on Smoking and Health, which leads strategic efforts to prevent tobacco use, encourages cessation, and attempts to eliminate health disparities by expanding research, building tobacco control programs, and working with other organizations to reduce the effects of tobacco on all Americans. (*From* Centers for Disease Control and Prevention.)

References

1. World Health Organization Tobacco Free Initiative: *Building Blocks for Tobacco Control: A Handbook.* Geneva: World Health Organization; 2004.

2. Doll R, Peto R, Boreham J, Sutherland I: Mortality in relation to smoking: 50 years' observations on male British doctors. *BMJ* 2004, 328:1519–1527.

3. Schoenborn CA, Adams PF, Barnes PM, *et al.*: Health behaviors of adults: United States 1999–2001. In *Vital Health Statistics*, vol 10. Hyattsville: National Center for Health Statistics; 2004.

4. Centers for Disease Control and Prevention: Cigarette smoking among adults: United States, 2002. *Morbid Mortal Wkly Rep* 2004, 53:427–431.

5. US Department of Health and Human Services: *Preventing Tobacco Use Among Young People: A Report of the Surgeon General.* Atlanta: Centers for Disease Control and Prevention, National Center for Chronic Disease Prevention and Health Promotion, Office on Smoking and Health; 1994.

6. Centers for Disease Control and Prevention: Cigarette use among high school students: United States, 1991–2003. *Morbid Mortal Wkly Rep* 2004, 53:499–502.

7. Centers for Disease Control and Prevention: State-specific prevalence of current cigarette smoking among adults: United States, 2002. *Morbid Mortal Wkly Rep* 2004, 52:1277–1280.

8. Mokdad AH, Marks JS, Stroup DF, Gerberding JL: Actual causes of death in the United States, 2000. *JAMA* 2004, 291:1238–1245.

9. Al-Delaimy WK, Manson JE, Solomon CG, *et al.*: Smoking and risk of coronary heart disease among women with type 2 diabetes mellitus. *Arch Intern Med* 2002, 162:273–279.

10. Biesenbach G, Zazgornik J: Influence of smoking on the survival rate of diabetic patients requiring hemodialysis. *Diabetes Care* 1996, 19:625–628.

11. Castelli WP: Cardiovascular disease: pathogenesis, epidemiology, and risk among users of oral contraceptives who smoke. *Am J Obstet Gynecol* 1999, 180:S349–S356.

12. Centers for Disease Control and Prevention: Annual smoking-attributable mortality, years of potential life lost, and economic costs: United States, 1995-1999. *Morbid Mortal Wkly Rep* 2002, 51:300–303.

13. Lopez AD, Collishaw NE, Piha T: A descriptive model of the cigarette epidemic in developed countries. *Tob Control* 1994, 3:242–247.

14. Jacobs DR, Adachi H, Mulder I, *et al.*: Cigarette smoking and mortality risk: twenty-five-year follow-up of the Seven Countries Study. *Arch Intern Med* 1999, 159:733–740.

15. Yu PB, Pasternak RC, Rigotti NA: Smoking cessation. In *Clinical Trials in Heart Disease.* Edited by Manson JE, Buring JE, Ridker PM, Gaziano JM. Philadelphia: Elsevier-Saunders; 2004:297–314.

16. Kawachi I, Colditz G, Stampfer MJ, et al.: Smoking cessation and time course of decreased risks of coronary heart disease in middle-aged women. *Arch Intern Med* 1994, 154:169–175.

17. LaCroix AZ, Lang J, Scherr P, *et al.*: Smoking and mortality among older men and women in three communities. *N Engl J Med* 1991, 324:1619–1625.

18. Wilson K, Gibson N, Willan A, Cook D: Effect of smoking cessation on mortality after myocardial infarction: meta-analysis of cohort studies. *Arch Intern Med* 2000, 160:939–944.

19. Fiore MC, Bailey WC, Cohen SJ, *et al.*: Treating Tobacco Use and Dependence: Clinical Practice Guideline. Rockville: US Department of Health and Human Services: Public Health Service; 2000.

20. Rigotti NA: Treatment of tobacco use and dependence. *N Engl J Med* 2002, 346:506–512.

21. Silagy C, Lancaster T, Stead L, *et al.*: Nicotine replacement therapy for smoking cessation. *Cochrane Database Syst Rev* 2004, 3:CD000146.

22. Hurt RD, Sachs D, Glover ED, *et al.*: A comparison of sustained-release bupropion and placebo for smoking cessation. *N Engl J Med* 1997, 337:1195–1202.

23. Hays JT, Hurt RD, Rigotti NA, *et al.*: Sustained-release bupropion for pharmacologic relapse prevention after smoking cessation: a randomized, controlled trial. *Ann Intern Med* 2001, 135:423–433.

24. US Department of Health and Human Services: *Smoking and Health: Report of the Advisory Committee to the Surgeon General of the Public Health Service.* Washington, DC: Department of Health, Education, and Welfare, Public Health Service, Center for Disease Control; 1964.

25. US Department of Health and Human Services: *The Health Consequences of Smoking: A Report of the Surgeon General.* Atlanta: US Department of Health and Human Services; 2004.

26. Fichtenberg CM, Glantz SA: Association of the California Tobacco Control Program with declines in cigarette consumption and mortality from heart disease. *N Engl J Med* 2000, 343:1772–1777.

27. Schroeder SA: Tobacco control in the wake of the 1998 Master Settlement Agreement. *N Engl J Med* 2004, 350:293–301.

28. US Department of Health and Human Services: *Healthy People 2010. With Understanding and Improving Health and Objectives for Improving Health.* Washington, DC: US Department of Health and Human Services; 2000.

29. Proctor RN: The global smoking epidemic: a history and status report. *Clin Lung Cancer* 2004, 5:371–376.

30. World Health Organization: *Framework Convention on Tobacco Control.* Geneva: World Health Organization; 2003.

31. Centers for Disease Control and Prevention: Smoking-attributable mortality, morbidity and economic costs (SAMMEC): adult SAMMEC software, 2002. Available at http://www.cdc.gov/tobacco/sammec.

32. Gu D, Wu X, Reynolds K, *et al.*: Cigarette smoking and exposure to environmental tobacco smoke in China: the international collaborative study of cardiovascular disease in Asia. *Am J Public Health* 2004, 94:1972–1976.

33. *The Cochrane Library 2004, Issue 4.* Chichester, UK: John Wiley & Sons, Ltd; 2004.

Hypertension Management

Paul K. Whelton and Jiang He

Cardiovascular disease (CVD) is the most common cause of death in economically developed countries and in the industrialized nations of eastern Europe. CVD is also a rapidly evolving cause of mortality and morbidity in almost all economically developing countries. Based on current trends, it is projected that ischemic heart disease will be the most important, and stroke the fourth most important, contributor to disability-adjusted years of life lost on a worldwide basis. A natural response to the epidemic of CVD is to ensure availability of care for patients with clinical manifestations of CVD such as coronary heart disease, congestive heart failure, stroke, and renal insufficiency. Unfortunately, two major barriers limit the effectiveness of this approach. First, CVD often manifests as sudden death, with little opportunity for a treatment intervention. Second, it is difficult to reverse the underlying pathophysiology of CVD once it has developed. To produce a meaningful reduction in morbidity and mortality, management of patients with existing CVD must be coupled with treatment and prevention of major modifiable risk factors for CVD. Currently, we have only a rudimentary knowledge of the genetic underpinning of CVD, and gene therapy for common forms of CVD is almost nonexistent. In contrast, several major, modifiable environmental risk factors for CVD are well established, and most appear to influence the risk of coronary heart disease, stroke, congestive heart failure, and renal insufficiency. High blood pressure is among the most important of these modifiable risk factors.

In this chapter, the authors present selected observations from studies that have identified the prevalence of hypertension in different populations, the risk of developing hypertension during adulthood, the risk of cardiovascular and renal complications in persons with different levels of blood pressure at baseline, and the capacity of nonpharmaclogic interventions and drug therapy to prevent and control high blood pressure.

Classification of Adults According to Average Level of Systolic and Diastolic Blood Pressure

BP classification	Systolic BP, *mm Hg*	Diastolic BP, *mm Hg*
Normal	< 120	And < 80
Prehypertension	120–139	Or 80–89
Stage 1 hypertension	140–159	Or 90–99
Stage 2 hypertension	160 or greater	Or 100 or greater

Figure 7-1.

Classification of adults according to average level of systolic and diastolic blood pressure. This table displays current criteria for classification of adults according to their average level of blood pressure [1]. Using these criteria, adults can be classified as having a normal blood pressure, prehypertension, or hypertension (stage 1 or stage 2). Classification should be based on an average of two or more blood pressure readings obtained on two or more occasions using standard measurement techniques [1]. The prevalence of hypertension in a population is dependant on the criteria chosen for classification as well as the methods used for measurement of blood pressure (including choice of instruments and training of observers) and the population studied (probability sample of the general population or selected sample). All of the prevalence estimates presented in this chapter are from studies of general populations in which blood pressure measurements were obtained by trained observers, usually using the auscultatory method of measurement. (*Adapted from* Chobanian *et al.* [1].)

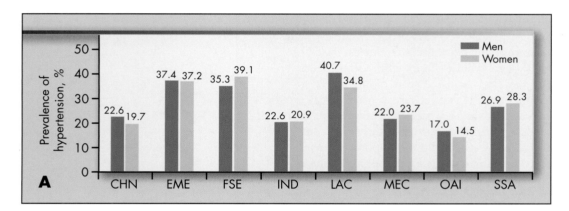

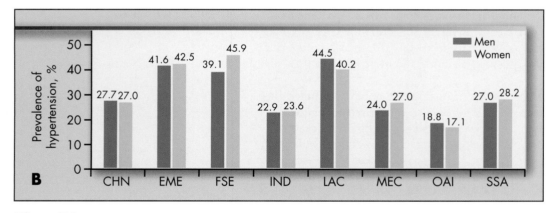

Figure 7-2.

Prevalence of hypertension in adults aged 20 years and older by world region in 2000. Hypertension is an important worldwide public health challenge because of its high prevalence and concomitant increases in risk of cardiovascular and kidney disease. Hypertension has been identified as the leading global risk factor for mortality and is ranked third as a cause of disability-adjusted life years. In a recent study, estimates of the prevalence of hypertension from different world regions were pooled [2]. World regions were defined by the World Bank as China (CHN), countries with established market economies (EME), countries of the former socialist economies of Europe (FSE), India (IND), Latin America and the Caribbean (LAC), the Middle Eastern crescent (MEC), other Asia and Islands (OAI), and sub-Saharan Africa (SSA).

Hypertension was defined as a systolic blood pressure of 140 mm Hg or greater, a diastolic blood pressure of 90 mm Hg or greater, or use of antihypertensive medication. **A,** Prevalence estimates by gender and world region for 2000. The overall worldwide pooled estimate of prevalence for adults was 26.4% (95% CI: 26.0%–26.8%), 26.6% in men (95% CI: 26.0%–27.2%), and 26.1% in women (95% CI: 25.5%–26.6%). Based on current trends, the authors projected that the worldwide prevalence of hypertension is likely to increase to 29.2% (95% CI: 28.8%–29.7%) by 2025 (**B**), 29.0% in men (95% CI: 28.6%–9.4%), and 29.5% in women (95% CI: 29.1%–29.9%).

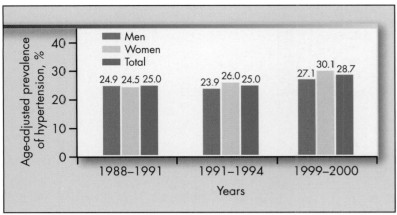

Figure 7-3.
Temporal trends in age-adjusted prevalence of hypertension in the general adult population of the United States: 1988–2000. The prevalence of hypertension in the general population of the United States has been repeatedly examined in the US National Health and Nutrition Examination Surveys (NHANES). The NHANES estimates are based on use of a stratified multistage probability sample of the civilian noninstitutionalized US population. The third NHANES was conducted in two phases between 1988 and 1994; the first phase was during 1988–1991 (n = 9901) and the second phase was during 1991–1994 (n = 9717). The most recent NHANES was conducted in 1999 and 2000 (n = 5448). In a recent analysis, experience from these three surveys was used to explore temporal trends in prevalence of hypertension among US adults [3].

In each survey, an individual's blood pressure was calculated on the basis of an average of several readings obtained by trained observers using a mercury sphygmomanometer and a standardized measurement procedure. The average was based on readings obtained during a home interview (up to three) and a visit at a mobile examination center (up to three). Hypertension was defined as a systolic blood pressure 140 mm Hg or greater, a diastolic blood pressure 90 mm Hg or greater, or use of antihypertensive medication. In 1999 to 2000, 28.7% of US adults (27.1% men and 30.1% women) aged 18 years and older had hypertension, reflecting a significant increase from the corresponding estimate of 25.0% (24.9% in men and 24.5% in women) obtained during 1988 to 1991. (*Adapted from* Hajjar and Kotchen [3].)

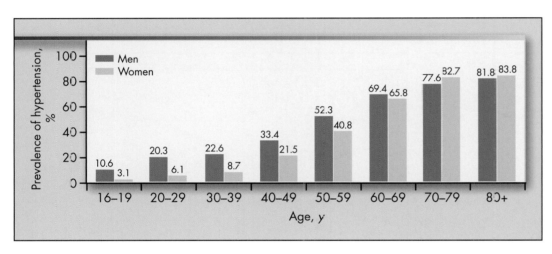

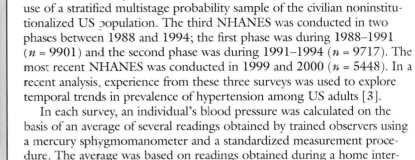

Figure 7-4.
Prevalence of hypertension by age and gender in the 1998 Health Survey for England. The 1998 Health Survey for England was a cross-sectional study conducted in a random, nationally representative sample of 11,529 noninstitutionalized adults (16 years and older) living in England [4]. Three right arm blood pressure readings were obtained using the Dinamap 8100 (GE Healthcare, Chicago, IL) automatic blood pressure recorder after a 5 minute period of rest. Hypertension has been defined as a systolic blood pressure 140 mm Hg or greater, a diastolic blood pressure 90 mm Hg or greater, or use of antihypertensive medication. The overall prevalence of hypertension was 41.5% in men and 33.3% in women. The prevalence of hypertension rose with age across the entire range and was higher in men than in women until 70+ years of age. (*Adapted from* Primatesta *et al.* [4].)

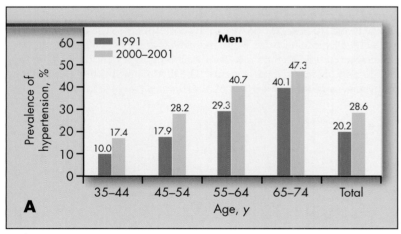

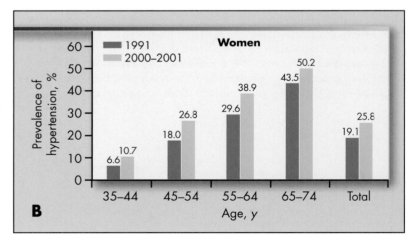

Figure 7-5.
A and **B**, Age-specific and age-adjusted prevalence of hypertension among Chinese adults aged 35 to 74 years in 1991 and 2000–2001. The prevalence of hypertension was examined in the International Collaborative Study of Cardiovascular Disease in ASIA (InterASIA), which was conducted in a nationally representative sample of 15,540 adults, aged 35 to 74 years between 2000 and 2001 [5]. Three blood pressure measurements were obtained in the seated position by a trained observer using a standard mercury sphygmomanometer after a 5-minute period of rest. Information on history of hypertension and use of antihypertensive medication was obtained by means of a standard questionnaire. Hypertension has been defined as a systolic blood pressure of 140 mm Hg or greater, a diastolic blood pressure of 90 mm Hg or greater, or use of antihypertensive medication. Overall, 27.2% of the adult Chinese population aged 35 to 74 years had hypertension, representing a total of 129,824,000 persons [6]. Compared with national estimates obtained in 1991 [7], the prevalence of hypertension in 2000 to 2001 was 42% higher in men (20.2%–28.6%) and 35% higher in women (19.1%–25.8%). (*Adapted from* He *et al.* [5] and Gu *et al.* [6].)

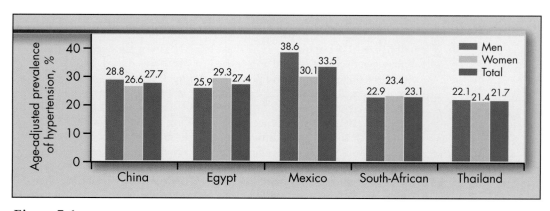

Figure 7-6.

Age-adjusted prevalence of hypertension in five economically developing countries. The prevalence of hypertension has been examined recently in five economically developing countries [8]. In each country, the prevalence estimate was based on findings in a national probability survey, which used a large sample size (China, *n* = 15,854; Egypt, *n* = 6733; Mexico, *n* = 14,657; South African, *n* = 13,802; and Thailand, *n* = 5350) and standard methods for blood pressure measurement.

Hypertension was defined as a systolic blood pressure 140 mm Hg or greater, a diastolic blood pressure 90 mm Hg or greater, or use of anti-hypertensive medication. When the estimates were standardized to the 1990 world population, age-adjusted prevalence of hypertension varied from 22.1% and 21.4% in Thailand to 38.6% and 30.1% in Mexico, for men and women, respectively. The prevalence of hypertension was as high in these economic developing countries as it is in more economically developed nations. (*Adapted from* Kearney *et al.* [8].)

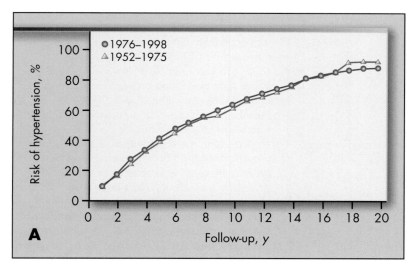
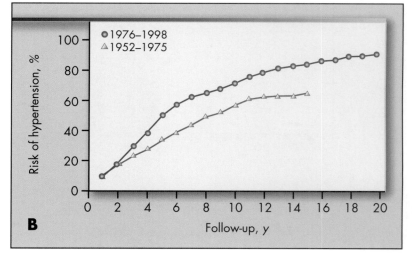

Figure 7-7.

A and **B**, Residual lifetime risk of hypertension in women and men aged 65 years in the Framingham Heart Study. Lifetime risk for development of hypertension was estimated among 1298 Framingham Heart Study participants who were aged 55 to 65 years and free of hypertension at a baseline examination between 1976 and 1998 [9]. For those who were 55 years old at entry, the cumulative risk for developing hypertension was calculated through age 80 years, and for those who were 65 years old at

entry, the cumulative risk for developing hypertension was calculated through age 85 years. These follow-up time intervals (25 years for 55-year-olds and 20 years for 65-year-olds) correspond to the current mean residual life expectancies for white individuals at these two ages in the United States. The lifetime risks for developing hypertension were 90% in the 55- and 65-year-old participants. The lifetime probability of receiving antihypertensive medication was 60%. (*Adapted from* Vasan *et al.* [9].)

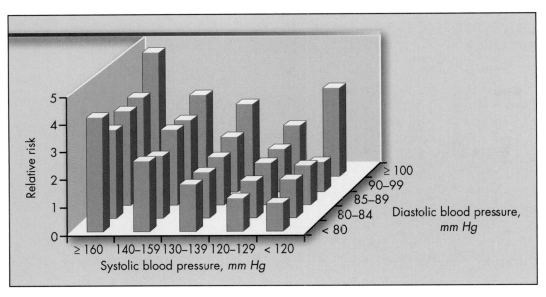

Figure 7-8.

Multivariate-adjusted relative risks of coronary heart disease death according to baseline systolic and diastolic blood pressure in men screened for the Multiple Risk Factor Intervention Trial (MRFIT). Results from prospective cohort studies indicate that elevated blood pressure levels are associated with an increased risk of coronary heart disease. This increased risk is continuous throughout a wide range of blood pressure, even in "normal" level, and is independent of other established cardiovascular risk factors.

Furthermore, the association of systolic blood pressure with cardiovascular disease is stronger than that of diastolic blood pressure. The MRFIT screened patient cohort consists of 347,978 men, 35 to 57 years of age, who were screened for possible entry into the MRFIT between 1973 and 1975 and did not report a previous hospitalization for coronary heart disease or stroke. Given the large sample size of the MRFIT screened patient cohort, it was possible to evaluate the relationship of systolic and diastolic blood pressure to coronary heart disease and stroke while concurrently stratifying for level of blood pressure. This experience is depicted in the figure. Compared with men with a systolic/diastolic blood pressure of less than 120/80 mm Hg, all other strata were at a greater risk of subsequent coronary heart disease [10]. Furthermore, a higher systolic blood pressure was related to a higher risk of coronary heart disease in a continuous and graded fashion at almost every level of diastolic blood pressure. Although the risk of coronary heart disease also tended to increase with progressively higher levels of diastolic blood pressure at every level of systolic blood pressure, the increase was not as steep or as consistent as that for systolic blood pressure. (*Adapted from* Stamler *et al.* [10].)

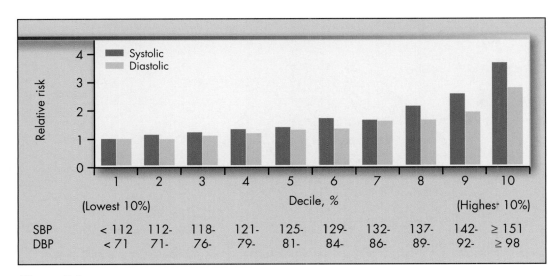

Figure 7-9.

Multivariate-adjusted relative risks of coronary heart disease death according to deciles of baseline systolic (SBP) and diastolic blood pressure (DBP) in men screened for the Multiple Risk Factor Intervention Trial (MRFIT). To compare the relative risks of coronary heart disease associated with corresponding levels of systolic and diastolic blood pressure, the range of systolic and diastolic blood pressure in MRFIT screened patient cohort members was divided into deciles [10]. As shown in the figure, the risk of coronary heart disease was higher for systolic compared with diastolic blood pressure at each corresponding decile of blood pressure. For example, in a comparison of the highest versus the lowest decile of blood pressure, the relative risks associated with systolic and diastolic blood pressure were 3.7 and 2.8, respectively. (*Adapted from* Stamler *et al.* [10].)

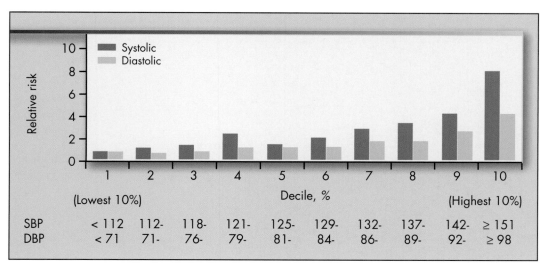

Figure 7-10.
Multivariate-adjusted relative risks of stroke death according to deciles of baseline systolic (SBP) and diastolic blood pressure (DBP) in men screened for the Multiple Risk Factor Intervention Trial (MRFIT). Prospective cohort studies have documented that progressively higher levels of systolic or diastolic blood pressure are strongly, continuously, and independently associated with an increasing risk of stroke. The association between systolic blood pressure and risk of stroke is stronger than that for corresponding differences in diastolic blood pressure. To compare the relative risk of stroke for corresponding levels of systolic and diastolic blood pressure, baseline blood pressure levels in the MRFIT- screened patient cohort were divided into deciles. At every decile, systolic blood pressure was more strongly related to risk of stroke than was the case for the corresponding level of diastolic blood pressure [10]. For example, in a comparison of the highest versus the lowest decile of blood pressure, the relative risks of stroke associated with systolic and diastolic blood pressure were 8.2 and 4.4, respectively. (*Adapted from* Stamler *et al.* [10].)

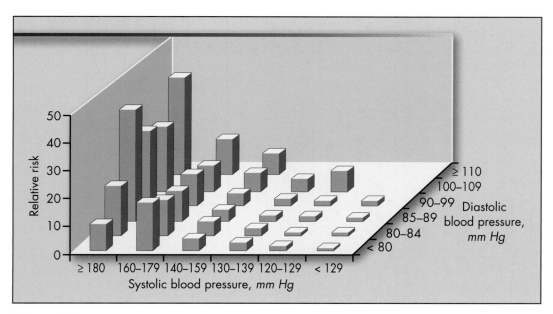

Figure 7-11.
Age-adjusted relative risks of end-stage renal disease according to baseline levels of systolic and diastolic blood pressure in men screened for the Multiple Risk Factor Intervention Trial (MRFIT). Prospective cohort studies have documented a strong, graded, and independent relationship between systolic and diastolic blood pressure and risk of end-stage renal disease. The effect of systolic and diastolic blood pressure on the age-adjusted relative risk of end-stage renal disease was examined in the MRFIT screened patient cohort [11]. The difference in relative risks of end-stage renal disease associated with variations in systolic blood pressure within each stratum of diastolic blood pressure was far greater than that for the corresponding variations in diastolic blood pressure within each stratum of systolic blood pressure. For example, among the men in whom the diagnosis of stage 1 hypertension was based on a systolic blood pressure between 140 and 159 mm Hg, the relative risks for the four lower categories of diastolic blood pressure were similar. In contrast, for the men in whom the diagnosis of stage 1 hypertension was based on a diastolic blood pressure between 90 and 99 mm Hg, the relative risks of end-stage renal disease for increasing levels of systolic blood pressure rose sharply from 1.8 to 27.1. Indeed, the increase in risk was present even across the three categories of systolic blood pressure within the normotensive range. (*Adapted from* Klag *et al.* [11].)

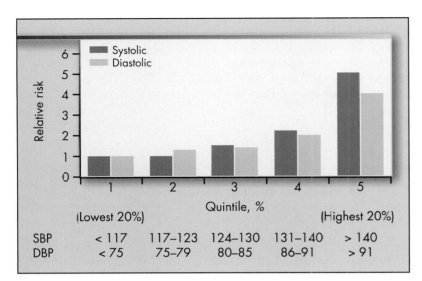

	Quintile, %				
	(Lowest 20%)				(Highest 20%)
SBP	< 117	117–123	124–130	131–140	> 140
DBP	< 75	75–79	80–85	86–91	> 91

Figure 7-12.

Multivariate-adjusted relative risks of end-stage renal disease according to quintiles of baseline systolic (SBP) and diastolic blood pressure (DBP) in men screened for the Multiple Risk Factor Intervention Trial. A comparison of the relative risk of end-stage renal disease by quintile of systolic and diastolic blood pressure in the Multiple Risk Factor Intervention Trial screened patient cohort demonstrated that systolic blood pressure was a quantitatively more important predictor of subsequent end-stage renal disease than diastolic blood pressure [11]. For example, the relative risk (95% CI) in the highest compared with the lowest quintile was 5.0 (3.7– 6.7) for systolic and 4.0 (3.0–5.2) for diastolic blood pressure, respectively. (*Adapted from* Klag *et al.* [11].)

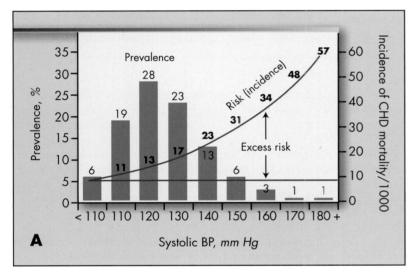

Figure 7-13.

A and **B**, Excess risk of blood pressure (BP)-related coronary heart disease (CHD) during an average follow-up of 11.6 years in 347,978 adults who were screened for participation in the Multiple Risk Factor Intervention Trial (MRFIT). As shown in *panel A*, there was a progressive increase in absolute and excess risk of CHD with increasing level of systolic BP at baseline [10]. The minority of the population with the most elevated levels of BP was exposed to the highest risk of CHD, but an increased risk of CHD was observed even in the large number with a baseline BP that would be classified as normotensive. Population excess risk can be estimated by summing the excess risk of CHD at each level of BP. *Panel B* presents the estimated distribution of BP-related CHD by baseline level of systolic BP. The approximately 5% of the population with a baseline BP in excess of 160 mm Hg account for almost a quarter (24%) of all BP-related CHD. The 24% with a baseline systolic BP in excess of 140 mm Hg account for approximately two thirds (67%) of all BP-related CHD. Almost one third (32%) of all BP-related CHD is the result of excess risk in the residual 76% of the population with a "normal" level of BP at baseline. These epidemiologic results underscore the potential for disproportional benefit after successful treatment of hypertension in those with the highest levels of BP. However, they also underscore the importance of treating the much larger number of individuals in the population with a less severe elevation of BP to achieve a meaningful reduction in the population burden of BP-related CHD. These data also underscore the value of preventing hypertension and its associated high risk of BP-related CHD. (*Adapted from* Stamler *et al.* [10].)

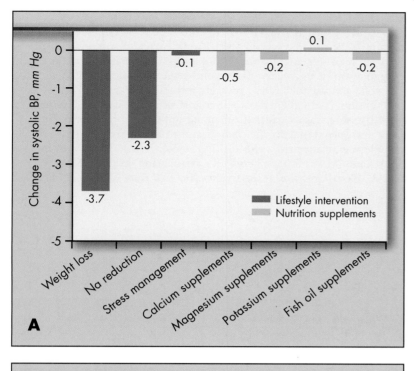

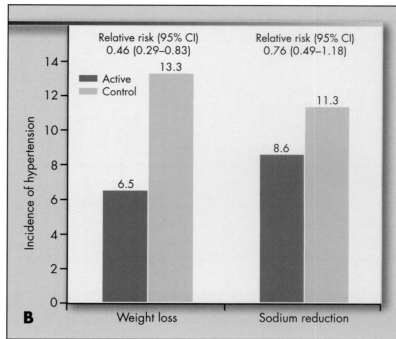

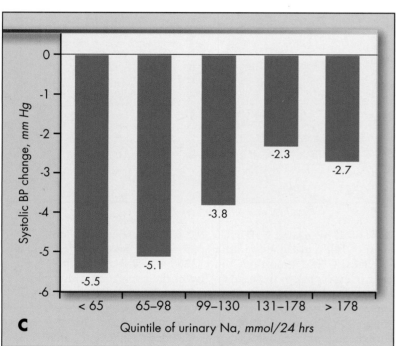

Figure 7-14.

Efficacy of three lifestyle change and four nutrition supplement interventions used to prevent hypertension in middle-aged adults with high-normal blood pressure (BP). The Trials of Hypertension Prevention (TOHP) has been by far the largest and most prolonged randomized controlled trial to evaluate the efficacy of interventions aimed at prevention of hypertension. TOHP was conducted in two phases. In the first phase, behavioral interventions aimed at encouraging weight loss and sodium reduction proved to be the two most promising interventions. Weight loss and sodium reduction resulted in significant net decreases in average systolic BP of 3.7 and 2.3 mm Hg, respectively, at 6 months (**A**) [12]. The corresponding average reduction in incidence of new-onset hypertension during 18 months of follow-up was 54% for the weight loss group (**B**) [13]. The capacity of sodium reduction to prevent hypertension also seemed promising but did not reach significance in this exploratory phase. There was a dose-response relationship between BP reduction and level of urinary sodium and body weight (pattern for sodium reduction [**C**]) [14]. In a second phase, conducted in 2382 adults over 2 years, weight loss and sodium reduction reduced the incidence of hypertension by approximately 20% [15]. (*Panel A adapted from* TOHP Collaborative research group [12]; *panel B adapted from* Whelton *et al.* [13]; *panel C adapted from* Kumanyika *et al.* [14].)

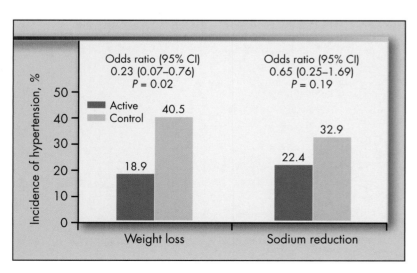

Figure 7-15.

Long-term effectiveness of behavioral interventions aimed at prevention of hypertension. The long-term impact of behavioral interventions aimed at prevention of hypertension was explored in a 7-year follow-up of 181 adults who had participated in phase I of the Trials of Hypertension Prevention. A total of 53 participants who had been assigned to counseling in weight loss and 58 participants who had been assigned to counseling in sodium reduction were included in the study group. After 7 years of follow-up, the incidence of hypertension was 77% lower in the 53 individuals who had been counseled in weight loss compared with 42 counterparts who had been in the usual care group [16]. There was a corresponding trend toward a reduction in incidence of hypertension in the 58 participants who had been assigned to counseling in sodium reduction compared with 70 counterparts who had been in the usual care group, but, in this small study, it did not reach statistical significance. (*Adapted from* He *et al.* [16].)

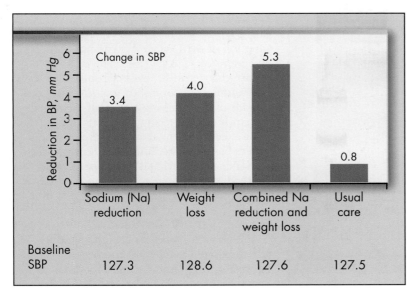

Figure 7-16.

Efficacy of nonpharmacologic intervention in patients being treated with antihypertensive medication. The Trial of Nonpharmacologic Intervention in the Elderly was the largest randomized controlled trial to have assessed the efficacy of weight loss and sodium reduction in reducing blood pressure (BP) among patients already receiving antihypertensive drug therapy. Despite an average starting level of systolic blood pressure (SBP) of approximately 128 mm Hg, both interventions resulted in a significant reduction in BP. The average reduction for those who were assigned to counseling in weight loss and sodium reduction was 5.3 mm Hg compared with 0.8 mm Hg for their counterparts assigned to usual care [17]. (*Adapted from* Whelton *et al.* [17].)

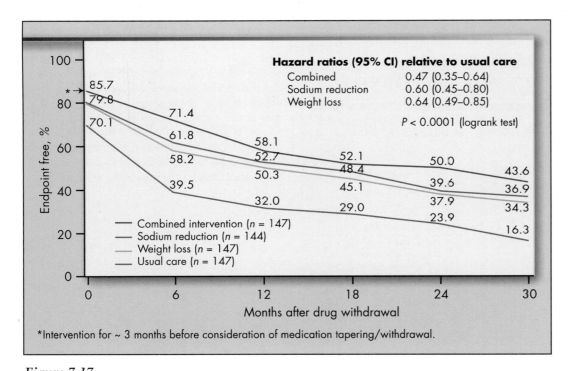

Figure 7-17.

Efficacy of nonpharmacologic interventions in patients being treated with antihypertensive medication. The Trial of Nonpharmacologic Intervention in the Elderly (TONE) explored the capacity for withdrawal of antihypertensive medication in persons assigned to a lifestyle intervention aimed at weight loss, sodium reduction, or a combination of weight loss and sodium reduction. Medication withdrawal was attempted after approximately 90 days on nonpharmacologic intervention provided the participant's blood pressure was controlled and his/her primary care physician agreed [17]. Participants were observed carefully for evidence of the primary endpoint (recurrent hypertension) over 30 months of follow-up. Recurrent hypertension requiring antihypertensive medication was reported in almost all of the usual care participants. In contrast, many of those assigned to an active intervention—especially the combined intervention—continued to achieve good blood pressure control without the need for antihypertensive medication. These results underscore the effectiveness of weight loss and sodium reduction in reducing the need for antihypertensive medication but indicate the importance of prolonged careful monitoring in those who are initially successful. (*Adapted from* Whelton *et al.* [17].)

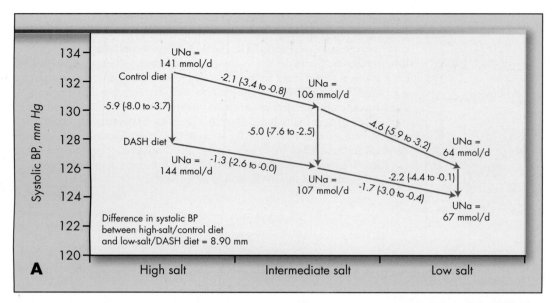

A

Figure 7-18.

A and **B**, Blood pressure (BP) lowering after adoption of the Dietary Approaches to Stop Hypertension (DASH) diet. The effect of dietary change on BP has been studied in several randomized controlled trials in which participants were given most or all of their foods at a study center (feeding studies). Among the most effective of the diets tested in feeding studies has been the DASH diet [18]. In the DASH-Sodium trial, 412 participants were assigned to be fed for approximately 30 days with a control (standard American) diet or a DASH diet (high in fruit and vegetable content and in low-fat dairy products) [19].

Within each treatment arm, participants were randomly assigned to three levels of sodium intake (high, intermediate, and low). At each level of sodium intake, the DASH diet resulted in a significantly lower level of BP compared with the control group. Likewise, for both assigned groups BP was progressively lower with decreasing intake of sodium. The best (lowest) BP was attained in those assigned to the DASH diet at the lowest level of sodium intake and the worst (highest) BP was experienced by those assigned to the control diet at the highest level of sodium intake. Given its well-proven efficacy, there was no attempt to test the effect of a concurrent change in body weight in this trial. (*Adapted from* Appel *et al.* [18] and Sacks *et al.* [19].)

B. Effects of Three Levels of Sodium Intake on Control and Combination Diet (Dietary Approaches to Stop Hypertension [DASH])

Nutrition goal	Control diet	DASH diet
Fat, *% kcal*	37	27
Saturated fat, *% kcal*	16	6
Cholesterol, *mg*	300	150
Protein, *% kcal*	15	18
Fiber, *g/d*	9	31
Potassium, *mg/d*	1700	4700
Magnesium, *mg/d*	165	500
Calcium *mg/d*	450	1240

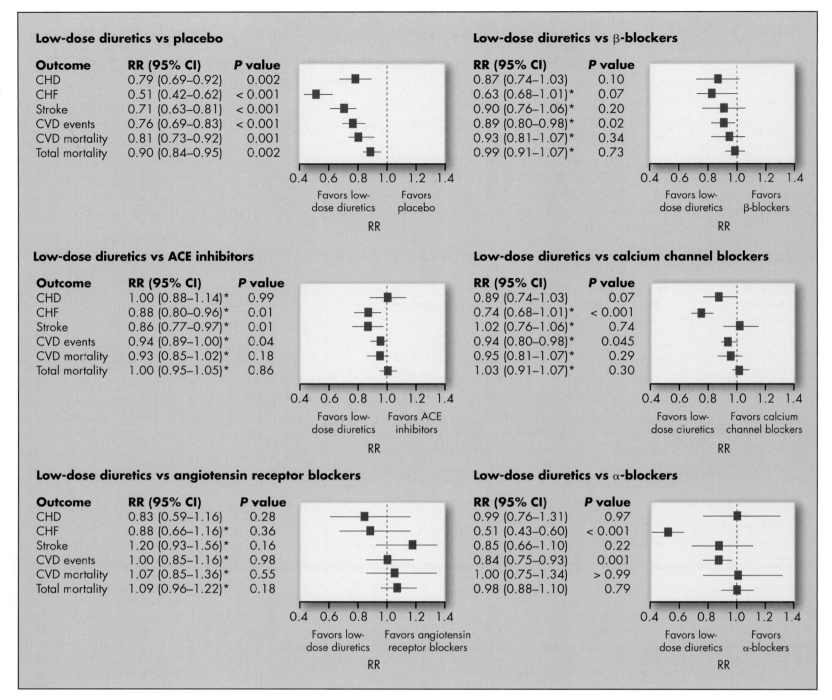

Low-dose diuretics vs placebo

Outcome	RR (95% CI)	P value
CHD	0.79 (0.69–0.92)	0.002
CHF	0.51 (0.42–0.62)	< 0.001
Stroke	0.71 (0.63–0.81)	< 0.001
CVD events	0.76 (0.69–0.83)	< 0.001
CVD mortality	0.81 (0.73–0.92)	0.001
Total mortality	0.90 (0.84–0.95)	0.002

Favors low-dose diuretics / Favors placebo
RR

Low-dose diuretics vs β-blockers

RR (95% CI)	P value
0.87 (0.74–1.03)	0.10
0.63 (0.68–1.01)*	0.07
0.90 (0.76–1.06)*	0.20
0.89 (0.80–0.98)*	0.02
0.93 (0.81–1.07)*	0.34
0.99 (0.91–1.07)*	0.73

Favors low-dose diuretics / Favors β-blockers
RR

Low-dose diuretics vs ACE inhibitors

Outcome	RR (95% CI)	P value
CHD	1.00 (0.88–1.14)*	0.99
CHF	0.88 (0.80–0.96)*	0.01
Stroke	0.86 (0.77–0.97)*	0.01
CVD events	0.94 (0.89–1.00)*	0.04
CVD mortality	0.93 (0.85–1.02)*	0.18
Total mortality	1.00 (0.95–1.05)*	0.86

Favors low-dose diuretics / Favors ACE inhibitors
RR

Low-dose diuretics vs calcium channel blockers

RR (95% CI)	P value
0.89 (0.74–1.03)	0.07
0.74 (0.68–1.01)*	< 0.001
1.02 (0.76–1.06)*	0.74
0.94 (0.80–0.98)*	0.045
0.95 (0.81–1.07)*	0.29
1.03 (0.91–1.07)*	0.30

Favors low-dose diuretics / Favors calcium channel blockers
RR

Low-dose diuretics vs angiotensin receptor blockers

Outcome	RR (95% CI)	P value
CHD	0.83 (0.59–1.16)	0.28
CHF	0.88 (0.66–1.16)*	0.36
Stroke	1.20 (0.93–1.56)*	0.16
CVD events	1.00 (0.85–1.16)*	0.98
CVD mortality	1.07 (0.85–1.36)*	0.55
Total mortality	1.09 (0.96–1.22)*	0.18

Favors low-dose diuretics / Favors angiotensin receptor blockers
RR

Low-dose diuretics vs α-blockers

RR (95% CI)	P value
0.99 (0.76–1.31)	0.97
0.51 (0.43–0.60)	< 0.001
0.85 (0.66–1.10)	0.22
0.84 (0.75–0.93)	0.001
1.00 (0.75–1.34)	> 0.99
0.98 (0.88–1.10)	0.79

Favors low-dose diuretics / Favors α-blockers
RR

Figure 7-19.

Comparison of cardiovascular disease (CVD) and total mortality during first-line treatment with various classes of antihypertensive drug therapy. The relative benefit of treatment with different classes of antihypertensive drug therapy has been tested in a series of randomized controlled trials, beginning with a landmark study conducted by the Veterans Administration Cooperative Study Group on Antihypertensive Agents. Pooling of the experience in different trials provides the most precise estimates of relative benefit and risk. This figure displays the pooled

relative risks (RR) and corresponding 95% CI for seven classes of antihypertensive drug therapy studied in a network meta-analysis of 42 clinical trials that included 192,478 study participants [20]. In this analysis, low-dose diuretics appeared to be the most effective therapy for prevention of cardiovascular disease and total mortality. ACE—angiotensin-converting enzyme; CHD—coronary heart disease; CHF—congestive heart failure. (*Adapted from* Psaty *et al.* [20].)

Effects of Different Blood Pressure–Lowering Regimens on Major Cardiovascular Disease

| Outcomes | Trials, n | Events/participants | | Difference in blood pressure, *mean mm Hg* | Relative risk (95% CI) | P Value |
		First listed	Second listed			
Stroke						
ACEI vs placebo	5	473/9111	660/9118	-5/-2	0.72 (0.64–0.81)	0.33
CCB vs placebo	4	76/3794	119/3688	-8/-4	0.62 (0.47–0.82)	0.90
More vs less	4	140/7494	261/13,394	-4/-3	0.77 (0.63–0.95)	0.15
Coronary heart disease						
ACEI vs placebo	5	667/9111	834/9118	-5/-2	0.80 (0.73–0.88)	0.91
CCB vs placebo	4	125/3794	156/3688	-8/-4	0.78 (0.62–0.99)	0.34
More vs less	4	274/7494	348/13,394	-4/-3	0.95 (0.81–1.11)	0.26
Heart failure						
ACEI vs placebo	5	219/8233	269/8246	-5/-2	0.82 (0.69–0.98)	0.60
CCB vs placebo	3	104/3382	88/3274	-8/-4	1.21 (0.93–1.58)	0.17
More vs less	4	54/7494	72/13,394	-4/-3	0.84 (0.59–1.18)	0.11
Major cardiovascular events						
ACEI vs placebo	5	1283/9111	1648/9118	-5/-2	0.78 (0.73–0.83)	0.42
CCB vs placebo	3	280/3382	337/3274	-8/-4	0.82 (0.71–0.95)	0.54
More vs less	4	482/8034	719/13,948	-4/-3	0.85 (0.76–0.95)	0.27
Cardiovascular death						
ACEI vs placebo	5	488/9111	614/9118	-5/-2	0.80 (0.71–0.89)	0.29
CCB vs placebo	4	107/3382	135/3274	-8/-4	0.78 (0.61–1.00)	0.43
More vs less	5	209/8034	271/13,948	-4/-3	0.93 (0.77–1.11)	0.15
Total mortality						
ACEI vs placebo	5	839/9111	951/9118	-5/-2	0.88 (0.81–0.96)	0.54
CCB vs placebo	4	239/3794	263/3688	-8/-4	0.89 (0.75–1.05)	0.99
More vs less	5	404/8034	549/13,948	-4/-3	0.96 (0.84–1.09)	0.09

Figure 7-20.

Effects of different blood pressure–lowering regimens on major cardiovascular disease outcomes. Experience from a prospectively designed overview of randomized controlled trials. The relative benefit of lowering blood pressure with newer classes of antihypertensive drug therapy compared with placebo and more versus less intense treatment has been tested in a prospectively designed overview of experience from randomized controlled trials [21]. This figure displays results from pooling of five trials that compared treatment with an angiotensin-converting enzyme inhibitor (ACEI) or placebo (n = 18,229), four trials that compared treatment with a calcium channel blocker (CCB) or placebo (n = 7482), and four trials that compared more versus less intensive reduction in blood pressure (n = 21,982). Compared with placebo, ACEI and CCB reduced the risk of cardiovascular disease and total mortality. Likewise, the risk was lower with more versus less intensive reduction in blood pressure. (*Adapted from* Blood Pressure Lowering Treatment Trialists Collaboration [21].)

Effects of Different Blood Pressure–lowering Regimens on Major Cardiovascular Disease

Outcomes	Trials, n	Events/participants		Difference in blood pressure, *mean mm Hg*	Relative risk (95% CI)	P Value
		First listed	Second listed			
Stroke						
ACEI vs D/BB	5	984/20,195	1178/26,358	+2/0	1.09 (1.00–1.18)	0.13
CCB vs D/BB	9	999/31,031	1358/37,418	+1/0	0.93 (0.86–1.00)	0.67
ACEI vs CCB	5	701/12,562	622/12,541	+1/+1	1.12 (1.01–1.25)	0.20
Coronary heart disease						
ACEI vs D/BB	5	1172/20,195	1658/26,358	+2/0	0.98 (0.91–1.05)	0.21
CCB vs D/BB	9	1394/31,031	1840/37,418	+1/0	1.01 (0.94–1.08)	0.48
ACEI vs CCB	5	907/12,562	948/12,541	+1/+1	0.96 (0.88–1.04)	0.01
Heart failure						
ACEI vs D/BB	3	547/12,498	809/18,652	+2/0	1.07 (0.96–1.19)	0.43
CCB vs D/BB	7	732/23,425	850/29,734	+1/0	1.33 (1.21–1.47)	0.92
ACEI vs CCB	4	502/10,357	609/10,345	+1/+1	0.82 (0.73–0.92)	0.75
Major cardiovascular events						
ACEI vs D/BB	6	2581/20,631	3450/26,799	+2/0	1.02 (0.98–1.07)	0.31
CCB vs D/BB	9	2998/31,031	3839/37,418	+1/0	1.04 (1.00–1.09)	0.92
ACEI vs CCB	5	1953/12,562	2011/12,541	+1/+1	0.97 (0.92–1.03)	0.22
Cardiovascular death						
ACEI vs D/BB	6	1061/20,631	1440/26,799	+2/0	1.03 (0.95–1.11)	0.36
CCB vs D/BB	9	1237/31,031	1584/37,418	+1/0	1.05 (0.97–1.13)	0.33
ACEI vs CCB	5	870/12,562	840/12,541	+1/+1	1.03 (0.94–1.13)	0.56
Total mortality						
ACEI vs D/BB	6	2176/20,631	3067/26,799	+2/0	1.00 (0.95–1.05)	0.76
CCB vs D/BB	9	2527/31,031	3437/37,418	+1/0	0.99 (0.95–1.04)	0.71
ACEI vs CCB	6	1763/12,998	1683/12,758	+1/+1	1.04 (0.98–1.10)	0.68

Figure 7-21.

Effects of different blood pressure–lowering regimens on major cardiovascular disease outcomes. Experience from a prospectively designed overview of randomized controlled trials. The relative benefit of lowering blood pressure with newer classes of antihypertensive drug therapy such as angiotensin-converting enzyme inhibitors (ACEI) or calcium channel blockers (CCB) compared with the traditional "gold standard" of therapy (diuretics or β-blockers [D/BB]) has been tested in a prospectively designed overview of experience from randomized controlled trials [21]. This figure displays results from pooling of six trials that compared treatment with an ACEI versus traditional therapy (*n* = 47,430), nine trials that compared treatment with a CCB versus traditional therapy (*n* = 68,449), and six trials that compared ACEI versus CCB (*n* = 25,756). There were no significant differences between the treatment approaches for all major cardiovascular disease events, cardiovascular death, or total mortality. There were, however, differences in cause-specific outcomes, especially heart failure (restricted to heart failure resulting in death or hospitalization). (*Adapted from* Blood Pressure Lowering Treatment Trialist's Collaboration [21].)

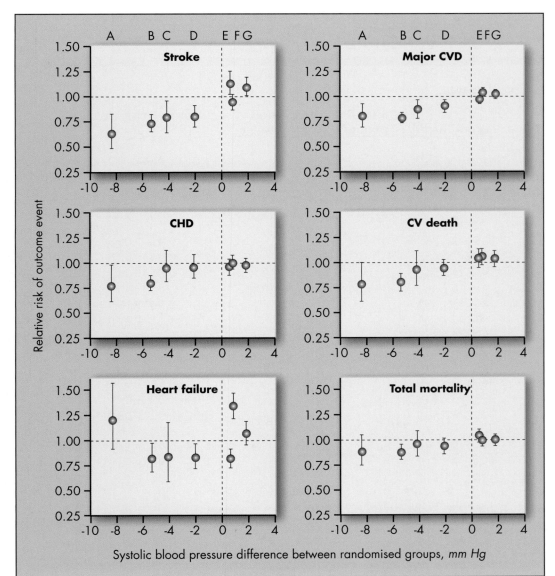

Figure 7-22.
Association between difference in blood pressure between treatment regimens and risk of major cardiovascular disease (CVD) outcomes and total mortality. Experience from a prospectively designed overview of randomized controlled trials. The association between differences in blood pressure for seven treatment comparisons and risk of major CVD complications and total mortality has been tested in a prospectively designed overview of experience from 29 randomized controlled trials (n = 162,341 participants). This figure displays the relative risk and corresponding 95% CI for the association between differences in blood pressure during treatment with seven contrasting regimens and five CVD outcomes and total mortality [21]. From left to right, the treatment comparisons were calcium channel blocker (CCB) versus placebo (*A*), angiotensin-converting enzyme inhibitor (ACEI) versus placebo (*B*), more intensive versus less intensive reduction in blood pressure (*C*), angiotensin receptor blocker versus control (*D*), ACEI versus CCB (*E*), CCB versus diuretic or β-blocker (*F*), and ACEI versus diuretic or β-blocker (*G*). For all seven comparisons, the weighted mean differences among the treatment groups were directly associated with corresponding differences in risks of stroke, coronary heart disease (CHD), major cardiovascular (CV) events, CV death, and total mortality. In contrast, blood pressure differences were not associated with risk of heart failure, suggesting that this effect may be mediated through a drug-specific effect. (*Adapted from* Blood Pressure Lowering Treatment Trialist's Collaboration [21].)

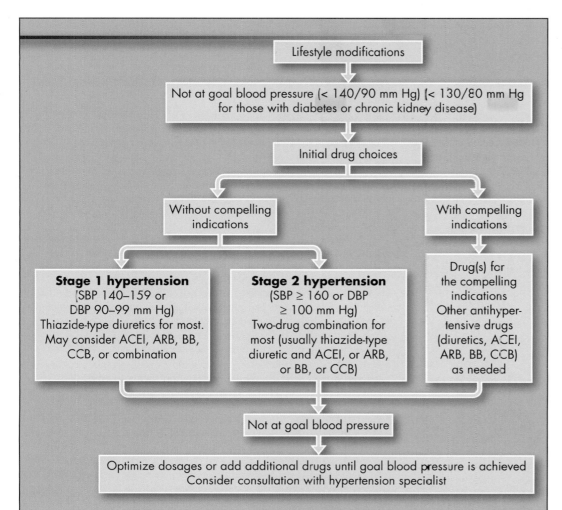

Figure 7-23.
Algorithm for treatment of hypertension recommended in the Seventh Report of the Joint National Committee on Prevention, Detection, Evaluation, and Treatment of High Blood Pressure (JNC 7). For more than three decades, the National High Blood Pressure Education Program of the National Heart, Lung, and Blood Institute has produced the most widely used consensus guidelines for prevention, detection, evaluation, and treatment of hypertension. In the most recent JNC 7 guidelines, lifestyle modification was recommended as the initial approach to therapy in patients with hypertension [1]. For those who do not achieve satisfactory blood pressure control (systolic/diastolic blood pressure < 140/90 mm Hg) with attempts to modify lifestyle, thiazide-type diuretics were recommended as initial drug therapy as monotherapy or in combination with an agent from one of the other major classes of antihypertensive drug therapy (angiotensin-converting enzyme inhibitors [ACEI], calcium channel blockers [CCB], angiotensin receptor blockers [ARB], or β-blockers [BB]). Use of more than two drugs was recommended in patients who fail to achieve satisfactory blood pressure control while observing lifestyle modification recommendations and taking full doses of drugs from two classes of antihypertensive drug therapy. DBP—diastolic blood pressure; SBP—systolic blood pressure. (*Adapted from* Chobanian *et al.* [1].)

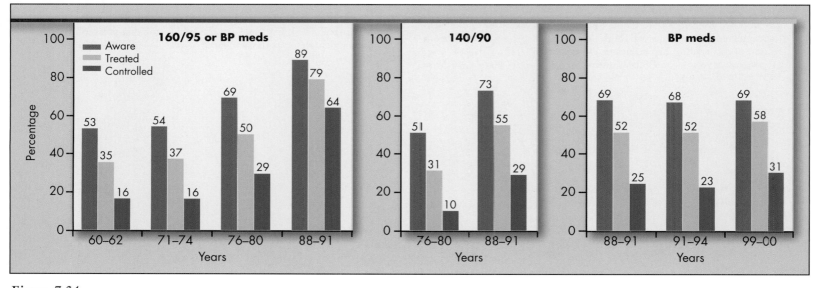

Figure 7-24.
Temporal trends in awareness, treatment, and control of hypertension in the noninstitutionalized adult population of the United States. During the 1960s and early 1970s, the systolic/diastolic cut points for diagnosis of hypertension were 160/95 mm Hg, and control of hypertension was defined by achievement of a systolic blood pressure < 160 mm Hg and a diastolic blood pressure < 95 mm Hg. Using these criteria, awareness, treatment, and control of hypertension improved progressively among adults in the US general population [22]. As shown in the *left panel*, almost 90% of all adults with this severity of hypertension between 1988 and 1991 were aware of their diagnosis, nearly 80% were being treated with antihypertensive medication, and almost two thirds (64%) had a systolic/diastolic blood pressure less than 160/95 mm Hg. The current

criteria for diagnosis of hypertension (systolic blood pressure 140 mm Hg or greater, diastolic blood pressure 90 mm Hg or greater, or use of antihypertensive medication) was introduced in the early 1970s. Although the prevalence of awareness, treatment and control for the 140/90 mm Hg cut-point was less impressive, the pattern in the *middle panel* indicates there was an impressive trend toward improvement between 1976 to 1980 and 1988 to 1991 [22]. More recent surveys (*right panel*) have identified no further improvement in awareness of hypertension, and only modest improvement in rates of treatment and control [3]. National surveys also point to a disturbing increase in the prevalence of high blood pressure in adolescents and children [23]. BP—blood pressure. (*Adapted from* Hajjar and Kotchen [3] and Muntner *et al.* [23].)

Hypertension Management

References

1. Chobanian AV, Bakris GL, Black HR, *et al.*: Seventh report of the Joint National Committee on Prevention, Detection, Evaluation, and Treatment of High Blood Pressure. *Hypertension* 2003, 42:1206–1252.

2. Kearney PM, Whelton M, Reynolds K, et al.: Global burden of hypertension: analysis of worldwide data. *Lancet* 2005, 365:217–223.

3. Hajjar I, Kotchen TA: Trends in prevalence, awareness, treatment, and control of hypertension in the United States, 1988–2000. *JAMA* 2003, 290:199–206.

4. Primatesta P, Brookes M, Poulter NR: Improved hypertension management and control: results from the Health Survey for England 1998. *Hypertension* 2001, 38:827–832.

5. He J, Neal B, Gu D, *et al.*: International Collaborative Study of Cardiovascular Disease in Asia (InterASIA): design, rationale, and preliminary results. *Ethn Dis* 2004, 14:260–268.

6. Gu D, Reynolds K, Wu X, *et al.*: Prevalence, awareness, treatment, and control of hypertension in China. *Hypertension* 2002, 40:920–927.

7. Wu X, Duan X, Gu D, *et al.*: Prevalence of hypertension and its trends in Chinese populations. *Int J Cardiol* 1995, 52:39–44.

8. Kearney PM, Whelton M, Reynolds K, *et al.*: Worldwide prevalence of hypertension: a systematic review. *J Hypertens* 2004, 22:11–19.

9. Vasan RS, Beiser A, Seshadri S, *et al.*: Residual lifetime risk for developing hypertension in middle-aged women and men: The Framingham Heart Study. *JAMA* 2002, 287:1003–1010.

10. Stamler J, Stamler R, Neaton JD: Blood pressure, systolic and diastolic, and cardiovascular risks. US population data. *Arch Intern Med* 1993, 153:598–615.

11. Klag MJ, Whelton PK, Randall RL, *et al.*: Blood pressure and end-stage renal disease in men. *N Eng J Med* 1996, 334:13–18.

12. Trials of Hypertension Prevention (TOHP) Collaborative Research Group: The effects of nonpharmacologic interventions on blood pressure of persons with high normal levels: results of the Trials of Hypertension Prevention, Phase I. *JAMA* 1992, 267:1213–1220.

13. Whelton PK, Kumanyika SK, Cook NR, *et al.*: Efficacy of non-pharmacologic intervention in adults with high normal blood pressure: results from phase I of the Trials of Hypertension Prevention (TOHP). Trials of Hypertension Prevention Collaborative Research Group. *Am J Clin Nutr* 1997, 65:652S–660S.

14. Kumanyika SK, Hebert PR, Cutler JA, *et al.*: Feasibility and efficacy of sodium reduction in the Trials of Hypertension Prevention, phase I. Trials of Hypertension Prevention Collaborative Research Group. *Hypertension* 1993, 22:502–512.

15. The Trials of Hypertension Prevention Collaborative Research Group: The effect of weight loss and sodium reduction on blood pressure and hypertension incidence in overweight non-hypertensive persons: final results of the Trials of Hypertension Prevention, Phase II. *Arch Intern Med* 1997, 157:657–667.

16. He J, Whelton PK, Appel LJ, *et al.*: Long-term effects of weight loss and dietary sodium reduction on incidence of hypertension. *Hypertension* 2000, 35:544–549.

17. Whelton PK, Appel LA , Espeland MA, *et al.*: Sodium reduction and weight loss in the treatment of hypertension in older persons: a randomized, controlled trial of non-pharmacologic interventions in the elderly (TONE). *JAMA* 1998, 279:839–846.

18. Appel LJ, Moore TJ, Obarzanek E, *et al.*: A clinical trial of the effects of dietary patterns on blood pressure. *N Engl J Med* 1997, 336:1117–1124.

19. Sacks FM, Svetkey LP, Vollmer WM, *et al.*: Effects on blood pressure of reduced dietary sodium and the Dietary Approaches to Stop Hypertension (DASH) diet. DASH-Sodium Collaborative Research Group. *N Engl J Med* 2001, 344:3–10.

20. Psaty BM, Lumley T, Furberg CD, *et al.*: Health outcomes associated with various antihypertensive therapies used as first-line agents: a network meta-analysis. *JAMA* 2003, 289:2534–2544.

21. Blood Pressure Lowering Treatment Trialists' Collaboration: Effects of different blood-pressure-lowering regimens on major cardiovascular events: results of prospectively-designed overviews of randomized trials. *Lancet* 2003, 362:1527–1535.

22. Burt VL, Cutler JA, Higgins M, *et al.*: Trends in the prevalence, awareness, treatment and control of hypertension in the adult U.S. population: data from health examination surveys 1960–1991. *Hypertension* 1995, 26:60–69.

23. Muntner P, He J, Cutler JA, *et al.*: Trends in blood pressure among children and adolescents in the United States. *JAMA* 2004, 291:2107–2113.

Dyslipidemia

Heather L. Gornik and Jorge Plutzky

Lipids, lipoproteins, and their components, including cholesterol, are essential for life. Lipids play a crucial role in vital physiologic processes, including maintenance of cell membranes, provision of energy resources, generation of intracellular signals, transport of materials, absorption of nutrients, and synthesis of hormones. Given their complexity and importance, it is not surprising that dysregulation of lipid metabolism contributes to so many pathologic conditions. Fortunately, scientific insight into abnormalities of lipid metabolism has combined with advances in drug therapy to yield major clinical benefits. Cholesterol has been suggested as the most decorated molecule in existence given the number of Nobel Prizes awarded for its study.

Cholesterol and lipids arise from exogenous (*ie*, dietary) or endogenous (primarily hepatic) sources. Distinct but overlapping mechanisms exist for cholesterol, triglyceride, fatty acids, and phospholipids uptake, transport, and delivery—a particular challenge given the hydrophobicity of many of these molecules. The major circulating lipoproteins—low-density lipoprotein (LDL), high-density lipoprotein (HDL), very low-density lipoprotein (VLDL), and chylomicrons—vary in terms of their relative percentage of different lipid components. LDL is a cholesterol-enriched lipoprotein that helps deliver cholesterol to distant sites, such as adrenal glands and sex organs, for hormone biosynthesis. HDL is considered the primary lipoprotein involved in reverse cholesterol transport, helping move lipids and cholesterol from the periphery back to the liver. VLDL (from the liver) and chylomicrons (from the gut) are triglyceride-enriched molecules, thus serving as a valuable energy resource through fatty acid delivery.

Extensive epidemiologic data have established the strong relationship between lipids and cardiovascular events, such as myocardial infarction, stroke, and peripheral arterial disease. Many different genotypes contribute to alterations in circulating lipoproteins that contribute to or directly account for the association between lipid abnormalities and vascular disease. "Western" lifestyle also can result in significant differences in lipoproteins that may contribute to atherosclerosis [1]. For LDL, a linear relationship exists around the world between cardiovascular mortality and increasing levels of LDL [2]. Although numerous therapeutic and even surgical approaches to lowering LDL have existed for some time, the discovery of 3-hydroxy-3-methylglutaryl coenzyme A reductase inhibitors, known commonly as "statins," was the major breakthrough in preventive medicine, offering the ability to lower LDL levels by 30% to 60%. Multiple studies have established a decrease in cardiovascular events in individuals with and without prior cardiovascular events in response to statin therapy [3]. This has been found to be true independent of baseline LDL in recent studies [4,5], prompting revisions of current guidelines as to the appropriate target LDL level [6]. With the development of more potent statins and newer agents, such as cholesterol absorption inhibitors, it is increasingly possible to achieve even greater degrees of LDL lowering. The strong and steep inverse relationship between HDL levels and cardiac events has drawn attention to options for raising HDL, with established medicines like niacin, as well as new pharmacologic agents under study [7]. Finally, evidence continues to accumulate regarding the role of triglyceride levels in atherosclerosis, especially in settings such as diabetes mellitus and the metabolic syndrome. Even with decades of remarkable progress, many unresolved issues and therapeutic opportunities persist in the field of lipoprotein metabolism and dyslipidemia.

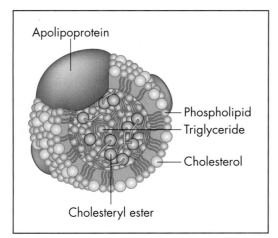

Figure 8-1.
Lipoproteins and their structure. Lipoproteins provide an essential function by packaging and allowing systemic transport of molecules essential for life. These molecular components (*see* Fig. 8-2), many of which are hydrophobic, are critical to cellular structure, energy balance, and biologic signaling. As such, it is not surprising that abnormalities in lipoproteins contribute to so many pathologic conditions. The ultimate disposition of each lipoprotein particle is determined by the specific apolipoproteins that are present on the surface of the lipoprotein particle. The apolipoproteins function as a zip code of sorts, directing lipoproteins to specific cellular and tissue locales through an intricate series of enzymatic interactions and ligand-receptor binding. Each lipoprotein is composed of a hydrophobic lipid core filled with esterified cholesterol molecules and triglycerides. Phospholipid, free cholesterol, and a specific panel of apolipoproteins form the outer surface of the lipoprotein particles. The relative concentration of each of these components varies depending on the lipoprotein subclass [8].

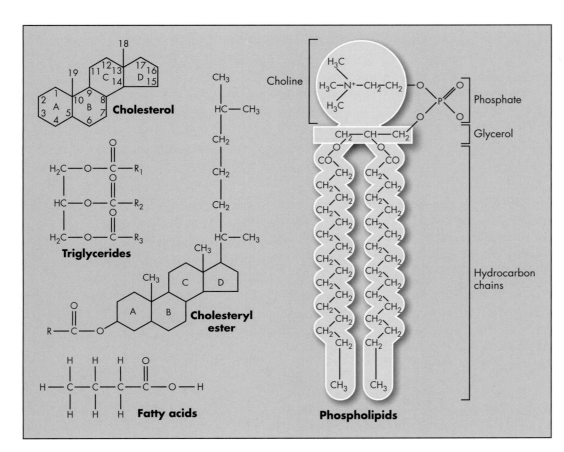

Figure 8-2.
Biochemical structures of the major components of lipoproteins [1,9]. Lipoproteins contain various amounts of cholesterol, cholesterol ester, triglycerides, and phospholipids. Cholesterol can be stored as cholesteryl ester in the lipid core of a lipoprotein or as free cholesterol in the more hydrophilic outer surface of circulating lipoproteins. Cholesterol is an important component of all cellular membranes, is involved in nutrient absorption as a part of bile, and is a precursor for the synthesis of steroid hormones. Triglycerides are composed of three long-chain fatty acids attached to a monoacylglycerol backbone. These fatty acids, released enzymatically, are a critical energy resource. Phospholipids, a key component of cell membranes, are composed of two fatty acid chains linked to a glycerol backbone. One carbon molecule in the glycerol backbone contains a phosphate molecule that carries a distinct head group of choline, ethanolamine, serine, or inositol. Pictured here is the phospholipid phosphatidyl choline or lecithin.

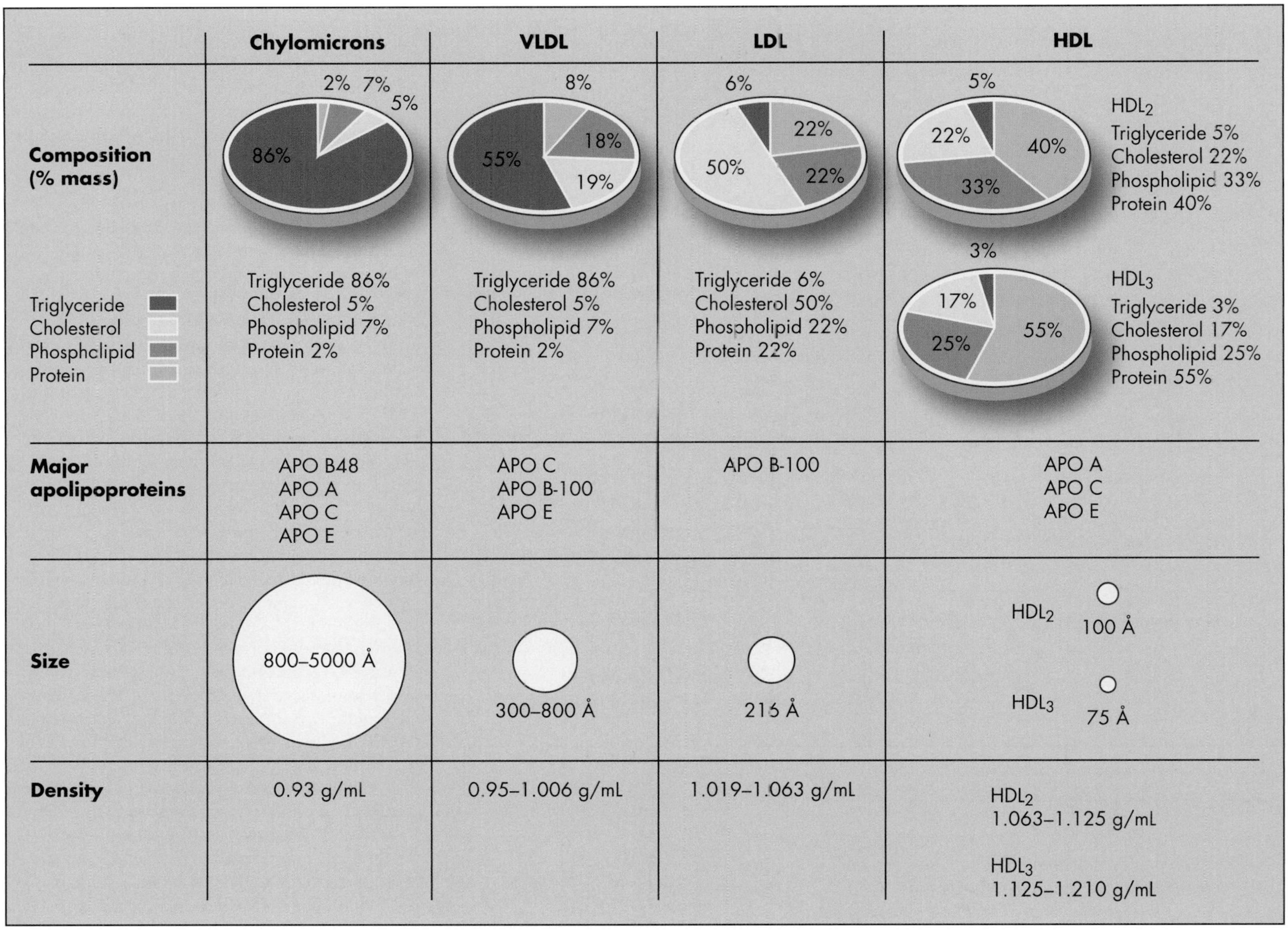

	Chylomicrons	VLDL	LDL	HDL
Composition (% mass)	2% 7% 5% 86%	8% 18% 19% 55%	6% 22% 22% 50%	HDL₂ 5% 22% 40% 33% — HDL_2 Triglyceride 5% Cholesterol 22% Phospholipid 33% Protein 40%; HDL₃ 3% 17% 25% 55% — HDL_3 Triglyceride 3% Cholesterol 17% Phospholipid 25% Protein 55%
Legend: Triglyceride, Cholesterol, Phospholipid, Protein	Triglyceride 86% Cholesterol 5% Phospholipid 7% Protein 2%	Triglyceride 86% Cholesterol 5% Phospholipid 7% Protein 2%	Triglyceride 6% Cholesterol 50% Phospholipid 22% Protein 22%	
Major apolipoproteins	APO B48 APO A APO C APO E	APO C APO B-100 APO E	APO B-100	APO A APO C APO E
Size	800–5000 Å	300–800 Å	216 Å	HDL_2 100 Å; HDL_3 75 Å
Density	0.93 g/mL	0.95–1.006 g/mL	1.019–1.063 g/mL	HDL_2 1.063–1.125 g/mL; HDL_3 1.125–1.210 g/mL

Figure 8-3.

Characteristics of the major lipoproteins [1,8,9]. The major circulating lipoprotein classes include chylomicrons, very low-density lipoprotein (VLDL), low-density lipoprotein (LDL), and high-density lipoprotein (HDL). Within each class, there is a spectrum of size, which varies as a function of lipoprotein content. Chylomicrons are large, triglyceride-rich particles with low protein content and low density that are derived from intestinal sources and contain APO B48. VLDL is also triglyceride-rich, but derived from the liver, and contains apolipoprotein (APO) B100. HDL particles are protein-rich, have low buoyancy, and are small in diameter. HDL can be characterized by its APOs AI and AII. Distinct HDL subclasses exist, with HDL_2 containing a larger core of cholesteryl esters, and HDL_3 smaller and less buoyant than HDL_2. APO B–containing lipoproteins include LDL. Each LDL particle contains only one single APO B, thus allowing APO B levels to serve as an indicator of total particle number. The pattern of APOs expressed on the surface of the lipoproteins determines its metabolism and destination. Each lipoprotein class plays a distinct role in lipid metabolism and physiology, as well as pathology.

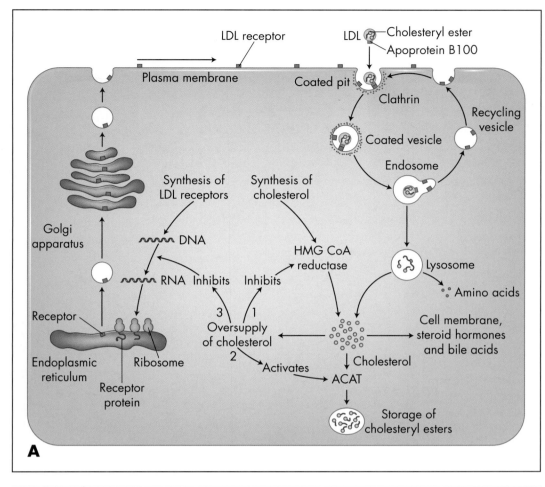

A

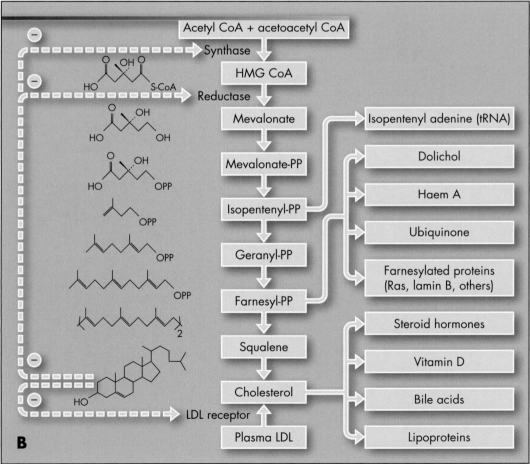

B

Figure 8-4.
Cholesterol synthesis and metabolism: the low-density lipoprotein (LDL) pathway. The supply of cholesterol to peripheral cells is determined by two distinct processes: the delivery of existing cholesterol into cells by LDL particles and the de novo synthesis of cholesterol by the mevalonate pathway.

A, The LDL receptor pathway is a key element of cholesterol metabolism [10–12]. The LDL receptor is synthesized in the rough endoplasmic reticulum and processed in the golgi apparatus before insertion into the cell membrane within clathrin-coated pits. The LDL receptors bind cholesterol-rich LDL particles through the interaction of apoprotein B100 and the LDL receptor. Receptor-bound LDL is then carried into the cell via endocytosis. LDL dissociates from the receptor, which is recycled to the cell surface. Cholesteryl esters are hydrolyzed within intracellular lysosomes. These cholesterol molecules can then be utilized as substrate in various biosynthetic pathways or for cell membranes. The cholesterol produced from hydrolysis of LDL particles exerts a negative feedback effect on de novo cholesterol synthesis by mevalonate pathway (*see panel B*), as well on the synthesis of new LDL receptors. Intracellular cholesterol also stimulates activation of the enzyme acetyl-coenzyme A (CoA): cholesteryl acyltransferase (ACAT), which helps to re-esterify cholesterol for intracellular storage [11].

B, The mevalonate pathway [13]. De novo synthesis of cholesterol occurs via a series of biochemical reactions that begin with the synthesis of mevalonate from acetyl-CoA and acetoacetyl-CoA by the enzymes 3-hydroxy-3-methylglutaryl (HMG)-CoA synthase and HMG-CoA reductase. Endogenous intracellular cholesterol, obtained from plasma LDL, inhibits both of these enzymes, thus regulating de novo cholesterol synthesis. Low levels of mevalonate continue to be produced, however, to maintain a supply of the non-sterol isoprenoids, such as ubiquinone and other farnesylated proteins. In the presence of LDL cholesterol and excess mevalonate, this pathway is shut off entirely [13]. The mechanism of action of the statin drugs is the inhibition of the enzyme HMG-CoA reductase, the rate-limiting step in this process. In response to inhibition of HMG-CoA reductase, hepatocytes increase expression of LDL receptors.

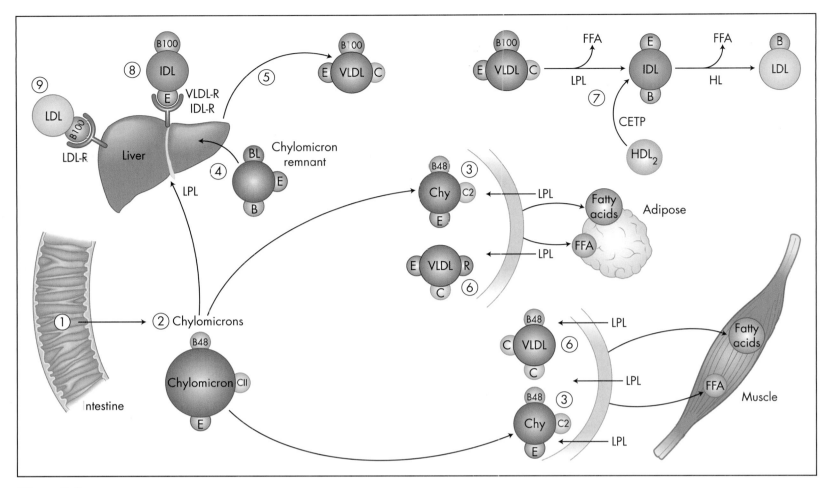

Figure 8-5.

Transport of the lipid rich proteins: triglycerides and very low-density lipoproteins (VLDL) [1,9]. 1) Fatty acids, cholesterol, lipids, and other nutrients contained in food are absorbed in the small intestine after enzymatic breakdown of dietary fats and emulsification with bile salts, ultimately forming micelles. 2) Within the enterocytes, fatty acids are re-esterified into triglycerides and packaged into chylomicrons (apolipoprotein [apo] B48–containing) for transport through the lymphatics into the portal circulation. 3) The enzyme lipoprotein lipase (LPL), present on endothelial cells, acts on circulating chylomicrons and VLDL to liberate fatty acids from each triglyceride molecule. These fatty acids are then combusted, through β-oxidation, to generate energy for tissues such as muscle, or are taken up into adipose tissue for storage. Fatty acids can also be used for synthesis of VLDL particles by the liver. 4) The progressive liberation of fatty acid and depletion of triglycerides from a given lipoprotein particle over time leads to a cholesterol-ester enriched chylomicron remnant particle, which can be taken up by the liver. The apo are recycled. 5) An analogous system exists in the liver through the synthesis of triglyceride-rich VLDL particles, thus ensuring fatty acids can be delivered to peripheral tissues even in the fasting state. VLDL particles are similar in structure to chylomicrons, but contain relatively less triglyceride, more cholesteryl esters, and apo B100. 6) VLDL delivers fatty acids to adipose tissue and muscle as its triglycerides are hydrolyzed by lipoprotein lipase. VLDL also receives cholesteryl esters from high-density lipoprotein (HDL) particles via cholesteryl ester transfer protein (CETP) to ultimately become intermediate-density lipoprotein (IDL) (7). IDL can be taken up by the liver via the apo E receptor (8). Alternatively, IDL can be further metabolized by hepatic lipase to LDL cholesterol, which is returned to the liver and peripheral cells by the LDL receptor via apo B100 (9).

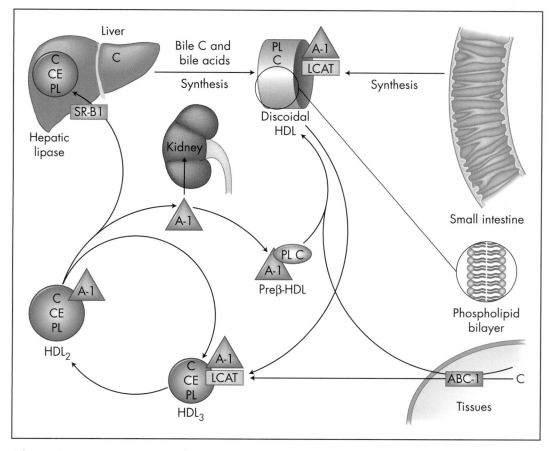

the liver. This mechanism offers a plausible explanation for the strong inverse relationship between HDL levels and cardiovascular events. 1) Lipid-free apolipoprotein A1 (Apo A1) is secreted by the liver into the circulation. 2) By interacting with the cholesterol effluxing adenosine triphosphate (ATP)-binding cassette transporter 1 (ABCA1), Apo A-1 scavenges free cholesterol (C) and phospholipids (PL) from the peripheral tissues, becoming nascent or pre-β-HDL in the process. Pre-β-HDL acquires additional free cholesterol from peripheral cells, ultimately forming mature α-HDL as its cholesterol is esterified (CE) in the lipid core by lecithin-cholesterol acyltransferase (LCAT) (3). The spherical α-HDL particle is known as HDL_3. Apo A1 is a cofactor in the LCAT reaction. As more cholesterol is esterified in the lipid core of the α-HDL particle, it becomes larger and more buoyant (HDL_2) (4). Mature α-HDL_2 has two fates. Its cholesteryl esters can be taken up by hepatocyes or other steroidogenic cells through the hepatic scavenger receptor class B (SR-B1) (5). The cholesteryl esters are then used for steroid synthesis, very low-density lipoprotein (VLDL) synthesis, or are secreted into bile. Alternatively (6), mature α-HDL can transfer its cholesteryl esters to VLDL, intermediate-density lipoprotein, and LDL by the cholesterol ester transfer protein (CETP). These lipoproteins are then taken up by the LDL receptor via Apo B-100.

Figure 8-6.
Reverse cholesterol transport and high-density lipoprotein (HDL) [1,7,9]. HDL is the central lipoprotein in the postulated mechanism of reverse cholesterol transport, moving various lipoproteins from peripheral tissues, such as atherogenic macrophages in the arterial wall, back to

The Fredrickson/World Health Organization Classification System of Hyperlipidemias

Type	Standing plasma appearance	Elevated particles	Plasma total cholesterol	Plasma triglycerides
I	Creamy top layer; clear infranatant	Increased chylomicrons	Normal	↑↑
IIA	Clear	Increased LDL; normal VLDL	↑↑	Normal
IIB	Clear or slightly turbid	Increased LDL; increased VLDL	↑↑	↑
III	Faint creamy top layer; turbid infranatant	Increased IDL	↑	↑
IV	Turbid	Increased VLDL	Normal or slight ↑	↑↑
V	Prominent creamy top layer; turbid infranatant	Increased VLDL; increased chylomicrons	↑	↑↑

Figure 8-7.
The Fredrickson/World Health Organization Classification system of hyperlipidemias [14]. This system, originally proposed in 1967 by Fredrickson and adopted by the World Health Organization, classifies the lipid disorders by plasma analysis. The initial characterization is based on visual inspection of a fasting plasma sample after 18 to 24 hours of refrigeration. Triglyceride-rich chylomicrons, when present, give plasma a milky appearance and rise to a top layer of "cream." Very low-density lipoprotein (VLDL) gives the plasma a cloudy or turbid appearance. The secondary classification is based on lipoprotein electrophoresis. Although less often invoked currently, the Fredrickson classification system represents crucial early and enduring insight into the spectrum of lipid disorders. Of note, abnormalities of high-density lipoprotein (HDL) cholesterol are not included in this classification system. IDL—intermediate-density lipoprotein; LDL—low-density lipoprotein.

Genetic Low-density Lipoprotein Cholesterol Disorders

Familial hypercholesterolemia
  Autosomal dominant disorder
  Genetic mutation in LDL receptor impairs cellular LDL uptake
  Multiple (> 100) mutations described
  Homozygotes (total cholesterol > 500 mg/dL) present in childhood with
      cardiovascular events
  Heterozygous patients present in adulthood
  HMG-CoA reductase inhibitors (statins) first-line therapy
Familial defective apo B100
  Defective apo B100 prohibits binding to LDL receptor
  Elevated LDL levels
  Patients are typically of European descent
Sitosterolemia
  Autosomal recessive disorder
  Mutations of genes for ABCG8 and ABCG5 transporters on chromosome 2p21
  Abnormal intestinal transporters absorb large quantities of plant sterols
  Decreased biliary section of plant sterols
  Sterols are taken up into lipoprotein particles
  Similar phenotype as familial hypercholesterolemia
  Treated with diet, bile acid resins, ezetimibe
Lipoprotein(a)
  Formed by linkage of apo B100 of the LDL particle to lipoprotein(a)
  Structural homology to fibrinogen
    Elevated lipoprotein(a) levels associated with premature atherosclerosis and thrombosis
  Treated with high-dose niacin therapy

Figure 8-8.
Selected genetic disorders of low-density lipoprotein (LDL) cholesterol [15]. A list of the most common genetic abnormalities of LDL cholesterol is provided. Heterozygous familial hypercholesterolemia (FH) is the most prevalent of these disorders. Up to 5% of myocardial infarction survivors have heterozygous FH, with an even greater prevalence of cardiac events among younger individuals [15]. Homozygous FH can present in dramatic fashion, with myocardial infarction occurring as early as 2 years of age. The discovery that genetic defects in the LDL receptor, of which over 100 have now been described, led to Brown and Goldstein receiving the Nobel Prize. Familial defective apolipoprotein B100 (apo B100) and sitosterolemia are rare disorders. Lipoprotein(a), although not a true disorder of LDL cholesterol, has received increasing attention as an emerging risk factor for coronary artery disease [16]. HMG-CoA— 3-hydroxy-3-methylglutaryl coenzyme A.

Genetic High-density Lipoprotein Disorders

Familial hypoalphalipoproteinemia
  Autosomal recessive disorder related to mutations in apo AI gene
  Decreased apo AI production causes very low HDL cholesterol levels
  Associated with premature atherosclerosis
Tangier disease
  Caused by a mutation in ATP binding cassette (*ABCA1*) gene
  Abnormal intracellular trafficking of cholesterol and processing with apo AI
  Very low serum HDL and total cholesterol
  Engorgement of reticuloendothelial system with lipids
    Hepatosplenomegaly
    Lymphadenopathy
    Massively enlarged, orange-colored tonsils
  Associated with premature atherosclerosis and peripheral neuropathy
Familial HDL deficiency
  Also associated with mutations of the *ABCA1* gene
  Very low serum HDL and total cholesterol, premature coronary artery disease
  Not associated with the reticuloendothelial engorgement of Tangier disease
Apo AI-Milano
  Initially reported in a Northern Italian family
  Very low HDL levels (typically < 15 mg/dL) and moderately elevated triglycerides
  Beneficial phenotype protective against atherosclerosis
  Allelic variant of Apo I protein with cysteine residue substituted for arginine at
      position 173

Figure 8-9.
Selected genetic disorders of high-density lipoprotein (HDL) cholesterol [15]. Most but not all genetic disorders resulting in low HDL cholesterol are associated with premature atherosclerosis and early cardiovascular events. Multiple genetic disorders have been identified, including mutations of the apolilpoprotein AI (apo AI) gene. Isolated low HDL level is referred to as hypoalphalipoproteinemia, and is among the most common abnormalities found in young patients with coronary artery disease. In the case of Apo AI-Milano, a rare "disorder" of HDL initially reported in a Northern Italian family [18], a single amino acid substitution in the Apo-I protein is associated with low HDL cholesterol but a decreased incidence of cardiovascular events, a likely result of increased ability to flux cholesterol through reverse cholesterol transport. Indeed, early studies suggest injection of synthetic Apo AI-Milano may decrease plaque volume over a relatively short time period [19]. ATP—adenosine triphosphate.

Genetic Disorders of Triglycerides

LPL deficiency
  Caused by absence (class I) or defective (class II or III) LPL activity
  Multiple genetic mutations of LPL gene (8p22) identified
  Presents with eruptive xanthomas, recurrent pancreatitis
  Associated with low HDL cholesterol
  Association with cardiovascular disease controversial
  Can be successfully managed with low-fat diet, abstinence from alcohol
Apo CII deficiency
  Mutation in *APOC2* gene (19q13.2) causes absent or defective Apo CII
  Chylomicrons cannot be processed by LPL because of deficient Apo CII
  Clinically mimics LPL deficiency
  Can be successfully managed with low-fat diet, abstinence from alcohol
Familial hypertriglyceridemia
  Common disorder
  Fredrickson class IV phenotype
  Genetics not fully established
  Likely caused by hepatic VLDL overproduction
  Phenotype associated with environmental factors (*eg*, obesity, diabetes, alcohol consumption)
  VLDL, triglycerides are moderately to severely elevated; LDL cholesterol is normal
  Associated with cardiovascular disease
  Not associated with eruptive xanthomas or pancreatitis

Figure 8-10.
Selected genetic disorders of triglycerides [15]. Lipoprotein lipase (LPL) deficiency and apolipoprotein CII (Apo CII) deficiency are rare disorders associated with markedly elevated levels of serum triglycerides (often > 1000 mg/dL). These disorders often present with abdominal pain related to pancreatitis and eruptive xanthomas, rather than premature cardiovascular events. Familial hypertriglyceridemia is a common disorder associated with moderately elevated levels of serum very low-density lipoprotein (VLDL) cholesterol and triglycerides and normal low-density lipoprotein (LDL) cholesterol. HDL—high-density lipoprotein.

Causes of Secondary Hypertriglyceridemia

Disorders and drugs causing hypertriglyceridemia	Disorders and drugs causing hypertriglyceridemia and hypercholesterolemia
Diseases	
Uncontrolled diabetes mellitus	Type 2 diabetes mellitus
Chronic renal failure	Ethanol excess
Peritoneal dialysis	Renal transplantation
Septicemia	Dysgammaglobulinemia
Hepatocellular disease	Hemodialysis
Systemic lupus erythematosus	Monoclonal gammopathies
Acromegaly	
Gaucher's disease	
Tay Sachs disease	
Partial lipodystrophy	
Drugs	
β-Adrenoreceptor blockers	Glucocorticoids
Anabolic steroids	Phenytoin
Oral contraceptives	
Oestrogens	
Isoretinoin	
HIV protease inhibitors	
Diuretics, especially thiazides	

Figure 8-11.
Secondary causes of hypertriglyceridemia [8]. Every patient found to have hypertriglyceridemia requires a thorough evaluation for potential reversible secondary causes. Hypothyroidism, can contribute to elevated triglycerides, as well as elevated low-density lipoprotein levels, and will respond rapidly to thyroid repletion therapy. Thiazide diuretics can cause elevated triglycerides, although this has not been associated with adverse cardiovascular sequelae in antihypertensive clinical trials [21]. Other potential contributors to hypertriglyceridemia are shown (*Adapted from* Bhatnagar [8].)

Diabetic Dyslipoproteinemia

Low HDL cholesterol
Elevated triglycerides
Elevated VLDL cholesterol
Moderately elevated total and LDL cholesterol

Figure 8-12.
Features of diabetes-associated dyslipidemia. Type 2 diabetes mellitus (T2DM) confers a significantly increased risk of atherosclerotic complications, even to the extent of now being considered as having the same risk for future cardiovascular events as having survived a prior myocardial infarction. The low-density lipoprotein (LDL) of T2DM is often not particularly elevated although these LDL particles are often smaller, denser, more prone to oxidation, and hence more atherogenic. More typically patients with T2DM have elevated triglycerides and a lower high-density lipoprotein (HDL). This pattern is encountered in the metabolic syndrome, the constellation of central obesity, hypertension, procoagulant state, insulin resistance with hyperinsulinemia and impaired fasting glucose, and dyslipidemia. The metabolic syndrome often precedes the development of frank diabetes and, frequently, cardiovascular disease. Aggressive glycemic control may improve this lipid profile, particularly serum triglycerides. Insulin sensitizers also have been shown to improve this dyslipidemia, as do fibrates. Niacin may be effective as well, but may be associated with worsened glucose control. Statins remain first-line therapy for the management of diabetic dyslipidemia, given the benefits seen in the diabetes subgroup of large clinical trials independent of baseline LDL [22]. Adjunctive therapies may include niacin or a fibrate to lower triglycerides and raise HDL cholesterol levels. VLDL—very low-density lipoprotein.

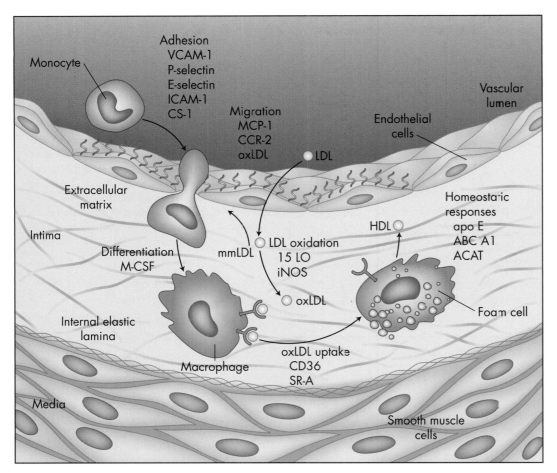

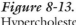

Figure 8-13.

Hypercholesterolemia and the initiation of atherogenesis. After uptake into the arterial wall, low-density lipoprotein (LDL) cholesterol is thought to undergo oxidation within the subendothelial space (*eg*, from inducible nitric oxide synthase [iNOS], myeloperoxidase [MPO], and 15-lipoxygenase [15-LO]). Oxidized LDL (oxLDL) is proatherogenic. Components of oxLDL increase expression of adhesion molecules on the endothelium, such as vascular cell adhesion molecule-1 (VCAM), stimulating entry of monocytes into the subendothelial space. Inflammatory cytokines (macrophage colony-stimulating factor [M-CSF]) promote differentiation of monocytes into macrophages. These cells ultimately become foam cells by uptake of oxLDL, forming the early fatty streak. Oxidized LDL cholesterol can be returned to the liver via reverse cholesterol transport by high-density lipoprotein (HDL). Early fatty streaks progress to become complex atherosclerotic plaques as lymphocytes and macrophages secrete pro-inflammatory cytokines and smooth muscle cells migrate into the arterial media to form a fibrous cap. Apo E—apolipoprotein E; CCR-2—chemokine receptor-2; MCP-1—monocyte chemoattractant protein-1; mmLDL—minimally modified LDL. (*Adapted from* Glass and Witztum [23].)

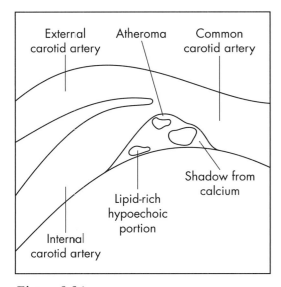

Figure 8-14.

Carotid atheroma. Duplex ultrasound of an atherosclerotic plaque (atheroma) at the origin of the right internal carotid artery in a patient with hypercholesterolemia and transient ischemic attacks (TIAs). The carotid bifurcation is the most common location for accumulation of atherosclerotic plaque in the cerebrovasculature, with the potential for development of significant stenosis. The plaque is heterogeneous in appearance. There is an echolucent component, as well as significant calcification. Oxidized lipids within activated macrophages, known as foam cells, form the core of such atheromas. This plaque encroaches on the lumen of the vessel and was associated with a hemodynamically significant stenosis of 60% to 65%. The patient was referred for carotid revascularization.

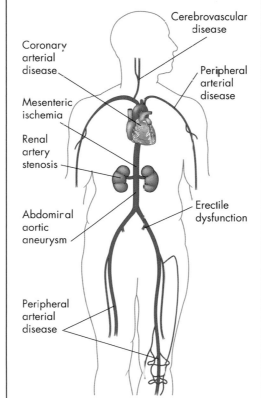

Figure 8-15.

Atherosclerosis is a systemic process. Although the most commonly recognized and life-threatening manifestations of atherosclerosis are coronary artery disease and cerebrovascular disease, any vascular bed can be affected. Renovascular disease may present with uncontrolled hypertension, renal insufficiency, or recurrent pulmonary edema. Mesenteric ischemia may cause postprandial abdominal pain and weight loss, although it is often asymptomatic. Atherosclerotic arterial occlusive disease is a common cause of erectile dysfunction. Atherosclerosis is a contributing factor in the pathogenesis of abdominal aortic aneurysm. The prevalence of peripheral arterial disease has been traditionally underappreciated. Recent studies have suggested that 29% of the elderly population has evidence of peripheral artery disease, as manifest by an abnormal ankle-brachial index [24]. Many of these patients are asymptomatic. All of these systemic manifestations of atherosclerosis can be driven in part by hypercholesterolemia and dyslipidemia.

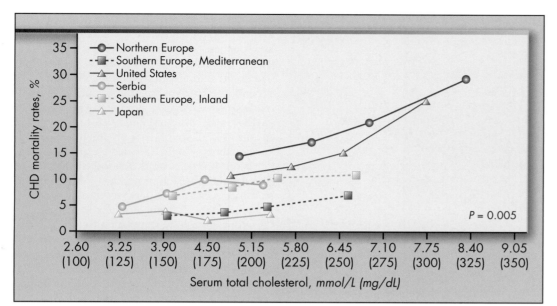

Figure 8-16.
Worldwide relationship between total cholesterol levels and cardiovascular mortality: data from the Seven Countries Study [2]. Over a wide range of cultures, elevated total cholesterol was predictive of cardiovascular death during extended follow-up. The original Seven Countries Study, led by Dr. Ancell Keys, included 12,763 men between the ages of 40 and 59 years and helped frame the cholesterol hypothesis. Data shown are from subsequent 25 year follow-up. Coronary heart disease (CHD) mortality rates have been adjusted for age, cigarette smoking, and systolic blood pressure. (*Adapted from* Verschuren *et al.* [2].)

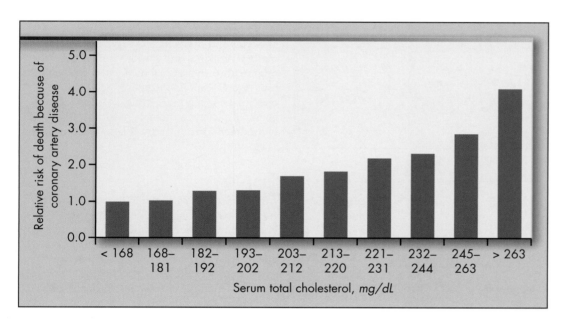

Figure 8-17.
Elevated total cholesterol increases risk of death from coronary artery disease in a continuous fashion: data from the Multiple Risk Factor Intervention Trial (MRFIT) [25]. MRFIT observed 356,222 men between the ages of 35 to 57 years for the development of cardiovascular events over 6 years of follow-up. In this cohort of patients, the risk of death from coronary artery disease increased in a continuous fashion with increasing levels of total cholesterol. Elevated total cholesterol is primarily a marker of increased low-density lipoprotein cholesterol. The relative risk of coronary death increased for all patients beyond those in the lowest decline of total cholesterol measurement (< 167 mg/dL). The relative risk of death from coronary artery disease was 4.13 for patients in the highest decline of total cholesterol.

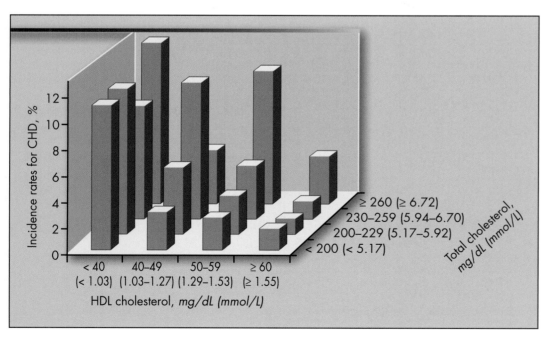

Figure 8-18.
Low high-density lipoprotein (HDL) cholesterol is an independent predictor of coronary events: data from the Framingham Study [26]. The original Framingham cohort was composed of men and women from a single community between the ages of 49 and 82 years. Shown are the rates of incident coronary events over a period of 4 years among patients stratified by baseline total and HDL cholesterol levels. Among patients with normal total cholesterol (< 200 mg/dL) and low HDL cholesterol (< 40 mg/dL), the risk of a cardiac event was the same or higher than for patients with normal HDL (> 40 mg/dL) and elevated total cholesterol (> 230 mg/dL). CHD—coronary heart disease. (*Adapted from* Castelli *et al.* [26].)

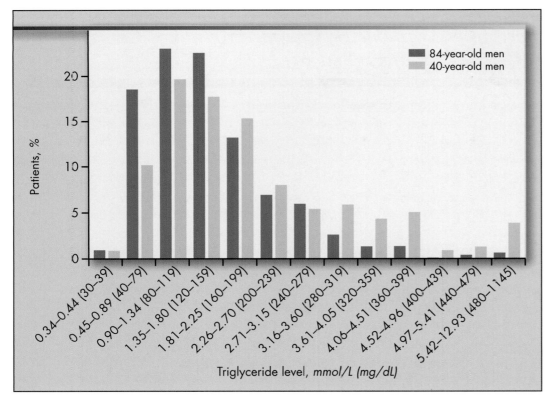

Figure 8-19.
Hypertriglyceridemia and the risk of myocardial infarction. The link between elevated triglycerides and cardiovascular events had been controversial. Although a linear relationship exists between triglycerides and cardiovascular events, this relationship weakens or disappears in multivariate analysis [27]. This issue is confounded by the strong relationship between triglycerides and most, if not at all, other cardiovascular risk factors. For example, there is a tight inverse biologic relationship between triglycerides and high-density lipoprotein (HDL). Within patients with the same total cholesterol:HDL ratio, the presence of increased triglycerides often identifies a further increase in risk. In this case-control analysis of data from the Physicians' Health Study of male subjects 40 to 84 years old, increased baseline serum triglyceride level was significantly associated with the risk of myocardial infarction (relative risk 1.40 per 100 mg/dL increase in triglycerides) [28]. Similarly, in a meta-analysis of 17 epidemiologic studies, there was a significant association of hypertriglyceridemia and incident cardiovascular events, with an adjusted relative risk of 1.14 in men and 1.37 in women for each 1 mmol/L (88.6 mg/dL) increase in baseline triglyceride levels [29]. (*Adapted from* Stampfer *et al.* [28].)

Medical Therapies for Dyslipidemia

Increased LDL	Decreased HDL	Increased triglycerides
HMG-CoA reductase inhibitors (statins)	Nicotinic acid	Fibrates
Ezetimibe	Fibrates	Nicotinic acid
Fibrates	Statins	Statins
Nicotinic acid	Lifestyle modification	Lifestyle modification
Plant stanol and sterol esters	Weight loss	Weight loss
Bile-acid binding resins	Exercise	Reduced carbohydrate diet
Dietary modification	Red wine	
Low fat	Monounsaturated fats	
Low trans-fatty acid		
Soluble dietary fiber		
Plasmapheresis (refractory hypercholesterolemia)		

Figure 8-20.
Overview of medical therapies for the major categories of dyslipidemia. Dietary modification, exercise, and weight loss are recommended for all patients over the entire spectrum of lipid disorders, and these recommendations clearly have independent benefit on overall cardiovascular risk. Pharmacotherapy is tailored to the predominant lipid abnormality. 3-Hydroxy-3-methylglutaryl coenzyme A (HMG-CoA) reductase inhibitors (*ie*, statins) are recommended across the spectrum of lipid disorders, given their well-established tolerability and proven cardiovascular risk reduction. Statins should be the agents of first choice for the management of elevated low-density lipoprotein (LDL) cholesterol. Statins also have modest effects on triglycerides and high-density lipoprotein (HDL) cholesterol. Certain statins are more effective than others in terms of their non-LDL cholesterol activity. Ezetimibe is discussed in detail herewith. The mechanism of action for nicotinic acid remains incompletely understood but may work by inhibiting free fatty acid mobilization from adipose tissue, thus decreasing available substrate for hepatic very low-density lipoprotein (VLDL) production [30,31]. It also may decrease VLDL conversion to LDL, and it increases HDL cholesterol by mechanisms that have not been well established. Nicotinic acid is the only known pharmacotherapy for elevated lipoprotein(a) cholesterol. Fibrates increase the oxidation of fatty acids and reduce hepatic synthesis of VLDL and triglycerides [31]. They also enhance VLDL catabolism by lipoprotein lipase. Fibrates lower triglycerides and raise HDL but have a variable effect on LDL cholesterol. In addition, fibrates raise HDL cholesterol by inducing transcription of the apolipoprotein-A1 and -AII lipoproteins. The fibrate mechanism of action is thought to be activation of the nuclear receptor/ transcription factor peroxisome proliferators-activated receptor-a.

Characteristics of the Six Commercially Available Hydroxymethylglutaryl Coenzyme A Reductase Inhibitors (Statins)

	Lovastatin	Pravastatin	Simvastatin	Fluvastatin	Abvastatin	Rosuvastatin
Year FDA-approved	1987	1991	1991	1993	1996	2003
Maximum approved dose, *mg*	80	80	80	40	80	40
Maximum serum LDL cholesterol reduction, %	40	34	47	24	60	55
Maximum serum HDL cholesterol increase, %	9	12	12	8	6	10
Maximum serum triglyceride reduction, %	16	24	18	10	29	26
Mechanism of metabolism	CYP P450 3A4	Sulfation	CYP P450 3A4	CYP P450 2C9	CYP P450 3A4	Negligible CYP P450 metabolism
Elimination half-life, $T_{1/2}$	3	1.8	2	1.2	14	19
Optimal timing of administration	With meals; morning or evening	Bedtime	Evening	Dosed twice daily; extended-release preparation taken at bedtime	Evening	No difference

Figure 8-21.

Characteristics of the six commercially available hydroxymethylglutaryl coenzyme A reductase inhibitors (statins) [31–33]. A seventh statin, pitavastatin, is currently undergoing phase III clinical trials, but is not yet available in the United States. In general, initiation of statin therapy at a standard starting dose is associated with a 30% to 40% reduction in low-density lipoprotein (LDL) cholesterol. Doubling of the statin dose typically results in an additional 6% reduction in LDL cholesterol. The statins vary in terms of maximal LDL cholesterol reduction and effects on serum high-density lipoprotein (HDL) cholesterol and triglycerides. The short elimination half-life of fluvastatin requires twice-daily dosing or prescription of an extended release preparation. Extensive clinical trial data has established a decrease in cardiovascular events in large clinical trials of many of these agents.

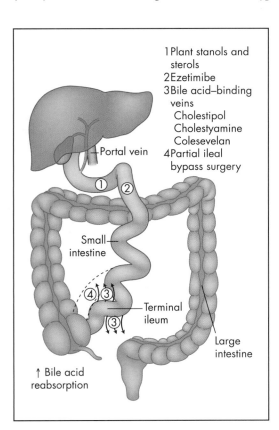

1 Plant stanols and sterols
2 Ezetimibe
3 Bile acid–binding veins
   Cholestipol
   Cholestyamine
   Colesevelan
4 Partial ileal bypass surgery

Portal vein

Small intestine

Terminal ileum

Large intestine

↑ Bile acid reabsorption

Figure 8-22.

Therapies to alter cholesterol absorption. Given the substantial flux of cholesterol through the enterohepatic circulation, attention has long focused on the intestines and the biliary system as a means of lowering cholesterol by increasing cholesterol excretion. Plant stanol and sterol esters decrease small intestine absorption of cholesterol by displacing cholesterol from micelles during enterocyte absorption. These compounds, available in the form of diet supplements (margarines) or in pill form, can reduce low-density lipoprotein (LDL) cholesterol by up to 10% if taken at high doses (2 g/day) [34] The discovery of ezetimibe was a major recent advance in cholesterol metabolism, with a significant (but still much smaller than statin) reduction of cholesterol aborportion across the brush border of enterocytes of the small intestine through blockade of a transporter protein. These drugs are used as an adjunct to statins to further lower LDL levels or in patients who are statin intolerant. Bile acid sequestrants (resins) block enterohepatic circulation of bile acids, which would otherwise be absorbed into the portal circulation via the terminal ileum. These drugs, once the mainstay of therapy for dyslipidemia, are now used as adjunctive therapy for patients with severely elevated LDL cholesterol. Constipation is a common side effect of the bile acid–binding resins. Partial ileal bypass, a surgical procedure that involves bypass of the distal one third of the small intestine, prevents reabsorption of cholesterol in much the same way. One of the earliest demonstrations of lipid-lowering therapy for the secondary prevention of cardiovascular events was a randomized trial of diet versus partial ileal bypass surgery in survivors of myocardial infarction [35].

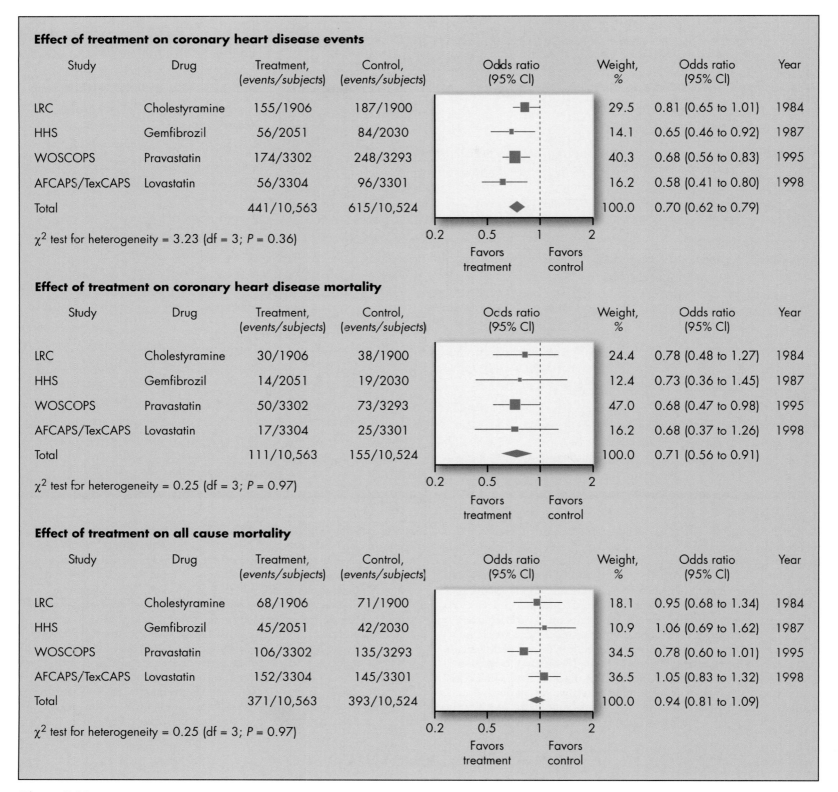

Effect of treatment on coronary heart disease events

Study	Drug	Treatment, (events/subjects)	Control, (events/subjects)	Odds ratio (95% CI)	Weight, %	Odds ratio (95% CI)	Year
LRC	Cholestyramine	155/1906	187/1900		29.5	0.81 (0.65 to 1.01)	1984
HHS	Gemfibrozil	56/2051	84/2030		14.1	0.65 (0.46 to 0.92)	1987
WOSCOPS	Pravastatin	174/3302	248/3293		40.3	0.68 (0.56 to 0.83)	1995
AFCAPS/TexCAPS	Lovastatin	56/3304	96/3301		16.2	0.58 (0.41 to 0.80)	1998
Total		441/10,563	615/10,524		100.0	0.70 (0.62 to 0.79)	

χ^2 test for heterogeneity = 3.23 (df = 3; P = 0.36)

Effect of treatment on coronary heart disease mortality

Study	Drug	Treatment, (events/subjects)	Control, (events/subjects)	Odds ratio (95% CI)	Weight, %	Odds ratio (95% CI)	Year
LRC	Cholestyramine	30/1906	38/1900		24.4	0.78 (0.48 to 1.27)	1984
HHS	Gemfibrozil	14/2051	19/2030		12.4	0.73 (0.36 to 1.45)	1987
WOSCOPS	Pravastatin	50/3302	73/3293		47.0	0.68 (0.47 to 0.98)	1995
AFCAPS/TexCAPS	Lovastatin	17/3304	25/3301		16.2	0.68 (0.37 to 1.26)	1998
Total		111/10,563	155/10,524		100.0	0.71 (0.56 to 0.91)	

χ^2 test for heterogeneity = 0.25 (df = 3; P = 0.97)

Effect of treatment on all cause mortality

Study	Drug	Treatment, (events/subjects)	Control, (events/subjects)	Odds ratio (95% CI)	Weight, %	Odds ratio (95% CI)	Year
LRC	Cholestyramine	68/1906	71/1900		18.1	0.95 (0.68 to 1.34)	1984
HHS	Gemfibrozil	45/2051	42/2030		10.9	1.06 (0.69 to 1.62)	1987
WOSCOPS	Pravastatin	106/3302	135/3293		34.5	0.78 (0.60 to 1.01)	1995
AFCAPS/TexCAPS	Lovastatin	152/3304	145/3301		36.5	1.05 (0.83 to 1.32)	1998
Total		371/10,563	393/10,524		100.0	0.94 (0.81 to 1.09)	

χ^2 test for heterogeneity = 0.25 (df = 3; P = 0.97)

Figure 8-23.
Cholesterol-lowering therapy for the primary prevention of death and cardiovascular events. Meta-analysis of four major randomized clinical trials of primary prevention [36]. Each trial enrolled patients with hypercholesterolemia (initial mean cholesterol 220–290 mg/dL) without known atherosclerotic vascular disease. Patients were randomized to dietary modification plus cholesterol-lowering therapy or dietary modification plus placebo. Patients were followed for 5 to 7 years for the occurrence of major cardiovascular endpoints. Mean total cholesterol was reduced by 8.5% to 20%, with the highest levels of cholesterol reduction achieved in the two statin trials. The studies consistently demonstrate a reduction in coronary artery disease events (*eg*, myocardial infarction) and mortality related to coronary artery disease among patients randomized to cholesterol-lowering therapy of approximately 30%. There is no consistent reduction in all-cause mortality demonstrated in these trials. These findings have formed the basis for clinical guidelines for lipid-lowering therapy in patients with primary hypercholesterolemia who have not yet had a cardiovascular event. AFCAPS/TexCAPS–Air Force/Texas Coronary Atherosclerosis Prevention Study; HHS–Helsinki Heart Study; LRC–Lipid Research Clinics Coronary Primary Prevention Trial; WOSCOPS–West of Scotland Coronary Prevention Study. (*Adapted from* Pignone *et al.* [36].)

Recent Large-scale Randomized Trials of Cholesterol Lowering in the Secondary Prevention of Cardiovascular Disease

Study	Year	Baseline LDL cholesterol, *mg/dL*	Study population	Intervention	Duration, *y*	LDL reduction, %	CVD event reduction: relative risk (95% CI)	Overall mortality: relative risk (95% CI)
4S	1994	187	4444 men and women, mean age 59	Simvastatin, titration	5.4	35	0.58 (0.46–0.73)	0.70 (0.58–0.85)
CARE	1996	139	4159 men and women, mean age 59	Pravastatin 40 mg	5.0	28	0.76 (0.64–0.91)	0.91 (0.74–1.12)
LIPID	1998	150	9014 men and women, age 31–75	Pravastatin 40 mg	6.1	25	0.76 (0.65–0.88)	0.78 (0.69–0.87)
HPS	2002	132	20,526 men and women, age 40–80	Simvastatin 40 mg	5.5	29	0.83 (0.75–0.91)	0.87 (0.81–0.94)
PROSPER	2002	147	5804 men and women, age 70–82	Pravastatin 40 mg	3.2	34	0.85 (0.74–0.97)	—
GREACE	2002	180	1600 men and women, mean age 58	Atorvastatin 10–80 mg	3.0	46	0.49 (0.27–0.73)	0.57 (0.39–0.78)
ASCOT	2003	133	19.342 men and women, age 40–79	Atorvastatin 10 mg	3.3	29	0.64 (0.50–0.83)	0.87 (0.71–1.06)

Figure 8-24.

Major randomized clinical trials of cholesterol-lowering therapy with statins in the secondary prevention of cardiovascular events among stable patients with atherosclerotic vascular disease. These trials have studied the effect of low-density lipoprotein (LDL) cholesterol-lowering therapy with statins on the prevention of recurrent cardiovascular events relative to placebo and dietary counseling. Patients with documented atherosclerotic vascular disease were enrolled, primarily patients with coronary artery disease and prior myocardial infarction, but also patients with stroke or symptomatic peripheral arterial disease, depending on the trial. Patients were observed for an extended period of time (3–6 years) for the development of recurrent vascular events or death. Each of these clinical trials demonstrated a significant reduction in the relative risk of death or a recurrent cardiovascular event among patients randomized to active therapy. In general, the magnitude of reduction in LDL cholesterol correlates with increasing reduction in relative risk of death or a major cardiovascular event. In one meta-analysis of the published primary and secondary prevention trials of cholesterol-lowering therapy (including statins, diet, and other pharmacologic agents), it was estimated that for every 10 percentage points of cholesterol lowering, there is an associated 15% reduction in death from coronary artery disease and an 11% reduction in all cause mortality [37]. 4S–Scandinavian Simvastatin Survival Study; ASCOT—Anglo-Scandinavian Cardiac Outcomes Trial-Lipid Lowering Arm; CARE—Coronary Events after Myocardial Infarction in Patients with Average Cholesterol Levels; CVD—cardiovascular disease; GREACE—Greek Atorvastatin and Coronary Heart Disease Evaluation; HPS—Heart Protection Study; LIPID—Long-Term Intervention with Pravastatin in Ischemic Disease; PROSPER—Prospective Study of Pravastatin in the Elderly at Risk. (*Adapted from* Scranton and Gaziano [3].)

Results of the Heart Protection Study: Low-density Lipoprotein Cholesterol

Presenting feature	Simvastatin-allocated	Placebo-allocated	Heterogeneity or trend χ_2
LDL cholesterol, *mg/dL*			
< 116	598/3389 (17.6%)	756/3404 (22.2%)	0.10
116 to < 135	484/2549 (19.0%)	646/2514 (25.7%)	
135 or greater	951/4331 (22.0%)	1183/4349 (27.2%)	

Figure 8-25.

Statins reduce risk of a first major vascular event in high-risk patients regardless of baseline low-density lipoprotein (LDL) cholesterol: results of the Heart Protection Study [38]. Twenty thousand five hundred and eight-six patients were enrolled on the basis of one or more of the following high-risk features: coronary artery disease, cardiovascular disease, peripheral artery disease, diabetes mellitus (type 1 or type 2), or hypertension in elderly men. Patients were enrolled regardless of LDL cholesterol level, as long as their total cholesterol was greater than 135 mg/dL. Patients were randomized to receive simvastatin 40 mg daily or placebo, as well as antioxidant vitamins or placebo, in a two-by-two factorial design. Patients were observed for a median of 5 years. Among patients randomized to simvastatin, there was a 13% reduction in all-cause mortality and a 17% reduction in vascular death. Overall, there was a significant 24% reduction in the incidence of first major vascular event (*ie*, myocardial infarction, stroke, or revascularization) among patients randomized to simvastatin. As illustrated in this figure, the benefit of simvastatin for the prevention of first major vascular event was present regardless of baseline LDL cholesterol level at the time of enrollment. Based on these data, it is recommended that all patients with atherosclerotic vascular disease, diabetes mellitus, or high-risk cardiovascular profile be treated with statins for the prevention of cardiovascular events, regardless of baseline LDL cholesterol level. (*Adapted from* [38].)

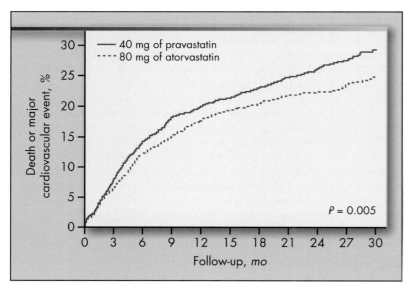

Figure 8-26.

Intensive lipid-lowering therapy with atorvastatin prevents recurrent cardiovascular events in patients with acute coronary syndromes (Pravastatin or Atorvastatin Evaluation and Infection Therapy [PROVE IT]–Thrombolysis in Myocardial Infarction [TIMI]-22 trial) [5]. The extensive statin database has formulated a number of new questions, including that of the ideal low-density lipoprotein (LDL) level in a patient post-myocardial infarction. In this study, 4162 patients were enrolled within 10 days of an acute coronary syndrome (*ie*, high-risk unstable angina, ST or non-ST segment elevation myocardial infarction), regardless of baseline cholesterol values or whether or not they were currently taking a statin drug. Patients were randomized to receive pravastatin 40 mg daily or atorvastatin 80 mg day and were observed for 24 months for the development of one of the following clinical events: death, myocardial infarction, unstable angina, coronary revascularization (30 days after randomization), and stroke. Mean on-treatment LDL cholesterol levels were 95 mg/dL in the pravastatin group and 62 mg/dL in the atorvastatin group. After a mean 24 months of follow-up, patients randomized to atorvastatin had a 16% reduction in the incidence of major cardiovascular events (26.3% pravastatin vs 22.4% atorvastatin). Given the findings of this trial and other new data, such as the findings of the Heart Protection Study, the National Cholesterol Education Program (NCEP) has recommended intensive therapy with statins to a target LDL cholesterol of less than 70 mg/dL for high-risk patients, including those with recent acute coronary syndrome [6]. (*Adapted from* Cannon et al. [5].)

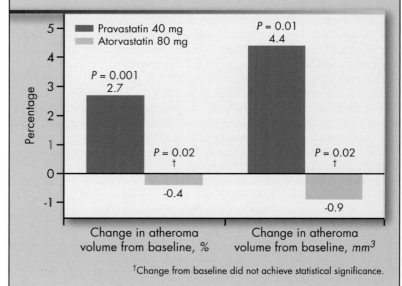

†Change from baseline did not achieve statistical significance.

Figure 8-27.

Intensive lipid-lowering therapy with atorvastatin reduces progression of coronary atherosclerosis: results of the Reversal of Atherosclerosis with Aggressive Lipid Lowering (REVERSAL) trial [39]. In this study, 654 patients with symptomatic coronary artery disease who underwent coronary angiography were randomized to receive pravastatin 40 mg daily or atorvastatin 80 mg daily. Patients underwent coronary intravascular ultrasound (IVUS) assessment at baseline and after 18 months of drug therapy. IVUS images were available for 502 patients. After 18 months of drug therapy, the median low-density lipoprotein (LDL) cholesterol in the pravastatin group was 110 mg/dL, compared with 79 mg/dL in the atorvastatin group. The primary endpoint of the study was the percent change in coronary atheroma volume, as determined by IVUS. Although there was significant progression in atheroma volume among patients randomized to pravastatin, patients randomized to atorvastatin did not have progressive atheroma. A subset of patients randomized to atorvastatin demonstrated significant regression of coronary atheroma. This study provides evidence to support the recommendation of a target LDL cholesterol of less than 70 mg/dL for patients with stable coronary artery disease, although clinical outcome trials in this population are ongoing. (*Adapted from* Nissen et al. [39].)

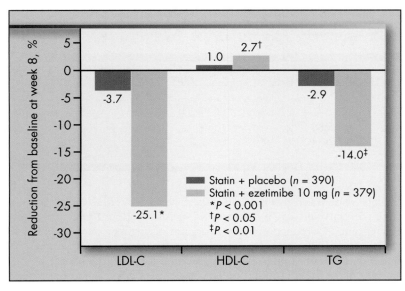

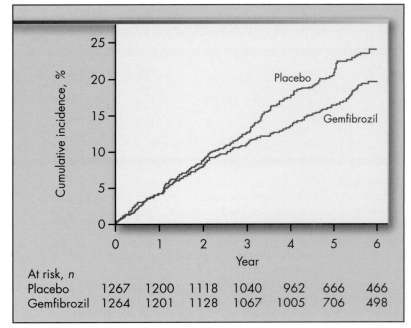

Figure 8-28.

Combination therapy with ezetimibe and statin further reduces low-density lipoprotein (LDL) cholesterol compared with statin monotherapy [40]. In this randomized trial, 769 patients with primary hypercholesterolemia who failed to meet LDL cholesterol treatment goal after at least 6 weeks of statin monotherapy were randomized to combination therapy with ezetimibe (10 mg) or placebo. Patients were observed for a total of 8 weeks. Combination therapy with statin and ezetimibe was associated with a highly statistically significant reduction in LDL cholesterol of an additional 25.1%. There was also a substantial reduction in triglycerides and a modest increase in HDL cholesterol with combination therapy. In a second placebo-controlled trial of placebo, ezetimibe, simvastatin, or combination therapy in patients with primary hypercholesterolemia, ezetimibe monotherapy was associated with a 19.1% reduction in LDL cholesterol compared with placebo [41]. To date, no trials have demonstrated a clinical benefit of ezetimibe in terms of prevention of cardiovascular events (*ie*, myocardial infarction, stroke, or mortality). As such, ezetimibe should be considered as an adjunctive therapy for patients who have not achieved target LDL cholesterol despite adequate doses of statins, or for patients who are intolerant of statins due to documented adverse events. (*Adapted from* Gagne *et al.* [40].)

Figure 8-29.

Gemfibrozil prevents recurrent cardiovascular events among patients with coronary artery disease and low high-density lipoprotein (HDL) cholesterol, results of the Veterans Affairs HDL Intervention Trial (VA-HIT) study [42]. Two thousand five hundred and thirty-one male Veterans with coronary artery disease and HDL cholesterol less than 40 mg/dL were randomized to receive gemfibrozil (600 mg twice daily) or placebo and observed for a median of 5.1 years. Patients were required to have a low-density lipoprotein (LDL) cholesterol of less than 140 mg/dL. Among patients randomized to gemfibrozil, there was a 22% reduction in the relative risk of death from coronary heart disease or non-fatal myocardial infarction. The mean HDL cholesterol was 32 mg/dL in the placebo and gemfibrozil groups at baseline. HDL cholesterol increased by only 6% in the gemfibrozil group (to 34 mg/dL), despite the substantial decrease in the incidence of cardiovascular events. There was no significant change in LDL cholesterol among patients randomized to gemfibrozil. (*Adapted from* Rubins *et al.* [42].)

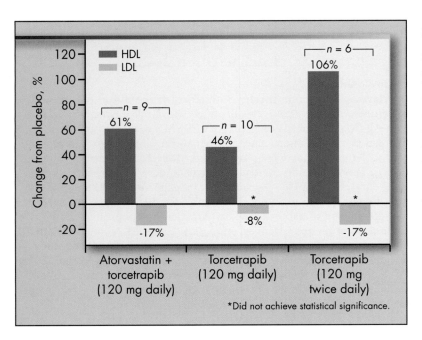

Figure 8-30.

The cholesteryl ester transfer protein (CETP) inhibitor torcetrapib increases high-density lipoprotein (HDL) cholesterol alone or in combination with atorvastatin [43]. Nineteen nonsmokers (mean age 50 years) with low HDL cholesterol (mean 33 mg/dL) were enrolled in this single-blind crossover study. Patients received torcetrapib (120 mg daily) for 4 weeks after a 4-week placebo phase. Patients with low-density lipoprotein (LDL) cholesterol greater than 160 mg/dL also received atorvastatin 20 mg daily. A subset of patients who did not require atorvastatin received high-dose torcetrapib (120 mg twice daily) for an additional 4 weeks. Torcetrapib was associated with a dramatic and highly statistically significant increase in HDL cholesterol compared with placebo. Torcetrabip also significantly increased levels of apolipoprotein AI and AII. The clinical impact of this change in HDL is not yet established. This drug, which is not yet commercially available, is currently undergoing clinical trials.

Treatment Goals for Hypercholesterolemia from the National Cholesterol Education Program Expert Panel on Detection, Evaluation, and Treatment of High Blood Pressure in Adults

Risk category	LDL-C goal	Initiate TLC	Consider drug therapy
High risk: CHD or CHD risk equivalents	< 100 mg/dL (optional goal: < 70 mg/dL)	100 mg/dL or greater	100 mg/dL or greater (< 100 mg/dL: consider drug options)
Moderately high risk: Two or more risk factors (10-year risk 10% to 20%)	< 130 mg/dL	130 mg/dL or greater	130 mg/dL or greater (100–129 mg/dL: consider drug options)
Moderate risk: Two or more risk factors (10-year risk < 10%)	< 130 mg/dL	130 mg/dL or greater	160 mg/dL or greater
Low risk: 0 to one risk factor	< 160 mg/dL	160 mg/dL or greater	190 mg/dL or greater (160–189 mg/dL: LDL-lowering drug optional)

Figure 8-31.

Updated treatment goals for hypercholesterolemia from the National Cholesterol Education Program (NCEP) Expert Panel on Detection, Evaluation, and Treatment of High Blood Pressure in Adults (Adult Treatment Panel III 2004 update) [6,44]. Coronary heart disease (CHD) includes myocardial infarction, unstable angina, stable angina, prior coronary artery revascularization procedure, or evidence of significant myocardial ischemia (eg, by noninvasive testing). CHD risk equivalents include diabetes mellitus and significant atherosclerotic vascular disease in non-coronary arterial beds (eg, peripheral artery disease, cardiovascular disease, abdominal aortic aneurysm). Risk factors for cardiovascular disease include tobacco smoking, hypertension, low high-density lipoprotein (HDL) cholesterol, family history of premature coronary artery disease, and advanced age (mean ages 45 and older, women ages 55 and older). For patients at the highest risk of a cardiovascular event, particularly those patients with recent acute coronary syndrome, the low-density lipoprotein cholesterol (LDL-C) target should be less than 70 mg/dL. Ten-year risk of a cardiovascular event can be calculated using the Framingham Risk Score or the European Risk Score [45,46]. TLC—therapeutic lifestyle changes. (*Adapted from* Grundy *et al.* [6] and the National Cholesterol Education Program [44].)

References

1. Genest J, Libby P, Gotto AM: Lipoprotein disorders and cardiovascular disease. In *Braunwald's Heart Disease: A Textbook of Cardiovascular Medicine.* Philadelphia: Elsevier-Saunders; 2005.

2. Verschuren WM, Jacobs DR, Bloemberg BP, *et al.*: Serum total cholesterol and long-term coronary heart disease mortality in different cultures. Twenty-five-year follow-up of the seven countries study. *JAMA* 1995, 274:131–136.

3. Scranton R, Gaziano J: Cholesterol reduction. In *Clinical Trials in Heart Disease: A Companion to Braunwald's Heart Disease.* Edited by Manson J. Philadelphia: Elsevier-Saunders; 2004.

4. Heart Protection Study Collaborative Group: MRC/BHF Heart Protection Study of cholesterol lowering with simvastatin in 20,536 high-risk individuals: a randomised placebo-controlled trial. *Lancet* 2002, 360:7–22.

5. Cannon CP, Braunwald E, McCabe CH, *et al.*: Intensive versus moderate lipid lowering with statins after acute coronary syndromes. *N Engl J Med* 2004, 350:1495–1504.

6. Grundy SM, Cleeman JI, Merz CN, *et al.*: Implications of recent clinical trials for the National Cholesterol Education Program Adult Treatment Panel III guidelines. *Circulation* 2004, 110:227–239.

7. Brewer HB Jr: Increasing HDL cholesterol levels. *N Engl J Med* 2004, 350:1491–1494.

8. Bhatnagar D: Hypertriglyceridemia. In *Lipoproteins in Health and Disease.* Edited by Betteridge DJ, Illingworth DR, and Shepherd J. London: Oxford University Press; 1999.

9. Galton D, Krone W: *Hyperlipidemia in Practice.* London: Gower Medical Publishing; 1991.

10. Brown MS, Goldstein JL: Receptor-mediated endocytosis: insights from the lipoprotein receptor system. *Proc Natl Acad Sci U S A* 1979, 76:3330–3337.

11. Brown MS, Goldstein JL: How LDL receptors influence cholesterol and atherosclerosis. *Sci Am* 1984, 251:58–66.

12. Brown MS, Goldstein JL: The LDL receptor and the regulation of cellular cholesterol metabolism. *J Cell Sci Suppl* 1985, 3:131–137.

13. Brown MS, Goldstein JL: Regulation of the mevalonate pathway. *Nature* 1990, 343:425–430.

14. Beaumont JL, Cooper GR, Fejfar Z, *et al.*: Classification of hyperlipidemias and hyperlipoproteinemias. *Bull World Health Organ* 1970, 43:891–915.

15. Online Mendelian Inheritance in Man, OMIM. McKusick-Nathans Institute for Genetic Medicine, Johns Hopkins University, Baltimore, MD, and National Center for Biotechnology Information, National Library of Medicine, Bethesda, MD; 2000. Available at http://www.ncbi.nlm.nih.gov/omim/.

16. Craig WY, Neveux LM, Palomaki GE, *et al.*: Lipoprotein(a) as a risk factor for ischemic heart disease: metaanalysis of prospective studies. *Clin Chem* 1998, 44:2301–2306.

17. Winder AF, Jolleys JC, Day LB, Butowski PF: Corneal arcus, case finding and definition of individual clinical risk in heterozygous familial hypercholesterolemia. *Clin Genet* 1998, 54:497–502.

18. Franceschini G, Sirtori CR, Capurso A II, *et al.*: A-IMilano apoprotein. Decreased high density lipoprotein cholesterol levels with significant lipoprotein modifications and without clinical atherosclerosis in an Italian family. *J Clin Invest* 1980, 66:892–900.

19. Nissen SE, Tsunoda T, Tuzcu EM, *et al.*: Effect of recombinant ApoA-I Milano on coronary atherosclerosis in patients with acute coronary syndromes: a randomized controlled trial. *JAMA* 2003, 290:2292–2300.

20. Singaraja RR, Brunham LR, Visscher H, *et al.*: Efflux and atherosclerosis: the clinical and biochemical impact of variations in the ABCA1 gene. *Arterioscler Thromb Vasc Biol* 2003, 23:1322–1332.

21. ALLHAT Officers and Coordinators for the ALLHAT Collaborative Research Group. The Antihypertensive and Lipid-Lowering Treatment to Prevent Heart Attack Trial: Major outcomes in high-risk hypertensive patients randomized to angiotensin-converting enzyme inhibitor or calcium channel blocker vs diuretic: the Antihypertensive and Lipid-Lowering Treatment to Prevent Heart Attack Trial (ALLHAT). *JAMA* 2002, 288:2981–2997.

22. MRC/BHF Heart Protection Study of cholesterol lowering with simvastatin in 20,536 high-risk individuals: a randomised placebo-controlled trial. *Lancet* 2002, 360:7–22.

23. Glass CK, Witztum JL: Atherosclerosis: the road ahead. *Cell* 2001, 104:503–516.

24. Hirsch AT, Criqui MH, Treat-Jacobson D, *et al.*: Peripheral arterial disease detection, awareness, and treatment in primary care. *JAMA* 2001, 286:1317–1324.

25. Stamler J, Wentworth D, Neaton JD: Is relationship between serum cholesterol and risk of premature death from coronary heart disease continuous and graded? Findings in 356,222 primary screenees of the Multiple Risk Factor Intervention Trial (MRFIT). *JAMA* 1986, 256:2823–2828.

26. Castelli WP, Garrison RJ, Wilson PW, *et al.*: Incidence of coronary heart disease and lipoprotein cholesterol levels. The Framingham Study. *JAMA* 1986, 256:2835–2838.

27. Criqui MH, Heiss G, Cohn R, *et al.*: Plasma triglyceride level and mortality from coronary heart disease. *N Engl J Med* 1993, 328:1220–1225.

28. Stampfer MJ, Krauss RM, Ma J, *et al.*: A prospective study of triglyceride level, low-density lipoprotein particle diameter, and risk of myocardial infarction. *JAMA* 1996, 276:882–888.

29. Hokanson JE, Austin MA: Plasma triglyceride level is a risk factor for cardiovascular disease independent of high-density lipoprotein cholesterol level: a meta-analysis of population-based prospective studies. *J Cardiovasc Risk* 1996, 3:213–219.

30. Opie L, Gersh BJ: *Drugs for the Heart*. Philadelphia: WB Saunders; 2001.

31. Knopp RH: Drug treatment of lipid disorders. *N Engl J Med* 1999, 341:498–511.

32. Jones PH, Davidson MH, Stein EA, *et al.*: Comparison of the efficacy and safety of rosuvastatin versus atorvastatin, simvastatin, and pravastatin across doses (STELLAR* Trial). *Am J Cardiol* 2003, 92:152–160.

33. Schachter M: Chemical, pharmacokinetic and pharmacodynamic properties of statins: an update. *Fundam Clin Pharmacol* 2005, 19:117–125.

34. Katan MB, Grundy SM, Jones P, *et al.*: Efficacy and safety of plant stanols and sterols in the management of blood cholesterol levels. *Mayo Clin Proc* 2003, 78:965–978.

35. Buchwald H, Varco RL, Matts JP, *et al.*: Effect of partial ileal bypass surgery on mortality and morbidity from coronary heart disease in patients with hypercholesterolemia. Report of the Program on the Surgical Control of the Hyperlipidemias (POSCH). *N Engl J Med* 1990, 323:946–955.

36. Pignone M, Phillips C, Mulrow C: Use of lipid lowering drugs for primary prevention of coronary heart disease: meta-analysis of randomised trials. *BMJ* 2000, 321:983–936.

37. Gould AL, Rossouw JE, Santanello NC, *et al.*: Cholesterol reduction yields clinical benefit: impact of statin trials. *Circulation* 1998, 97:946–952.

38. MRC/BHF Heart Protection Study of antioxidant vitamin supplementation in 20,536 high-risk individuals: a randomised placebo-controlled trial. *Lancet* 2002, 360:23–33.

39. Nissen SE, Tuzcu EM, Schoenhagen P, *et al.*: Effect of intensive compared with moderate lipid-lowering therapy on progression of coronary atherosclerosis: a randomized controlled trial. *JAMA* 2004, 291:1071–1080.

40. Gagne C, Bays HE, Weiss SR, *et al.*: Efficacy and safety of ezetimibe added to ongoing statin therapy for treatment of patients with primary hypercholesterolemia. *Am J Cardiol* 2002, 90:1084–1091.

41. Davidson MH, McGarry T, Bettis R, *et al.*: Ezetimibe coadministered with simvastatin in patients with primary hypercholesterolemia. *J Am Coll Cardiol* 2002, 40:2125–2134.

42. Rubins HB, Robins SJ, Collins D, *et al.*: Gemfibrozil for the secondary prevention of coronary heart disease in men with low levels of high-density lipoprotein cholesterol. Veterans Affairs High-Density Lipoprotein Cholesterol Intervention Trial Study Group. *N Engl J Med* 1999, 341:410–418.

43. Brousseau ME, Schaefer EJ, Wolfe ML, *et al.*: Effects of an inhibitor of cholesteryl ester transfer protein on HDL cholesterol. *N Engl J Med* 2004, 350:1505–1515.

44. National Cholesterol Education Program: *Third Report of the Expert Panel on Detection, Evaluation, and Treatment of High Blood Cholesterol in Adults (Adult Treatment Panel III) Executive Summary*. Bethesda: National Heart, Lung, and Blood Institute; 2001.

45. Wilson PW, D'Agostino RB, Levy D, *et al.*: Prediction of coronary heart disease using risk factor categories. *Circulation* 1998, 97:1837–1847.

46. Conroy RM, Pyorala K, Fitzgerald AP, *et al.*: Estimation of ten-year risk of fatal cardiovascular disease in Europe: the SCORE project. *Eur Heart J* 2003, 24:987–1003.

Diabetes/Diabetes Prevention

Karin Nelson, Gayle Reiber, and Edward Boyko

Diabetes is an increasingly common disorder in the United States, affecting almost 5% of the adult population. Type 2 diabetes accounts for over 90% of all cases and is linked to the epidemic of obesity in the United States [1]. Coronary heart disease (CHD) is the number one cause of mortality among individuals with diabetes [2]. Diabetes predisposes to worse outcomes when cardiovascular (CV) complications occur, with increased mortality of patients with acute myocardial infarction and heart failure [3]. In-hospital and long-term mortality rates after acute myocardial infarction are twice as high among individuals with diabetes as among those without diabetes [4]. This excess risk may be in part from the increased prevalence of other CHD risk factors.

Individuals with diabetes have higher incidence of known CV risk factors, including dyslipidemia, hypertension, obesity, and renal insufficiency. In the past decade CV risk factor profiles have worsened, with increased rates of obesity, high blood pressure, and high blood cholesterol among individuals with diabetes [5]. Hypertension affects more than 60% of individuals with type 2 diabetes, with multiple factors, including obesity, insulin resistance, hyperinsulinemia, and renal disease contributing to the increased incidence [6].

Recent evidence has provided strong support for more aggressive management of CV disease risk factors for the primary prevention of CHD among individuals with diabetes [7]. Several interventions, including pharmacotherapy for controlling blood pressure and cholesterol values, and aspirin, can lower the risk for CV disease. Behavioral interventions, such as diet, physical activity, and cessation of smoking, are also extremely important. Cigarette smoking is strongly associated with an increased risk of CHD among individuals with diabetes, even more so than individuals without diabetes, and quitting smoking decreases this excess risk substantially [8]. The majority of patients with type 2 diabetes are overweight [9]. Although it is widely accepted that most patients with type 2 diabetes need to lose weight, there is no universal agreement on the most desirable or efficacious diet prescription [9]. Moderate levels of physical activity are associated with a decreased risk of CV disease among individuals with diabetes [10,11].

Clinical trials of lipid management and blood pressure control suggest that the benefit of treatment may be greater for individuals with diabetes than those without diabetes. Lipid-lowering with pharmacologic treatment can decrease CV events 22% to 24%, with higher absolute risk reductions among those with known CHD [12]. A recent meta-analysis of pharmacologic lipid-lowering therapy found a significant reduction for the primary prevention of cardiovascular outcomes (relative risk 0.78, 95% CI 0.67–0.89) [12]. In addition, the Heart Protection Study (HPS) has shown that simvastatin significantly reduced the risk of major vascular events for diabetic individuals without coronary disease at normal initial low-density lipoprotein (LDL) concentrations [13]. Because of this and other recent studies, the presence of diabetes has recently been added to the National Cholesterol Education Program (NCEP) as an independent risk factor for CV disease [14]. Although the NCEP recommends treating to an LDL of less than 100 mg/dL, the clinical trial data does not clearly support this level [12]. The benefits of the statins, or 3- hydroxymethylglutaryl coenzyme A reductase inhibitors, may not be mediated through lowering LDL cholesterol levels, leading some authors to question whether goals of treatment should be expressed in LDL cholesterol concentrations, or whether a fixed dose of a statin should be given [15]. Some experts suggest that all patients with type 2 diabetes should be given a statin, regardless of their cholesterol value [16]. Most studies do not address whether treating the common combination of high triglycerides and low high-density lipoprotein (HDL) cholesterol levels in addition to LDL provides additional benefit. A subgroup analysis of a study of gemfibrozil compared with placebo suggests that raising HDL cholesterol and lowering triglycerides also has a beneficial role in preventing coronary artery disease in patients with low HDL and elevated triglycerides, lipid abnormalities common among individuals with type 2 diabetes [17].

Hypertension is a major risk factor for diabetic complications and blood pressure control is one of the most important components of therapy. Multiple studies have shown that treatment of hypertension is efficacious [18,19]. A recent meta-analysis of blood pressure–lowering trials among individuals with diabetes found a large, significant effect (relative risk 0.73, 95% CI 0.57–0.94) for aggregate cardiovascular events (CHD death and nonfatal myocardial infarction) [20]. The United Kingdom Prospective Diabetes Study (UKPDS) among over 3600 patients with type 2 diabetes showed an inverse correlation between the mean systolic blood pressure and aggregate endpoints related to diabetes [21]. The UKPDS trial demonstrated that a 10-point reduction in systolic blood pressure, from 154 mm Hg to 144 mm Hg, led to a substantial decrease in diabetes related mortality. The Hypertension Optimal Treatment (HOT) trial demonstrated improved outcomes in patients assigned to lower diastolic blood

pressure targets. A four-point difference in diastolic blood pressure, from 85 mm Hg to 81 mm Hg, resulted in a 50% decrease in risk for CV events in patients with diabetes [22]. Based on this strong clinical trial data, the recommended target blood pressure goal is between 135/80 and 130/80 mm Hg for individuals with diabetes [18,23], although systolic targets have not been as rigorously evaluated as diastolic targets [24].

Diabetes-specific CHD risk factors include the duration of disease, microalbuminuria and possibly hyperglycemia. Microalbuminuria is considered an early manifestation of diabetic nephropathy and screening for albuminuria identifies individuals at high risk for CV events [25]. Because diabetes is considered an independent risk factor for coronary disease, most patients should be on a daily aspirin. The American Diabetes Association currently recommends aspirin as a primary prevention strategy in men and women with diabetes who are at increased CV risk, including those over the age of 40 years or who have additional CV risk factors [26]. Although a recent meta-analysis of observational studies suggests a modest relationship between HbA_{1c} and CV disease, the role of intensive glucose lowering in the primary prevention of CV events remains unclear [27].

Despite the proven benefit of CV risk factor reduction, there is evidence of poor risk factor control and lifestyle modifications among individuals with diabetes [28,29]. A recent national survey reported that over 35% of individuals with diabetes had a blood pressure over 140/90 mm Hg and 58% had LDL cholesterol levels over 130 mg/dL [30]. Only 7% of individuals with diabetes had achieved the recommended level for blood pressure, lipids, and glucose control [28]. According to US data, a gap exists between recommended diabetes care and the care patients actually receive [30]. Future challenges will include translating important research findings about multiple risk factor control into general clinical practice to improve health outcomes of individuals with diabetes.

Prevalence/Incidence

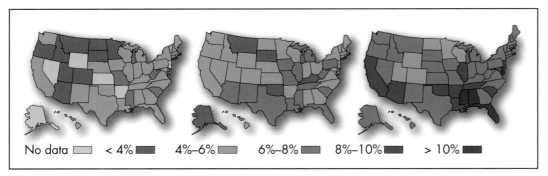

No data ▢   < 4% ▣   4%–6% ▣   6%–8% ▣   8%–10% ▣   > 10% ▣

Figure 9-1. Increasing prevalence of diabetes in the United States, 1990 to 2001. Data from this figure, obtained from the Centers for Disease Control, show the dramatic increase in rates of diabetes over the past decade. Although the magnitude of the increase varied, the prevalence of diagnosed diabetes among adults increased in every state in the United States. Type 2 diabetes is one of the most common chronic medical conditions and accounts for over 90% of the cases of diabetes. Studies of estimates of type 1 diabetes are limited and do not show a consistent pattern of increase or decrease in prevalence [2]. The rise in the rates of diabetes has mirrored the sharp increase in rates of obesity in the United States [1]. Obesity and lifestyle factors, especially excess calorie and fat intake and low levels of physical activity, are considered central causes of type 2 diabetes [31].

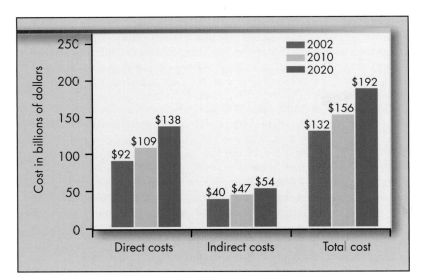

Figure 9-2.
Economic burden of diabetes. In 2002, per capita medical expenditures total $13,243 for people with diabetes and $2560 for people without diabetes. When adjusting for differences in age, gender, and race/ethnicity between the populations with and without diabetes, people with diabetes spend 2.4 to 2.6 times more in medical costs than does a person without diabetes [32]. Adults with diabetes have high rates of other comorbid diseases, such as hypertension and dyslipidemia, and higher rates of cardiovascular disease than the general population. Excess health care expenditures in individuals with diabetes are largely related to treating these long-term complications. Using current diabetes prevalence rates applied to Census Bureau populations projections, the national cost of diabetes could grow to $156 billion by 2010 and $192 billion by 2020, as shown in this figure. (*Adapted from* Hogan *et al.* [33].)

Associated Risk

Increased Rates of Cardiovascular Risks Among Individuals with Diabetes

Risk factor	Undiagnosed diabetes	IPH	No diabetes
Age, *y*	57.8	62.4	53.7
Total cholesterol, *mg/dL*	216	230	215
HDL, *mg/dL*	41	51	51
LDL, *mg/dL*	131	139	137
TG, *mg/dL*	245	199	143
HbA$_{1c}$, %	7.1	5.6	5.3
BMI, *kg/m²*	31.5	29.1	27.0

Figure 9-3.
Increased rates of cardiovascular risks among individuals with diabetes. Individuals with diabetes and impaired glucose tolerance have higher rates of other cardiovascular disease risk factors than nondiabetic individuals. This table presents data from the Third National Health and Nutrition Examination Survey, a nationally representative sample of US adults. Values shown are the weighted mean levels of HbA$_{1c}$ and established cardiovascular disease risk factors among people with undiagnosed diabetes (fasting glucose 126 mg/dL or greater), isolated postchallenge hyperglycemia ([IPH] fasting glucose < 126 mg/dL and oral glucose tolerance test > 200 mg/dL), and nondiabetic individuals. Individuals with diabetes and IPH have unfavorable lipid profiles, glycemic control, and body mass index (BMI) values compared with individuals without diabetes. HDL—high-density lipoprotein; LDL—low-density lipoprotein; TG—triglycerides. (*Adapted from* Resnick *et al.* [34].)

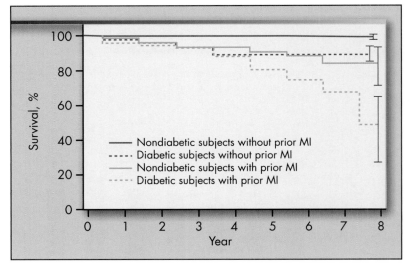

Figure 9-4.
Increased mortality from myocardial infarction (MI) among individuals with diabetes. Diabetes is now considered an independent risk factor for cardiovascular disease. This figure shows data from a study by Haffner *et al.* [4], which compared the 7-year incidence of MI (fatal and nonfatal) among 1373 nondiabetic subjects with the incidence among 1059 diabetic subjects, all from a Finnish population-based study. The 7-year incidence rates of MI in nondiabetic subjects with and without prior MI at baseline were 18.8% and 3.5%, respectively (*P* < 0.001). The 7-year incidence rates of MI in diabetic subjects with and without prior MI at baseline were 45.0% and 20.2%, respectively (*P* < 0.001). The hazard ratio for death from coronary heart disease for diabetic subjects without prior MI compared with nondiabetic subjects with prior MI was not significantly different from 1.0 (hazard ratio 1.4; 95% CI, 0.7–2.6) after adjustment for age and gender, suggesting similar risks of infarction in the two groups. After further adjustment for total cholesterol, hypertension, and smoking, this hazard ratio remained close to 1.0 (hazard ratio, 1.2; 95% CI, 0.6–2.4). These data make a strong case for diabetes as an independent risk factor for coronary artery disease. (*Adapted from* Haffner *et al.* [4].)

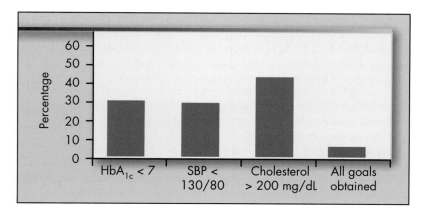

Figure 9-5.
Evidence for poor cardiovascular risk factor control among individuals with diabetes. Individuals with diabetes have higher rates of cardiovascular risk factors, and there is evidence to suggest poor cardiovascular risk factor control. This figure presents data from the National Health and Nutrition Examination Survey (NHANES), a population-based US sample. In NHANES 1999 to 2000, only 37.0% of participants achieved the target goal of HbA_{1c} level less than 7.0%, and 37.2% of participants were greater than the recommended "take action" HbA_{1c} level of greater than 8.0%. Only 35.8% of participants achieved the target of systolic blood pressure (SBP) less than 130 mm Hg and diastolic blood pressure (DBP) less than 80 mm Hg, and 40.4% had SBP greater than 140 mm Hg or DBP greater than 90 mmHg. Over half (51.8%) of the participants in NHANES 1999 to 2000 had total cholesterol levels of 200 mg/dL or greater.

Overall, the percentage of adults with diagnosed diabetes who achieved currently recommended goals of HbA_{1c} level, blood pressure, and total serum cholesterol was only 7.3%. (*Adapted from* Saydah *et al.* [28].)

Benefits of Intervention

Lifestyle

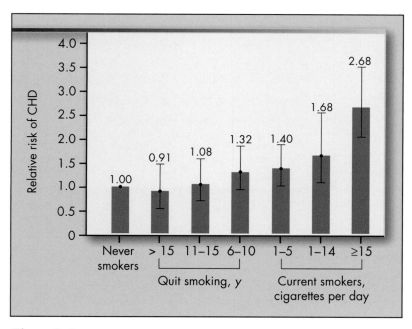

Figure 9-6.
Multivariate-adjusted relative risk of coronary heart disease (CHD) according to smoking status and duration of quitting smoking among diabetic women. All patients with diabetes who smoke should be strongly counseled about smoking cessation, because the adverse effects of smoking on CHD risk diminish over time. This figure shows the multivariate-adjusted relative risk of CHD according to smoking status from the Nurses' Health Study, a prospective cohort study of 121,700 female nurses surveyed in 11 states and observed from 1976 to 1996. This survey involved 6547 women with type 2 diabetes. This observational evidence and extrapolation from studies of individuals without diabetes suggest that smoking cessation is likely to reduce cardiovascular events among individuals with diabetes. (*Adapted from* Al-Delaimy *et al.* [8].)

	Fasting Plasma Lipids Comparing American Diabetes Association Diet with High-fiber Diet		
Variable	**ADA Diet, *mg/dL***	**High-fiber diet, *mg/dL***	**Differences between diets (95% CI)**
Total cholesterol	210	196	-14 (-27 to -2)*
Triglycerides	205	184	-21 (-37 to -4)*
VLDL	40	35	-5 (-9 to -1)*
LDL	142	133	-9 (-22 to 3)
HDL	29	28	-1 (-4 to 3)
*$P < 0.05$.			

Figure 9-7.
Dietary management. Dietary changes also are important to manage cardiovascular risk factors. For individuals with type 2 diabetes, the American Diabetes Association (ADA) recommends a diet low in saturated fat and high in fiber, similar to diets recommended to treat hyperlipidemia and hypertension. A high intake of dietary fiber has been shown to improve glycemic control and decrease insulin levels and plasma lipid concentrations in patients with type 2 diabetes. The data in this figure are from a small randomized trial in which participants were assigned to a diet containing moderate amounts of fiber (24 g), as recommended by the ADA, or a high-fiber diet (50 g). Both diets, prepared in a research kitchen, had the same macronutrient and energy content. The high-fiber diet reduced plasma total cholesterol concentrations by 6.7% ($P = 0.02$), triglyceride concentrations by 10.2% ($P = 0.02$), and very low-density lipoprotein (VLDL) cholesterol concentrations by 12.5% ($P = 0.01$). HDL—high density lipoprotein; LDL—low-density lipoprotein. (*Adapted from* Chandalia *et al.* [35].)

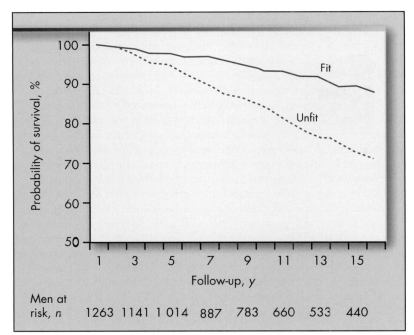

Men at
risk, n   1263 1141 1 014 887   783   660   533   440

Figure 9-8.
Survival curves for all-cause mortality by cardiorespiratory fitness
category. Several observational cohort studies have concluded that moderate levels of physical activity are associated with a decreased risk of cardiovascular disease among individuals with diabetes. This figure shows
data from a prospective cohort study conducted in a preventive medicine
clinic. Data are from 1263 men with type 2 diabetes, with 180 all-cause
deaths during 14,777 years of observation from 1970 to 1994.
Measurements were made by a maximal exercise test, self-reported physical inactivity at baseline, and subsequent death determined by using the
National Death Index. After adjustment for age, baseline cardiovascular
disease, fasting plasma glucose level, high cholesterol level, overweight,
current smoking, high blood pressure, and parental history of cardiovascular disease, men in the low-fitness group had an adjusted risk for all-
cause mortality of 2.1 (95% CI, 1.5–2.9) compared with fit men. Men
who reported being physically inactive had an adjusted risk for mortality
that was 1.7-fold (CI, 1.2-fold to 2.3-fold) higher than that in men who
reported being physically active. (*Adapted from* Wei *et al.* [11].)

Pharmacotherapy

Summary Statistics of the Effectiveness of Lipid-lowering Therapy in Diabetes

Category	Studies, *n*	Relative risk for CHD events (95% CI)	Absolute risk reduction in CHD events (95% CI)	Number needed to treat for benefit
Primary prevention	6	0.78 (0.67 to 0.89)	0.03 (0.01 to 0.04)	34.5
Secondary prevention	8	0.76 (0.59 to 0.93)	0.07 (0.03 to 0.12)	13.8

Figure 9-9.
Effectiveness of lipid-lowering therapy in diabetes. Based on a recent
systematic review of the evidence, the American College of Physicians
adopted several recommendations for the treatment of hyperlipidemia
among individuals with type 2 diabetes based on the evidence
presented in this table. The recommendations are 1) lipid-lowering
therapy should be used for secondary prevention of coronary artery disease for all patients with diabetes mellitus and coronary artery disease;
2) statins should be used for primary prevention against macrovascular

complications in patients with type 2 diabetes and other cardiovascular
risk factors; and 3) patients with diabetes should be taking at least a
moderate dose of a statin. These recommendations are based on the
data in this table, which found a pooled relative risk deduction of 22%
for primary prevention and 24% for secondary prevention, among studies of lipid-lowering therapy in diabetes. CHD—coronary heart disease.
(*Adapted from* Vijan *et al.* [12].)

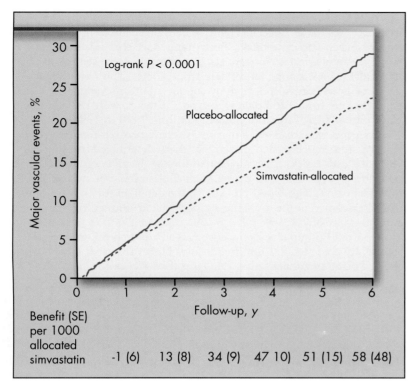

| Benefit (SE) per 1000 allocated simvastatin | -1 (6) | 13 (8) | 34 (9) | 47 10) | 51 (15) | 58 (48) |

Figure 9-10.

Cholesterol lowering. The results of the landmark Heart Protection Study are shown in this figure. Most other randomized controlled trials of primary prevention of cardiovascular disease enrolled few subjects with diabetes. This randomized controlled trial is the largest to date, enrolling over 5900 patients over age 40 with diabetes and a total cholesterol of 135 mg/dL or greater. Participants were randomized to receive placebo or simvastatin. The graph plots the effects of simvastatin allocation on percentages of diabetic participants having major vascular events. Approximately 25% of the placebo-allocated participants had a first major vascular event during 5 years of follow-up, compared with only 20% of those allocated to simvastatin. There was a relative risk reduction in the simvastatin group of 26% for major coronary events. The reduction in cardiovascular disease was similar across all low-density lipoprotein (LDL) subcategories, including among those with LDL cholesterol levels of less than 116 mg/dL. This study provides evidence that cholesterol-lowering therapy is beneficial for people with diabetes for primary prevention of coronary artery disease, even if they do not have high LDL cholesterol concentrations. It is clear that any lowering of LDL or total cholesterol should be attempted in most patients with diabetes. This large clinical trial solidifies the evidence for treating almost all individuals with diabetes with a statin and has generated debate about the need for cholesterol measurement and treatment targets. (*Adapted from* Heart Protection Study Collaborative Group [13].)

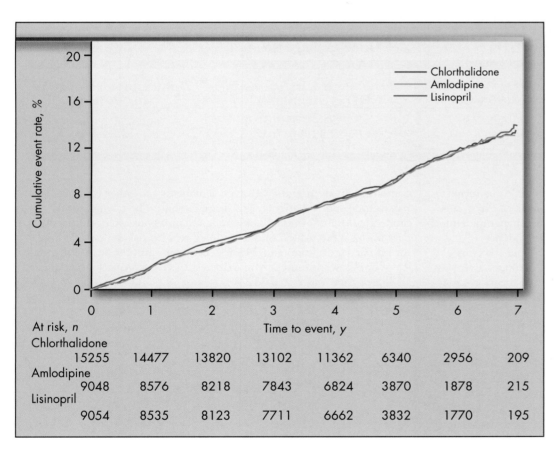

At risk, n							
Chlorthalidone							
15255	14477	13820	13102	11362	6340	2956	209
Amlodipine							
9048	8576	8218	7843	6824	3870	1878	215
Lisinopril							
9054	8535	8123	7711	6662	3832	1770	195

Figure 9-11.

Treatment of hypertension. Large, randomized, controlled trials including individuals with diabetes have found significant benefit to control diastolic pressures less than 80 mm Hg or less to reduce major cardiovascular events.

Systematic reviews and randomized controlled trials have found that angiotensin-converting enzyme inhibitors, diuretics, β-blockers, and calcium channel blockers all reduce cardiovascular comorbidity and mortality, but have different side effect profiles. No lower threshold for treatment of high blood pressure has been firmly identified. Most trials suggest that more than one agent is necessary. The Antihypertensive and Lipid-Lowering Treatment to Prevent Heart Attack Trial (ALLHAT) is the largest study to date (*n* = 12,063) of people with diabetes (out of a total study population of *n* = 33,657, or 36% of the total study population). ALLHAT found that there were no significant differences between lisinopril, amlodipine, or chlorthalidone in 6-year rates of combined fatal coronary heart disease or nonfatal myocardial infarction. (*Adapted from* ALLHAT Officers and Coordinators for the ALLHAT Collaborative Research Group [36].)

Events in Patients with Diabetes Mellitus at Baseline in Relation to Target Blood Pressure Groups*

Event	Events, n	Events per 1000 patient-years	P value	Comparison	Relative risk (95% CI)
Major cardiovascular events					
90 mm Hg or less	45	24.4		90 vs 85	1.32 (0.84–2.06)
85 mm Hg or less	34	18.6		85 vs 80	1.56 (0.91–2.67)
80 mm Hg or less	22	11.9	0.005	90 vs 80	2.06 (1.24–3.44)
Cardiovascular mortality					
90 mm Hg or less	21	11.1		90 vs 85	0.99 (0.54–1.82)
85 mm Hg or less	21	11.2		85 vs 80	3.0 (1.29–7.13)
80 mm Hg or less	7	3.7	0.016	90 vs 80	3.0 (1.28–7.08)

*n = 501.501 and 499 in target groups< 90 mm Hg, < 85 mm Hg, and < 80 mm Hg, respectively.

Figure 9-12.

Target blood pressure. The United Kingdom Prospective Diabetes Study compared moderate reductions in blood pressure (< 180/105) to tighter control (< 150/85), and found that tighter control reduced rates of cardiovascular disease and stroke. The Systolic Hypertension in the Elderly Program study compared use of chlorthalidone, atenolol, and reserpine among older diabetic patients, and found a 34% risk reduction for 5-year rates of major cardiovascular disease among those in treatment groups compared with control subjects. This slide displays results from the Hypertension Optimal Treatment (HOT) study.

Patients with diabetes in the HOT trial experienced a 51% reduction in the relative risk of major cardiovascular events when randomized to a diastolic blood pressure of less than 80 mm Hg compared with less than 90 mm Hg. There was also a significant reduction in cardiovascular mortality. In this study, felodipine was given as the baseline therapy, with the addition of other agents, according to a five-step regimen that included angiotensin-converting enzyme inhibitors, β-blockers, and diuretics. In addition, half of the patients were assigned to receive aspirin or placebo. (*Adapted from* Hansson *et al.* [22].)

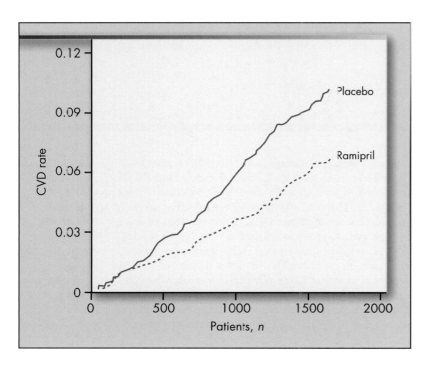

Figure 9-13.

Use of angiotensin-converting enzyme (ACE) inhibitors. The Heart Outcomes Prevention Evaluation (HOPE) study demonstrated the positive impact of ACE inhibitors on cardiovascular and microvascular outcomes in 3577 individuals with diabetes aged 55 years or older who had a previous cardiovascular event or at least one other cardiovascular risk factor, no clinical proteinuria, heart failure, or low ejection fraction, and who were not taking ACE inhibitors. These subjects were randomly assigned to the ACE inhibitor ramipril (10 mg/d) or placebo and vitamin E or placebo, according to a two-by-two factorial design. The combined primary outcome was myocardial infarction, stroke, or cardiovascular death. Cardiovascular death rates are shown in the figure, with placebo as *solid line* and ramipril as *dashed line*. Ramipril lowered the risk of the combined primary outcome by 25% (95% CI, 12–36, $P = 0.0004$), myocardial infarction by 22% (6–36), stroke by 33% (10–50), cardiovascular death by 37% (21–51), total mortality by 24% (8–37), revascularisation by 17% (2–30), and overt nephropathy by 24% (3–40, $P = 0.027$). After adjustment for the changes in systolic (2.4 mm Hg) and diastolic (1.0 mm Hg) blood pressures, ramipril still lowered the risk of the combined primary outcome by 25% (12–36, $P = 0.0004$). The relative effect of ramipril was present in all subgroups regardless of hypertensive status, microalbuminuria, type of diabetes, or type of diabetes treatment. CVD—cardiovascular disease. (*Adapted from* [37].)

Cost Efficacy

Incremental Cost Effectiveness by Intervention

	Cost, $§				Remaining life-years (not discounted)	QALYs	Incremental cost effective ratio (total cost/QALY), $
	Standard treatment	Complications	Intervention	Total			
Intensive glycemic control*							
Conventional glycemic control (standard)	10,741	37,602	0	48,343	17.2067	11.8791	
Intervention	10,785	33,271	12,213	56,270	17.5240	12.0707	
Incremental	44	-4330	12,213	7927	0.3173	0.1915	41,384
Intensive hypertension control†							
Moderate hypertension control (standard)	10,679	33,738	0	44,417	14.4380	10.3990	
Intervention	11,030	28,902	3708	43,641	14.9124	10.7952	
Incremental	351	-4836	3708	-776	0.4744	0.3962	-1959
Reduction in serum cholesterol level‡							
Standard	10,353	34,819	0	45,171	16.3187	11.4690	
Intervention	10,756	36,505	15,942	63,204	16.9909	11.8165	
Incremental	404	1687	15,942	18,033	0.6722	0.3475	51,889

*All patients who were newly diagnosed as having type 2 diabetes.
†All patients who were newly diagnosed as having type 2 diabetes and hypertension.
‡All patients who were newly diagnosed as having type 2 diabetes and greater than normal serum cholesterol level.
§Discounted at 3% annual rate. Costs are for patient's lifetime (1997 dollars).

Figure 9-14.
Cost effectiveness of diabetes interventions. This figure presents the results of a cost effectiveness analysis of a hypothetical cohort of individuals living in the United States, aged 25 years or older, with newly diagnosed type 2 diabetes. The results of the United Kingdom Prospective Diabetes Study and other studies were used to create a model of disease progression and treatment patterns. Costs were based on those used in US community practices. The interventions studied included insulin or sulfonylurea therapy for intensive glycemic control; angiotensin-converting enzyme inhibitor or β-blocker for intensified hypertension control; and pravastatin for reduction of serum cholesterol level. The incremental cost effectiveness ratio for intensive glycemic control is $41,384 per quality-adjusted life-year (QALY); this ratio increased with age at diagnosis from $9614 per QALY for patients aged 25 to 34 years to $2.1 million for patients aged 85 to 94 years. For intensified hypertension control, the cost effectiveness ratio is -$1959 per QALY. The cost effectiveness ratio for reduction in serum cholesterol level is $51,889 per QALY; this ratio varied by age at diagnosis and is lowest for patients diagnosed between the ages of 45 and 84 years. The study showed that intensified hypertension control reduces costs and improves health outcomes. Intensive glycemic control and reduction in serum cholesterol level increase costs and improve health outcomes. The cost effectiveness ratios for these interventions are comparable with those of several other frequently used health care interventions. (*Adapted from* CDC Diabetes Cost-effectiveness Group [38].)

Annual Costs of Statin Treatment Per Patient with Diabetes and for the US Population with Diabetes by Baseline LDL Cholesterol Level

	LDL 100–129 mg/dL	LDL 130–149 mg/dL	LDL 150–169 mg/dL	LDL 170–189 mg/dL	LDL 90 mg/dL or greater
Population estimates, n	3,023,000	2,243,000	2,300,000	702,000	675,000
Atorvastatin	10 mg	20 mg	**20 mg**	**40 mg**	**80 mg**
Costs per patient per year	$900	$1300	**$1300**	**$1400**	**$1400**
Total costs in population (in billions of dollars)	$2.66	$2.83	**$2.91**	**$0.95**	**$0.92**
Simvastatin	10 mg	20 mg	40 mg	80 mg	
Cost per patient per year	$1000	$1600	$1600	$1600	—
Total costs in population (in billions of dollars)	$2.91	$3.67	$3.76	$1.15	—
Lovastatin	20 mg	40 mg	80 mg		
Costs per patient per year	$600	$1100	$2100	—	—
Total costs in population (in billions of dollars)	$1.90	$2.46	$4.89	—	—
Fluvastatin	**40 mg**	**80 mg**			
Costs per patient per year	**$600**	**$700**	—	—	—
Total costs in population (in billions of dollars)	**$1.75**	**$1.68**	—	—	—
Pravastatin	20 mg	40 mg			
Costs per patient per year	$1000	$1600	—	—	—
Total costs in population (in billions of dollars)	$3.17	$3.62	—	—	—

Goal or LDL cholesterol—lowering (> 100 mg/dL) cannot be achieved. *Bolded entries* in the table indicated the least expensive statin for each LDL cholesterol stratum.

Figure 9-15.

Cost effectiveness of statin therapy for primary prevention of major coronary events in individuals with type 2 diabetes. Brandle *et al.* [39] performed cost effectiveness analyses using US population estimates from the National Health and Nutrition Examination Survey III, cost estimates from a health system perspective, statin low-density lipoprotein (LDL)-lowering effectiveness from several clinical trials, and treatment effectiveness from subgroups of individuals with diabetes participating in the Heart Protection Study. The authors reported over 8.2 million Americans with diabetes and LDL cholesterol levels greater than 100 mg/dL and no evidence of cardiovascular disease. Costs were computed to treat these individuals with statins. This included the medication, monitoring, and adverse events. Also computed was the total cost to the patient and population per year. Sensitivity analyses were performed to assess the impact of plausible changes in underlying assumptions on the results.

Treatment of LDL cholesterol between 100 and 129 mg/dL to achieve LDL cholesterol levels less than 100 mg/dL cost $600 to $1000 per patient per year, with the annual per capita therapy cost ranging from $700 to $2100 in the groups with LDL cholesterol levels greater than 130 mg/dL. Statin therapy could prevent 71,000 major coronary events in this population. The cost savings would be $7.4 billion if statin therapy were used for type 2 diabetes and mildly elevated (100–129 mg/dL) LDL cholesterol with no clinical evidence cardiovascular disease. (*Adapted from* Brandle *et al.* [39].)

Guidelines/Recommendations

Target Levels of Risk Factors in Patients with Diabetes

Blood pressure < 130/80 mm Hg
Lipids
  LDL cholesterol < 100 mg/dL
  HDL cholesterol > 40 mg/dL
  Triglycerides < 150 mg/dL
HbA_{1c} < 7%

Figure 9-16.

American Diabetes Association (ADA) recommendations for risk factor control. This figure outlines recommendations from the ADA for risk factor reduction among individuals with diabetes. The order of priorities the ADA defines for lipid management are the following: 1) low-density lipoprotein (LDL) cholesterol-lowering with lifestyle interventions and treatment with 3-hydroxy-3-methylglutaryl coenzyme A reductase inhibitor (statin) as the preferred agent; 2) increase high-density lipoprotein (HDL) cholesterol with lifestyle interventions and nicotinic acid or fibrates as needed; and 3) triglyceride-lowering with lifestyle interventions, glycemic control, and fibric acid derivatives (gemfibrozil), niacin, or high-dose statin (in those who require statins for LDL cholesterol treatment).

American Diabetes Association Guidelines for Treatment of Hypertension

	Systolic, mm Hg	Diastolic, mm Hg
Goal	< 130	< 80
Behavioral therapy alone (maximum 3 months), then add pharmacologic treatment	130–139	80–89
Behavior therapy plus pharmacologic treatment	140 or greater	90 or greater

Figure 9-17.

Treatment of hypertension. Current guidelines from the American Diabetes Association for the management of hypertension among individuals with diabetes include the following: 1) blood pressure should be measured at every routine diabetes visit. Patients should be treated to a systolic blood pressure of less than 130 mm Hg and a diastolic of less than 80 mm Hg. 2) Patient with borderline readings up to 139 or 89 mm Hg should receive lifestyle and behavioral therapy for 3 months. If blood pressures are over 140 mm Hg systolic or 90 mm Hg diastolic, patients should receive pharmacotherapy. Multiple drugs are usually required to achieve blood pressure targets. 3) One of these medications should probably be an angiotensin-converting enzyme inhibitor or an angiotensin receptor blocker. (*Adapted from* Arauz-Pacheco *et al.* [23].)

Future Challenges

Much is known about interventions to reduce mortality and probably improve quality of life in persons with diabetes. Lifestyle interventions have great promise at reducing these endpoints, but pose particular challenges with regard to implementation. Effective treatment of hyperglycemia, hypertension, and dyslipidemia will improve survival and decrease morbidity. Substantial under-treatment of these problems still exists, and better methods to improve achievement of treatment targets is needed to achieve the full potential benefits that have thus far been elusive. For persons with diabetes, there are other obstacles to effective treatment. Figure 9-19 demonstrates that in the United Kingdom

Prospective Diabetes Study, hyperglycemia as measured by HbA_{1c} continues to worsen over time in the intensive treatment and control groups. By approximately 6 years of follow-up, the HbA_{1c} levels in the intensive treatment group have returned to the baseline value. Thus, diabetes appears to continually worsen even when under an intensive treatment program. Weight also continues to increase, which may lead to worsening of hyperglycemia and other cardiovascular disease risk factors (Fig. 9-20). Another challenge will be to find a means to halt the progression of hyperglycemia and overweight in order to obtain a sustained effect of diabetes treatment on reduction in cardiovascular disease risk.

At risk, n
Conventional therapy: 80 72 70 63 59 50 44 41 13
Intensive therapy: 80 78 74 71 66 63 61 59 19

A

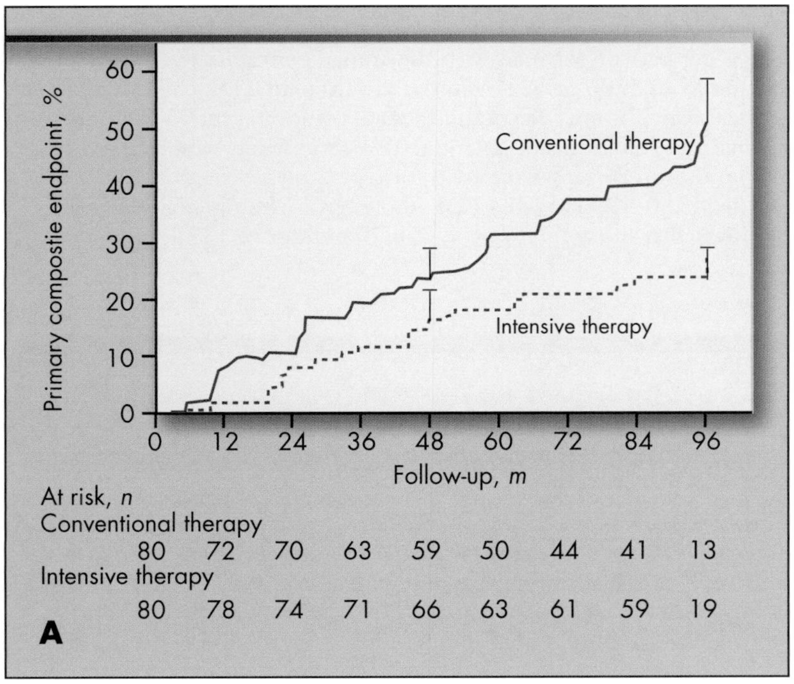

Figure 9-18.

A and **B**, Multifactorial risk factor reduction. This figure shows the results from a study by Gaede *et al.* [7] that compared the effect of a targeted, intensified, multifactorial intervention with that of conventional treatment on modifiable risk factors for cardiovascular disease in patients with type 2 diabetes and microalbuminuria. The primary endpoint of this open, parallel trial was a composite of death from cardiovascular causes, nonfatal myocardial infarction, nonfatal stroke, revascularization, and amputation. The intensive treatment group received a stepwise implementation of behavior modification and pharmacologic therapy that targeted hyperglycemia, hypertension, dyslipidemia, and microalbuminuria, along with secondary prevention of cardiovascular disease with aspirin. Patients receiving intensive therapy also had a significantly lower risk of cardiovascular disease (hazard ratio, 0.47; 95% CI, 0.24–0.73), nephropathy (hazard ratio, 0.39; 95% CI, 0.17–0.87), retinopathy (hazard ratio, 0.42; 95% CI, 0.21–0.86), and autonomic neuropathy (hazard ratio, 0.37; 95% CI, 0.18–0.79). (*Adapted from* Gaede *et al.* [7].)

(*continued on next page*)

Figure 9-18. *continued*

Variable	Relative risk (95% CI)	P value
Nephropathy	0.39 (0.17–0.87)	0.003
Retinopathy	0.42 (0.71–0.86)	0.02
Autonomic neuropathy	0.37 (0.18–0.79)	0.002
Peripheral neuropathy	1.09 (0.54–2.22)	0.66

B

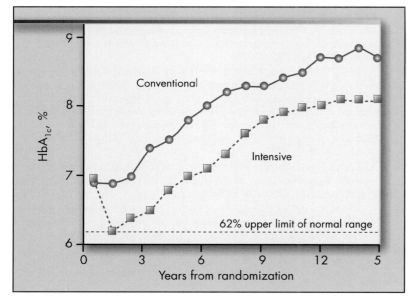

Figure 9-19.
Glucose control during the United Kingdom Prospective Diabetes Study.

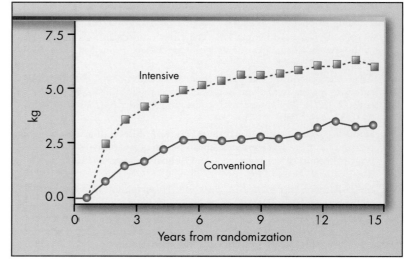

Figure 9-20.
Change in body weight in the United Kingdom Prospective Diabetes Study.

References

1. Mokdad AH, Bowman BA, Ford ES, *et al.*: The continuing epidemics of obesity and diabetes in the United States. *JAMA* 2001, 286:1195–1200.

2. Engelgau MM, Geiss LS, Saaddine JB, *et al.*: The evolving diabetes burden in the United States. *Ann Intern Med* 2004, 140:945–950.

3. Mukamal KJ, Nesto RW, Cohen MC, *et al.*: Impact of diabetes on long-term survival after acute myocardial infarction: comparability of risk with prior myocardial infarction. *Diabetes Care* 2001, 24:1422–1427.

4. Haffner SM, Lehto S, Ronnemaa T, *et al.*: Mortality from coronary heart disease in subjects with type 2 diabetes and in nondiabetic subjects with and without prior myocardial infarction. *N Engl J Med* 1998, 339:229–234.

5. Okoro CA, Mokdad AH, Ford ES, *et al.*: Are persons with diabetes practicing healthier behaviors in the year 2001? Results from the Behavioral Risk Factor Surveillance System. *Prev Med* 2004, 38:203–208.

6. Redberg RF, Greenland P, Fuster V, *et al.*: Prevention Conference VI: diabetes and cardiovascular disease. Writing Group III: risk assessment in persons with diabetes. *Circulation* 2002, 105:144e–152e.

7. Gaede P, Vedel P, Larsen N, *et al.*: Multifactorial intervention and cardiovascular disease in patients with type 2 diabetes. *N Engl J Med* 2003, 348:383–393.

8. Al-Delaimy WK, Manson JE, Solomon CG, *et al.*: Smoking and risk of coronary heart disease among women with type 2 diabetes mellitus. *Arch Intern Med* 2002, 162:273–279.

9. Grundy SM, Garber A, Goldberg R, *et al.*: Prevention Conference VI: diabetes and cardiovascular disease. Writing Group IV: lifestyle and medical management of risk factors. *Circulation* 2002, 105:153e–158e.

10. Hu FB, Stampfer MJ, Solomon C, *et al.*: Physical activity and risk for cardiovascular events in diabetic women. *Ann Intern Med* 2001, 134:96–105.

11. Wei M, Gibbons LW, Kampert JB, *et al.*: Low cardiorespiratory fitness and physical inactivity as predictors of mortality in men with type 2 diabetes. *Ann Intern Med* 2000, 132:605–611.

12. Vijan S, Hayward RA: Pharmacologic lipid-lowering therapy in type 2 diabetes mellitus: background paper for the American College of Physicians. *Ann Intern Med* 2004, 140:650–658.

13. Heart Protection Study Collaborative Group: MRC/BHF Heart Protection Study of cholesterol lowering with simvastatin in 20,536 high-risk individuals: a randomised placebo-controlled trial. *Lancet* 2002, 360:7–22.

14. Expert Panel on Detection E, and Treatment of High Blood Cholesterol in Adults: Executive Summary of the Third Report of the National Cholesterol Education Program (NCEP) Expert Panel on Detection, Evaluation, and Treatment of High Blood Cholesterol in Adults (Adult Treatment Panel III). *JAMA* 2001 2001, 285:2486–2497.

15. Gami AS, Montori VM, Erwin PJ, *et al.*: Systematic review of lipid lowering for primary prevention of coronary heart disease in diabetes. *BMJ* 2003, 326:528–529.

16. Lindholm LH: Major benefits from cholesterol-lowering in patients with diabetes. *Lancet* 2003, 361:2000–2001.

17. Rubins HB, Robins SJ, Collins D, *et al.*: Gemfibrozil for the secondary prevention of coronary heart disease in men with low levels of high-density lipoprotein cholesterol. *N Engl J Med* 1999, 341:410–418.

18. Snow V, Weiss KB, Mottur-Pilson C: The evidence base for tight blood pressure control in the management of type 2 diabetes mellitus. *Ann Intern Med* 2003, 138:587–592.

19. Curb JD, Pressel SL, Cutler JA, *et al.*: Effect of diuretic-based antihypertensive treatment on cardiovascular disease risk in older diabetic patients with isolated systolic hypertension. Systolic Hypertension in the Elderly Program Cooperative Research Group. *JAMA* 1996, 276:1886–1892.

20. Huang ES, Meigs JB, Singer DE: The effect of interventions to prevent cardiovascular disease in patients with type 2 diabetes mellitus. *Am J Med* 2001, 111:633–642.

21. Adler AI, Stratton IM, Neil HA, *et al.*: Association of systolic blood pressure with macrovascular and microvascular complications of type 2 diabetes (UKPDS 36): prospective observational study. *BMJ* 2000, 321:412–419.

22. Hansson L, Zanchetti A, Carruthers SG, *et al.*: Effects of intensive blood-pressure lowering and low-dose aspirin in patients with hypertension: principal results of the Hypertension Optimal Treatment (HOT) randomised trial. *Lancet* 1998, 351:1755–1762.

23. Arauz-Pacheco C, Parrott MA, Raskin P: Hypertension management in adults with diabetes. *Diabetes Care* 2004, 27(suppl):S65–S67.

24. Vijan S, Hayward RA: Treatment of hypertension in type 2 diabetes mellitus: blood pressure goals, choice of agents, and setting priorities in diabetes care. *Ann Intern Med* 2003, 138:593–602.

25. Gerstein HC, Mann JFE, Yi Q, *et al.*: Albuminuria and risk of cardiovascular events, death, and heart failure in diabetic and nondiabetic individuals. *JAMA* 2001, 286:421–426.

26. Colwell JA, American Diabetes Association: Aspirin therapy in diabetes. *Diabetes Care* 2004, 27(suppl):72S–73S.

27. Selvin E, Marinopoulos S, Berkenblit G, *et al.*: Meta-analysis: glycosylated hemoglobin and cardiovascular disease in diabetes mellitus. *Ann Intern Med* 2004, 141:421–431.

28. Saydah SH, Fradkin J, Cowie CC: Poor control of risk factors for vascular disease among adults with previously diagnosed diabetes. *JAMA* 2004, 291:335–342.

29. Nelson KM, Rieber G, Boyko EJ: Diet and exercise among adults with type 2 diabetes; data from NHANES III. *Diabetes Care* 2002, 25:1722–1728.

30. Saaddine JB, Engelgau MM, Beckles GL, *et al.*: A diabetes report card for the United States: quality of care in the 1990s. *Ann Intern Med* 2002, 136:565–574.

31. Barrett-Connor E: Epidemiology, obesity, and non-insulin-dependent diabetes mellitus. *Epidemiol Rev* 1989, 11:172–181.

32. Zhang P, Engelgau MM, Norris SL, *et al.*: Application of economic analysis to diabetes and diabetes care. *Ann Intern Med* 2004, 140:972–997.

33. Hogan P, Dall T, Nikolov P, American Diabetes Association: Economic costs of diabetes in the US in 2002. *Diabetes Care* 2003, 26:917–932.

34. Resnick HE, Harris MI, Brock DB, Harris TB: American Diabetes Association diabetes diagnostic criteria, advancing age, and cardiovascular disease risk profiles: results from the Third National Health and Nutrition Examination Survey. *Diabetes Care* 2000, 23:176–180.

35. Chandalia M, Garg A, Lutjohann D, *et al.*: Beneficial effects of high dietary fiber intake in patients with type 2 diabetes mellitus. *N Engl J Med* 2000, 342:1392–1398.

36. ALLHAT Officers and Coordinators for the ALLHAT Collaborative Research Group: The Antihypertensive and Lipid-Lowering Treatment to Prevent Heart Attack Trial: major outcomes in high-risk hypertensive patients randomized to angiotensin-converting enzyme inhibitor or calcium channel blocker vs. diuretic. The Antihypertensive and Lipid-Lowering Treatment to Prevent Heart Attack Trial (ALLHAT). *JAMA* 2002, 288:2981–2997.

37. Effects of ramipril on cardiovascular and microvascular outcomes in people with diabetes mellitus: results of the HOPE study and MICRO-HOPE substudy. *Lancet* 2000, 355:253–259.

38. CDC Diabetes Cost-effectiveness Group: Cost-effectiveness of intensive glycemic control, intensified hypertension control, and serum cholesterol level reduction for type 2 diabetes. *JAMA* 2002, 287:2542–2551.

39. Brandle M, Davidson MB, Schriger DL, *et al.*: Cost effectiveness of statin therapy for the primary prevention of major coronary events in individuals with type 2 diabetes. *Diabetes Care* 2003, 26:1796-1801.

Obesity and Weight Loss

Shari S. Bassuk and JoAnn E. Manson

Although viewed more as a cosmetic rather than a health concern by the general public and some health care professionals, excess body weight is a major risk factor for chronic disease and other medical complications. Recent epidemiologic research has quantified the impact of overweight and obesity on premature mortality, cardiovascular disease (CVD), type 2 diabetes mellitus, cancer, respiratory disorders, and other adverse outcomes [1].

Direct, dose-dependent relationships between increasing body mass index and lifetime risks of cardiovascular and other conditions have been observed in nationally representative samples, such as the National Health and Nutrition Examination Surveys (NHANES) [2] and the Behavioral Risk Factor Surveillance System surveys [3], and in large cohorts observed for long periods of time, such as the Nurses' Health Study [4] and the Framingham Heart Study [5]. Data from the national Healthcare for Communities survey indicate that, in the United States, obesity is associated with greater morbidity and poorer health-related quality of life than smoking, problem drinking, or poverty [6].

One conservative estimate, derived from five long-term cohort studies, is that obesity accounts for 300,000 deaths per year in the United States [7] and will overtake smoking as the primary cause of preventable death if current trends continue [8]. Data from the Framingham Heart Study [9] and NHANES III [10] indicate that even a moderate amount of excess weight confers a measurable diminution in life expectancy and that, as degree of overweight increases, a steady contraction of lifespan occurs. For example, in the Framingham Heart Study, 40-year-old overweight but not obese nonsmokers without a history of CVD lived an average of 3 years less than their normal-weight counterparts, and obese 40-year-olds lived 6 to 7 years less than those with normal weight [9]. In NHANES III, the number of years of life lost because of severe obesity (body mass index 45 kg/m^2 or greater) was estimated to be 13 years for 20- to 30-year-old white men and 8 years for their female counterparts [10]. Obesity costs the United States an estimated \$98 billion to \$129 billion per year, including direct (preventive, diagnostic, and treatment services, including doctor visits, medications, hospitalizations) and indirect costs (value of lost wages and productivity because of illness or premature mortality) [11]. The direct medical costs of obesity constitute 9% of US health care expenditures [12].

In randomized clinical trials, modest weight loss (5%–15% of excess body weight) among overweight and obese individuals has been associated with favorable changes in cardiovascular risk factors, including lipoproteins, blood pressure, glucose tolerance, and markers of inflammation and hemostasis. Although few trials have examined whether intentional weight loss reduces the risk of CVD or mortality, data from observational studies, as well as scientific plausibility, suggest this link.

The substantial morbidity and mortality associated with overweight and obesity underscore the pressing need to educate the public and medical communities about the hazards of excess weight and to remove the barriers to healthy eating and greater physical activity. The alarming increase in the prevalence of obesity, along with a concurrent rise in that of type 2 diabetes, threaten to undermine advances in the prevention and treatment of CVD thought to be responsible for the striking decline in cardiovascular mortality that occurred during the latter half of the 20th century in the United States and other developed countries.

NHLBI/WHO BMI Guidelines

BMI	Classification
< 18.5 kg/m^2	Underweight
18.5–24.9 kg/m^2	Normal weight
25.0–29.9 kg/m^2	Overweight
≥ 30 kg/m^2	Obese

Figure 10-1.
Definition of overweight and obesity. Obesity, or excess body fat, is operationally defined in terms of body mass index (BMI), calculated by dividing an individual's weight in kilograms by the square of height in meters. The National Heart, Lung, and Blood Institute (NHLBI) and the World Health Organization (WHO) define overweight as a BMI of 25 to 29.9 kg/m^2 and obesity as a BMI of 30 kg/m^2 or greater [13].

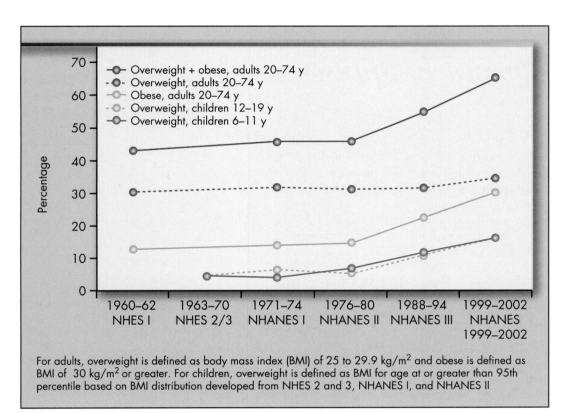

For adults, overweight is defined as body mass index (BMI) of 25 to 29.9 kg/m^2 and obese is defined as BMI of 30 kg/m^2 or greater. For children, overweight is defined as BMI for age at or greater than 95th percentile based on BMI distribution developed from NHES 2 and 3, NHANES I, and NHANES II

Figure 10-2.
Prevalence of obesity in the United States. The prevalence of obesity has increased dramatically in recent years. Nearly two of three US adults are overweight or obese [14]. Although the percentage of adults classified as overweight but not obese has been stable since the 1960s, the prevalence of obesity doubled between 1980 and 2002, rising from 14.5% to 30.4% [14,15]. In addition, the prevalence of extreme obesity (*ie*, body mass index 40 kg/m^2 or greater) more than tripled, increasing from 1.3% to 4.9% during this period. The proportion of US children and adolescents who are overweight is also increasing. In 2002, the prevalence of overweight among those aged 2 to 5 years, 6 to 11 years, and 12 to 19 years was 10.3%, 15.8%, and 16.1%, respectively, compared with 7.2%, 11.3%, and 10.5% in 1994 [14,16]. International data indicate that similar trends are occurring in many developed and developing countries. NHANES—National Health and Nutrition Examination Survey; NHES—National Health Examination Survey. (*Data from* Hedley *et al.* [14]; Flegal *et al.* [15]; and Ogden *et al.* [16].)

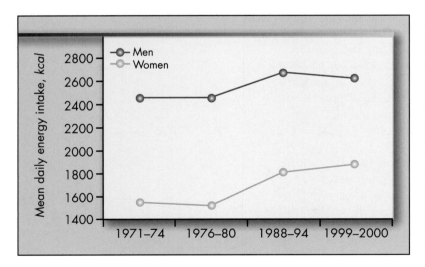

Figure 10-3.
Mean daily energy intake among US adults aged 20 to 74 years, 1971 to 2000: National Health and Nutrition Examination Surveys. Overweight and obesity result from the interaction of many factors, including genetic, metabolic, behavioral, and environmental influences. Heritability estimates for body mass index range from 0.40 to 0.80 [17,18]. However, the rapid rise in obesity prevalence in recent years suggests that behavioral and environmental factors, rather than biologic changes, have fueled the epidemic. Increasing calorie intakes, decreasing energy expenditures, or a combination has led to a positive energy balance and a marked increase in weight. Data from the National Health and Nutrition Examination Surveys suggest that average calorie intake increased between 1971 and 2000 [19]. From 1971 to 2000, the daily caloric intake of the typical woman rose 22%, from 1542 to 1877 kilocalories (kcal), while the typical man increased his intake by 7%, from 2450 to 2618 kcal. (*Data from* Centers for Disease Control and Prevention [19].)

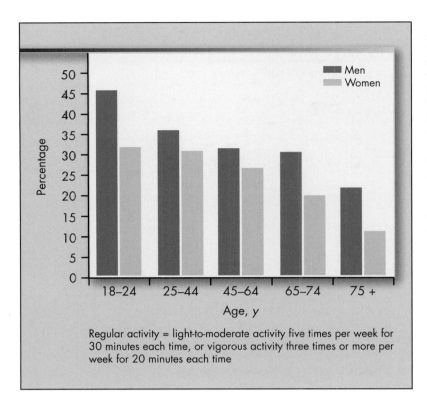

Regular activity = light-to-moderate activity five times per week for 30 minutes each time, or vigorous activity three times or more per week for 20 minutes each time

Figure 10-4.
Percent of US adults engaging in regular leisure-time physical activity, by gender and age, 1997 to 1998: National Health Interview Survey. Although rigorous data on national trends in overall physical activity during the past three decades are lacking, the amount of activity expended in work and daily living has been declining for several generations. Advances in technology have largely obviated reliance on walking and cycling for transportation. Household and occupational energy requirements have also decreased because of labor-saving devices and, in general, jobs have become more sedentary. Despite a widely publicized 1995 recommendation by the Centers for Disease Control and the American College of Sports Medicine that adults engage in 30 minutes of moderate-intensity physical activity on most, preferably all, days of the week (or vigorous exercise for at least 20 minutes three times per week) [20], data from the National Health Interview Survey indicate that 73% of women and 66% of men fail to meet this guideline; and 41% of women and 35% of men engage in no leisure-time physical activity at all [21]. (*Data from* Schoenborn and Barnes [21].)

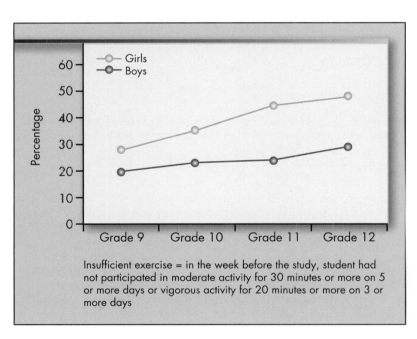

Insufficient exercise = in the week before the study, student had not participated in moderate activity for 30 minutes or more on 5 or more days or vigorous activity for 20 minutes or more on 3 or more days

Figure 10-5.
Percent of students achieving insufficient exercise: Youth Risk Behavior Surveillance Survey. The national Youth Risk Behavior Surveillance Survey conducted by the Centers for Disease Control found that a large percentage of adolescents also fail to meet the aforementioned physical activity guideline (*see* Fig. 10-4) [22]. The prevalence of insufficient physical activity rises steadily from the first to the fourth year of high school, a trend that is especially pronounced among girls. The decline in the prevalence of enrollment in daily physical education classes during the high school years is striking, with nearly one of every two ninth graders but only one of four male twelfth graders and one of seven female twelfth graders enrolled [22]. (*Data from* Grunbaum *et al.* [22].)

Obesity and Weight Loss

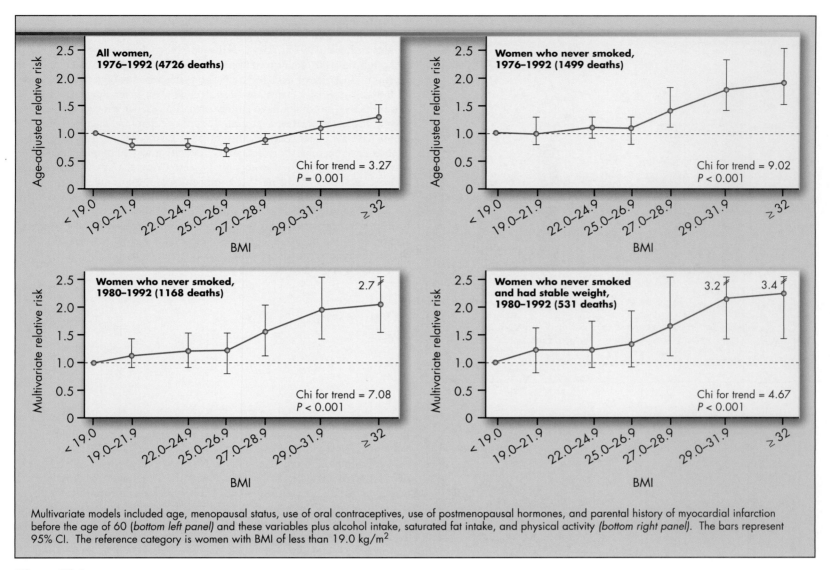

Multivariate models included age, menopausal status, use of oral contraceptives, use of postmenopausal hormones, and parental history of myocardial infarction before the age of 60 (*bottom left panel*) and these variables plus alcohol intake, saturated fat intake, and physical activity (*bottom right panel*). The bars represent 95% CI. The reference category is women with BMI of less than 19.0 kg/m²

Figure 10-6.
The influence of increasing control for methodologic bias on the shape of the curve describing the relation between body mass index (BMI) and mortality: Nurses' Health Study. Many epidemiologic studies report U- or J-shaped relationships between BMI and morbidity or mortality, with disease or death rates elevated in persons with very low and high relative body weights. Although extremes of adiposity or leanness are clearly deleterious, pinpointing the precise range of weights associated with optimal health or minimal mortality has been controversial, primarily because of methodologic problems that can distort inferences about the role of weight in health outcomes. These methodologic problems include failure to control for cigarette smoking (smoking tends to be more prevalent among lean individuals and is also a strong independent risk factor for diseases such as cardiovascular disease and cancer; failure to adjust for its effect will produce artificially inflated disease or mortality rates among the lean); inappropriate statistical control for biologic consequences of obesity such as hypertension, dyslipidemia,

or hyperglycemia (thus eliminating at least some of the physiologic pathways by which obesity mediates morbidity and mortality risk and attenuating observed associations); and failure to consider weight loss caused by preclinical disease (potential for reverse causation because of preclinical disease) [23]. These biases account for the J- or U-shaped relationship between BMI and mortality observed in many studies and to a systematic underestimate of the impact of obesity on premature mortality. In the Nurses' Health Study, a cohort of 115,195 women aged 30 to 55 years followed for 16 years, age-adjusted analyses suggested a J-shaped relation between BMI and mortality (*top left panel*) [23]. An increasingly direct association was observed when the analysis was restricted to women who never smoked (*top right panel*), when early deaths were excluded (*bottom left panel*), and when only women with stable weight in the previous 4 years were included (*bottom right panel*). (*From* Manson *et al.* [23]; with permission.)

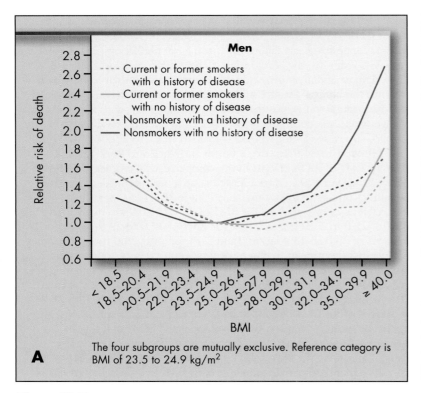

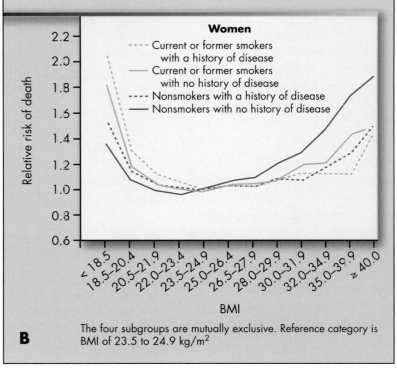

Figure 10-7.
Multivariate relative risk of all-cause mortality among men (**A**) and women (**B**) according to body mass index (BMI), smoking status, and disease status: Cancer Prevention Study II. An analysis of an American Cancer Society cohort of more than 1 million adults with 14 years of follow-up also shows a more direct relationship between increasing weight and mortality among participants with no history of smoking, cancer, cardiovascular disease, respiratory disease, or recent weight loss than among other participants [24]. In individuals meeting these criteria, the lowest mortality occurred at a BMI of 23.5 to 24.9 kg/m² for men and 22.0 to 23.4 kg/m² for women. These results are in agreement with observations from other large cohort studies, including a 27-year follow-

up of 19,000 middle-aged men in the Harvard Alumni Study, a 10-year follow-up of 40,000 middle-aged men in the Health Professionals Follow-up Study, a 5-year follow-up of 85,000 middle-aged and elderly men from the Physicians' Health Study enrollment cohort, a 12-year follow-up of 20,000 nonsmoking Seventh Day Adventists in the Adventist Health Study, a 13-year follow-up of 10,000 Canadians in the nationally representative Canada Fitness Survey, and a 22-year follow-up of more than 2 million Norwegian men and women. Taken as a whole, these studies support current guidelines that set the healthy weight range for adults at BMIs between 18.5 and 25 kg/m². (*From* Calle *et al.* [24]; with permission.)

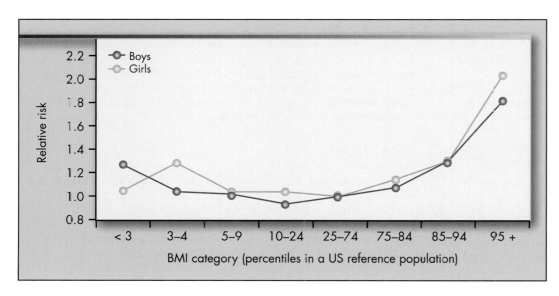

Figure 10-8.
Relative risk of death, according to body mass index (BMI) during adolescence (age 14 to 19) in a Norwegian cohort observed for 32 years. Weight in childhood has been less extensively studied than weight in adulthood as a predictor of subsequent health outcomes. However, a recent investigation of 227,000 Norwegian adolescents aged 14 to 19 years who were observed for 32 years found that a high BMI was strongly associated with premature mortality [25]. Compared with those whose baseline BMI was in the 25th to 75th percentile of a US reference population, males with baseline BMI in the 85th to 95th percentile and those with BMI above the 95th percentile were 29% and 82% more likely to die in early to middle adulthood, respectively. The corresponding risk increases among females were 31% and 103%. (*Data from* Engeland *et al.* [25].)

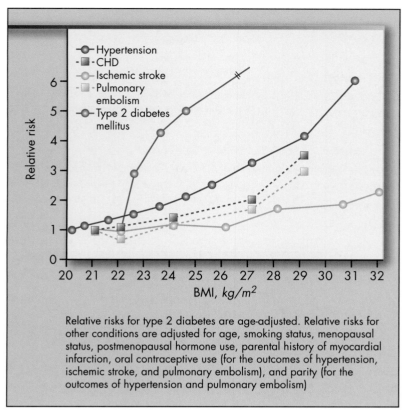

Figure 10-9.
Relative risks of hypertension, coronary heart disease (CHD), ischemic stroke, pulmonary embolism, and type 2 diabetes mellitus, according to body mass index (BMI) up to 32 kg/m² , after 14 to 16 years of follow-up: Nurses' Health Study. Studies of total mortality, compared with studies of disease-specific outcomes, are relatively insensitive in pinpointing the weight range associated with optimal health because obesity, similar to virtually every other risk factor, is unlikely to influence all causes of death. In large investigations of multiple health outcomes, the relative risks associated with high BMI tend to be lower for all-cause mortality than for the incidence of specific conditions such as myocardial infarction, ischemic stroke, and type 2 diabetes. Similarly, although only limited data support the hypothesis that intentional weight loss reduces total mortality, such weight loss has conclusively been shown to reduce several disease-specific risks. Moreover, focusing only on mortality overlooks the considerable morbidity associated with obesity-related illnesses.

Although linked with cardiovascular disease for centuries, obesity was named a major modifiable coronary risk factor by the American Heart Association only within the past decade [26]. In long-term prospective

cohort studies, excess body weight has been associated with an increased risk of CHD, hypertension, stroke, type 2 diabetes, venous thromboembolism, congestive heart failure [27], and atrial fibrillation [28]. For many of these conditions, the relationship is linear, with even individuals of average weight at midlife at increased risk compared with their leaner counterparts. In the Nurses' Health Study, after adjustment for age, smoking status, menopausal status, postmenopausal hormone use, and parental history of myocardial infarction, the relative risk of developing CHD over 14 years of follow-up was 1.19 for women with BMI of 21 to 22.9 kg/m², 1.46 for BMI of 23 to 24.9 kg/m², 2.06 for BMI of 25 to 28.9 kg/m², and 3.56 for BMI of 29 kg/m² or more, compared with women with BMI below 21 kg/m² [29]. . The adjusted relative risks of incident hypertension after 16 years of follow-up were 1.00 for BMI less than 20 kg/m² (the referent category), 1.15 for BMI of 20.0 to 20.9 kg/m², 1.36 for BMI of 21.0 to 21.9 kg/m², 1.57 for BMI of 22.0 to 22.9 kg/m², 1.82 for BMI of 23.0 to 23.9 kg/m², and 2.15 for BMI 24.0 to 24.9 kg/m². Relative risks continued to climb with increasing degrees of overweight, reaching 6.31 for BMI of 31 kg/m² or greater [30]. Being overweight was also predictive of an increased risk of ischemic stroke, with adjusted 16-year relative risks of 1.75 among women with BMI of 27.0 to 28.9 kg/m², 1.90 for BMI of 29.0 to 31.9 kg/m², and 2.37 for BMI of 32 kg/m² or greater, compared with women with a BMI of less than 21 kg/m² [31]. The adjusted risk of primary pulmonary embolism over 16 years of follow-up was threefold higher among women with BMI of at least 29 kg/m² compared with those with BMI below 21 kg/m² [32].

Obesity, especially abdominal obesity, causes insulin resistance and compensatory hyperinsulinemia, which in turn are implicated in the development of type 2 diabetes, a disease designated as a CHD risk equivalent by the National Cholesterol Education Program because of the very high risk of new coronary disease it confers within 10 years [33]. The marked rise in obesity among US adults during the past decade has been accompanied by a 61% increase in diabetes prevalence, and the number of Americans with diagnosed diabetes is projected to more than double by 2050 [34]. Observed increases in type 2 diabetes have been especially marked in younger age groups; indeed, if current trends continue, more than one in three individuals born in 2000 will develop the condition during their lifetime [35]. In the Nurses' Health Study, the age-adjusted risk of incident type 2 diabetes over 14 years of follow-up was more than 40-fold higher for participants with a BMI of 31 kg/m² or greater compared with those with a BMI of less than 22 kg/m² [36]. Even a BMI in the high-normal range (23.0 to 24.9 kg/m²) was associated with a four- to fivefold increase in risk over that experienced by women with BMI of less than 22.0 kg/m². Of five lifestyle variables examined—obesity, physical inactivity, poor diet, current smoking, and alcohol abstinence—excess body weight was by far the single most powerful predictor of diabetes onset [37]. (*Data from* Willett *et al.* [29]; Huang *et al.* [30]; Rexrode *et al.* [31]; Goldhaber *et al.* [32]; and Colditz *et al.* [36].)

Figure 10-10.
Weight change and risk of coronary heart disease (CHD), hypertension, stroke, and diabetes: Nurses' Health Study. In the Nurses' Health Study, weight gain between age 18 and midlife was associated in a dose-dependent manner with increased risks of CHD [29], hypertension [30], ischemic stroke [31], and type 2 diabetes [36]. Compared with women with stable weight, women who gained 5 to 7.9 kg were 25% more likely to develop CHD, and those who gained 20 kg or more were 165% more likely to do so [29]. More than one fourth (27%) of the overall incidence of CHD in this cohort could be accounted for by weight gains of 5 kg or more. Compared with women with stable weight, women who gained 5.0 to 7.9 kg from early to mid-adulthood had a near doubling of risk of diabetes over a 14-year follow-up, and women who gained 20.0 kg or more had more than a 12-fold risk increase [36].

However, because the number of CHD cases among women who lost a large amount of weight (11 kg or more) was small (36 cases), the relative risk estimates are unstable. Moreover, because intentionality of weight loss was not assessed, the potential for confounding by the presence of subclinical disease cannot be eliminated. (*Data from* Willett *et al.* [29]; Huang *et al.* [30]; Rexrode *et al.* [31]; Goldhaber *et al.* [32]; and Colditz *et al.* [36].)

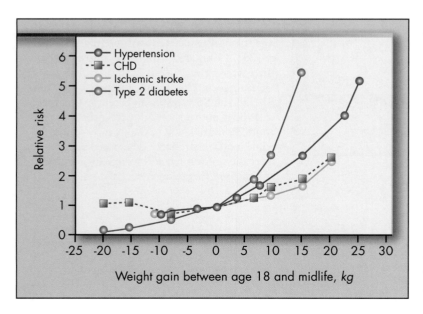

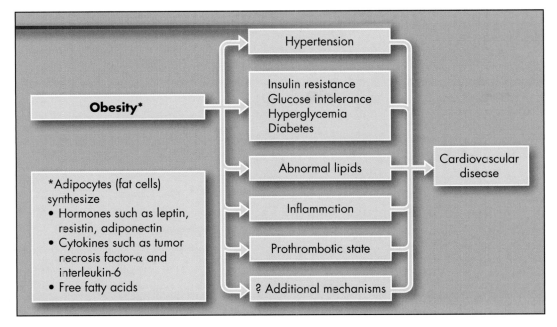

Figure 10-11.
Mechanisms by which obesity raises risk of cardiovascular disease (CVD). Obesity raises the risk for CVD partly through its effects on established vascular risk factors such as hypercholesterolemia, hypertension, and hyperglycemia. Excess weight is also associated with several novel risk factors, including atherogenic dyslipidemia (*ie*, elevated triglycerides, apolipoprotein B, small low-density

lipoprotein particles, low high-density lipoprotein cholesterol); insulin resistance; elevations in thrombotic markers, such as fibrinogen and plasminogen activator inhibitor-1; and increases in inflammatory markers, such as interleukin-6 and C-reactive protein [38]. Once viewed as inert storage depots, adipocytes are now known to synthesize hormones such as leptin, resistin, and adiponectin, which may play important regulatory roles in lipid and glucose metabolism and insulin action; cytokines such as tumor necrosis factor-α and interleukin-6; and free fatty acids [39]. Independent of its effect on established and novel cardiovascular risk factors, obesity also appears to have a residual impact on risk of CVD itself, a finding that is most pronounced in prospective studies with long follow-up periods. For example, a 26-year follow-up of 5200 participants in the Framingham Heart Study showed that high relative weight at baseline was directly associated with coronary heart disease and coronary mortality independent of age, cholesterol level, systolic blood pressure, smoking, and other cardiovascular risk factors, but the association did not emerge until after 8 years of observation [5].

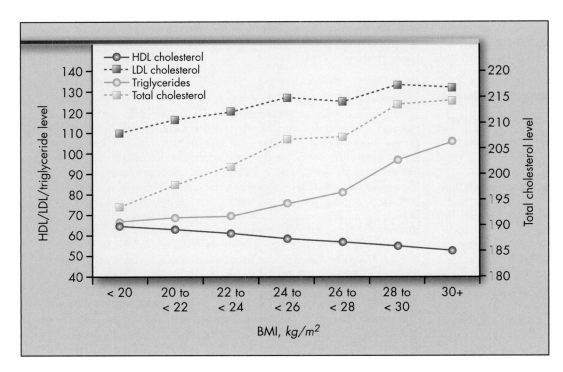

Figure 10-12.
Age-adjusted means for coronary heart disease risk factors by body mass index (BMI): Marks and Spencer Cardiovascular Risk Factor Study. Consistent with the excess coronary heart disease risk observed even among persons at the upper limit of the healthy weight range, the prevalence and incidence of many cardiovascular risk factors rise rapidly at BMI greater than 20 kg/m^2. In a study of 14,000 healthy, middle-aged female employees of the British company Marks and Spencer, marked age-adjusted increases in systolic and diastolic blood pressure, serum total cholesterol, low-density lipoprotein (LDL) cholesterol, triglycerides, and fasting blood glucose, as well as significant decreases in high-density lipoprotein (HDL) cholesterol, were observed across seven categories of BMI ranging from less than 20 to greater than 30 kg/m^2 [40]. (*Data from* Ashton *et al.* [40].)

Relative Risks of Cardiovascular Risk Factors, According to Overweight Status, Among 5- to 17-year-old Children and Adolescents: Bogalusa Heart Study

Risk factor	Relative risk* (95% CI)
Total cholesterol > 200 mg/dL	2.4 (2.0–3.0)
Triglycerides > 130 mg/dL	7.1 (5.8–8.6)
LDL cholesterol > 130 mg/dL	3.0 (2.4–3.6)
HDL cholesterol < 35 mg/dL	3.4 (2.8–4.2)
Insulin level ≥ 95th percentile of sample distribution	12.6 (10–16)
High systolic blood pressure†	4.5 (3.6–5.8)
High diastolic blood pressure†	2.4 (1.8–3.0)

*Relative risk comparing overweight (BMI ≥ 95% of US reference population) versus nonoverweight children. Relative risks are adjusted for race, gender, and age.
†Defined in a manner comparable with that used by the National High Blood Pressure Education Program. Regression models containing race, gender, age, age^2, height, height^2, and various product terms were used to predict blood pressure. Individuals with residuals greater than 95th percentile from these models were considered to have high blood pressure.

Figure 10-13.

Relationship between overweight and cardiovascular risk factors among 5- to 17-year-old participants in the Bogalusa Heart Study. Strong associations between relative body weight and cardiovascular risk factors also have been observed in children and adolescents. In the Bogalusa Heart Study, which examined 9157 Louisiana children aged 5 to 17 years, lipid, insulin, and blood pressure levels did not vary with body mass index (BMI) at levels below the 85th percentile of a national reference population [41]. However, the probability of having an adverse lipid, blood pressure, or insulin profile was substantially higher in children with BMI above the 95th percentile than in children with BMI below the 85th percentile. Overweight children were 2.4, 3.0, 3.4, 7.1, and 12.6 times more likely than normal-weight children to have a total cholesterol level greater than 200 mg/dL, low-density lipoprotein (LDL) cholesterol greater than 130 mg/dL, high-density lipoprotein (HDL) cholesterol less than 35 mg/dL, triglycerides of 130 mg/dL or higher, and fasting insulin at or above the 95th percentile, respectively. Overweight children were also 4.5 times more likely to have an elevated systolic blood pressure and 2.4 times more likely to have an elevated diastolic blood pressure than their normal-weight counterparts. (*Data from* Freedman *et al.* [41].)

Metabolic Syndrome: National Cholesterol Education Program's Adult Treatment Panel III Report

Components

Abdominal obesity
Atherogenic dyslipidemia (elevated triglycerides, low HDL cholesterol, other lipoprotein abnormalities)
Raised blood pressure
Insulin resistance ± glucose intolerance
Proinflammatory state (elevated C-reactive protein)
Prothrombotic state (increased plasminogen activator inhibitor-1 and fibrinogen)

Clinical identification

Presence of three or more of the following:
  Waist circumference
    Men > 40 inches
    Women > 35 inches
  Triglycerides ≥ 150 mg/dL
  HDL cholesterol
    Men < 40 mg/dL
    Women < 50 mg/dL
  Blood pressure ≥ 130/85 mm Hg
  Fasting glucose ≥ 110 mg/dL

Prevalence in the United States

Adults: 27.0%
Adolescents (aged 12–19 years): 10.0%

Figure 10-14.

Abdominal obesity and the metabolic syndrome. Adipose tissue in the waist, abdomen, and upper body is more metabolically active than that in the hip, thigh, or buttocks, and abdominal fat accumulation appears to be a stronger predictor than gluteofemoral fat of atherogenic dyslipidemia, hypertension, type 2 diabetes, and coronary heart disease. The heightened sensitivity of abdominal fat cells to lipolytic agents and the subsequent direct delivery of free fatty acids and glycerol to the liver, which can induce insulin resistance, are possible pathophysiologic explanations for these associations [42]. Abdominal adiposity is often estimated using waist circumference or waist-to-hip ratio. The National Heart, Lung, and Blood Institute recommends that a waist circumference of more than 88 cm (> 35 inches) in women or more than 102 cm (> 40 inches) in men, or, alternatively, a waist-to-hip ratio higher than 0.80 in women or 0.95 in men, be used as an adjunct to body mass index to classify "high-risk" obesity [13]. Abdominal obesity is a prominent component of the clustering of metabolic abnormalities known as the metabolic syndrome. Defined by the National Cholesterol Education Program as the presence of at least three of the following: abdominal obesity, hypertriglyceridemia, low high-density lipoprotein (HDL) cholesterol, hypertension, and fasting hyperglycemia [33,43], the metabolic syndrome, a powerful risk factor for diabetes and cardiovascular disease, is present in an estimated 27% of US adults [44] and 10% of US adolescents aged 12 to 19 years [45].

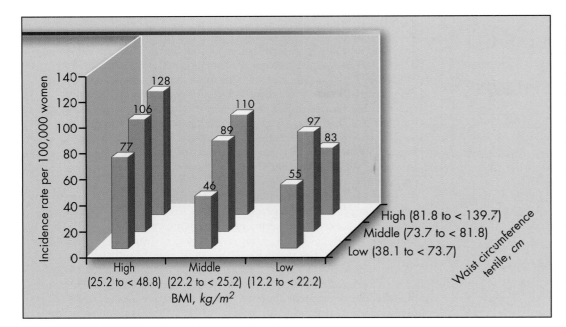

Figure 10-15.
Age-adjusted incidence rates for coronary heart disease according to body mass index (BMI) and waist circumference tertiles: Nurses' Health Study. The joint contribution of amount of and regional distribution of excess fat to coronary risk can be seen in an 8-year follow-up of Nurses' Health Study participants [46]. A higher waist circumference was associated with an increased risk of coronary heart disease, regardless of BMI tertile. Within each BMI tertile, women in the highest waist circumference tertile had a twofold higher incidence of coronary heart disease than did women in the lowest waist circumference tertile. Within each waist circumference tertile, higher BMI was generally associated with increased risk. (*From* Rexrode *et al.* [46]; with permission.)

Weight Loss and All-cause Mortality

American Cancer Society's Cancer Prevention Study I

Twelve-year follow-up of 93,000 never-smoking, overweight (BMI ≥ 27 kg/m²) men and women aged 40 to 64 years

Intentional weight loss was associated with a 20% reduction in mortality among women with obesity-related comorbidities at baseline; intentional weight loss was not predictive of mortality among women without comorbidities and among men

National Health Interview Survey

Nine-year follow-up of 6391 overweight (BMI ≥ 25 kg/m²) men and women aged 35 years and older (mean age, 54 years)

Respondents reporting intentional weight loss experienced a 24% reduction in mortality, whereas those reporting unintentional weight loss had a 31% increase in mortality, compared with individuals not trying to lose weight and reporting no weight change

Lower mortality was also observed among persons who attempted to lose weight than among persons who did not attempt to do so, independent of actual weight change; respondents trying to lose weight and reporting no weight change experienced a 19% reduction in mortality compared with individuals not trying to lose weight and reporting no weight change

Figure 10-16.
Intentional weight loss and mortality. The association between intentional weight loss and mortality was examined among nearly 93,000 never-smoking, overweight (body mass index [BMI] 27 kg/m² or greater) men and women aged 40 to 64 years observed for 12 years as part of the American Cancer Society's Cancer Prevention Study I [47,48]. Among women with obesity-related health conditions at baseline, intentional weight loss was associated with a 20% reduction in all-cause mortality. However, in women without obesity-related illnesses and in men, there was little association between intentional weight loss and all-cause mortality. In a 9-year follow-up of 6391 overweight (BMI 25 kg/m² or greater) men and women in the National Health Interview Survey, persons reporting intentional weight loss experienced a 24% reduction in mortality, whereas those reporting unintentional weight loss had a 31% increase in mortality, compared with persons not trying to lose weight and reporting no weight change [49]. However, lower mortality was also observed among persons who attempted to lose weight than among persons who did not attempt to do so, independent of actual weight change. Compared with persons not trying to lose weight and reporting no weight change, persons trying to lose weight had the following relative risks: no weight change, 0.80; gained weight, 0.94; and lost weight, 0.76. This suggests that attempted weight loss, as a marker of healthy behavior, may be an important predictor of longevity.

Weight Loss and Cardiovascular Risk Factors

Framingham Heart Study

A 5-pound weight loss over 16 years lowered the sum of five cardiovascular risk factors—highest quintile of systolic blood pressure, triglycerides, blood glucose, and serum total cholesterol, plus lowest quintile of high-density lipoprotein cholesterol—by 48% in men and 40% in women; conversely, a 5-pound weight gain was associated with a 20% increase in the cardiovascular risk factor sum in men and a 37% increase in women

Randomized clinical trials

Modest weight loss (5%–15% of excess weight) among overweight and obese individuals has been associated with favorable changes in cardiovascular risk factors, including lipoprotein profile, blood pressure, glucose tolerance, and markers of inflammation and hemostasis

Figure 10-17.

Weight change and cardiovascular risk factor profile. Few data are available regarding the long-term benefits of intentional weight loss on incidence of cardiovascular disease. In the observational Framingham Heart Study, a 2.25-kg weight loss over 16 years lowered the sum of five cardiovascular risk factors (highest quintile of systolic blood pressure, triglycerides, blood glucose, and serum total cholesterol, plus lowest quintile of high-density lipoprotein cholesterol) by 48% in men and 40% in women; conversely, a 2.25-kg weight gain was associated with a 20% increase in the cardiovascular risk factor sum in men and a 37% increase in women [50]. In randomized trials, modest weight loss (*ie*, 5%–15% of excess body weight) among overweight and obese individuals has been associated with favorable changes in cardiovascular risk factors, including lipoprotein profile, blood pressure, glucose tolerance and diabetes incidence, and markers of inflammation and hemostasis [13,51–57]. For example, a National Heart, Lung, and Blood Institute review of 14 diet and exercise trials ranging from 12 weeks to 1 year in duration concluded that weight loss achieved through lifestyle modification, particularly an increase in physical activity, reduces serum triglycerides and increases high-density lipoprotein cholesterol and, to a lesser degree, lowers low-density lipoprotein and total cholesterol [13]. Although no summary statistics were computed, intervention versus control group comparisons showed net reductions in body weight from 5% to 13% and changes in lipid parameters as follows: triglycerides, -2% to -44%; high-density lipoprotein cholesterol, -7% to +27%; low-density lipoprotein cholesterol, -3% to -22%; and total cholesterol, 0% to -18%.

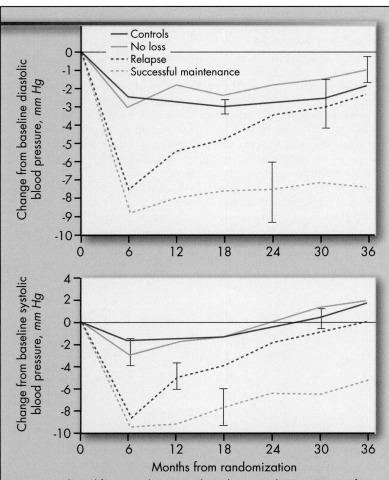

Data are adjusted for age, ethnicity, and gender, according to patterns of weight change. Usual-care control subjects were not assigned to intervention. Participants with successful maintenance of weight loss were defined as those who lost 4.5 kg or more at 6 months and maintained at least 4.5 kg of weight loss at 36 months. Participants with relapse were defined as those who lost at least 4.5 kg at 6 months, but whose weight loss at 36 months was less than 2.5 kg. Participants with no weight loss were defined as those with weight loss of 2.5 kg or less at 6 and 36 months. Error bars represent 95% CI

Figure 10-18.

Mean change in diastolic (*top*) and systolic (*bottom*) blood pressure: Trials of Hypertension Prevention II. A meta-analysis of 25 randomized trials with a total of 4874 participants (mean body mass index = 30.7 kg/m^2) and mean duration of 67 weeks found that a net weight reduction of 5.1 kg (5.8% of initial body weight) by means of caloric restriction, increased physical activity, or both was associated with a reduction of 4.44 mm Hg in systolic blood pressure and 3.57 mm Hg in diastolic blood pressure [51]. After control for the amount of intervention-associated weight loss, the reduction in diastolic blood pressure was significantly larger in trials that included a physical activity component than in trials of caloric restriction only, a finding that suggests that exercise lowers blood pressure in part by mechanisms that are unrelated to weight change. On average, maximal blood pressure benefits were observed midway through the course of treatment. A likely explanation for this pattern is decreasing compliance with the intervention. In the Trials of Hypertension Prevention [58], one of the largest (*n* = 1191) and longest (3 years) studies of weight loss and blood pressure, mean weight change in the intervention group (members were assigned to a program of group and individual counseling sessions focused on dietary change, physical activity, and social support) was -4.4 kg at 6 months, -2.0 kg at 18 months, and -0.2 kg at 36 months, compared with mean weight change of +0.1, +0.7, and +1.8 kg in the usual-care control group. Assignment to the intervention was associated with a reduced risk of hypertension, with relative risks of 0.58, 0.78, and 0.81 at 6, 18, and 36 months, respectively. There was a direct dose-response relationship between weight loss and blood pressure reduction. Combining the data from the intervention and control groups, participants in the quintile of greatest weight loss (> 4.4 kg) had reductions in systolic and diastolic blood pressure of 7.0 and 5.0 mm Hg, whereas those who lost the least amount of weight (*ie*, those who gained 4.2 kg or more) had decreases of 2.4 and 0.7 mm Hg. Similarly, parsing the intervention group by patterns of weight loss showed that intervention participants who sustained a loss of at least 4.5 kg experienced a substantial reduction in blood pressure through 36 months compared with members of the usual-care group, the no-loss intervention group, and the relapse intervention group. Indeed, the reduction in risk (compared with the usual-care group) was much more dramatic among the successful-maintenance intervention group (relative risk, 0.35) than among the intervention group as a whole (relative risk, 0.81). (*From* Stevens *et al.* [58]; with permission.)

Randomized Trials of Diet/Exercise and Incidence of Type 2 Diabetes Mellitus

Study	Study population	Intervention(s)	Length, y	Reduction in risk of type 2 diabetes in intervention group(s) compared with control group
Da Qing Impaired Glucose Tolerance and Diabetes Study	577 men and women with impaired glucose tolerance; mean age, 45 years; mean BMI, 25.8 kg/m^2	Diet only; exercise only; diet plus exercise; control	6	Diet only: 31% ($P < 0.03$) Exercise only: 46% ($P < 0.0005$) Diet plus exercise: 42% ($P < 0.005$)
Finnish Diabetes Prevention Trial	522 men and women with impaired glucose tolerance; mean age, 55 years; mean BMI, 31 kg/m^2	Lifestyle modification program (goal of weight loss = 5%; diet composed of < 30% kcal from fat, < 10% kcal from saturated fat, and ≥ 15 g fiber/1000 kcal; moderate-intensity exercise ≥ 30 min/day) or control	3.2	58% ($P < 0.001$)
US Diabetes Prevention Program	3234 men and women with elevated fasting and post-load glucose; mean age, 51 years; mean BMI, 34 kg/m^2	Lifestyle modification program (goal of weight loss ≥ 7% and exercise ≥ 150 min/wk); or metformin (850 mg twice daily); or placebo	2.8	Lifestyle modification: 58% (95% CI, 48%–66%) Metformin: 31% (95% CI; 17%–43%)

Figure 10-19.

Lifestyle intervention trials and diabetes incidence. Although the data are not entirely consistent, metabolic benefits of weight loss have been observed in population-based observational studies. Among more than 200,000 overweight participants in the American Cancer Society's Cancer Prevention Study I, a history of intentional weight loss at baseline, compared with a history of stable weight, was associated with a reduction in diabetes incidence of 28% in women and 21% in men over 13 years of follow-up, after adjustment for pre-baseline body mass index (BMI) and other metabolic risk factors [59]. On average, for every 20 pounds lost, the risk of diabetes fell by 17% in women and by 11% in men. Among the 4970 overweight participants with diabetes, intentional weight loss (average amount lost, 24 pounds) was associated with a 28% reduction in mortality from diabetes or cardiovascular disease and a 25% reduction in total mortality [60].

Randomized trials demonstrate that even modest weight loss reduces diabetes incidence. In the Da Qing Impaired Glucose Tolerance and Diabetes Study, 577 middle-aged Chinese men and women with impaired glucose tolerance were randomized to one of three treatment groups—diet only, exercise only, or diet plus exercise—or to a control group [52]. Over 6 years, the three interventions were associated with statistically significant reductions of 31%, 46%, and 42% in diabetes risk, respectively In the Finnish Diabetes Prevention Study, 522 middle-aged, overweight men and women with impaired glucose tolerance were randomly assigned to an intensive lifestyle intervention designed to promote healthy eating and exercise patterns or to a control group [53].

Members of the diet and exercise intervention group lost significantly more weight than did the control group (3.5 vs 0.8 kg) and reduced their risk of developing diabetes by 58% over a 3-year interval. The US Diabetes Prevention Program, a 3-year follow-up of 3234 overweight individuals aged 25 to 85 with impaired glucose tolerance, also reported a 58% reduction in diabetes risk among the intervention group, whose members, on average, exercised 30 minutes per day and lost 5% to 7% of their body weight during the course of the trial [54]. An ongoing large-scale randomized intervention, the Look AHEAD (Action For Health in Diabetes) trial funded by the National Institute of Diabetes and Digestive and Kidney Diseases, should provide valuable data on the long-term (10 years or longer) effects of sustained weight loss through decreased caloric intake and exercise on the risk of cardiovascular disease and other chronic conditions in obese diabetic individuals [61].

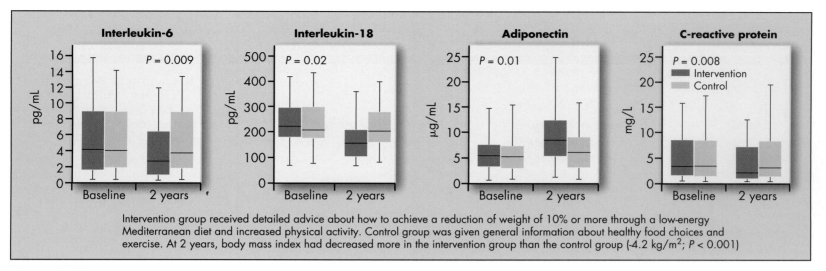

Intervention group received detailed advice about how to achieve a reduction of weight of 10% or more through a low-energy Mediterranean diet and increased physical activity. Control group was given general information about healthy food choices and exercise. At 2 years, body mass index had decreased more in the intervention group than the control group (-4.2 kg/m²; P < 0.001)

Figure 10-20.

Effect of weight loss and lifestyle changes on serum concentrations of cytokines and C-reactive protein: a 2-year randomized trial. In a recent randomized trial, obese premenopausal women assigned to a 2-year weight-loss program that emphasized a low-energy Mediterranean-style diet and moderate physical activity experienced favorable changes in proinflammatory cytokine and C-reactive protein levels compared with women in the control group who were given general information about healthy food choices and exercise [55]. Mean body mass index decreased more in the intervention than in control group

(-4.2 kg/m², P < 0.001), as did serum concentrations of interleukin-6 (-1.1 pg/mL; P = 0.009), interleukin-18 (-57 pg/mL, P = 0.02), and C-reactive protein (-1.6 mg/L, P = 0.008), whereas concentrations of adiponectin increased (+2.2 µg/mL, P = 0.01). Weight loss achieved by caloric restriction alone has also been shown to lower C-reactive protein levels in obese postmenopausal women [56]. Whether these effects translate into a reduced risk of subsequent cardiovascular events has not yet been determined. (*From* Esposito *et al.* [55]; with permission.)

Weight Loss Drugs

Drug	Dosage	Action	Adverse effects
Sibutramine	5, 10, 15 mg; 10 mg orally each day to start, may be increased to 15 mg or decreased to 5 mg	Norepinephrine, dopamine, and serotonin reuptake inhibitor	Increase in heart rate and blood pressure
Orlistat	120 mg; 120 mg orally three times daily before meals	Inhibits pancreatic lipase, decreases fat absorption	Decrease in absorption of fat-soluble vitamins; soft stools and anal leakage

Figure 10-21.

Pharmacologic approaches to weight loss. Two medications—orlistat and sibutramine—are approved by the US Food and Drug Administration for long-term (more than 1 year) use in the treatment of obesity (body mass index 30 kg/m² or greater, or 27 kg/m² or greater with comorbidity). In randomized trials, these medications promote modest weight loss (mean, 3 to 5 kg) beyond that of controls, and prolonged treatment helps maintain at least part of the weight loss for up to 2 years [62,63].

Phentermine, which stimulates the release of norepinephrine and dopamine from nerve terminals, has similar efficacy with respect to weight loss as do orlistat and sibutramine, but is approved only for short-term use (3 months or less) because of a paucity of long-term efficacy and safety data. It is the most commonly prescribed weight loss drug in the United States. Whether these drugs reduce the incidence of cardiovascular disease is not known.

Orlistat reduces fat absorption by inhibiting gastrointestinal lipases. In the 4-year XENDOS (XENical [Roche Pharmaceuticals, Basel, Switzerland] in the prevention of Diabetes in Obese Subjects) trial, 3305 obese subjects aged 30 to 60 years with normal or impaired glucose tolerance were randomized to orlistat (120 mg three times daily) or placebo [64]. All participants were prescribed a reduced-calorie diet and encouraged to walk at least one extra kilometer per day. Mean weight loss was greater in the orlistat than in the placebo group (5.8 vs 3.0 kg, P < 0.001). The cumulative incidence of diabetes was 6.2% in

the orlistat group versus 9% in the placebo group, corresponding to a risk reduction of 37.3% (P = 0.003). Orlistat was also associated with early and significant improvements in cardiovascular risk factors that were sustained throughout the study, including blood pressure and lipid profile (reductions in total cholesterol, low-density lipoprotein cholesterol, and low- to high-density lipoprotein cholesterol ratio).

Gastrointestinal events such as fatty stool, fecal urgency, and oily spotting were the main side effects. Orlistat-treated patients also experienced decreases in levels of the fat-soluble vitamins A, D, E, and K₁, though mean levels remained within their reference ranges. Although XENDOS is the only trial of pharmacologic weight loss to examine incident diabetes as an endpoint, other trials have confirmed the beneficial effect of orlistat on other cardiovascular risk factors [62].

Sibutramine, which is a norepinephrine and serotonin reuptake inhibitor, inhibits appetite and increases satiety. In randomized trials, sibutramine has been associated with an improved lipid profile, although the findings are not entirely consistent. However, sibutramine adversely affects heart rate (mean increase of 4 beats/min) and blood pressure (mean increase of 2–4 mm Hg). Other side effects include dry mouth, constipation, and insomnia. The use of sibutramine is contraindicated in patients with cardiovascular disease or uncontrolled hypertension, or with concomitant use of monoamine oxidase inhibitors or other serotonin reuptake inhibitors. (*Adapted from* National Heart, Lung, and Blood Institute [65].)

Bariatric Surgery: Effects on Weight Loss and Cardiovascular Risk Factors

Weight loss	
Absolute weight loss, *kg*	39.7
BMI decrease, *kg/m²*	14.2
Percent of initial weight lost	32.6
Percent of excess weight lost	61.2
Cardiovascular risk factors	
Diabetes resolved, %	76.8
Hyperlipidemia improved, %	79.3
Hypertension resolved, %	61.7
Hypertension resolved or improved, %	78.5
Obstructive sleep apnea resolved or improved, %	83.6

Figure 10-22.

Surgical approaches to weight loss. Bariatric surgery is the most effective weight-loss therapy available for people who are extremely obese. A recent meta-analytic review of studies of varying design (10,172 patients in total) found that the mean percentage of excess weight lost after bariatric surgery was 61% [66]. Although average duration of follow-up was not reported, the reviewers wrote that "weight-loss outcomes did not differ significantly for assessments at 2 years or less compared with those at more than 2 years." Surgically induced weight loss leads to rapid and dramatic improvements in glucose metabolism, lipid profile, blood pressure, and pulmonary disease. In the meta-analysis, 86% of surgical patients with diabetes experienced amelioration or resolution of this condition; the corresponding figures for dyslipidemia, hypertension, and obstructive sleep apnea were 79%, 78%, and 84%, respectively [66]. The Swedish Obese Subjects study, which is examining long-term outcomes, including mortality and cardiovascular disease incidence, of surgically induced weight loss in middle-aged obese individuals (mean initial body mass index [BMI], 41 kg/m²), found that, over a 10-year period, rates of recovery from diabetes, hypertriglyceridemia, low levels of high-density lipoprotein cholesterol, hypertension, and hyperuricemia were more favorable in the surgical group than in the control group [67]. The widely anticipated final results of this study are not yet available. However, a Canadian study of 1035 bariatric surgery patients (initial BMI 38 kg/m² or greater) and 5746 age- and gender-matched obese control subjects found that the surgery patients, who on average lost 67% of their excess weight and reduced their initial body mass index by 35%, were much less likely than control subjects to die (relative risk, 0.11) or to develop cardiovascular disease (relative risk, 0.18), respiratory disorders (relative risk, 0.24), and other health conditions during 5 years of follow-up [68]. Risks of bariatric surgery include a 30-day mortality rate of approximately 1%, with approximately 75% of deaths caused by anastomotic leaks and peritonitis and 25% by pulmonary embolism [69]; iron and vitamin B12 deficiency; and gastrointestinal symptoms such as nausea, bloating, diarrhea, and colic. (*Data from* Buchwald *et al.* [67].)

Economic Burden of Obesity

Economic burden of overweight/obesity in US adults
 Total cost = $117 billion
 Direct cost (health care spending for preventive, diagnostic, and treatment services, including outpatient visits, medications, and hospitalizations) = $61 billion
 Indirect cost (value of lost wages and productivity) = $56 billion

Direct cost of obesity represents
 9% of total health care spending
 17% of health care spending to treat cardiovascular disease

Economic burden of overweight/obesity in US children and adolescents
 Annual hospital costs for obesity-related diagnoses rose from $35 million in 1979–1981 to $127 million in 1997–1999

Figure 10-23.

Economic burden of obesity. Estimates of the economic burden of overweight and obesity among US adults range from $98 billion to $129 billion per year, with a roughly even split between direct costs (preventive, diagnostic, and treatment services, including doctor visits, medications, and hospitalizations) and indirect costs (value of lost wages and productivity because of illness or premature death) [8,11]. Direct costs related to overweight and obesity account for an estimated 9% of total health care spending [12] and an estimated 17% of health care spending for the treatment of cardiovascular disease [69,70]. Among US children, annual hospital costs for obesity-related diagnoses have more than tripled in recent years, rising from $35 million between 1979 and 1981 to $127 million between 1997 and 1999 [71].

Although many studies have examined the relationship between obesity and health care costs, few have focused on the economic consequences of weight gain per se. However, in a recent study of initially overweight men and women aged 35 to 65 years in a large US health maintenance organization, the 3-year increase in health care costs was $561 greater for individuals who gained 20 or more pounds during this period than for their weight-stable counterparts, after adjustment for age, gender, and baseline body mass index, comorbid health conditions, and costs [72]. In analyses limited to individuals with baseline comorbidities, the corresponding statistic was $711. The demonstration that weight gain is accompanied by high-er medical expenses even in the relatively short term provides a strong economic incentive for weight maintenance or obesity prevention initiatives.

A systematic review of the cost-effectiveness of weight-loss treatments is beyond the scope of this chapter. Although recommending intensive counseling and behavior therapy for obese patients, the United States Preventive Services Task Force reported that such therapy may require "a large amount of time and substantial staffing commitment" [73]. Estimates of the incremental economic benefit gained by adding pharmacologic therapies to diet and exercise for the treatment of obesity vary widely depending on model assumptions and populations studied (most studies have been conducted in Europe). Findings from a recent US study suggest that the addition of orlistat to established therapies may be economically beneficial among overweight patients with type 2 diabetes, with a cost-effectiveness ratio of US $8327 per event-free life-year gained [74]. The large Canadian study described in the legend to figure 10-22 found that bariatric surgery led to decreased health care costs during a 5-year follow-up period [75]. Although health care costs were higher among bariatric surgery patients than among other obese patients in the first year of the study, the reverse was true in later years. Over 5 years, the annualized cost advantage attributable to bariatric surgery was estimated to be $1150 (Canadian dollars) per patient. (*Data from* US Department of Health and Human Services [8]; Finkelstein *et al.* [12]; and Wang *et al.* [70,71].)

US Preventive Services Task Force Findings

The US Preventive Services Task Force concluded that high-intensity counseling and behavioral interventions for obesity typically result in weight loss of 3 to 5 kg within 1 year; however, the evidence was not sufficient to determine whether moderate- to low-intensity counseling together with behavioral interventions leads to sustained weight loss or increased physical activity

This underscores the need for rigorous long-term randomized clinical trials of behavioral interventions for weight loss and increased physical activity

Figure 10-24.
Lifestyle interventions for weight loss. In 1998, the National Heart, Lung, and Blood Institute reviewed randomized clinical trials on the efficacy of lifestyle interventions for weight loss [13]. In 34 trials of caloric restriction (1000–1200 kcal/day) for weight reduction, an average weight loss of 8% of initial body weight was obtained over 3 to 12 months. In most of these studies, a low-fat diet was promoted as a practical way to reduce calories. Ten of 12 randomized trials of physical activity (primarily aerobic exercise performed in 30- to 60-minute sessions, three to seven times per week, for 16 weeks to 1 year) for weight reduction showed a benefit, with a mean weight loss of 2.4 kg in the exercise group compared with the control group. In 12 of 15 trials that directly compared caloric restriction only, exercise only, or a combination intervention, the latter approach produced greater weight loss than diet alone (mean difference, 1.9 kg) or exercise alone (5.3 kg). The addition of behavior therapy to help patients acquire the skills and supports needed to change eating patterns and to become physically active is also beneficial. In its 2003 review, the US Preventive Services Task Force concluded that high-intensity counseling and behavioral interventions for obesity typically result in weight loss of 3 to 5 kg within 1 year (*high-intensity* was defined as two or more sessions per month for at least the first 3 months of a given intervention) [76]. Because of a dearth of research, the US Preventive Services Task Force was unable to evaluate whether moderate- or low-intensity counseling leads to sustained weight loss [75] or increased physical activity [77], underscoring the need for rigorous long-term randomized trials of these interventions.

Descriptive studies of formerly obese individuals suggest that permanent weight reduction requires long-term adherence to a maintenance program. In the National Weight Control Registry, a sample of 629 women and 155 men who lost an average of 30 kg and maintained a minimum weight loss of 13.6 kg for 5 years, respondents reported daily energy intakes of 1300 to 1500 kcal, and daily energy expenditures of 2500 kcal (women) and 3300 kcal (men), exercise levels that correspond to 1 to 1.5 hours per day of moderate-intensity exercise such as brisk walking [78]. Findings from this study also suggest that low-fat diets are more effective than low-carbohydrate diets for maintaining weight loss, but randomized trials comparing isocaloric diets of differing composition for weight control are sparse. Importantly, although low-fat diets have been associated with favorable health effects in long-term studies, the health consequences of low-carbohydrate diets are not known.

The shape of the dose-response curve between physical activity and body weight also remains unclear. As reported in figure 10-4, the Centers for Disease Control (CDC) and American College of Sports Medicine (ACSM) have recommended that adults engage in 30 minutes of moderate-intensity physical activity on most, and preferably all, days of the week [20], a standard also endorsed by the US Surgeon General [79]. The CDC/ACSM and Surgeon General's guidelines, developed in the 1990s, focused on multiple health outcomes rather than on weight control specifically. In 2002, the Institute of Medicine doubled the daily goal to 60 minutes of moderate-intensity exercise, arguing that lesser amounts of activity have not been consistently shown to ensure weight maintenance within the healthy body mass index range of 18.5 to 25.0 kg/m^2 or to promote weight loss in the absence of curtailing caloric intake [80]. In 2005, the US Department of Health and Human Services and the US Department of Agriculture, while concurring with the CDC/ACSM and Surgeon General's recommendations of 30 minutes of daily activity for disease risk reduction, also espoused a 60- to 90-minute per day goal for weight control [81]. Several lines of evidence do suggest that an hour of activity per day may be necessary to control weight without also practicing dietary restraint. In an Institute of Medicine–compiled database of 407 healthy stable-weight adults whose energy expenditures had been estimated with the doubly-labeled water method, considered the gold standard of energy expenditure measurement, persons with body mass index between 18.5 and 25.0 kg/m^2 expended a daily energy equivalent of at least 1 hour of moderate activity. Studies such as the National Weight Control Registry also suggest that 80 minutes per day of moderately intense activity (or 35 minutes per day of vigorous activity) are required for long-term weight-loss maintenance. However, findings from recent randomized trials of exercise in overweight, sedentary individuals who were asked to adhere to their usual diet indicate that lesser amounts of physical activity can also have a beneficial effect on weight control [82]. (*Data from* US Preventive Services Task Force [76,77].

Figure 10-25.

Clinician counseling. Although the most effective weight loss programs combine calorie control with increased physical activity, only 20% of US adults attempting to lose weight reported using the recommended combination of eating fewer calories and engaging in at least 150 minutes of moderate-intensity activity per week [83]. By reinforcing the importance of dietary moderation and physical activity, clinicians can play an important role in reducing the epidemic of obesity. The US Preventive Services Task Force recommends that clinicians screen all adult patients for obesity and offer high-intensity counseling and behavioral interventions to promote sustained weight loss for those who are obese [76]. However, national studies find that many clinicians do not routinely assess weight and physical activity or offer advice on these factors. Data from the Behavioral Risk Factor Surveillance Survey indicate that less than one half (42%) of obese adults who had visited their physicians for a routine check-up reported receiving advice to lose weight [84]. Moreover, despite the fact that more than two of three adults do not exercise enough to meet the 30-minute per day guideline, data from the National Health Interview Survey indicate that just one of three adults who saw a physician in the prior year were counseled about physical activity at their last visit [85]. These trends are generally attributed to lack of training, lack of time for counseling in practice settings, a dearth of appropriate patient materials, and little or no reimbursement. Although intensive intervention may be ideal for obese patients, simply acknowledging the problem and providing straightforward suggestions for remedies are excellent starting points that require little training or time.

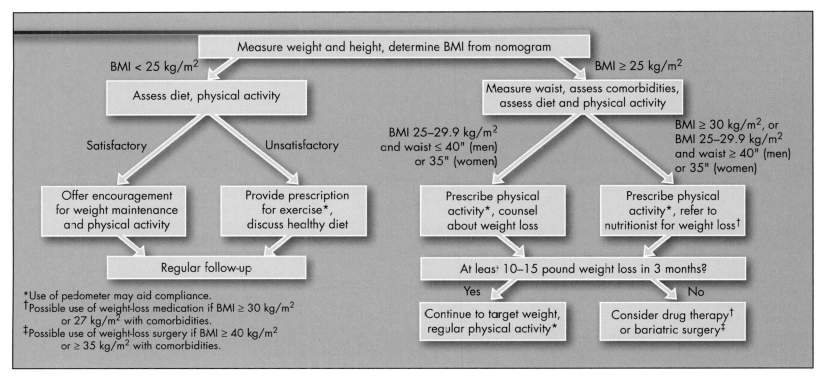

Figure 10-26.

Flow chart for the evaluation and counseling of an individual regarding weight and physical activity during the patient encounter. A strategy based on guidelines on obesity developed by the National Heart, Lung, and Blood Institute [13,65] and the US Surgeon General's reports on obesity [8] and physical activity [79] offers a blueprint for clinicians who are perplexed about how to incorporate counseling about weight and physical activity into their daily practices [86]. Similar guidelines have been endorsed by the American Heart Association [69] and jointly by the American Diabetes Association, North American Association for the Study of Obesity, and American Society for Clinical Nutrition [87]. BMI—body mass index. (*From* Manson *et al.* [86]; with permission.)

Possible Elements for a "Prescription" for Weight Loss or Maintenance

Diet	Exercise
Pay attention to portions; avoid "super-sizing"; when eating out, consider splitting an entrée	Take the stairs whenever possible
Set regular times to eat: three meals and no more than two snacks per day	Purchase a pedometer and aim for 10,000 steps per day
Limit saturated and trans fat	Display "exercise prescription" in a visible place
Increase daily intake of fruits and vegetables: at least five, but aim for seven to nine servings	If you drive to work or stores, park in a space far away from the door and walk
Because fiber can increase the feeling of fullness, aim for two to three servings of whole grain food per day	If you take public transportation, get off a stop early and walk
Limit sweet beverages; drink water or nonfat or 1% milk	Walk on your lunch break
	Try exercising with friends or a group
	Consider strength training for 20 minutes two to three times per week

Figure 10-27.

Elements that may be used in a "prescription" for weight loss or maintenance. A loss of 5% of initial body weight at a rate of 0.5 to 0.9 kg (1 to 2 pounds) per week over a 6-month period is a reasonable goal for most patients and can generally be accomplished with an energy deficit of 500 to 1000 kcal/day that is best achieved by restricting intake through smaller portion sizes; minimizing snacks, desserts, sugar-sweetened sodas, and other sugar-laden beverages; lowering the energy density of the diet (*eg*, by increasing fruit and vegetable intakes and limiting foods that are high in fat); and increasing physical activity. Although target calorie intakes vary by baseline body weight, weight-loss diets should generally supply 1000 to 1200 kcal/day for women and 1200 to 1600 kcal/day for men. Physical activity is an important component of any weight-management program. The National Heart, Lung, and Blood Institute recommends an initial goal of 30 to 45 minutes of moderate-intensity aerobic physical activity 3 to 5 days per week [65]. Programs to help sedentary patients work up to 30 minutes of activity per day over the course of several weeks are available from the American Heart Association [88,89] and the National Institute on Aging [90]. Data from randomized trials suggest that so-called "lifestyle activity" interventions, which encourage patients to incorporate short bouts of physical activity in their daily life (*eg*, taking short walks during lunch breaks; doing yard work or gardening; and using the stairs instead of the elevator), can be more effective than traditional exercise programs (*eg*, structured workout sessions at the gym) in boosting activity levels and improving physical fitness and cardiovascular risk profiles [91]. The use of self-monitoring strategies such as a pedometer or exercise diaries may also encourage daily activity [92]. Greater activity levels (*ie*, at least 60 minutes of moderate activity per day, or 30 minutes of vigorous activity) may be needed for long-term weight loss without sufficient reduction in caloric intake. Strength training should also be included in a physical activity prescription; the associated increase in resting metabolic rate may contribute to weight loss. (*From* Manson *et al.* [86]; with permission.)

Guide to Treating Overweight/Obesity

Therapy	BMI Category, kg/m^2				
	25–26.9	27–29.9	30–34.9	35–39.9	≥ 40
Diet, physical activity, and behavior therapy to achieve weight loss*	WC	WC	+	+	+
Pharmacotherapy†	NR	WC	+	+	+
Surgery	NR	NR	NR	WC	+

*Prevention of weight gain with lifestyle therapy is indicated in any patient with BMI 25 or greater even without comorbidities, whereas weight loss is not necessarily recommended for those with BMI 25–29.9, unless they have two or more comorbidities. Combined therapy with lower calorie diet, increased physical activity, and behavior therapy provides the most successful intervention for weight loss and maintenance.

†Consider pharmacotherapy only if patient has not lost four pounds per month after 3 to 6 months of combined lifestyle therapy.

Figure 10-28.

Guide to treating overweight/obesity. Patients with body mass index (BMI) of 30 kg/m^2 or greater, or with BMI of 27 kg/m^2 or greater and comorbidities, may be candidates for pharmacotherapy with orlistat, sibutramine, or phentermine. If concerted efforts of lifestyle modification and pharmacotherapy have failed, bariatric surgery may be an option for patients with BMI of 40 kg/m^2 or greater, or with BMI of 35 kg/m^2 or greater and comorbidities. Comorbidities such as hypertension and hyperlipidemia should be intensively managed. +—consider use of indicated treatment regardless of comorbidities; NR—not recommended; WC—with comorbidities. (*Adapted from* National Heart, Lung, and Blood Institute [65].)

Community-level Interventions

Federal government	Industry and media	State and local government	Community and nonprofit organizations	State and local education authorities
Develop nutrition standards for foods and beverages sold in schools	Develop healthier food and beverage products and packaging innovations	Expand and promote opportunities for physical activity through changes to ordinances, capital improvement programs, and other planning practices	Provide opportunities for healthful eating and physical activity in existing and new community programs, particularly for high-risk populations	Improve nutritional quality of foods and beverages served and sold in schools
Fund state-based nutrition and physical-activity grants with strong evaluation components	Expand consumer nutrition information			Increased opportunities for frequent, more intensive physical activity during or after school
Develop guidelines for advertising and marketing to children	Provide clear and consistent media messages	Work with communities to support partnerships and networks that expand availability and access to healthful foods		Implement school-based interventions to reduce children's screen time
Expand funding for prevention intervention research, experimental research, and community-based population research; and evaluation efforts				Develop, implement, evaluate innovative pilot programs for teaching about healthful eating and physical activity

Figure 10-29.

Community-level interventions. Clinicians can also be influential by endorsing government, community, school, and workplace policies that promote healthy weight, increased physical activity, and disease prevention. A partial list of such policies is provided by the Institute of Medicine in its 2005 report *Preventing Childhood Obesity: Health in the Balance* [11]. Although interventions to foster preferences for healthy foods and physical activity appear to be most effective in early life, many of these policies are likely to benefit people of all ages [93]. A growing body of evidence links food advertising, which overwhelmingly favors foods of poor nutritional quality (in the United States, the average child views 10,000 food ads on television per year, with 90%–95% of these for sugared cereals, fast food, soft drinks, and candy [93]), and unhealthful food consumption patterns [94]. Data from the National Health and Nutrition Examination Survey indicate that one third of the calories consumed by adults are from sweets, alcoholic beverages, and sodas, with the latter alone contributing approximately 7% of calories [95]. Although direct regulation of such advertising would be optimal, allotting equal time for pro-nutrition messages may be more politically feasible. Other potential obesity-prevention policies include prohibiting the sale of fast foods and soft drinks in schools; subsidizing the sale of healthy foods and taxing unhealthy foods; increasing mandatory physical education requirements in schools; and providing resources for physical activity in communities and workplaces. Although additional studies are urgently needed to determine whether these and other community-level interventions foster lasting improvements in nutrition and physical activity behaviors, there are data to suggest that these policies are effective. For example, a recent randomized trial has shown that a school-based educational program aimed at reducing soda consumption led to a significant decline in the number of overweight and obese children [96]. (*From* Institute of Medicine [11]; with permission.)

Future Challenges

For basic researchers:
  To develop an increased understanding of the pathophysiology of obesity (interrelationship between obesity, metabolic syndrome, and cardiovascular disease)
For health care providers and policymakers:
  To determine how best to promote healthy diet and physical activity levels to patients and the general public, respectively

Figure 10-30.

Future challenges. Despite recent advances in basic and clinical research, our understanding of the connection between obesity, the metabolic syndrome, and cardiovascular disease remains incomplete. Obesity influences multiple metabolic pathways and has been linked to so many potential cardiovascular risk factors that scientists to date have not yet fully disentangled the more important and the less important mechanisms by which obesity raises cardiovascular risk. Unraveling the pathophysiologic complexity of obesity may lead to the discovery of new therapeutic targets to prevent its cardiovascular sequelae. However, regardless of whether a complete understanding of the pathophysiology of obesity is ultimately achieved, the core challenge for health care providers and policymakers is determining how best to promote healthy diet and physical activity levels to their patients and to the general public, respectively. Given the soaring prevalence of obesity, helping even a small percentage of overweight or obese individuals reach a lower weight would substantially reduce cardiovascular morbidity and mortality, as would helping those already in the healthy weight range avoid future weight gain.

References

1. Willett WC, Dietz WH, Colditz GA: Guidelines for healthy weight. *N Engl J Med* 1999, 341:427–434.

2. Must A, Spadano J, Coakley EH, *et al.*: The disease burden associated with overweight and obesity. *JAMA* 1999, 282:1523–1529.

3. Mokdad AH, Ford ES, Bowman BA, *et al.*: Prevalence of obesity, diabetes, and obesity-related health risk factors, 2001. *JAMA* 2003, 289:76–79.

4. Field AE, Coakley EH, Must A, *et al.*: Impact of overweight on the risk of developing common chronic diseases during a 10-year period. *Arch Intern Med* 2001, 161:1581–1586.

5. Hubert HB, Feinleib M, McNamara PM, Castelli WP: Obesity as an independent risk factor for cardiovascular disease: a 26-year follow-up of participants in the Framingham Heart Study. *Circulation* 1983, 67:968–977.

6. Sturm R, Wells KB: Does obesity contribute as much to morbidity as poverty or smoking? *Public Health* 2001, 115:229–235.

7. Allison DB, Fontaine KR, Manson JE, *et al.*: Annual deaths attributable to obesity in the United States. *JAMA* 1999, 282:1530–1538.

8. US Department of Health and Human Services: *The Surgeon General's Call to Action to Prevent and Decrease Overweight and Obesity*. Rockville: US Department of Health and Human Services, Public Health Service, Office of the Surgeon General; 2001.

9. Peeters A, Barendregt JJ, Willekens F, *et al.*: Obesity in adulthood and its consequences for life expectancy: a life-table analysis. *Ann Intern Med* 2003, 138:24–32.

10. Fontaine KR, Redden DT, Wang C, *et al.*: Years of life lost due to obesity. *JAMA* 2003, 289:187–193.

11. Institute of Medicine: *Preventing Childhood Obesity: Health in the Balance*. Washington DC: National Academies Press; 2005.

12. Finkelstein EA, Fiebelkorn IC, Wang G: National medical spending attributable to overweight and obesity: how much, and who's paying? *Health Aff (Millwood)* 2003, W3:219–226.

13. National Heart Lung and Blood Institute: *Clinical Guidelines on the Identification, Evaluation, and Treatment of Overweight and Obesity in Adults: The Evidence Report*. Washington DC: NIH Publication Number 98-4083; 1998. Available at http://www.nhlbi.nih.gov/guidelines/obesity/ob_gdlns.htm.

14. Hedley AA, Ogden CL, Johnson CL, *et al.*: Prevalence of overweight and obesity among US children, adolescents, and adults, 1999–2002. *JAMA* 2004, 291:2847–2850.

15. Flegal KM, Carroll MD, Ogden CL, Johnson CL: Prevalence and trends in obesity among US adults, 1999–2000. *JAMA* 2002, 288:1723–1727.

16. Ogden CL, Flegal KM, Carroll MD, Johnson CL: Prevalence and trends in overweight among US children and adolescents, 1999–2000. *JAMA* 2002, 288:1728–1732.

17. Brown WM, Beck SR, Lange EM, *et al.*: Age-stratified heritability estimation in the Framingham Heart Study families. *BMC Genet* 2003, 4(suppl 1):S32.

18. Bulik CM, Sullivan PF, Kendler KS: Genetic and environmental contributions to obesity and binge eating. *Int J Eat Disord* 2003, 33:293–298.

19. Centers for Disease Control and Prevention: Trends in intake of energy and macronutrients—United States, 1971–2000. *MMWR Morbid Mortal Wkly Rep* 2004, 53:80–82.

20. Pate RR, Pratt M, Blair SN, *et al.*: Physical activity and public health: a recommendation from the Centers for Disease Control and Prevention and the American College of Sports Medicine. *JAMA* 1995, 273:402–407.

21. Schoenborn CA, Barnes P: *Leisure-time Physical Activity Among Adults, US 1997–98. Advance Data from Vital and Health Statistics*, no. 325. Hyattsville MD: National Center for Health Statistics; 2002.

22. Grunbaum JA, Kann L, Kinchen SA, *et al.*: Youth risk behavior surveillance—United States, 2001. *MMWR Surveill Summ* 2002, 51:1–62.

23. Manson JE, Willett WC, Stampfer MJ, *et al.*: Body weight and mortality among women. *N Engl J Med* 1995, 333:677–685.

24. Calle EE, Thun MJ, Petrelli JM, *et al.*: Body-mass index and mortality in a prospective cohort of U.S. adults. *N Engl J Med* 1999, 341:1097–1105.

25. Engeland A, Bjorge T, Sogaard AJ, Tverdal A: Body mass index in adolescence in relation to total mortality: 32-year follow-up of 227,000 Norwegian boys and girls. *Am J Epidemiol* 2003, 157:517–523.

26. Eckel RH, Krauss RM: American Heart Association call to action: obesity as a major risk factor for coronary heart disease. AHA Nutrition Committee. *Circulation* 1998, 97:2099–2100.

27. Kenchaiah S, Evans JC, Levy D, *et al.*: Obesity and the risk of heart failure. *N Engl J Med* 2002, 347:305–313.

28. Wang TJ, Parise H, Levy D, *et al.*: Obesity and the risk of new-onset atrial fibrillation. *JAMA* 2004, 292:2471–2477.

29. Willett WC, Manson JE, Stampfer MJ, *et al.*: Weight, weight change, and coronary heart disease in women: risk within the 'normal' weight range. *JAMA* 1995, 273:461–465.

30. Huang Z, Willett WC, Manson JE, *et al.*: Body weight, weight change, and risk for hypertension in women. *Ann Intern Med* 1998, 128:81–88.

31. Rexrode KM, Hennekens CH, Willett WC, *et al.*: A prospective study of body mass index, weight change, and risk of stroke in women. *JAMA* 1997, 277:1539–1545.

32. Goldhaber SZ, Grodstein F, Stampfer MJ, *et al.*: A prospective study of risk factors for pulmonary embolism in women. *JAMA* 1997, 277:642–645.

33. Expert Panel on Detection Evaluation and Treatment of High Blood Cholesterol in Adults: Executive summary of the Third Report of the National Cholesterol Education Program (NCEP) Expert Panel on Detection, Evaluation, and Treatment of High Blood Cholesterol in Adults (Adult Treatment Panel III). *JAMA* 2001, 285:2486–2497.

34. Centers for Disease Control and Prevention: *Diabetes: Disabling, Deadly, and on the Rise: 2004*. Atlanta: Centers for Disease Control and Prevention; 2004.

35. Narayan KM, Boyle JP, Thompson TJ, *et al.*: Lifetime risk for diabetes mellitus in the United States. *JAMA* 2003, 290:1884–1890.

36. Colditz GA, Willett WC, Rotnitzky A, Manson JE: Weight gain as a risk factor for clinical diabetes mellitus in women. *Ann Intern Med* 1995, 122:481–486.

37. Hu FB, Manson JE, Stampfer MJ, *et al.*: Diet, lifestyle, and the risk of type 2 diabetes mellitus in women. *N Engl J Med* 2001, 345:790–797.

38. Grundy SM: What is the contribution of obesity to the metabolic syndrome? *Endocrinol Metab Clin North Am* 2004, 33:267–282.

39. Rajala MW, Scherer PE: Mini-review: The adipocyte—at the crossroads of energy homeostasis, inflammation, and atherosclerosis. *Endocrinology* 2003, 144:3765–3773.

40. Ashton WD, Nanchahal K, Wood DA: Body mass index and metabolic risk factors for coronary heart disease in women. *Eur Heart J* 2001, 22:46–55.

41. Freedman DS, Dietz WH, Srinivasan SR, Berenson GS: The relation of overweight to cardiovascular risk factors among children and adolescents: the Bogalusa Heart Study. *Pediatrics* 1999, 103:1175–1182.

42. Reaven GM: Banting lecture 1988. Role of insulin resistance in human disease. *Diabetes* 1988, 37:1595–1607.

43. Grundy SM, Brewer HB Jr, Cleeman JI, *et al.*: Definition of metabolic syndrome: report of the National Heart, Lung, and Blood Institute/American Heart Association conference on scientific issues related to definition. *Circulation* 2004, 109:433–438.

44. Ford ES, Giles WH, Mokdad AH: Increasing prevalence of the metabolic syndrome among U.S. adults. *Diabetes Care* 2004, 27:2444–2449.

45. de Ferranti SD, Gauvreau K, Ludwig DS, *et al.*: Prevalence of the metabolic syndrome in American adolescents: findings from the third National Health and Nutrition Examination Survey. *Circulation* 2004, 110:2494–2497.

46. Rexrode KM, Carey VJ, Hennekens CH, *et al.*: Abdominal adiposity and coronary heart disease in women. *JAMA* 1998, 280:1843–1848.

47. Williamson DF, Pamuk E, Thun M, *et al.*: Prospective study of intentional weight loss and mortality in never-smoking overweight US white women aged 40–64 years. *Am J Epidemiol* 1995, 141:1128–1141.

48. Williamson DF, Pamuk E, Thun M, *et al.*: Prospective study of intentional weight loss and mortality in overweight white men aged 40–64 years. *Am J Epidemiol* 1999, 149:491–503.

49. Gregg EW, Gerzoff RB, Thompson TJ, Williamson DF: Intentional weight loss and death in overweight and obese U.S. adults 35 years of age and older. *Ann Intern Med* 2003, 138:383–389.

50. Wilson PW, Kannel WB, Silbershatz H, D'Agostino RB: Clustering of metabolic factors and coronary heart disease. *Arch Intern Med* 1999, 159:1104–1109.

51. Neter JE, Stam BE, Kok FJ, *et al.*: Influence of weight reduction on blood pressure: a meta-analysis of randomized controlled trials. *Hypertension* 2003, 42:878–884.

52. Pan XR, Li GW, Hu YH, *et al.*: Effects of diet and exercise in preventing NIDDM in people with impaired glucose tolerance. The Da Qing IGT and Diabetes Study. *Diabetes Care* 1997, 20:537–544.

53. Tuomilehto J, Lindstrom J, Eriksson JG, *et al.*: Prevention of type 2 diabetes mellitus by changes in lifestyle among subjects with impaired glucose tolerance. *N Engl J Med* 2001, 344:1343–1350.

54. Diabetes Prevention Program Research Group: Reduction in the incidence of type 2 diabetes with lifestyle intervention or metformin. *N Engl J Med* 2002, 346:393–403.

55. Esposito K, Pontillo A, Di Palo C, *et al.*: Effect of weight loss and lifestyle changes on vascular inflammatory markers in obese women: a randomized trial. *JAMA* 2003, 289:1799–804.

56. Tchernof A, Nolan A, Sites CK, *et al.*: Weight loss reduces C-reactive protein levels in obese postmenopausal women. *Circulation* 2002, 105:564–569.

57. Van Gaal LF, Wauters MA, De Leeuw IH: The beneficial effects of modest weight loss on cardiovascular risk factors. *Int J Obes Relat Metab Disord* 1997, 21(suppl 1):S5–S9.

58. Stevens VJ, Obarzanek E, Cook NR, *et al.*: Long-term weight loss and changes in blood pressure: results of the Trials of Hypertension Prevention, phase II. *Ann Intern Med* 2001, 134:1–11.

59. Will JC, Williamson DF, Ford ES, *et al.*: Intentional weight loss and 13-year diabetes incidence in overweight adults. *Am J Public Health* 2002, 92:1245–1248.

60. Williamson DF, Thompson TJ, Thun M, *et al.*: Intentional weight loss and mortality among overweight individuals with diabetes. *Diabetes Care* 2000, 23:1499–1504.

61. Ryan DH, Espeland MA, Foster GD, *et al.*: Look AHEAD (Action for Health in Diabetes): design and methods for a clinical trial of weight loss for the prevention of cardiovascular disease in type 2 diabetes. *Control Clin Trials* 2003, 24:610–628.

62. Padwal R, Li SK, Lau DC: Long-term pharmacotherapy for overweight and obesity: a systematic review and meta-analysis of randomized controlled trials. *Int J Obes Relat Metab Disord* 2003, 27:1437–1446.

63. Arterburn DE, Crane PK, Veenstra DL: The efficacy and safety of sibutramine for weight loss: a systematic review. *Arch Intern Med* 2004, 164:994–1003.

64. Torgerson JS, Hauptman J, Boldrin MN, Sjostrom L: XENical in the prevention of Diabetes in Obese Subjects (XENDOS) study: a randomized study of orlistat as an adjunct to lifestyle changes for the prevention of type 2 diabetes in obese patients. *Diabetes Care* 2004, 27:155–161.

65. National Heart Lung and Blood Institute, North American Association for the Study of Obesity: *The Practical Guide: Identification, Evaluation, and Treatment of Overweight and Obesity in Adults.* Washington DC: NIH Publication Number 00-4084, 2000. Available at http://www.nhlbi.nih.gov/guidelines/obesity/practgde.htm.

66. Sjostrom L, Lindroos AK, Peltonen M, *et al.*: Lifestyle, diabetes, and cardiovascular risk factors 10 years after bariatric surgery. *N Engl J Med* 2004, 351:2683–2693.

67. Buchwald H, Avidor Y, Braunwald E, *et al.*: Bariatric surgery: a systematic review and meta-analysis. *JAMA* 2004, 292:1724–1737.

68. Christou NV, Sampalis JS, Liberman M, *et al.*: Surgery decreases long-term mortality, morbidity, and health care use in morbidly obese patients. *Ann Surg* 2004, 240:416–423.

69. Klein S, Burke LE, Bray GA, *et al.*: Clinical implications of obesity with specific focus on cardiovascular disease: a statement for professionals from the American Heart Association Council on Nutrition, Physical Activity, and Metabolism: endorsed by the American College of Cardiology Foundation. *Circulation* 2004, 110:2952–2967.

70. Wang G, Zheng ZJ, Heath G, *et al.*: Economic burden of cardiovascular disease associated with excess body weight in U.S. adults. *Am J Prev Med* 2002, 23:1–6.

71. Wang G, Dietz WH: Economic burden of obesity in youths aged 6 to 17 years: 1979–1999. *Pediatrics* 2002, 109:E81.

72. Elmer PJ, Brown JB, Nichols GA, Oster G: Effects of weight gain on medical care costs. *Int J Obes Relat Metab Disord* 2004, 28:1365–1373.

73. McTigue KM, Harris R, Hemphill B, *et al.*: Screening and interventions for obesity in adults: summary of the evidence for the U.S. Preventive Services Task Force. *Ann Intern Med* 2003, 139:933–949.

74. Maetzel A, Ruof J, Covington M, Wolf A: Economic evaluation of orlistat in overweight and obese patients with type 2 diabetes mellitus. *Pharmacoeconomics* 2003, 21:501–512.

75. Sampalis JS, Liberman M, Auger S, Christou NV: The impact of weight reduction surgery on health-care costs in morbidly obese patients. *Obes Surg* 2004, 14:939–947.

76. US Preventive Services Task Force: Screening for obesity in adults: recommendations and rationale. *Ann Intern Med* 2003, 139:930–932.

77. US Preventive Services Task Force: Behavioral counseling in primary care to promote physical activity: recommendation and rationale. *Ann Intern Med* 2002, 137:205–207.

78. Hill J, Wing R: The National Weight Control Registry. *The Permanente Journal* 2003, 7:34–37. Available at http://xnet.kp.org/permanentejournal/sum03/registry.html.

79. US Department of Health and Human Services: *Physical Activity and Health: A Report of the Surgeon General.* Atlanta: US Department of Health and Human Services; 1996.

80. Institute of Medicine: *Dietary Reference Intakes for Energy, Carbohydrates, Fiber, Fat, Protein, and Amino Acids.* Washington DC: The National Academies Press; 2002.

81. US Department of Health and Human Services and US Department of Agriculture: *Dietary Guidelines for Americans*, edn 6. Washington, DC: US Government Printing Office; 2005.

82. Bassuk SS, Manson JE: Other risk interventions: exercise. In *Women and Heart Disease*, edn 2. Edited by Wenger NK, Collins P. London: Martin Dunitz; in press.

83. Serdula MK, Mokdad AH, Williamson DF, *et al.*: Prevalence of attempting weight loss and strategies for controlling weight. *JAMA* 1999, 282:1353–1358.

84. Galuska DA, Will JC, Serdula MK, Ford ES: Are health care professionals advising obese patients to lose weight? *JAMA* 1999, 282:1576–1578.

85. Wee CC, McCarthy EP, Davis RB, Phillips RS: Physician counseling about exercise. *JAMA* 1999, 282:1583–1588.

86. Manson JE, Skerrett PJ, Greenland P, VanItallie TB: The escalating pandemics of obesity and sedentary lifestyle: a call to action for clinicians. *Arch Intern Med* 2004, 164:249–258.

87. Klein S, Sheard NF, Pi-Sunyer X, *et al.*: Weight management through lifestyle modification for the prevention and management of type 2 diabetes: rationale and strategies: a statement of the American Diabetes Association, the North American Association for the Study of Obesity, and the American Society for Clinical Nutrition. *Diabetes Care* 2004, 27:2067–2073.

88. American Heart Association: *Exercise and Your Heart*. Dallas TX: American Heart Association, National Heart Lung and Blood Institute; 1999.

89. American Heart Association: *Choose To Move Handbook*. Dallas TX: American Heart Association; 2004.

90. National Institute on Aging: *Exercise: A Guide*. Bethesda: National Institute on Aging; 2004.

91. Pratt M: Benefits of lifestyle activity vs structured exercise. *JAMA* 1999, 281:375–376.

92. Speck BJ, Looney SW: Effects of a minimal intervention to increase physical activity in women: daily activity records. *Nurs Res* 2001, 50:374–378.

93. Wadden TA, Brownell KD, Foster GD: Obesity: responding to the global epidemic. *J Consult Clin Psychol* 2002, 70:510–525.

94. Caroli M, Argentieri L, Cardone M, Masi A: Role of television in childhood obesity prevention. *Int J Obes Relat Metab Disord* 2004, 28(suppl 3):S104–S108.

95. Block G: Foods contributing to energy intake in the US: data from NHANES III and NHANES 1999–2000. *J Food Composit Anal* 2004, 17:439–447.

96. James J, Thomas P, Cavan D, Kerr D: Preventing childhood obesity by reducing consumption of carbonated drinks: cluster randomized controlled trial. *BMJ* 2004, 328:1237.

Obesity and Weight Loss

Physical Inactivity/Exercise

Larry W. Gibbons and S. Michael Clark

In 1992, the American Heart Association designated physical inactivity as the fourth major risk factor for coronary heart disease, along with cigarette smoking, hypertension, and abnormal cholesterol profile. Despite the universal acceptance of the substantial benefits of exercise, the majority of adult Americans are still sedentary, adding to the burden of heart disease already firmly in control of the lead role in causes of death in the United States. Most Americans do not realize the significant danger associated with a sedentary lifestyle.

Approximately 70% of adult Americans get insufficient exercise. Inactivity is the most prevalent risk factor for coronary disease by a wide margin. Furthermore, inactivity is prevalent in adolescents as well, with declining participation in physical activity and physical education classes as high school graduation nears.

In addition to its direct effects on the heart, inactivity has substantial influence on hypertension, high-density lipoprotein cholesterol, overweight, and diabetes—major associated risks in heart disease incidence. The amount of exercise needed to bring about significant reductions in cardiovascular and all-cause mortality, as well as each of the major risk factors outlined herewith, is quite modest and well within the capacity of the vast majority of individuals. The total volume of exercise is more important than the intensity to reap the key health benefits. This required volume of activity is quite modest. Those who are unfit can reduce cardiovascular mortality by one-half in only 5 years by escaping the low-fit group. Furthermore, individuals who do not completely eliminate high blood pressure, abnormal cholesterol profile, diabetes, or overweight through beginning and maintaining an exercise program can still enjoy substantial reductions in mortality. All of this gives us some cause for encouragement.

The benefits of regular activity in the prevention of heart disease apply to all ages, all races, and men and women. Implementing an exercise program on an individual basis is not expensive. Membership in fitness centers is not necessary, and equipment needs for many of the most worthwhile kinds of physical activity are minimal.

Moreover, on a broader scale, it is estimated that if only an additional 10% of adults began a regular exercise program, $5.6 billion in heart disease–related cost would be saved. It is also estimated that a 10% weight loss in an overweight person would result in lifetime medical cost savings of $2200 to $5300. Lifetime medical costs of major diseases, including heart disease, hypertension, diabetes, stroke, and hypercholesterolemia among moderately obese people are $10,000 higher than among those at a healthy weight. Because physical activity is inexpensive or even free, the benefit versus cost comparison of implementing a good exercise program is overwhelmingly positive.

There are three different types of exercise training: endurance, strength, and flexibility. To enjoy all of the important benefits, one would need approximately 30 minutes of cardiovascular exercise on most days of the week, eight to 10 strength training exercises at least 2 days per week, approximately seven to eight different stretching exercises on most days of the week. The time required is less than 1 hour per day.

State by State Prevalence of Participation in Physical Activity

State	Regular Percentage	Regular 95% CI	Insufficient Percentage	Insufficient 95% CI	State	Regular Percentage	Regular 95% CI	Insufficient Percentage	Insufficient 95% CI
	Level of activity					Level of activity			
Alabama	23.5	±2.3	76.5	±2.3	Missouri	24.1	±2.5	75.9	±2.5
Alaska	32.9	±3.6	67.1	±3.6	Montana	28.1	±2.8	71.9	±2.8
Arizona	28.2	±2.9	71.8	±2.9	Nebraska	24.7	±2.2	75.3	±2.2
Arkansas	22.1	±2.3	77.9	±2.3	Nevada	31.7	±2.6	68.3	±2.6
California	29.7	±1.7	70.3	±1.7	New Hampshire	29.8	±2.6	70.2	±2.6
Colorado	32.8	±2.6	67.2	±2.6	New Jersey	26.7	±2.6	73.3	±2.6
Connecticut	34.1	±2.7	65.9	±2.7	New Mexico	35.4	±3.1	64.6	±3.1
Delaware	25.5	±2.2	74.5	±2.2	New York	20.9	±1.9	79.1	±1.9
District of Colombia	16	±2.3	84	±2.3	North Carolina	17.9	±1.9	82.1	±1.9
					North Dakota	27.1	±2.3	72.9	±2.3
Florida	32.2	±1.7	67.8	±1.7	Ohio	21.5	±2.5	78.5	±2.5
Georgia	25.5	±2.1	74.5	±2.1	Oklahoma	28.5	±2.4	71.5	±2.4
Hawaii	33.9	±2.5	66.1	±2.5	Oregon	35.7	±2.1	64.3	±2.1
Idaho	32.3	±2.8	67.7	±2.8	Pennsylvania	28.7	±1.7	71.3	±1.7
Illinois	23.9	±2.1	76.1	±2.1	South Carolina	21.7	±2.0	78.3	±2.0
Indiana	25	±2.0	75	±2.0	South Dakota	26.2	±2.3	73.8	±2.3
Iowa	23	±1.9	77	±1.9	Tennessee	22	±1.7	78	±1.7
Kansas	24.9	±2.6	75.1	±2.6	Texas	26.5	±2.7	73.5	±2.7
Kentucky	19.3	±1.9	80.7	±1.9	Utah	28.5	±2.3	71.5	±2.3
Louisiana	22.5	±2.3	77.5	±2.3	Vermont	34.5	±2.2	65.5	±2.2
Maine	18.5	±2.3	81.5	±2.3	Virginia	31.4	±2.5	68.6	±2.5
Maryland	25.8	±1.5	74.2	±1.5	Washington	33.4	±1.8	66.6	±1.8
Massachusetts	31.8	±2.6	68.2	±2.6	West Virginia	19.8	±2.0	80.2	±2.0
Michigan	29.1	±2.1	70.9	±2.1	Wisconsin	29.1	±2.8	70.9	±2.8
Minnesota	28.1	±1.6	71.9	±1.6	Wyoming	35.1	±3.3	64.9	±3.3
Mississippi	19.6	±2.3	80.4	±2.3					

Figure 11-1.

State by state prevalence of participation in physical activity. "Regular" indicates meeting the recommendation for regular vigorous physical activity (greater than 20 minutes per day of vigorous physical activity on 3 or more days per week) or the recommendation for regular sustained physical activity (average of 30 minutes or more per day of activity on 5 or more days per week). It can be seen that six states (five with the District of Columbia) show a prevalence of less than 20% of the population getting adequate exercise. Only 14 states have a percentage of individuals getting sufficient physical activity above 30% [1].

Prevalence of Adequate Physical Activity in Different Regions of the World

Men and Women	
Region	Exercise, %
Western Europe	38.4
Central and eastern Europe	11.3
Middle East	4.2
Africa	10.1
South Asia	37.1
China	20.3
Southeast Asia and Japan	31.4
Australia and New Zealand	23.8
South America	27.6
North America	25.6
Overall 1*	25.5
Overall 2†	12.2

*Adjusted for age, gender, and smoking status.
†Adjusted for all risk factors.

Figure 11-2.

The prevalence of adequate physical activity in different regions of the world. Study participants were recruited from 262 centers in 52 countries. These are men and women mostly in the 5th and 6th decades of life. Individuals were judged to be physically active if they were regularly involved in moderate (walking, gardening, or cycling) or strenuous exercise (jogging, football [soccer], and vigorous swimming) for 4 hours or more a week. This is a high standard to achieve. Not surprisingly, rates of activity across the world vary widely, from 4.2% in the Middle East to 38.4% in western Europe. With this standard, North America lags behind South America, South and Southeast Asia, and western Europe [2].

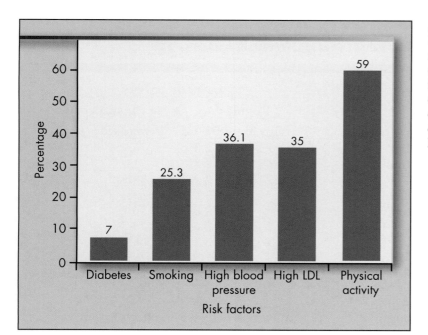

Figure 11-3.
Prevalence of major risk factors in the US population. Among the five major risk factors for coronary heart disease, lack of exercise dwarfs the other four in prevalence by a wide margin. Because the power of these five factors in the risk equation for coronary heart disease is approximately equal, there is a much greater opportunity to lower coronary heart disease rates by changing the activity patterns in the population than by lowering blood pressure, improving cholesterol profiles, treating diabetes, or helping people stop smoking [3]. LDL—low-density lipoprotein.

Coronary Heart Disease Attributable to Sedentary Lifestyle

State	CHD		Sedentary lifestyle			
	Deaths, *n*	Rate	Percentage	95% CI	PAR, %	Estimated preventable deaths, *n*
New York	55,702	229.5	73.7	±3.1	39.9	22,225
Ohio	28,522	209.6	63.2	±2.9	36.2	10,325
South Carolina	7155	204.6	65.9	±2.6	37.2	2662
Tennessee	12,283	204.2	67.3	±2.2	37.7	4631
Missouri	13,711	184.8	59	±3.0	34.6	4744
Florida	38,170	182.5	52.7	±2.9	32.2	12,290
Alabama	8472	169.9	57.8	±2.9	34.2	2897
Washington	8928	164.3	45.2	±3.0	28.9	2580

Figure 11-4.
Coronary heart disease (CHD) attributable to sedentary lifestyle. This figure shows state-specific age-adjusted (to the 1980 US population) coronary heart disease mortality, and prevalence of sedentary lifestyle with associated population-attributable risk. Even though these data were assembled a number of years ago, this figure gives a concrete example of the actual numbers of preventable deaths, if the population in selected states were to achieve recommended levels of activity. Because of the high prevalence of a sedentary lifestyle and its power as a risk factor, the potential is significant. These estimates come from the Behavioral Risk Factor Surveillance System (BRFSS), 1987 to 1988. PAR—population-attributable risk (prevalence estimates [PE] × [relative risk (RR) - 1]/PE × (RR - 1) +1). (*Adapted from* Centers for Disease Control and Prevention [4].)

Declining Percentage of High School Students Enrolled In, Attended, and Active During Physical Education

Characteristics	2003 data, % (95% CI)
Enrolled in physical education class	
9th Grade	71.0 (±6.9)
10th Grade	60.7 (±9.0)
11th Grade	45.7 (±8.8)
12th Grade	39.5 (±8.9)
Attended physical education class	
9th Grade	37.9 (±8.6)
10th Grade	31.3 (±8.0)
11th Grade	22.6 (±4.6)
12th Grade	18.2 (±4.0)
Physically active during physical education class	
9th Grade	49.5 (±5.1)
10th Grade	43.6 (±6.1)
11th Grade	31.1 (±4.6)
12th Grade	28.3 (±5.7)

Figure 11-5.
The declining percentage of high school students who were enrolled in, attended, and were physically active during physical education class from ninth through twelfth grade. As students approach high school graduation, fewer and fewer numbers enroll and participate in physical education classes at school. Seventy percent of ninth graders enrolled, but by the time students reached the twelfth grade, less than 40% were enrolled and less than 20% of those high school seniors attended physical education class daily. Schools are failing in promoting the healthy lifestyle of regular exercise in the captive audience of their students. Moreover, much of high school emphasis on activity centers on a minority of students who are involved in competitive athletics. This declining participation in exercise in youth sets the stage for a sedentary adult population [5].

Importance of Physical Activity Among Root Causes of Death in the United States, 1990 and 2000

Actual cause	1990, n (%)	2000, n (%)
Tobacco	400,000 (19)	435,000 (18.1)
Poor diet and physical activity	300,000 (14)	400,000 (16.6)
Alcohol consumption	100,000 (5)	85,000 (3.1)
Microbial agents	90,000 (4)	75,000 (2.3)
Toxic agents	60,000 (3)	55,000 (2.3)
Motor vehicle	25,000 (1)	43,000 (1.8)
Firearms	35,000 (2)	29,000 (1.2)
Sexual behavior	30,000 (1)	20,000 (0.8)
Illicit drug use	20,000 (< 1)	17,000 (0.7)
Total	1,060,000 (50)	1,159,000 (48.2)

Figure 11-6.
The importance of physical inactivity among root causes of death in the United States in 1990 and 2000. McGinnis and Foege [6] described the underlying root causes that contributed to death in the United States in 1990. Poor diet and physical inactivity were second only to tobacco as an actual cause of death that year. Mokdad *et al.* [7] reviewed the same factors in 2000. Although causes attributable to tobacco increased in number by 35,000, there was an actual 0.9% decrease that year. However, poor diet and physical activity showed an alarming increase in number by 33% to 400,000, with a relative percentage increase by 2.6%. Among associated risks of death, inactivity and poor diet are increasing much faster than any other category [6].

A. Studies of Estimated Summary of Relative Risks for Physical Inactivity in Canada

Disease, population	Sample size/studies, *n*	Activity level classification	Relative risk (95% CI)
CAD			
Meta-analysis [9]	9 studies	Low vs high	1.90 (1.60–2.20)
Stroke			
British men [10]	7735	None vs moderate	1.67 (0.67–5.00)
NHANEFS Men [11]	2368	Low vs moderate	1.24 (0.63–2.41)
NHANEFS Women [11]	2713	Low vs moderate	3.13 (0.95–10.32)
Honolulu Heart Study men [12]	7530	Low vs high tertile	3.70 (1.20–6.70)
Framingham Heart Study men [13]	1228	Tertile 1 vs tertile 2	2.44 (1.45–4.17)
Framingham Heart Study women [13]	1676	Tertile 1 vs tertile 2	1.03 (0.68–1.56)
Finnish men [14]	3978	None vs some leisure	1.00 (0.65–1.62)*
Finnish women [14]	3688	None vs some leisure	1.30 (0.73–2.16)*
Reykjavik men [15]	4484	None vs some after age 40	1.45 (0.99–2.13)
ARIC Women and men [16]	14,575	Low vs high quartile	1.12 (0.73–1.75)
Male physicians [17]	21,823	None vs vigorous exercise 2 to 4 times per week	1.25 (1.01–1.54)
Harvard University alumni [18]	11,130	< 4184 kj/wk vs 8368–12,548 kj/wk	1.85 (1.32–2.63)
Hypertension			
Harvard University alumni [19]	14,998	8368 kj/wk vs 8368 kj/wk or greater	1.30 (1.09–1.55)
Iowa women [20]	41,837	Low vs high tertile	1.43 (1.11–1.67)
Finnish men [21]	2840	Low vs high tertile	1.73 (1.13–2.65)
ARIC men [22]	7459	Low vs high quartile	1.52 (1.06–2.13)
Colon cancer			
Meta-analysis [23]	35 studies	Sedentary vs active	1.39 (1.27–1.51)
Breast cancer			
Meta-analysis [24]	13 studies	Sedentary vs active	1.22 (1.00–1.50)
Type 2 diabetes mellitus			
Female nurses [24]	87,253	None vs vigorous exercise once per week	1.45 (1.00–2.08)
Male physicians [25]	21,271	None vs vigorous exercise once per week	1.41 (1.10–1.79)
Finnish women [21]	2840	Low vs high tertile	2.64 (1.28–5.44)
Female nurses [26]	27,546	Low vs high quartile	1.35 (1.12–1.61)
Osteoporosis			
Nonblack women [27]	9704	< 1423 kj/wk vs > 9209 kj/wk	1.56 (1.12–2.22)
NHANEFS white women [28]	2143	None vs much or moderate exercise	1.90 (1.04–3.30)

*Estimates from 90% CI.

B. Summary of Relative Risks and Population-Attributable Risk Fractions

Disease	Relative risk, 95% CI	Population-attributable fraction, %
CAD	1.6–2.2	35.8
Stroke	1.2–1.5	19.9
Hypertension	1.2–1.6	19.9
Colon cancer	1.3–1.5	19.9
Breast cancer	1.0–1.5	11.0
Type 2 diabetes	1.2–1.6	19.9
Osteoporosis	1.2–2.2	27.1

Figure 11-7.

A and **B**, Studies of estimated summary relative risks for physical inactivity in Canada. Inactivity is not just a risk factor in heart disease. This table lists summary relative risks of physical inactivity for a number of major diseases in Canada. These associated risks of inactivity multiply the burden of a sedentary lifestyle. ARIC—Atherosclerotic Risk in Communities Study; CAD—coronary artery disease; NHANEFS—National Health and Nutrition Epidemiologic Follow-up Study. (*Adapted from* Katzmarzyk *et al.* [29].)

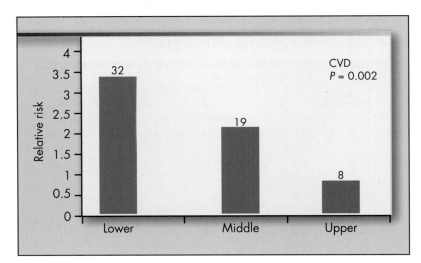

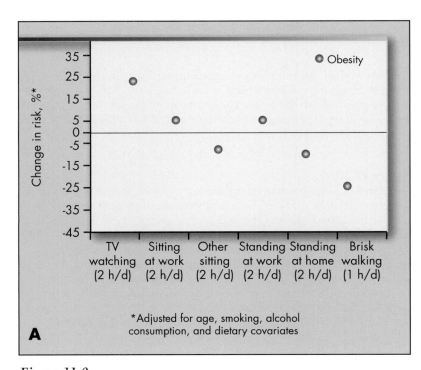

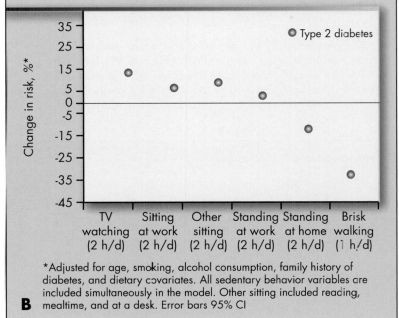

Figure 11-8.

Fitness and the metabolic syndrome. Relative risks of cardiovascular disease (CVD) mortality in men diagnosed as having the metabolic syndrome across baseline tertiles (lower, middle, and upper) of cardiorespiratory fitness in 3757 men aged 20 to 83 years from the Aerobics Center Longitudinal Study. Relative risks are adjusted for age, year of examination, smoking status, alcohol consumption, family history of CVD, and body mass index. Numbers atop the bars indicate the number of deaths; *P* values are for tests of linear trend across the cardiorespiratory fitness categories [29].

An important contributor to cardiovascular risk is the metabolic syndrome. In addition to the direct negative effects on the heart itself, physical inactivity has been shown to adversely affect components of the metabolic syndrome. Review of data from the Aerobics Center Longitudinal Study shows a very significant association of fitness with protection from cardiovascular disease mortality in men with the metabolic syndrome.

Figure 11-9.

Percentage changes in risk of developing obesity (**A**) among nonobese women and in risk of developing type 2 diabetes (**B**) among nondiabetic women associated with television watching, other sedentary behaviors, and walking. Obesity subjects were adjusted for age, smoking, alcohol consumption, and dietary covariates [9]. Diabetes subjects were adjusted for age, smoking, alcohol consumption, family history of diabetes, and dietary covariates. All sedentary behavior variables are included simultaneously in the model. Other sedentary behaviors included reading, mealtimes, and at a desk. Error bars have 95% CI [30]. A 6-year prospective cohort study of women in the Nurses' Health Study shows a correlation between various sedentary behaviors versus activity-related behaviors in the risk of developing obesity in nonobese women and type 2 diabetes in nondiabetic women.

Potential Mechanisms Through Which Exercise May Decrease Cardiovascular Events

Potential cardioprotective effects of regular physical activity

Anti-atherosclerotic	Psychologic	Anti-thrombotic	Anti-ischemic	Anti-arrhythmic
Improved lipids	Decreased depression	Decreased platelet adhesiveness	Decreased myocardial O_2 demand	Increased vagal tone
Improved blood pressure	Decreased stress	Increased fibrinolysis	Increased coronary flow	Decreased adrenergic activity
Reduced adiposity	Increased social support	Decreased fibrinogen	Decreased endothelial dysfunction	Increased heart rate variability
Increased insulin sensitivity		Decreased blood viscosity		
Increased inflammation				

Figure 11-10.

Potential mechanisms through which exercise may decrease cardiovascular events. These proven benefits of cardiovascular exercise, operating through different pathways, provide a variety of ways by which exercise may influence the onset or progression of cardiovascular disease [31].

Physical Inactivity/Exercise

The Importance of Fitness in Cardiovascular Disease Mortality

Mortality predictor	Subjects, n	Person-years of follow-up, n (%)	Deaths, n	Death rate per 10,000 person-years	Relative risk adjusted (95% CI)
Low fitness (20% least fit)	5223	54,729 (26)	111	20.0	1.70 (1.28–2.25)
Current or recent smoker	6730	60,829 (29)	82	16.6	1.57 (1.18–2.10)
Systolic blood pressure 140 mm Hg or greater	2759	26,398 (12)	87	19.5	1.34 (1.00–1.80)
Cholesterol 6.2 mmol/L or greater (24 mg/dL or greater)	6025	51,262 (24)	106	16.5	1.65 (1.26–2.15)
Parental history of death from coronary heart disease	6499	53,440 (25)	84	14.3	1.18 (0.89–1.57)
Body mass index 27 mg/m² or greater	8198	65,534 (31)	96	14.9	1.20 (0.91–1.58)
Fasting glucose 6.7 mmol/L or greater (120 mg/dL or greater)	1396	13,229 (6)	36	15.4	0.95 (0.66–1.37)

Figure 11-11.

The relative importance of fitness in cardiovascular disease mortality. From the Aerobics Center Longitudinal Study, 25,341 men were observed with average follow-up of 8.4 years. Data were adjusted for age, examination year, and each of the other variables in the table. Low fitness (least fit 20%) was more predictive than any of the other variables studied. All comparisons are dichotomies, with the referent category being the low-risk group (relative risk 1.00), and the high-risk group data shown in the table. These data show the substantial strength and independence of low cardiorespiratory fitness as a precursor of cardiovascular disease [32].

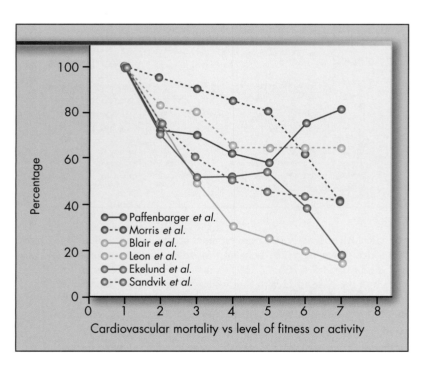

Figure 11-12.

The effect of fitness or activity on coronary disease mortality from six different landmark studies. These data from six prominent and frequently cited large studies (Harvard Alumni; British Civil Servants; Aerobics Center for Longitudinal Study; Multiple Risk Factor Intervention Trial; North American men; and Healthy Norwegian men), illustrate the widespread consistency and the strength of the association between fitness, activity, and reduced cardiovascular mortality. Values for more active or fit persons are expressed as the ratio of the event rate for more active or fit divided by the event rate for the least active or fit. The magnitude of the protective effect is impressive [33].

Role of Total Volume and Relative Intensity of Physical Activity in Reducing Cardiovascular Disease

Physical activity index, kcal/wk	Man-years, % death	CVD deaths, n	Per 10,000 CVD deaths	Relative risk	P value
< 1000	31	512	78.8	1.00	—
1000–2499	39	317	56.3	0.71	< 0.001
2500+	30	170	43.0	0.54	< 0.001
Sports play					
None	12	264	83.0	1.00	—
Light only	11	187	66.0	0.79	0.017
Moderately vigorous	77	506	52.4	0.63	< 0.001

Figure 11-13.

Total volume and relative intensity of physical activity play a significant role in reducing cardiovascular disease (CVD). These data come from 14,623 Harvard Alumni aged 45 to 84 years at entry observed for 12 years (1977–1988). Volume of exercise is measured in total kilocalories (kcal) expended per week. Intensity in this study is measured as no sports play, light only, or moderately vigorous. Light sports play is less than 4.5 metabolic equivalents. Moderately vigorous sports play, for example, is brisk walking, jogging, cycling, swimming, or squash. The data are standardized for age, cigarette smoking, hypertension, obesity, alcohol consumption, early parental mortality, and selected chronic diseases (coronary artery disease, stroke, chronic lung disease, diabetes, and cancer). There is a similar reduction in mortality rates for increased total volume of activity and increased intensity of activity, although volume is more protective [34].

Effect of Changes in Fitness on Cardiovascular Mortality

Physical fitness		Man-years of follow-up	Men, n	Deaths, n	Age-adjusted death rate per 10,000 man-years	Relative risk	95% CI
First examination	Second examination						
Unfit	Unfit	2826	356	15	65.0	1.00	
Unfit	Fit	4017	638	13	31.4	0.048	0.31–0.74
Fit	Unfit	1594	215	3	37.9	0.43	0.28–0.67
Fit	Fit	38,572	8432	56	14.2	0.22	0.12–0.39

Figure 11-14.

The effect of changes in fitness on cardiovascular mortality. These data address the question: "Can an unfit person who becomes fit change his cardiovascular risk?" From the Aerobic Center Longitudinal Study, 9777 men were given two separate examinations with a mean interval of 4.9 years who were then observed for a mean of an additional 5.1 years [35]. *Unfit* is defined as the least fit 20% of the population and *fit* is defined as all others. Men who improved from unfit to fit between the two examinations cut their risk in half (relative risk 1.0 to 0.48). Those who were fit at both examinations had the lowest relative risk (0.22). Further analysis of these data show that these findings applied to men of all ages including those over 60 years of age. After adjustment for potential confounders, each minute increase in treadmill time from the first to the subsequent visit was associated with a reduction in risk of mortality of 7.9%.

Women, Exercise, and Coronary Heart Disease

	Women, *n*	Cases of CHD, *n*	Age- and treatment-adjusted RR (95% CI)	Multivariable RR (95% CI)
Walking parameter				
Time spent walking per week				
Do not walk regularly	5826	68	1.00 (referent)	1.00 (referent)
1–59 minutes	6034	45	0.68 (0.46–0.62)	0.86 (0.57–1.29)
1.0–1.5 hours	4406	19	0.37 (0.22–0.62)	0.49 (0.28–0.86)
2 or more hours	6599	28	0.33 (0.21–0.52)	0.48 (0.29–0.78)
P value for trend			< 0.001	< 0.001
Usual walking pace, *km/h*				
Do not walk regularly	5826	68	1.00 (referent)	1.00 (referent)
< 3.2	2958	21	0.57 (0.35–0.93)	0.56 (0.32–0.97)
3.2–4.7	8356	50	0.50 (0.35–0.72)	0.71 (0.47–1.05)
4.8 or greater	5725	21	0.33 (0.20–0.54)	0.52 (0.30–0.90)
P value for trend			< 0.0001	0.02

Figure 11-15.

Women, exercise, and coronary heart disease (CHD) relative risks (RR) according to volume and intensity. Data are shown for women who reported no vigorous recreational activities requiring six or more metabolic equivalents (resting metabolic rate = 1 metabolic equivalent). Multivariable relative risks are adjusted for age, randomized treatment assignment, smoking status, consumption of alcohol, saturated fat, fiber, and fruits and vegetables, menopausal status, use of postmeno-pausal hormones, and parental history of myocardial infarction at < 60 years of age.

There is much more data on exercise and CHD in men than in women. These data in women come from the Nurses' Health Study and concern 37,372 women aged 45 or older with an average follow-up of 5 years. There were 244 confirmed CHD events. These data show that vigorous activity was not necessary for lower CHD rates. Time spent walking was more important than walking speed, but walking speed did lower CHD risk, although the association was not linear. These data support the conclusion that the protective effect of exercise is not limited to men [36].

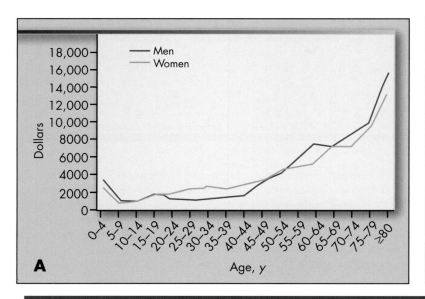

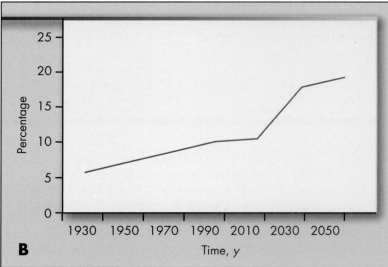

C. Growth in National Health Expenditure, 1980–2000

	1980	1993	1998	2000	2011 (estimated)
Total national health expenditure (B)	246	888	1150	1300	2815
Nursing home and home health care costs (B)	20	88	123	125	237
Per capita cost, $	1067	3371	4177	4637	9216
Gross Domestic Product, %	8.8	13.4	13.1	13.2	17

Figure 11-16.

Burden of health care expenses [37]. **A**, Estimated per capita health expenditures by age and gender, 1995. **B**, An aging population: percentage of US population over age 65. **C**, Growth in National Health Expenditure (NHE), 1980 to 2000. These three figures illustrate the rapidly expanding burden of health care expenses as the percentage of the population over 65 years of age increases. Regular physical activity becomes more important, not less important, with age. Regular activity could substantially reduce morbidity, mortality, and thus health care costs in the aging population. (*Panels A* and *B adapted from* McDevitt and Schieber [38]; *panel C adapted from* Levit *et al.* [39] and Heffler *et al.* [40].)

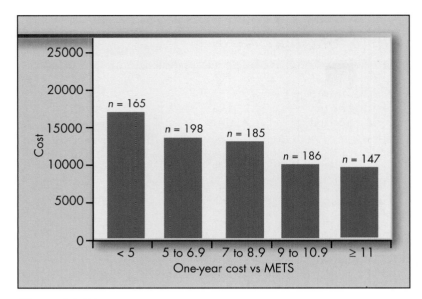

Figure 11-17.
Direct association of fitness with decrease in health care costs. In 881 patients treated at the Palo Alto Veterans Affairs Health Care Facility over a 1-year period, inpatient and outpatient costs were lower by an average of 5.4% per metabolic equivalent (METS) increase in treadmill time. This is just one small example of the favorable cost/benefit picture with physical activity and fitness. There is now a considerable body of data showing that health care costs are inversely associated with exercise capacity [41].

Recommendations for Cardiovascular Fitness, Muscular Fitness, and Flexibility

	Exercise recommendations
Cardiovascular fitness	30 minutes or more of moderate-intensity cardiovascular exercise on most (at least 5) days of the week
Muscular fitness	8 to 10 exercises using the major muscle groups, 8 to 12 repetitions each, moderate intensity, 2 days per week
Flexibility	10 repetitions of sustained (10 seconds) stretching exercises with particular focus on the lower back, hamstrings, calf and Achilles area, hips, quadriceps, shoulders, and neck; ideal is 6 to 7 days per week

Figure 11-18.
Recommendations for cardiovascular fitness, muscular fitness, and flexibility. Consensus public health recommendations for the three major categories of exercise.

Comparison of the Effects of Cardiovascular Exercise with Strength Training Exercise on Health and Fitness Variables

Variable	Aerobic exercise	Resistance exercise
Bone mineral density	↑↑	↑↑↑
Body composition		
Fat, %	↓↓	↓
Lean body mass	←→	↑↑
Strength	↑↑	↑↑↑
Glucose metabolism		
Insulin response to glucose challenge	↓↓	↓↓
Basal insulin levels	↓	↓
Insulin sensitivity	↑↑	↑↑
Serum lipids		
HDL cholesterol	↑↑	↑←→
LDL cholesterol	↓↓	↓←→
Resting heart rate	↓↓	←→
Stroke volume	↑↑	←→
Blood pressure at rest		
Systolic	↓↓	←→
Diastolic	↓↓	↓←→
VO_{2max}	↑↑↑	↑
Endurance time	↑↑↑	↑↑
Physical function	↑↑	↑↑↑
Basal metabolism	↑	↑↑

Figure 11-19.
Comparison of the effects of cardiovascular exercise with strength training exercise on a variety of health and fitness variables. (*Adapted from* Feigenbaum and Pollock [42].)

Variety of Exercise Benefits

Exercise	Aerobic benefits	Muscle strength	Weight control	Calories /hour
Jogging	4	2	4	600
Bicycling	4	2	3	500
Swimming	4	4	2	600
Handball, squash, racquetball	4	2	4	420
Cross-country skiing	4	3	4	600
Downhill skiing	2	3	2	410
Basketball	4	2	4	420
Tennis – singles	3	2	3	410
Aerobics	4	3	4	350
Calisthenics – nonaerobics	1	4	2	320
Walking	3	2	3	320
Golf (no carts)	2	2	1	320
Softball and baseball	2	2	1	264
Bowling	1	1	1	270

Figure 11-20.
A variety of exercise benefits. This figure compares the relative strength of a given activity in providing cardiovascular benefits versus benefits in weight control. An estimate of calories burned per hour for each activity is included. If an activity is very good for providing a given benefit, it rates a four (4); if weak for that benefit, it rates a one (1). This table may be helpful in matching an individual's goals for exercise with the benefits that are most important for him or her.

Cardiovascular Exercise Recommendations

Exercise	Advantages	Disadvantages	Minimum amount per day needed	METS	Other considerations
Walking	Natural, easy; no equipment; time to talk and think	Takes longer; should be brisk; weather may limit	45 minutes	5 to 7 (15 min/mile)	Age no barrier; orthopedic problems may limit
Running	Natural, easy; quick workout; exhilarating	May be hard on damaged, worn joints; less practical with aging	20 minutes	10 (10 min/mile)	Do not increase speed or distance > 10% per week; shoes and surface are important
Outdoor bicycling	Fresh air and scenery; easy skills; easy on joints	Weather may limit; safety a major issue; darkness and traffic may limit	30 minutes	7 (10 mph)	Helmet mandatory; participants must stay alert
Stationary bicycling	Not limited by weather, darkness or traffic; read or watch television during exercise; easy on joints	Non–weight-bearing; not exhilarating; need equipment	25 minutes	7 to 10	Recumbent bike style is an option
Treadmill	Versatile, soft surface; heart rate monitor available on some models; not limited by weather or darkness	Expensive; heavy; holding on for balance decreases the benefit	25 minutes	7 to 10	Variable elevation and speed a must; non-motorized models should be avoided
Swimming	Exercises most all muscle groups; all ages; helps lower back	Facilities may not be available; not as good as other activities for weight loss	25–30 minutes	8	Goggles helpful; ears may be at risk
Elliptical trainer	Easy and natural; upper and lower body; weight bearing without pounding	Expensive	25 minutes	7 to 10	Can watch television while exercising
Competitive sports (tennis, basketball, soccer, squash)	Enjoyable; competitive; excellent cardiovascular benefits	Requires opponents or team members; injury possible; weather may influence outdoor participation	60 minutes	7 to 12	Intensity may be variable and influence benefit; age may limit; orthopedic problems may limit

Figure 11-21.
Cardiovascular exercise recommendations. This figure provides some practical guidance for the most popular cardio-vascular exercises. An exercise plan should take into account the factors outlined, that is, time required, precautions, intensity required, and so forth. METS—metabolic equivalents.

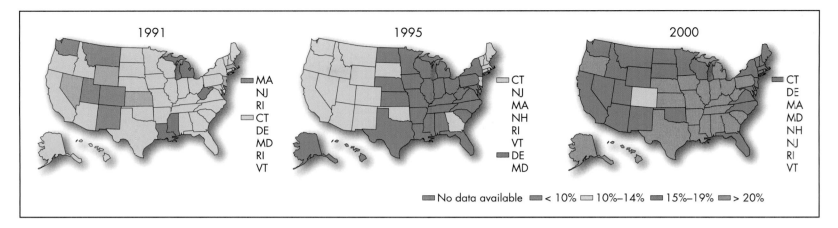

Figure 11-22.
Percentage of adults who report being obese by state. Obesity is defined as body mass index of 30 or greater or approximately 30 pounds overweight for a 5'4" individual. These data are based on self-reported weight and height. (*Adapted from* Centers for Disease Control and Prevention [43].)

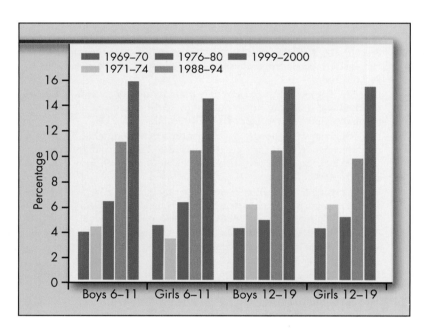

Figure 11-23.
Percentage of overweight children and teens. Childhood obesity has increased profoundly over the past four decades, and an alarmingly similar trend in the adult population has spread across the United States over the past 10 years. This epidemic of obesity relates to diet patterns and also to the sedentary lifestyle of youth and adults. A major challenge for the future is attacking and reversing this plague [44].

Challenges for the Present and Recommendations for the Future

Age group	Present challenges	Recommendations for the future
Elderly	Diminished capacity to perform activities of daily living, and to live independently and productively	Supervised activities improve cardiorespiratory fitness and functional status; modest participation in cardiovascular and strength training activity would bring about substantial improvement
Adult	Rising utilization and costs of medical care; decreasing levels of fitness; high prevalence of chronic disease morbidity and mortality related to sedentary life	Incorporate physical activity as an integral part of life; regular activity must become a higher priority
Youth	Increasing incidence of obesity and "adult-onset diabetes"	Participations in school-sponsored physical activity; provide education in types of activity useful in lifelong fitness
Everyone	Television, ease of transportation, lack of available facilities for daily exercise (including walking and biking trails)	More household, neighborhood, and community exercise-friendly environments

Figure 11-24.
Challenges for the present and recommendations for the future. This figure provides recommendations for using physical activity to meet some of the major health challenges facing youth, adults, and the elderly in the years to come.

References

1. Centers for Disease Control and Prevention: *Behavioral Risk Factor Surveillance System.* Available at http://www.cdc.gov/brfss.

2. Yusuf S, Hawken S, Ôunpuu S, *et al.*: Effect of potentially modifiable risk factors associated with myocardial infarction in 52 countries (the INTER-HEART study): case-control study. *Lancet* 2004, 364:937–952.

3. American Heart Association: *2004 Heart and Stroke Statistical Update.* Dallas: American Heart Association; 2000.

4. From the Centers for Disease Control and Prevention: coronary heart disease attributable to sedentary lifestyle—selected states, 1988. *JAMA* 1990, 264:1390–1392.

5. Centers for Disease Control: Participation in high school physical education: United States, 1991–2003. *MMWR Morbid Mortal Wkly Rep* 2004, 53:844–847.

6. McGinnis JM, Foege WH: Actual causes of death in the United States. *JAMA* 1993, 270:2207–2212.

7. Mokdad AH, Serdula MK, Dietz WH, *et al.*: The continuing epidemic of obesity in the United States. *JAMA* 2000, 284:1650–1651.

8. Hu FB, Li TY, Colditz GA, *et al.*: Television watching and other sedentary behaviors in relation to risk of obesity and type 2 diabetes mellitus in women. *JAMA* 2003, 289:1785–1791.

9. Berlin JA, Colditz GA: A meta-analysis of physical activity in the prevention of coronary heart disease. *Am J Epidemiol* 1990, 132:612–628.

10. Wannamethee G, Shaper AG: Physical activity and stroke in British middle aged men. *BMJ* 1992, 304:597–601.

11. Gillum RF, Mussolino ME, Ingram DD: Physical activity and stroke incidence in women and men. The NHANES I Epidemiologic Follow-up Study. *Am J Epidemiol* 1996, 143:860–869.

12. Abbott RD, Rodriguez BL, Burchfiel CM, Curb JD: Physical activity in older middle-aged men and reduced risk of stroke: the Honolulu Heart Program. *Am J Epidemiol* 1994, 139:881–893.

13. Kiely DK, Wolf PA, Cupples LA, *et al.*: Physical activity and stroke risk: the Framingham Study. *Am J Epidemiol* 1994, 140:608–620.

14. Salonen JT, Puska P, Tuomilehto J: Physical activity and risk of myocardial infarction, cerebral stroke and death: a longitudinal study in eastern Finland. *Am J Epidemiol* 1982, 115:526–537.

15. Agnarsson U, Thorgeirsson G, Sigvaldason H, Sigfusson N: Effects of leisure-time physical activity and ventilatory function on risk of stroke for men: the Reykjavik Study. *Ann Intern Med* 1999, 130:987–990.

16. Evenson KR, Rosamond WD, Cai J, *et al.*: Physical activity and ischemic stroke risk. The Atherosclerosis Risk in Communities Study. *Stroke* 1999, 30:1333–1339.

17. Lee IM, Hennekens CH, Berger K, *et al.*: Exercise and risk of stroke in male physicians. *Stroke* 1999, 30:1–6.

18. Lee IM, Paffenbarger RS Jr: Physical activity and stroke incidence: the Harvard Alumni Health Study. *Stroke* 1998, 29:2049–2054.

19. Paffenbarger RS Jr, Wing AL, Hyde RT, Jung DL: Physical activity and incidence of hypertension in college alumni. *Am J Epidemiol* 1983, 117:245–257.

20. Folsom AR, Prineas RJ, Kaye SA, Munger RG: Incidence of hypertension and stroke in relation to body fat distribution and other risk factors in older women. *Stroke* 1990, 21:701–706.

21. Haapanen N, Miilunpalo S, Vuori I, *et al.*: Association of leisure time physical activity with the risk of coronary heart disease, hypertension and diabetes in middle-aged men and women. *Int J Epidemiol* 1997, 26:739–747.

22. Pereira MA, Folsom AR, McGovern PG, *et al.*: Physical activity and incident hypertension in black and white adults: the Atherosclerosis Risk in Communities Study. *Prev Med* 1999, 28:304–312.

23. Shephard RJ, Futcher R: Physical activity and cancer: how may protection be maximized? [review]. *Crit Rev Oncog* 1997, 8:219–72.

24. Manson JE, Rimm EB, Stampfer MJ, *et al.*: Physical activity and incidence of non-insulin-dependent diabetes mellitus in women. *Lancet* 1991, 338:774–778.

25. Manson JE, Nathan DM, Krolewski AS, *et al.*: A prospective study of exercise and incidence of diabetes among US male physicians. *JAMA* 1992, 268:63–67.

26. Hu FB, Sigal RJ, Rich-Edwards JW, *et al.*: Walking compared with vigorous physical activity and risk of type 2 diabetes in women: a prospective study. *JAMA* 1999, 282:1433–1439.

27. Gregg EW, Cauley JA, Seeley DG, *et al.*: Physical activity and osteoporotic fracture risk in older women. Study of Osteoporotic Fractures Research Group. *Ann Intern Med* 1998, 129:81–88.

28. Farmer ME, Harris T, Madans JH, *et al.*: Anthropometric indicators and hip fracture. The NHANES I Epidemiologic Follow-up Study. *J Am Geriatr Soc* 1989, 37:9–16.

29. Katzmarzyk PT, Gledhill N, Shephard RJ: The economic burden of physical inactivity in Canada. *CMAJ* 2000, 163:1435–1440.

30. Katzmarzyk PT, Church TS, Blair SN: Cardiorespiratory fitness attenuates the effects of the metabolic syndrome on all-cause and cardiovascular disease mortality in men. *Arch Intern Med* 2004, 164:1092–1097.

31. Franklin BA, Kahn JK, Gordon NF, Bonow RO: A cardioprotective "polypill"? Independent and lifestyle modification. *Am J Cardiol* 2004, 94:162–166.

32. Blair SN, Kampert JB, Kohl HW III, *et al.*: Influences of cardiorespiratory fitness and other precursors on cardiovascular disease and all-cause mortality in men and women. *JAMA* 1996, 276:205–210.

33. Pate RR, Pratt M, Blair SN, *et al.*: Physical activity and public health: a recommendation from the Centers for Disease Control and Prevention and the American College of Sports Medicine. *JAMA* 1995, 273:402–408.

34. Paffenberger RS: *40 Years of Progress: Physical Activity, Health and Fitness.* 40th Anniversary Lecture presented at the Annual Meeting of the American College of Sports Medicine. Indianapolis, IN; June 1–4, 1994.

35. Blair SN, Kohl HW III, Barlow CE, *et al.*: Changes in physical fitness and all-cause mortality: a prospective study of healthy and unhealthy men. *JAMA* 1995, 273:1093–1098.

36. Lee IM, Rexrode KM, Cook NR, *et al.*: Physical activity and coronary heart disease in women: is "no pain, no gain" passé? *JAMA* 2001, 285:1447–1454.

37. Centers for Disease Control: Prevalence of disability and associated health conditions: United States, 1991–1992. *MMWR Morbid Mortal Wkly Rep* 1994, 43:730–731.

38. McDevitt RD, Schieber SJ: *From Baby Boom to Elder Boom: Providing Health Care for an Aging Population.* Washington, DC: Watson Wyatt Worldwide; 1996.

39. Levit K, Smith C, Cowan C, *et al.*: Inflation spurs health spending. *Health Aff* 2002, 21:172–181.

40. Heffler S, Smith S, Won G, *et al.*: Health spending projections for 2001–2011: the latest outlook. Faster health spending growth and a slowing economy drive the health spending projection for 2001 up sharply. *Health Aff* 2002, 21:207–218.

41. Weiss JP, Froelicher VF, Myers JN, Heidenreich PA: Health-care costs and exercise capacity. *Chest* 2004, 126:608–613.

42. Feigenbaum MS, Pollock ML: Prescription of resistance training for health and disease. *Med Sci Sports Exerc* 1999, 31:38–45.

43. Centers for Disease Control and Prevention, Department of Health and Human Services: Preventing chronic diseases: investing wisely in health. Preventing obesity and chronic diseases through good nutrition and physical activity. Available at http://www.cdc.gov/nccdphp/pe_fact-sheets/pe_pa.htm.

44. Ogden CL, Flegal KM, Carroll MD, Johnson CL: Prevalence and trends in overweight among US children and adolescents, 199–2000. *JAMA* 2002, 288:1728–1732.

Alcohol Consumption

Arthur L. Klatsky and
Natalia Udaltsova

A simple approach is precluded by disparities in relationships of alcohol drinking to various cardiovascular (CV) conditions [1,2], plus the basic disparity inherent in the difference between harmful effects of heavier drinking and probable beneficial effects of light to moderate drinking. Consideration of possible protection against atherothrombotic events by light to moderate drinking must account for interrelationships among various CV conditions and between alcohol drinking and other important risk factors. A good example is the strong correlation in many populations of alcohol drinking and cigarette smoking, with the latter established as a powerful predictor of several CV conditions. The imprecise nature and inaccuracy of much alcohol intake data create uncertainty about thresholds for effects. Further complexities are added by possible differences in effects of beverage types (*eg*, wine, beer, liquor) and the role of drinking pattern.

Alcoholic cardiomyopathy was perceived 150 years ago, but understanding was clouded by recognition of beriberi [3] and of synergistic toxicity from alcohol plus arsenic or cobalt [1,4–7]. The evidence is now strong that susceptible persons may suffer heart muscle damage from chronic use of large amounts of alcohol [8].

A report of a link between heavy drinking and hypertension in World War I French soldiers [9] was ignored for more than 50 years. This association is now firmly established by consistent epidemiologic data and clinical experiments, but a mechanism remains elusive [1,10–12].

Paroxysmal supraventricular rhythm disturbances in binge drinkers (the "holiday heart syndrome") were described 26 years ago [13]. Data remain sparse about the total role of heavier drinking in cardiac rhythm disturbances [1]. This topic will not be presented further here.

In 1786, Heberden [14] reported angina relief by alcohol and pathologists observed an inverse alcohol-atherosclerosis association early in the 20th century [15,16]. Since 1974 [17], an inverse relation of alcohol drinking to coronary heart disease (CHD) has been found in many population studies, as detailed in reviews [1,18–23]. Plausible mechanisms strengthen interpretation of these data as a causal protective effect of alcohol against CHD [1,18–23]. The high prevalence of CHD results in an impact by alcohol on total mortality statistics, so that light to moderate drinkers are at lower risk of death than abstainers [24–28]. International comparisons [29–31] and some population studies [28,32] suggest that wine drinkers may be more protected against CHD than liquor or beer drinkers. Reports of antioxidants, endothelial relaxant activity, and antithrombotic activity in wine, especially red wine [33–35], support the hypothesis of possible nonalcohol beneficial components in wine. These may hypothetically inhibit oxidation of low-density lipoprotein (LDL) cholesterol and thereby counteract a step in production of atherosclerotic plaques. Some see analogy to a diet high in fruits and vegetables, which is associated with lower CHD risk associated with a diet. Population studies show no consensus that wine is more protective [1,18–20,35]. Also relevant is that the favorable experience of wine drinkers in some studies could be related to a healthier pattern of drinking or to more favorable CHD risk traits in wine drinkers.

Relationships of alcohol drinking to types of stroke have been confusing and controversial. Consensus is growing that heavy drinking is related to higher risk of hemorrhagic stroke and that light to moderate drinking is associated with lower risk of the more common ischemic stroke [36–40].

Because definitions of moderate and heavy drinking are arbitrary, the operational boundary used here represents the level of drinking above which net harm is evident in most epidemiologic studies. Thus, three or more drinks per day is called "heavy" or "heavier" and lesser amounts "light," "lighter," or "moderate" drinking.

Standard–sized drinks of the three major beverage types are approximately equal. Individual factors, including gender and age, lower the boundary of safe drinking for some persons and raise it for others. In survey-based alcohol data, there is usually systematic underestimation, with some heavy drinkers alleging lighter intake. A common consequence of this underestimation is a lowering of the apparent threshold for harm.

Finally, the subject of advice to concerned persons will be considered in the context of how to best estimate individual risk-benefit factors in drinkers or potential drinkers.

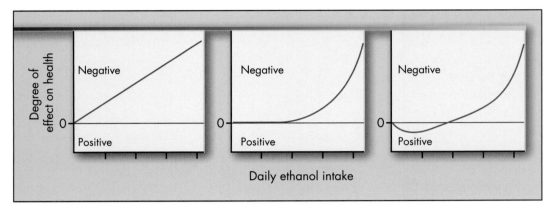

Figure 12-1.

Plausible alcohol-health relationships. Each panel of this figure could apply to an individual health measurement/outcome or to a composite of several outcomes. The *left panel* illustrates a linear relationship, such as may occur between amount of alcohol ingested and blood alcohol levels. Such a relationship is seldom, if ever, seen for adverse health outcomes in humans. The *middle panel* illustrates a threshold relationship, common for alcohol-health associations; the figure shows no apparent effect below the threshold dose but a logarithmically increasing effect greater than the threshold. This is commonly seen in population studies of alcohol and individual health outcomes (*eg*, liver cirrhosis). The *right panel* shows a beneficial effect below the threshold, but, again, a logarithmically increasing effect above the threshold. This is more typically seen in study of composite alcohol-health relationships (*eg*, total mortality or cardiovascular diseases in general).

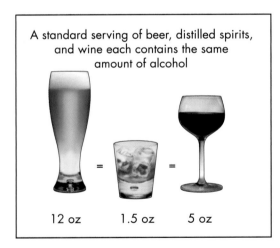

A standard serving of beer, distilled spirits, and wine each contains the same amount of alcohol

12 oz = 1.5 oz = 5 oz

Figure 12-2.

The "standard drink" and definition of moderate. The amount of alcohol is approximately the same in a standard-sized drink of each major beverage type. Thus, a 5-ounce glass of table wine at 12.5% alcohol contains 0.625 ounces of ethanol, 1.5 ounce of distilled spirits at 40% alcohol contains 0.60 ounces ethanol, and 12 ounces of beer at 5% alcohol contains 0.60 ounces ethanol. Usual packaging makes the can or bottle of beer the most standardized drink type. Larger (than standard) drinks are commonly taken by drinkers of distilled spirits. Because most people think in terms of "drinks" rather than milliliters or grams of alcohol, communication is best served by describing alcohol relations in terms of daily or weekly drinks. The clinician must inquire about drink size and number. A boundary of three standard drinks per day is used in this article to define "heavy" intake; some would set the upper limit of light to moderate intake at two standard drinks per day for men and one drink per day for women.

Alcoholic Cardiomyopathy

ACM was recognized in the 19th century, but later erroneously attributed by many to cardiovascular beriberi (deficiency of co-carboxylase, also called thiamine or vitamin B1)

Evidence is compelling that prolonged heavy alcohol drinking can cause dilated cardiomyopathy, but nonspecificity of the clinicopathologic picture impedes epidemiologic study [1]

Only a minority of heavy drinkers are afflicted, suggesting existence of risk traits and cofactors, *eg*, viral myocarditis and genetic predilection [41]

ACM from heavy alcohol intake for many years [8] regresses with abstinence or marked reduction in drinking [42]

Via acetaldehyde [43] or fatty acid ethyl esters [44], the mechanisms are unclear

Light to moderate drinking is not a proven factor in clinical heart failure or subclinical left ventricular dysfunction

Figure 12-3.

Alcoholic cardiomyopathy (ACM).

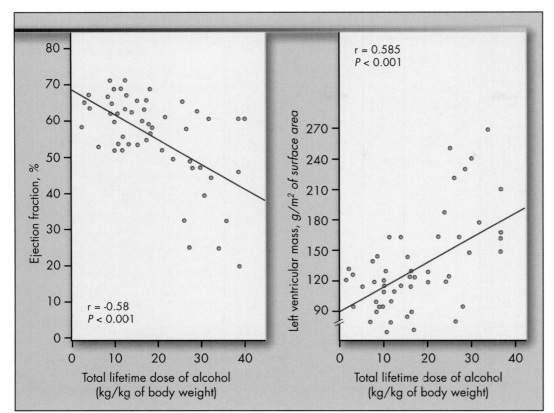

Figure 12-4.
Lifetime dose of alcohol versus ejection fraction and left ventricular (LV) mass. Good correlation (r = 0.46, *P* < 0.01) in 52 alcoholic subjects between total lifetime ethanol consumption and left ventricular ejection fraction (*left panel*) (LVEF). Good correlation in 52 alcoholic subjects between total lifetime ethanol consumption and LV mass (*right panel*) (r = 0.42, *P* < 0.01).

Using LVEF < 55% to define diminished function, all with diminished function reported at least 7 kg/kg of body weight lifetime alcohol, which approximates 200 mL (7 ounces) of 86-proof whiskey per day for 20 years in a 70-kg man. Type of beverage, age, nutritional status, and other covariates were not significantly related to lower LVEF or increased mass. Later work by this group suggests partial explanation by genetic susceptibility [41]. Historical episodes suggest synergistic toxicity with arsenic and cobalt but probably not with thiamine deficiency [1]. (*Adapted from* Urbano-Marquez *et al.* [8].)

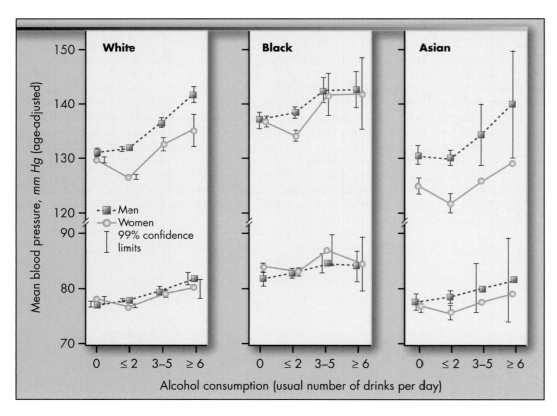

Figure 12-5.
Alcohol intake versus mean blood pressure (BP) in three races. Age-adjusted mean systolic BP (*upper portion of each panel*) and diastolic BP (*lower portion of each panel*) of 83,947 persons (32,449 white men, 4,449 black men, 1601 Asian men, 37,610 white women, 6026 black women, 1812 Asian women). Between 1964 and 1968, each individual had BP determinations at health examinations and supplied questionnaire responses classifying usual alcohol intake in the past year as none, less than two, three to five, or more than six drinks per day. The data show increased BP at three to five and more than six drinks per day in each gender and slightly lower BP among women reporting less than two drinks per day. By direct cross-classification, the relationships were independent of smoking, coffee, education, marital status, adiposity, and usual food salting habit. (*Adapted from* Klatsky *et al.* [45].)

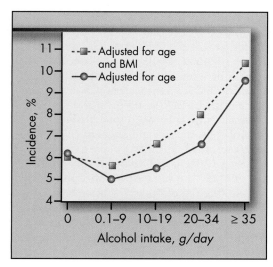

Figure 12-6.
Nurses' Health Study Prospective alcohol consumption/hypertension (HTN) relationship. Prospective 4-year cumulative incidence of HTN by level of alcohol consumption among 58,218 women ages 30 to 55. The *lower line* shows age-adjusted incidence of HTN; the *upper line* is also adjusted for body mass index (BMI). Up to approximately 20 g (two small drinks), there is no increased risk of HTN; however, beyond this amount of alcohol intake, there is progressively higher incident HTN. Similar results have been obtained in more than 10 other prospective studies. (*Adapted from* Witteman *et al.* [46].)

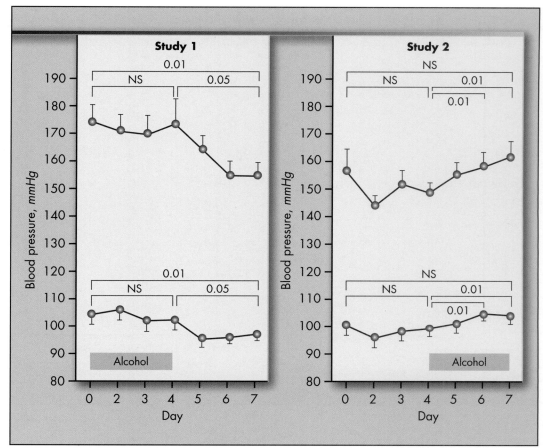

Figure 12-7.
Experimental alcohol-hypertension data [47]: data from an in-hospital study of 16 men with hypertension who usually drank up to 80 g of alcohol per day (equivalent to four pints of beer). Alcohol dose in the experiment was 1 g/kg/d (up to 80 g maximum) taken as beer over several hours. The *left panel* shows that there was little change over several days when alcohol was taken, but subsequent progressive drops in systolic and diastolic blood pressure (BP) over several days without alcohol. One patient had no drop in systolic BP and two had no drop in diastolic BP. The *right panel* shows a progressive rise in BP on resumption of alcohol, with an increase of systolic BP in seven patients and of diastolic BP in all eight patients. The increase in BP was gradual over 4 days. This study was one of the first of a number of reports with similar data in normotensive and hypertensive subjects. In these studies, no hypertensive effect of withdrawal was reported. A definitive mechanism remains elusive but a causal association is likely. NS—not significant. (*Adapted from* Potter and Beevers [47].)

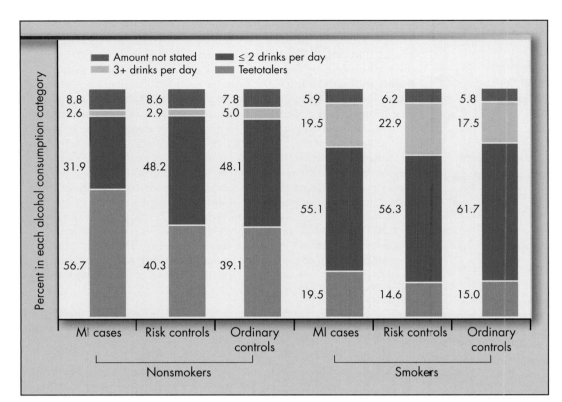

Figure 12-8.

Alcohol and myocardial infarction (MI) in smokers and nonsmokers: the relationship of previously reported alcohol intake to risk of hospitalization for acute MI in 464 smokers and nonsmokers. The proportion drinking various amounts in the MI patients is compared with two non-MI control groups. One group ("ordinary controls") was matched for age, gender, and ethnicity; the other "risk controls" group was matched additionally for smoking, blood pressure, blood cholesterol and glucose, ECG "abnormality," and skinfold thickness. The proportions of alcohol abstainers were higher in the subsequent MI patients than in each control group, indicating independence of the MI predictor (alcohol abstinence) from the established risk traits. The greater prevalence of alcohol abstinence in nonsmokers in the MI and control groups is evident, but MI subjects were more likely nondrinkers whether they smoked or not. There have been many subsequent reports indicating lower risk of fatal and nonfatal coronary heart disease (CHD) events in alcohol drinkers. Some early reports failed to allow for the drinking/smoking association, thus masking the lower CHD risk of alcohol drinkers because of confounding by the positive CHD association with smoking. (*Adapted from* Klatsky *et al.* [17].)

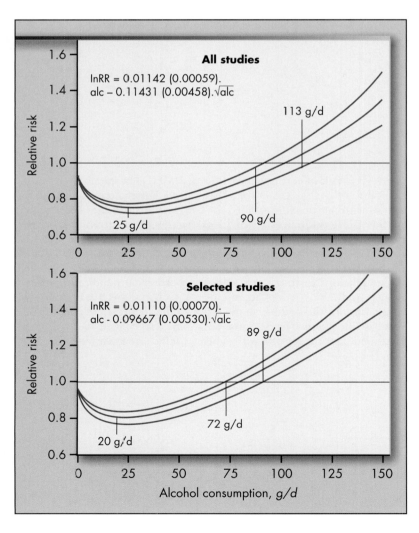

Figure 12-9.

Relative risks with 95% confidence intervals of coronary heart disease (CHD) according to alcohol intake in pooled studies published from 1966 through 1998. Studies for inclusion were selected by 15 defined quality criteria from 196 publications screened. The criteria included several relevant to freedom from bias, several relevant to alcohol categorization, and several relevant to control for potential confounders. The *upper panel* ("all studies") represents pooled data from all 51 studies that met inclusion criteria; it shows a J-shaped curve from abstinence to heavy drinking, with a nadir at 25 g alcohol (two drinks) per day, and protection up to a minimum of 90 g per day and a maximum of 113 g per day. The *lower panel* ("selected studies") represents 28 cohort studies judged to be of highest quality; in these the J-curve has a nadir at 20 g per day (relative risk = 0.80; 95% CI 0.78–0.83), with evidence of a protective effect up to 72 g per day (six drinks) and increased risk above 89 g per day. This may be considered a "conservative" estimate of the magnitude of CHD protection afforded by alcohol. Studies with fatal and nonfatal CHD events are included; *see* Figure 12-12 for further breakdown and comment. Taken as a whole, the apparent protective effect in reported studies is consistent, free of appropriately chosen confounders and prospectively ascertained. (*Adapted from* Corrao *et al.* [21].)

Alcohol Consumption

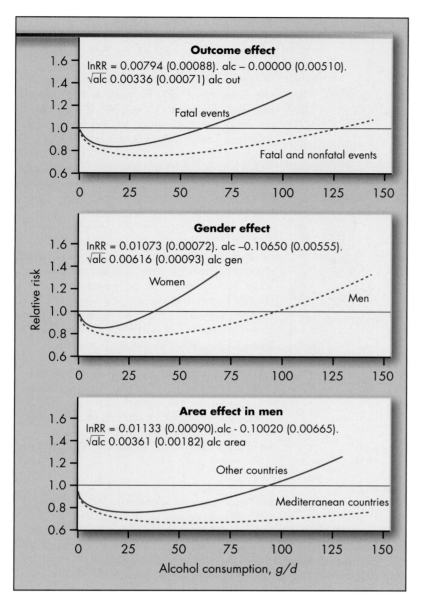

Figure 12-10.
These curves show that coronary heart disease (CHD) endpoint, gender, and geographic location interact with the alcohol-CHD curve in the meta-analysis by Corrao *et al.* [21]. The *top panel* shows that in studies with only fatal CHD events (vs those with fatal and nonfatal events combined), there is less protection at lighter drinking and a lowered threshold for evidence of harm. Some studies of nonfatal events show an L-shaped curve (*ie*, no upturn at heavy alcohol intake). Factors among heavy drinkers involved in this fatal/nonfatal CHD disparity may include greater severity of CHD, greater tendency to rhythm disturbances, misclassification of non-CHD as CHD deaths, higher blood pressure, and different effects on underlying mechanisms from those of lighter drinking. The *middle panel* shows that women are more susceptible at lower alcohol dosages to protective and harmful effects of alcohol on CHD. The *bottom panel* suggests that persons in Mediterranean countries had a greater protective effect of alcohol. This geographic phenomenon may reflect a more favorable drinking pattern (relatively constant daily alcohol amounts), the usual choice of beverage (wine), or dietary factors. (*Adapted from* Corrao *et al.* [21].)

Twelve-year Risk of Coronary Heart Disease Hospitalization According to Baseline Risk

Baseline total alcohol use	Baseline CHD risk	
	No (*n* = 1111)	Yes (*n* = 2758)
Abstainer	1.0 (referent)	1.0 (referent)
Ex-drinker	1.0	1.0
< Once per month	1.0	1.0
> Once per month; < one drink per day	0.8	0.9
One to two drinks per day	0.7*	0.7*
Three or more drinks per day	0.7†	0.7*

*P < 0.001.
†P < 0.01.

Figure 12-11.
Twelve-year risk of coronary heart disease (CHD) hospitalization according to baseline CHD risk. Data from a Kaiser Permanente cohort analysis with persons hospitalized for CHD subdivided into those with baseline CHD risk traits (any of 12 risk factors or symptoms) and those with no such traits. The Cox proportional hazards models were controlled for gender, age, race, smoking, and education. More than two thirds of the subjects had one or risk trait or symptom. The inverse alcohol relationship to risk was similar in both groups, indicating that changes in drinking habits because of risk or symptoms was an unlikely explanation for the finding. Some other studies entirely excluded those with baseline illness from the analyses. Some also controlled for dietary habits and physical activity, with similar results. (*Adapted from* Klatsky *et al.* [48].)

Mechanisms of Coronary Heart Disease Protection by Alcohol

Alcohol effects	Probable action
Increased HDL cholesterol	Removes and transports LDL cholesterol from vessel
Decreased blood LDL cholesterol	LDL level one of major CHD risk factors
Decreased LDL oxidation	LDL oxidation promotes plaque formation
Decreased blood fibrinogen	Risk of clot formation on atherosclerotic plaques
Other antithrombotic actions	
Decreased platelet stickiness	Risk of clot formation on atherosclerotic plaques
Decreased thromboxane A	
Increased prostacyclin	
Increased endogenous t-PA	
Decreased insulin resistance	Key factor in adult-onset diabetes mellitus and in atherosclerosis
Increased endothelial health	Key factors in atherothrombotic disease
Decreased intravascular inflammation	
Decreased psychosocial stress	Unclear, but widely believed a factor
Increased myocardial preconditioning	Resistance to damage by oxygen deprivation

Figure 12-12.

Mechanisms of coronary heart disease protection by alcohol. Supporting data for effect via high-density lipoprotein (HDL) is strong and includes experimental evidence. In several analyses, this results in approximately 50% decreased coronary heart disease risk [49–54]. Evidence for low-density lipoprotein (LDL) effect of alcohol is weak and it probably is not independent of diet. Effect via oxidation of LDL is hypothetical and not primarily an alcohol effect. Figures 12-17 and 12-20 discuss potential additional benefits of nonalcohol ingredients in wine. Evidence for antithrombotic effect via fibrinogen is moderately good [52]. Evidence for effect via other antithrombotic effects is inconsistent; these actions may be reversed by heavier or binge drinking. There is evidence for benefit via reduced insulin resistance in several studies; moderate alcohol intake may also reduce incidence of diabetes mellitus. Evidence of endothelial benefit and reduced intravascular inflammation by alcohol is growing. There are no good data showing coronary heart disease (CHD) benefit by alcohol via its sedative effect; this is an unlikely mechanism. There is preliminary evidence of possible direct myocardial preconditioning by alcohol. t-PA—tissue-type plasminogen activator.

Evidence that Lower Coronary Heart Disease Risk of Alcohol Drinkers Represents Causality

Criterion	Comment
Consistency	Dozens of virtually unanimous studies
Biologic plausibility	Good evidence via HDL cholesterol; antithrombotic and other mechanisms possible
Time sequence	A number of observational prospective studies
Specificity	Lower risk of light to moderate drinkers not a general alcohol-health phenomenon
Strength	Reduced risk approximately 20%–30% at moderate drinking; could be because of indirect (confounded) explanation
Dose response	Not linear; U- or J-curve (CHD mortality) or L-curve (nonfatal CHD)
Study design	No randomized controlled trial

Figure 12-13.

Evidence that lower coronary heart disease (CHD) risk of alcohol drinkers represents causality. Epidemiologic criteria strengthen probability of a causal association; no randomized controlled trials with coronary heart disease event endpoints have been reported. HDL—high-density lipoprotein.

Is Red Wine Best? The Beverage Choice Issue

Positives: evidence wine is better	Negatives: wine not clearly better
Decreased CHD mortality in wine-drinking countries vs liquor/beer-drinking countries (*see* Figs. 12-18 and 12-19)	No consensus in prospective studies [1,18–20,35]
Possible beneficial antioxidant and antithrombotic phenolics in red wine (*see* Fig. 12-21)	Evident CHD protection in beer-drinking populations [56,57]
Wine drinkers fare best in some prospective studies [28,49]	Confounding probably— apparent advantage for a beverage type could be the effect of the following: 1) associated traits; 2) associated drinking pattern; and 3) nonalcoholic ingredients; only 3 would be beverage-specific. Similar risk reductions for white and red wine [28] lessen probability that red wine phenolics explain benefit

Figure 12-14.

Is red wine best? The beverage choice issue. Reports from the US [55] and Denmark [56–58] show that wine drinkers have a healthier lifestyle. Higher socioeconomic status and favorable lifestyle traits tend to cluster. One US study [59] suggests that drinking frequency is more important than amount or beverage choice. CHD—coronary heart disease.

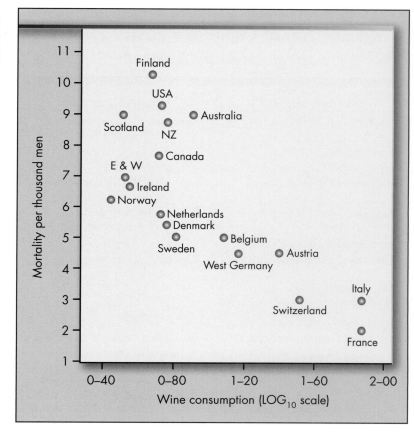

Figure 12-15.

International comparison of coronary heart disease (CHD) mortality and wine. The graph shows an excellent inverse correlation between mean wine consumption and mortality from CHD in the countries studied. This was the first of several international comparisons showing this correlation. These data do not study individuals—the comparisons of mean values are known to epidemiologists as "ecologic" studies. These comparisons also do not allow control for possible individual confounders, such as smoking. For several of the Mediterranean countries included, "wine" and "wine alcohol" are substantially synonymous. Because, especially in France, the prevalence of standard CHD risk traits has been thought high, the low CHD prevalence has become known as "The French Paradox." (*Adapted from* St. Leger *et al.* [29].)

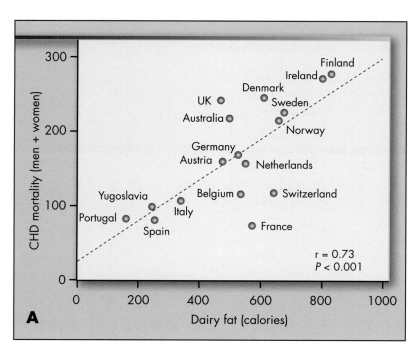

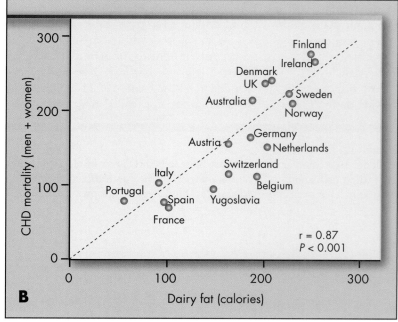

Figure 12-16.

Coronary heart disease (CHD) mortality versus dairy fat intake with and without control for alcohol. **A,** The expected generally good correlation between mean dairy fat intake in various countries and CHD mortality. France, with a high dairy intake and low CHD mortality rate, is an outlier. **B,** Adjustment for mean wine intake results in a better correlation. These ecologic data confirm a relationship between wine (or wine alcohol) intake and lower CHD mortality. (*Adapted from* Renaud and de Lorgeril [30].)

Atlas of Cardiovascular Risk Factors

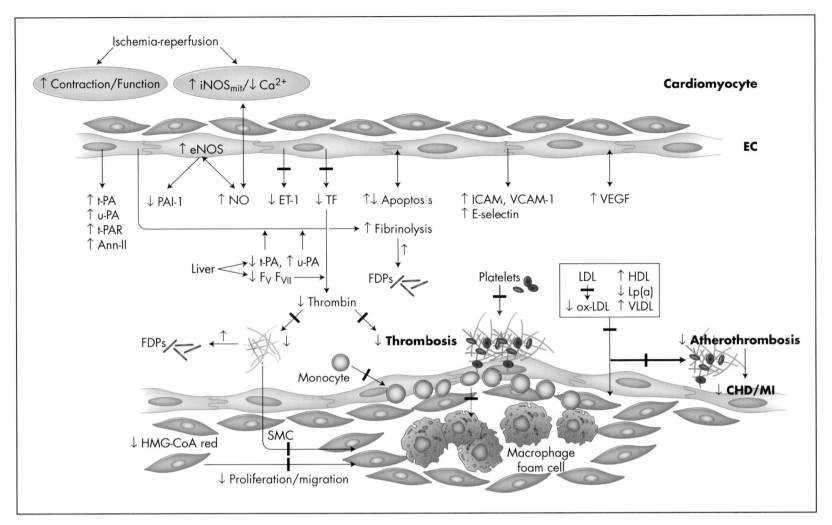

Figure 12-17.

Potential mechanisms of benefit by alcohol or other alcoholic beverage components (especially wine). Nitric oxide (NO) produced from endothelial NO synthase is a regulator of vascular homeostasis and is antithrombogenic. Red wine polyphenols increase NO and endothelial NO synthase (eNOS) in several studies. Decreased eNOS and NO are features in heart failure, diabetes, and hypertension. Endothelial cell (EC)–mediated fibrinolysis is regulated by fibrinolytic proteins (tissue-type plasminogen activator [t-PA], urokinase plasminogen activator [u-PA], and plaminogen activator inhibitor-1 [PAI-1]) and localized at the EC surface via specific receptors (Rs) for Pas (protease-activated receptor [PAR]) and circulating plasminogen (PmgRs). EC-mediated fibrinolysis requires complex multicomponent interactions of Pas PAI-1, PARs, and Pmg PmgRs to facilitate activation of EC-bound Pmg at the cell surface. Alcohol or red wine polyphenols (catechin, epicatechin, quercitin, resveratrol) components may alter one or more of these EC fibrinolytic components to increase fibrinolysis. Other possible antithrombotic actions of alcohol or red wine polyphenolics include decreased fibrinogen, factor V and VII (F_V and F_{VII}), decreased tissue factor (TF) activity, and decreased platelet aggregation. Alcohol or red wine phenolics may modulate other endovascular functions, including the inflammatory process, via intercellular adhesion molecule-1 (ICAM-1), vascular cell adhesion molecule-1 (VCAM-1), vascular endothelial growth factor (VEGF), and E-selectin. Atherosclerosis is associated with accumulation of oxidation products of low-density lipoproteins (ox-LDL) and other proteins. Wine polyphenols have potential robust antioxidant activity, although alcohol itself may have weak pro-oxidant effects. Moderate alcohol intake increases high-density lipoprotein cholesterol (HDL-C), an effect apparently responsible for approximately 50% of the reduced coronary heart disease (CHD). There may also be beneficial effects on lipoprotein(a) (Lp[a]) and very low-density lipoprotein (VLDL) cholesterol. Although some of these actions are only of hypothetic relevance at present, the concept is that overall cardioprotection may be mediated by some combination of diverse effects on vascular, cellular, and biologic functions [59,60]. These result in less smooth muscle cell (SMC) proliferation, less atherosclerotic plaque deposition, and, ultimately, fewer atherothrombotic events, such as myocardial infarction (MI). FDP—fibrinogen degradation product; HMG-CoA—3-hydroxy-3-methylglutaryl coenzyme A; ET-1—endothelin-1.

Type	Approximate total, %	Light to moderate drinking	Heavy drinking*
Hemorrhagic	15	Unresolved	Increased risk
Ischemic	85	Decreased risk	Unresolved

*Three or more standard drinks per day.

Figure 12-18.

Relationships of alcohol to major stroke types. Subarachnoid and intracerebral hemorrhage, pathogenetically distinct subsets of hemorrhagic stroke, have similar alcohol relationships with alcohol [36–38]. Heavier drinking increases risk in most studies, partially via alcohol-associated hypertension. Lighter intake increases risk in some studies, but has no relationship in others. Pathogenetically distinct subsets of ischemic stroke include intracerebral thrombosis, cardioembolic events, artery-to-artery emboli (*eg*, aorta or carotid to intracranial), and others. Available data suggest that light to moderate drinkers may have lower risk for each of these, but data are now robust for protection against the composite "ischemic stroke," the usual study endpoint [36,38–40]. Heavier drinkers are apparently at increased risk of ischemic stroke in some studies [61].

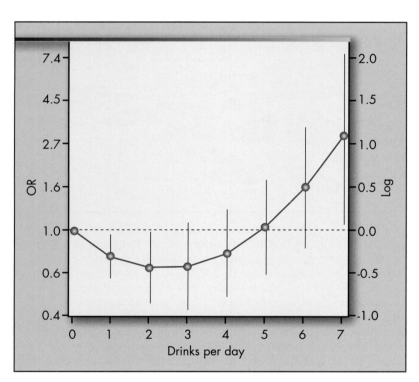

Figure 12-19.

Relationship of alcohol to risk of ischemic stroke. These data are from a case-control population-based study in Northern Manhattan, New York, with 677 ischemic stroke cases and 1139 community controls. Controls were matched for age, gender, and race/ethnicity. Odds ratios (OR) and 95% CIs (*vertical bars*) for risk of ischemic stroke by usual number of drinks per day versus those not drinking in the past year were also controlled for hypertension, diabetes mellitus, smoking, heart disease, and education. A J-shaped alcohol-ischemic stroke relationship is evident with reduced risk at one to four drinks per day and increased risk at more than six drinks per day. (*Adapted from* Gronbaek *et al.* [57].)

Condition	Amount of alcohol drinking		Comment
	Small	**Large**	
Dilated cardiomyopathy	No relation	One (of many) causes	Susceptibility cofactors (?); genetic, viral, etc.
Beri-beri	No relation	No direct relation	Thiamine deficiency
Arsenic or cobalt–beer disease	No relation	Synergistic	Probable examples of cardiomyopathy cofactors
Hypertension	Little or none	Probably causal factor	Mechanism unknown
Coronary disease	Protective	Unclear	Not beverage-specific; possible additional benefit from wine
Paroxysmal supraventricular arrhythmia	No relation	Binges probably causal	Susceptibility factors (?)
Hemorrhagic stroke	Unclear	Increased risk	Via higher blood pressure, antithrombotic actions
Ischemic stroke	Protective	Protective (?)	Complex interactions with other conditions

Figure 12-20.

Summary of relationships of alcohol drinking to various cardiovascular conditions.

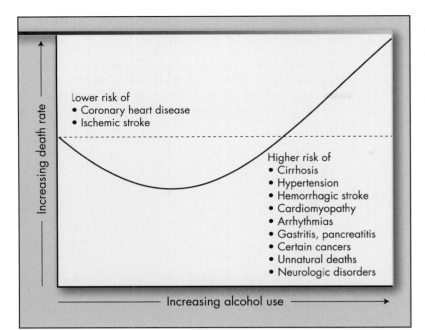

Figure 12-21.

The overall alcohol-health mortality risk is a J-shaped curve from abstinence to heavy drinking. The increased risk of heavier drinkers is due to
a variety of noncardiovascular and cardiovascular causes. The lower risk
to lighter drinkers is because of less risk of atherothrombotic causes,
primarily coronary heart disease.

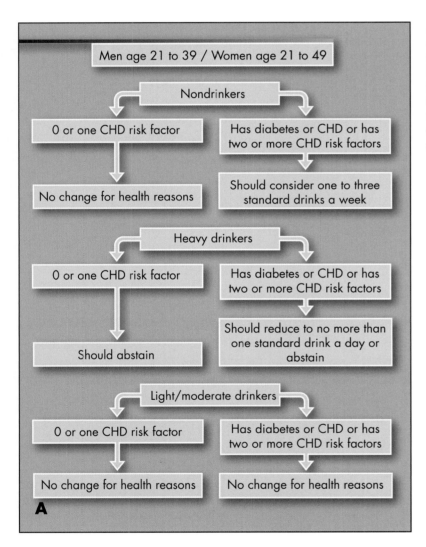

Figure 12-22.

A and **B**, These algorithms show the need for individualization of
advice about the risks and benefits of light to moderate alcohol drinking. Because of net medical and social harm, all heavy drinkers (> three
standard drinks per day for men; more than two per day for women)
should reduce or abstain from drinking. The majority of adults are light
to moderate drinkers and should be told they need no change,
especially if risk of coronary heart disease (CHD) is more than average
and risk of alcohol problems is less than average.

(*continued on next page*)

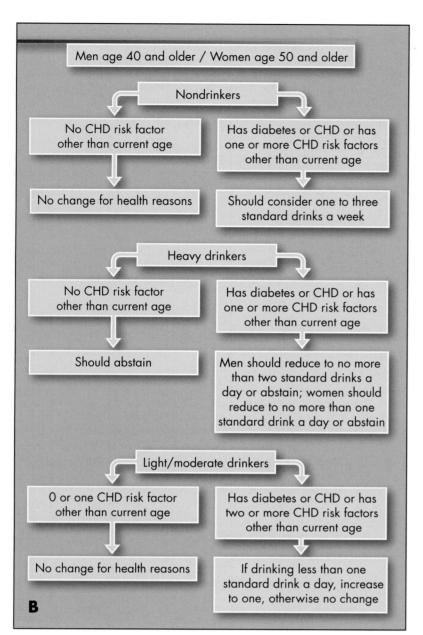

Men age 40 and older / Women age 50 and older

Nondrinkers

No CHD risk factor other than current age

Has diabetes or CHD or has one or more CHD risk factors other than current age

No change for health reasons

Should consider one to three standard drinks a week

Heavy drinkers

No CHD risk factor other than current age

Has diabetes or CHD or has one or more CHD risk factors other than current age

Should abstain

Men should reduce to no more than two standard drinks a day or abstain; women should reduce to no more than one standard drink a day or abstain

Light/moderate drinkers

0 or one CHD risk factor other than current age

Has diabetes or CHD or has two or more CHD risk factors other than current age

No change for health reasons

If drinking less than one standard drink a day, increase to one, otherwise no change

B

Figure 12-22. *continued*
Beverage choice is probably of minor importance, but a steady regular pattern of drinking small amounts of alcohol is optimal. Most abstainers have good reasons and other CHD risk management measures are more important than alcohol drinking. Some individual abstainers should be advised to drink moderately; most notable are established light drinkers with CHD who quit drinking under the mistaken impression that any alcohol was harmful.

References

1. Klatsky AL: Alcohol and cardiovascular health. *Integr Comp Biol* 2004, 44:58–62.

2. Klatsky AL: Drink to your health? *Scientific American* 2003, 288:74–81.

3. Aalsmeer WC, Wenckebach KF: Herz und Kreislauf bei der Beri-Beri Krankheit. *Wien Arch Inn Med* 1929, 16:193–272.

4. Reynolds ES: An account of the epidemic outbreak of arsenical poisoning occurring in beer drinkers in the North of England and the Midland Counties in 1900. *Lancet* 1901, i:166–170.

5. Royal Commission Appointed to Inquire into Arsenical Poisoning from the Consumption of Beer and other Articles of Food or Drink: *Final Report, Part I 1903*. London: Wyman and Sons; 1903.

6. Morin Y, Daniel P: Quebec beer-drinkers' cardiomyopathy: etiologic considerations. *Can Med Assoc J* 1967, 97:926–928.

7. Alexander CS: Cobalt and the heart. *Ann Intern Med* 1969, 70:411–413.

8. Urbano-Marquez A, Estruch R, Navarro-Lopez F, *et al.*: The effects of alcoholism on skeletal and cardiac muscle. *N Engl J Med* 1989, 320:409–415.

9. Lian C: L'alcoholisme cause d'hypertension arterielle. *Bull Acad Med (Paris)* 1915, 4:525–528.

10. MacMahon S: Alcohol consumption and hypertension. *Hypertension* 1987, 9:111–121.

11. Keil U, Swales JD, Grobbee DE: Alcohol intake and its relation to hypertension. In *Health Issues Related to Alcohol Consumption*. Edited by Verschuren PM. Washington, DC: ILSI Press; 1993:17–34.

12. Klatsky AL: Alcohol and hypertension. In *Hypertension*, edn 2. Edited by Operil, S, Weber M. Philadelphia: WB Saunders; 2000:211–220.

13. Ettinger PO, Wu CF, De La Cruz C Jr, *et al.*: Arrhythmias and the "holiday heart": alcohol-associated cardiac rhythm disorders. *Am Heart J* 1978, 95:555–562.

14. Heberden W: Some account of a disorder of the breast. *Med Trans R Col Physicians (London)* 1786, 2:59–67.

15. Cabot RC: The relation of alcohol to arteriosclerosis. *JAMA* 1904, 43:774–775.

16. Wilens SL: The relationship of chronic alcoholism to atherosclerosis. *JAMA* 1947, 135:1136–1138.

17. Klatsky AL, Friedman GD, Siegelaub AB: Alcohol consumption before myocardial infarction: results from the Kaiser Permanente Epidemiologic Study of Myocardial Infarction. *Ann Intern Med* 1974, 81:294–301.

18. Renaud S, Criqui MH, Farchi G, Veenstra J: Alcohol drinking and coronary heart disease. In *Health Issues Related to Alcohol Consumption*. Edited by Verschuren MP. Washington, DC: ILSI Press; 1993:43–80.

19. Grobbee DE, Rimm EB, Keil U, Renaud S: Alcohol and the cardiovascular system. In *Health Issues Related to Alcohol Consumption*. Edited by MacDonald I. Oxford, UK: Blackwell Science; 1999:125–180.

20. Paoletti R, Klatsky AL, Poli A, Zakhari S: *Moderate Alcohol Consumption and Cardiovascular Disease*. Dordrecht, the Netherlands: Kluwer Academic Publishers; 2000.

21. Corrao G, Rubbiati L, Bagnardi V, *et al.*: Alcohol and coronary heart disease: a meta-analysis. *Addiction* 2000, 95:1505–1523.

22. Marmot MG: Alcohol and coronary heart disease. *Int J Epidemiol* 2001, 30:724–729.

23. Hines LM, Rimm EB: Moderate alcohol consumption and coronary heart disease: a review. *Postgrad Med J* 2001, 77:747–752.

24. Boffetta P, Garfinkle A: Alcohol drinking and mortality among men enrolled in an American Cancer Society prospective study. *Epidemiology* 1990, 1:342–348.

25. Doll R, Peto R, Hall E, *et al.*: Mortality in relation to consumption of alcohol: 13 years' observations on British doctors. *BMJ* 1994, 309:911–918.

26. Klatsky AL, Armstrong MA, Friedman GD: Alcohol and mortality. *Ann Intern Med* 1992, 117:646–654.

27. Fuchs CS, Stampfer MJ, Colditz GA, *et al.*: Alcohol consumption and mortality among women. *N Engl J Med* 1995, 332:1245–1250.

28. Klatsky AL, Friedman GD, Armstrong MA, Kipp H: Wine, liquor, beer and mortality. *Am J Epidemiol* 2003, 158:585–595.

29. St. Leger AS, Cochrane AL, Moore F: Factors associated with cardiac mortality in developed countries with particular reference to the consumption of wine. *Lancet* 1979, i:1017–1020.

30. Renaud S, de Lorgeril M: Wine, alcohol, platelets, and the French paradox for coronary heart disease. *Lancet* 1992, 339:1523–1526.

31. Criqui MH, Ringel BL: Does diet or alcohol explain the French paradox? *Lancet* 1994, 344:1719–1723.

32. Gronbaek M, Becker U, Johansen D, *et al.*: Type of alcohol consumed and mortality from all causes, coronary heart disease, and cancer. *Ann Intern Med* 2000, 133:411–419.

33. Frankel EN, Kanner J, German JB, *et al.*: Inhibition of oxidation of human low-density lipoprotein by phenolic substances in red wine. *Lancet* 1993, 341:454–457.

34. Pace-Asciak CR, Hahn S, Diamandis EP, *et al.*: The red wine phenolics trans-resveratrol and quercetin block human platelet aggregation and eicosanoid synthesis: Implications for protection against coronary heart disease. *Clin Chim Acta* 1995, 235:207–219.

35. Rimm E, Klatsky A, Grobbee D, Stampfer MJ: Review of moderate alcohol consumption and reduced risk of coronary heart disease: Is the effect due to beer, wine, or spirits? *BMJ* 1996, 312:731–736.

36. Van Gign J, Stampfer MJ, Wolfe C, Algra A: The association between alcohol consumption and stroke. In *Health Issues Related to Alcohol Consumption*. Edited by Verschuren PM. Washington DC: ILSI Press; 1993:43–80.

37. Klatsky AL, Armstrong MA, Sidney S, Friedman GD: Alcohol drinking and risk of hemorrhagic stroke. *Neuroepidemiology* 2002, 21:115–122.

38. Camargo CA, Jr: Case-control and cohort studies of moderate alcohol consumption and stroke. *Clin Chim Acta* 1996, 246:107–119.

39. Stampfer MJ, Colditz GA, Willett WC, *et al.*: Prospective study of moderate alcohol consumption and the risk of coronary disease and stroke in women. *N Engl J Med* 1988, 319:267–273.

40. Klatsky AL, Armstrong MA, Sidney S, Friedman GD: Alcohol drinking and risk of ischemic stroke. *Am J Cardiol* 2001, 88:703–706.

41. Fernandez-Sola J, Nicolas JM, Oriola J, *et al.*: Angiotensin-converting enzyme gene polymorphism is associated with vulnerability to alcoholic cardiomyopathy. *Ann Intern Med* 2002, 137:321–326.

42. Nicolas JM, Fernandez-Sola J, Estruch R, *et al.*: The effect of controlled drinking in alcoholic cardiomyopathy. *Ann Intern Med* 2002, 136:192–200.

43. Zhang X, Li SY, Brown RA, Ren J: Ethanol and acetaldehyde in alcoholic cardiomyopathy: from bad to ugly en route to oxidative stress. *Alcohol* 2004, 32:175–186.

44. Laposata M, Hasaba A, Best CA, *et al.*: Fatty acid ethyl esters: recent observations. *Prostaglandins Leukot Essent Fatty Acids* 2002, 67:193–196.

45. Klatsky AL, Friedman GD, Siegelaub AB, Gerard MJ: Alcohol consumption and blood pressure. *N Engl J Med* 1977, 296:1194–2000.

46. Witteman JC, Willett WC, Stampfer MJ: Relation of moderate alcohol consumption and risk of systemic hypertension in women. *Am J Cardiol* 1990, 65:633–637.

47. Potter JF, Beevers DG: Pressor effect of alcohol in hypertension. *Lancet* 1984, 1:119–122.

48. Klatsky AL, Armstrong MA, Friedman GD: The relations of alcoholic beverage use to subsequent coronary artery disease hospitalization. *Am J Cardiol* 1986, 58:710–714.

49. Criqui, MH, Golomb BA: Epidemiologic aspects of lipid abnormalities. *Am J Med* 1998, 105:48S–57S.

50. Gaziano JM, Buring JM, Breslow JL, *et al.*: Moderate alcohol intake, increased levels of high density lipoprotein and its subfractions, and decreased risk of myocardial infarction. *N Engl J Med* 1993, 329:1829–1834.

51. Suh I, Shaten J, Cutler JA, Kuller L: Alcohol use and mortality from coronary heart disease: the role of high-density lipoprotein cholesterol. The Multiple Risk Factor Intervention Trial Research Group. *Ann Intern Med* 1992, 116:881–887.

52. Hendriks FJ, van der Gang MS: Alcohol, anticoagulation and fibrinolysis. In *Alcohol and Cardiovascular Diseases 1998*. Edited by Chadwick DJ, Goode JA. New York: Wiley; 1998:111–124.

53. Blackwelder WC, Yano K, Rhoads GG, *et al.*: Alcohol and mortality: the Honolulu Heart study. *Am J Med* 1980, 68:164–169.

54. Keil U, Chambless LE, Doring A, *et al.*: The relation of alcohol intake to coronary heart disease and all-cause mortality in a beer-drinking population. *Epidemiology* 1997, 8:150–156.

55. Klatsky AL, Armstrong MA, Kipp H: Correlates of alcoholic beverage preference: traits of persons who choose wine, liquor, or beer. *Br J Addict* 1990, 85:1279–1289.

56. Tjonneland A, Gronbaek M, Stripp C, Overvad K: Wine intake and diet in a random sample of 48,763 Danish men and women. *Am J Clin Nutr* 1999, 69:49–54.

57. Gronbaek M, Mortensen EL, Mygind K, *et al.*: Beer, wine, spirits and subjective health. *J Epidemiol Community Health* 1999, 53:721–724.

58. Mortensen EL, Jensen HH, Sanders SA, Reinisch JM: Better psychological functioning and higher social status may largely explain the apparent health benefits of wine: a study of wine and beer drinking in young Danish adults. *Arch Intern Med* 2001, 161:1844–1848.

59. Mukamal KJ, Conigrave KM, Mittleman MA, *et al.*: Roles of drinking pattern and type of alcohol consumed in coronary heart disease in men. *N Engl J Med* 2003, 348:109–118.

60. Booyse FM, Parks DA: Moderate wine and alcohol consumption: beneficial effects on cardiovascular disease. *Thromb Haemost* 2001, 86:517–528.

61. Sacco RL, Elkind M, Boden-Albala B, *et al.*: The protective effect of moderate alcohol consumption on ischemic stroke. *JAMA* 1999, 281:53–60.

Postmenopausal Estrogen Therapy

Francine Grodstein and JoAnn E. Manson

Several lines of evidence indicate that estrogen could protect against coronary heart disease (CHD). Women have lower rates of heart disease than men, which may be explained by differences in their estrogen levels. In addition, postmenopausal hormone therapy (HT) improves many intermediate markers of CHD, suggesting that it also may decrease the risk of CHD events; for example, in randomized clinical trials, hormone therapy raises high-density lipoproteins [1], lowers low-density lipoproteins [1], and decreases insulin and glucose [2]. However, HT also has adverse effects on some intermediate markers; for example, it leads to a rise in levels of C-reactive protein [3].

In epidemiologic studies of clinical events, observational studies, including the large Nurses' Health Study [4], have examined the relation of HT to major cardiovascular disease, as has a large randomized trial of primary prevention: the Women's Health Initiative (WHI) [5,6]. All of these studies consistently find that HT increases risk of stroke [4,6,7] and deep vein thrombosis [6,8,9]. However, observational studies of HT and CHD find that HT decreases risk of major coronary events [4], and randomized trials of HT and carotid atherosclerosis have shown that HT reduces progression of carotid atherosclerosis in young, healthy postmenopausal women [10]. In contrast, the WHI found that estrogen combined with progestin increased risk of major coronary disease [11] and unopposed estrogen use resulted in similar rates of CHD as placebo [6]. Numerous hypotheses have been suggested to explain these apparent discrepancies; the two primary hypotheses are 1) methodologic distinctions (primarily uncontrolled confounding in the observational studies), or 2) biologic differences between the populations in WHI and most observational investigations. In particular, the vast majority of subjects in WHI were older women, who may already have had underlying atherosclerosis. In observational studies, most women began hormone treatment near the onset of menopause. Although data are limited, mounting evidence suggests that HT has no coronary effects, or possibly harmful effects, specifically in older women with existing cardiovascular disease [12–16], but may have coronary benefits in younger, healthier women. Indeed, subgroup analyses in the WHI trials of estrogen alone and of combined therapy suggested that there may be an elevated risk of heart disease with combined hormone use starting at 10 or more years after onset of menopause [11], but a decreased risk of heart disease with use of unopposed estrogen at ages 50 to 59 years [6]. Nonetheless, the risks of HT are clear, with elevations in stroke, deep vein thrombosis, and possibly breast cancer; thus it is not recommended for chronic disease prevention at any age. Many alternate approaches to coronary health in postmenopausal women should be considered, including lifestyle modification, such as exercise, weight maintenance, avoidance of cigarette smoking, and a good diet, as well as pharmaceuticals such as antihypertensive and statin drugs.

Hormones and Cholesterol: PEPI Trial

	HDL, *mmol/L*	LDL, *mmol/L*
Placebo	-0.03	-0.11
Estrogen only	0.14	-0.37
E+ Cyclic MPA	0.04	-0.46
E+ Continuous MPA	0.03	-0.43
E+ Cyclic MP	0.11	-0.38

Figure 13-1.
Postmenopausal hormone therapy and cholesterol levels. Data from randomized trials have established that hormone therapy improves the lipid profile in postmenopausal women; cholesterol levels are an important risk factor for heart disease in women. In the Postmenopausal Estrogen and Progestin Intervention (PEPI) trial, 875 healthy postmenopausal women were assigned to one of five treatment arms: placebo, unopposed oral conjugated estrogen, estrogen (E) with cyclic medroxyprogesterone acetate (MPA), estrogen with continuous MPA, or estrogen with cyclic micronized progesterone (MP). For all four hormone regimens, there was a statistically significant increase in high-density lipoproteins (HDL) and decrease in low-density lipoproteins (LDL) compared with placebo. In addition, unopposed estrogen and estrogen with MP had significantly greater effects on HDL than estrogen with MPA. These trial data support the hypothesis that hormone use could provide coronary benefits. (*Adapted from* The Writing Group for the PEPI Trial [1].)

Hormone Therapy and Mean Change in Insulin and Glucose Over 3 Years; PEPI Trial

	Fasting insulin, %	Fasting glucose, *mmol/L*
Placebo	+15.3	-0.06
CEE	-5.6	-0.19
CEE + MPA cyclic	10.7	-0.24
CEE + MPA continuous	-9.3	-0.19
CEE + MP	-8.5	-0.16

Figure 13-2.
Postmenopausal hormone therapy and fasting insulin and glucose levels. In the same Postmenopausal Estrogen and Progestin Intervention (PEPI) trial, fasting insulin and glucose levels were also examined. After 3 years, across all the active treatment groups compared with placebo, mean insulin levels were 16% lower and mean glucose levels were 0.12 mmol/L lower ($P < 0.05$ for both). In general, effects were similar for all four active treatment regimens, although continuous medroxyprogesterone acetate (MPA) reduced fasting insulin to a greater extent than cyclic MPA. Thus, these data also support the hypothesis that hormone use could decrease heart disease because insulin is an important risk factor for coronary heart disease. CEE—conjugated equine estrogen; MP—micronized progesterone. (*Adapted from* Espeland *et al.* [2].)

Hormone Therapy and C-reactive Protein: PEPI Trial

	Baseline, *mgK*	At 36 months, *mgK*
Placebo	1.21	1.26
CEE	1.03	1.93
CEE + MPA Cyclic	1.23	2.52
CEE + MPA Continuous	1.28	2.28
CEE + MP	1.06	2.08

Average of 85% increase in active treatment groups.

Figure 13-3.
Postmenopausal hormone therapy and inflammatory markers. Hormone therapy does not have beneficial effects on all intermediate markers of coronary heart disease. For example, in the Postmenopausal Estrogen and Progestin Intervention (PEPI) trial, compared with placebo, all four active treatment regimens resulted in increased levels of high-sensitivity C-reactive protein, with an average 85% elevation in high-sensitivity C-reactive protein across the treatment groups. CEE—conjugated equine estrogen; MP—micronized progesterone; MPA—medroxyprogesterone acetate. (*Adapted from* Cushman *et al.* [3].)

Nurses' Health Study

Began in 1976
121,700 US registered nurses
11 States in the US
Age 30–55 years at entry
Biennial mailed questionnaires

Figure 13-4.
The Nurses' Health Study is one of the largest, long-term observational studies with substantial data on postmenopausal hormone therapy, and has contributed a substantial proportion of available information on the health effects of hormone use. This study includes 121,700 registered nurses from 11 states, who have been continuously observed since 1976; women ranged in age from 30 to 55 years when the study began, and thus are approximately aged 60 to 85 years currently. The subjects are sent mailed questionnaires every 2 years, providing extensive details on their health and lifestyle, including menopausal status, postmenopausal hormone use, and diagnosis of cardiovascular disease. Because the subjects are all health professionals, the women provide highly valid and reliable medical data. (*Adapted from* Grodstein *et al.* [4].)

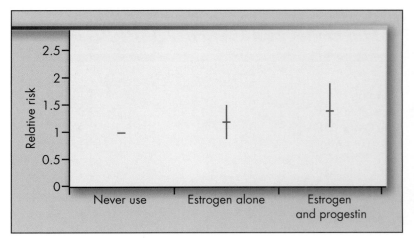

Figure 13-5.
The Women's Health Initiative is a randomized trial of postmenopausal hormone therapy, and is the only large-scale randomized study of the risks and benefits of hormone use in the primary prevention setting. There were two hormone components of the Women's Health Initiative: one of estrogen combined with progestin and one of unopposed estrogen. The combined hormone therapy trial included 16,608 women with a uterus randomized to oral conjugated estrogen with continuous medroxyprogesterone acetate or placebo. The trial ended after an average of 5.6 years of follow-up. The unopposed estrogen trial included 10,739 women without a uterus assigned to oral conjugated estrogen. The estrogen only trial ended after an average of 6.8 years of follow-up. In both components, subjects ranged from 50 to 79 years at randomization, although the majority was aged 60 years and older. (*Adapted from* Writing Group for the Women's Health Initiative Investigators [5] and The Women's Health Initiative Steering Committee [6].)

Figure 13-6.
Postmenopausal hormone therapy and stroke risk. These data from the Nurses' Health Study assess the risk of stroke in women who were currently using estrogen alone, or estrogen combined with progestin, compared with those who never used postmenopausal hormone therapy. The large majority of estrogen use in this study was oral conjugated estrogen, and the large majority of progestin use was medroxyprogesterone acetate. The relative risk of stroke for current users of estrogen alone was 1.18 (95% CI 0.95–1.46) and for estrogen with progestin was 1.45 (95% CI 1.10–1.92). These relative risks are controlled for differences between the hormone users and nonusers, including age, history of hypertension, high cholesterol, type 2 diabetes, family history of premature cardiovascular disease, body mass index, and cigarette smoking. (*Adapted from* Grodstein *et al.* [4].)

Figure 13-7.
Postmenopausal hormone therapy and stroke risk in the Women's Health Initiative. In the combined hormone therapy trial, there was a statistically significant 41% increase in the risk of stroke for women assigned to treatment compared with women assigned to placebo. Similarly, in the estrogen-only trial, there was a statistically significant 39% increase in the risk of stroke for women assigned to unopposed estrogen compared with placebo. These findings are virtually identical to those from the Nurses' Health Study. (*Adapted from* The Women's Health Initiative Steering Committee [6] and Wassertheil-Smoller *et al.* [7].)

Figure 13-8.
Postmenopausal hormone therapy and pulmonary embolism risk. These data from the Nurses' Health Study assess the risk of pulmonary embolism in women currently using hormone therapy (estrogen alone or estrogen combined with progestin) compared with those who never used postmenopausal hormone therapy. The relative risk (RR) of pulmonary embolism for current hormone users was 2.1 (95% CI 1.2–3.8). This RR was controlled for differences between the hormone users and nonusers, including age, history of hypertension, high cholesterol, type 2 diabetes, family history of premature cardiovascular disease, body mass index, and cigarette smoking. (*Adapted from* Grodstein *et al.* [8].)

Hormones and Deep Vein Thrombosis/Pulmonary Embolism: Women's Health Initiative Results

Estrogen with progestin trial:
  243 cases of DVT/PE
  RR of DVT/PE = 2.06 (95% CI 1.57–2.70)
Estrogen-only trial:
  179 cases of DVT/PE
  RR of DVT/PE = 1.33 (95% CI 0.99–1.79)

Figure 13-9.
Postmenopausal hormone therapy and risk of deep vein thrombosis (DVT) or pulmonary embolism (PE) from the Women's Health Initiative. In the combined hormone therapy trial, there was a statistically significant 2.1-fold higher rate of development of DVT or PE for women assigned to active treatment compared with women assigned to placebo. In the estrogen-only trial, this risk appeared somewhat lower, with a 33% increase, which was of borderline statistical significance for women assigned to unopposed estrogen compared with placebo. Again, as for stroke, these findings from the Women's Health Initiative trial are similar to the observational study data from the Nurses' Health Study. (*Adapted from* The Women's Health Initiative Steering Committee [6] and Cushman *et al.* [9].)

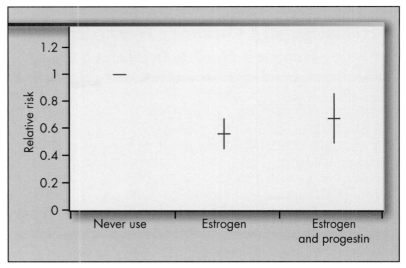

Figure 13-10.
Postmenopausal hormone therapy and coronary heart disease risk in the Nurses' Health Study. In these data from the Nurses' Health Study, as with data from many different observational studies of postmenopausal hormone therapy, women currently using hormone therapy had substantially lower rates of heart disease compared with women who never used hormone therapy. In the Nurses' Health Study, the relative risk for current use of estrogen with progestin was 0.64 (95% CI 0.49–0.85), and for estrogen alone was 0.55 (95% CI 0.45–0.68). The relative risks presented here were statistically controlled for differences in numerous cardiovascular risk factors between the hormone users and nonusers, including age, history of hypertension, high cholesterol, type 2 diabetes, family history of premature cardiovascular disease, body mass index, and cigarette smoking. (*Adapted from* Grodstein *et al.* [4].)

The Estrogen and Prevention of Atherosclerosis Trial

222 postmenopausal women aged 45+ years
No CVD, but LDL > 130 mg/dL
Randomized to 1 mg of oral estradiol or placebo

Figure 13-11.
Estrogen and atherosclerosis in women without existing heart disease. In randomized trials of generally healthy women, benefits of hormone therapy have also been found for carotid atherosclerosis. The Estrogen for the Prevention of Atherosclerosis (EPAT) trial examined subclinical atherosclerosis progression by carotid intima media thickness in 222 postmenopausal women without existing heart disease (but with low-density lipoprotein levels > 130 mg/dL). Subjects aged 45 years and older were assigned to 1 mg of oral micronized estradiol or to placebo and observed for 2 years. CVD—cardiovascular disease; LDL—low-density lipoprotein. (*Adapted from* Hodis *et al.* [10].)

The Estrogen and Prevention of Atherosclerosis Trial Results

Significantly less IMT progression of carotid artery for hormone-treated group over 2 years
Estrogen treatment:
  Average rate of progression = 0.0017 mm/year
Placebo:
  Average rate of progression = 0.0036 mm/year
P = 0.046

Figure 13-12.
Estrogen for the Prevention of Atherosclerosis (EPAT) trial results. The rate of change in intima media thickness (IMT) of the right distal common carotid artery far wall in computer image processed B-mode ultrasonograms was obtained at baseline and every 6 months during the 2-year trial. The average rate of progression of subclinical atherosclerosis was significantly lower in women assigned to unopposed estradiol than in those assigned to placebo (-0.0017 mm/year vs 0.0036 mm/year, P = 0.046). (*Adapted from* Hodis *et al.* [10].)

Hormones and Coronary Heart Disease: Women's Health Initiative

Estrogen with progestin trial:
RR of CHD = 1.25 (95% CI 1.00–1.54)
RR of CHD in year 1 = 1.81 (1.09–3.01)
RR of CHD in year 6+ = 0.70 (0.42–1.14)
Estrogen-only trial:
RR of CHD = 0.91 (95% CI 0.75–1.12)
RR of CHD in year 1 = 1.16; year 2 = 1.20, year 7+ = 0.42
From year 1 to end: *P* = 0.02

Figure 13-13.
Hormone therapy and coronary heart disease (CHD) in the Women's Health Initiative. In contrast to the studies of primary prevention, the Women's Health Initiative trial found no overall coronary benefits for subjects assigned to hormones relative to those assigned to placebo. For women given estrogen with progestin, there was a suggestion of a 24% higher rate of development of CHD for the treatment compared with placebo groups. In the estrogen only trial, rates of CHD were generally similar in the treatment compared with placebo groups. In both trial components, there appeared to be particular harm in the initial years of treatment. For estrogen with progestin, the relative risk in year 1 was 1.81 (95% CI 1.09–3.01) and in year 6 and later was 0.70 (95% CI 0.42–1.14). For unopposed estrogen, there was a trend of slightly elevated risk in years 1 and 2 (relative risk [RR] = 1.16 and 1.20, respectively) that diminished over time (RR = 0.42 in year 7 and later). (*Adapted from* The Women's Health Initiative Steering Committee [6] and Manson *et al.* [11].)

Possible Explanations for Apparent Discrepancies Between the Women's Health Initiative and Previous Primary Prevention Studies

Confounding: observation data are biased because of confounding
Populations: Women's Health Initiative data are largely based on women aged 60+ years (*ie*, with more CVD risk factors), but previous data generally based on hormone use in younger women (with fewer CVD risk factors)

Figure 13-14.
Apparent discrepancies between abservational and trial data. These apparent discrepancies in the effect of hormone therapy on coronary heart disease (CHD) between the Women's Health Initiative (WHI) and previous studies of primary prevention have resulted in substantial controversy. Many hypotheses have been proposed, but two primary explanations are most likely to explain these apparent differences. The first is that the observational data, which constitute the large majority of evidence on hormones and CHD, were invalid because of confounding. That is, women who choose to use hormone therapy are healthier than women who do not take hormones, and it is these health differences that made it spuriously appear that hormone use was beneficial.

A second explanation is differences in the populations in WHI and in previous studies of hormone therapy. The women recruited into WHI were generally older women (*eg*, in the combined therapy trial, two thirds of subjects were aged 60 years or older). In contrast, in most previous studies of hormone therapy, women taking hormones were much younger, near menopause (*eg*, in their late 40s and early 50s). It is possible that coronary effects of hormone therapy differ between older women, who likely have more cardiovascular disease (CVD) risk factors and underlying disease, compared with younger, healthier women.

Confounding

Many observational studies use select, homogenous populations (*eg*, nurses) that limit opportunities for confounding
Stroke and CHD share many risk factors, yet findings were identical for stroke in observational and trial data, suggesting confounding could not completely explain CHD findings

Figure 13-15.
The confounding hypothesis. Several lines of evidence suggest confounding likely does not completely explain apparent discrepancies between the trial data and observational data. First, the populations studied in many observational studies are relatively homogenous, for example, registered nurses in the Nurses' Health Study or residents of a high-income retirement community in the Leisure World Study. Such homogeneous populations reduce the potential for confounding as hormone users and nonusers in those studies would likely still have similar health care access and health habits (*see* Fig. 13-16 for example of risk factors in hormone users compared with nonusers in the Nurses' Health Study).

Second, the findings for stroke (as well as other cardiovascular outcomes such as deep vein thrombosis) in the WHI and in observational data were similar. Yet, stroke and coronary heart disease ([CHD] and likely deep vein thrombosis and CHD) share important risk factors; thus one would expect to see protection against stroke in the observational data if confounding by cardiovascular disease risk factors could completely explain the observed protection against CHD in the observational studies.

Characteristics of Hormone Users: Nurses' Health Study

	Never	Current
Parenteral MI < 60 years, %	30	21
HBP, %	33	31
Diabetes, %	6	3
High cholesterol, %	36	43
Moderate smoker, %	9	5
Mean BMI, %	26	25

Figure 13-16.
Cardiovascular disease risk factors in the Nurses' Health Study. This table demonstrates that, in a homogeneous population such as the Nurses' Health Study, there are limited differences in major cardiovascular disease risk factors between women who use hormone therapy and those who do not. For example, the prevalence of high blood pressure (HBP) and high cholesterol are quite similar in both groups. The modest differences in some risk factors (*eg*, 30% of women who never used hormones have a family history of premature heart disease vs 21% of women who use hormones) could not explain the 40% lower rates of heart disease in hormone users versus nonusers found in the Nurses' Health Study. BMI—body mass index; MI—myocardial infarction.

Cardiovascular Health Study

1636 postmenopausal women > 70 years of age
Vasodilation measured via brachial artery

Figure 13-17.
The Cardiovascular Health Study. To address the possibility that hormone use may affect subgroups of women differently, several studies have examined potential differences in the coronary effects of hormone therapy in healthier women compared to women with cardiovascular risk factors or disease. One of these was the Cardiovascular Health Study, which used ultrasound examinations to measure vasodilation in response to a flow stimulus (hyperemia) in 1636 older women. (*Adapted from* Herrington *et al.* [12].)

Cardiovascular Health Study Results

No CVD or risk factors:
  40% increase in vasodilator response for hormone users ($P = 0.01$)
CVD or risk factors:
  4% increase in vasodilator response for hormone users ($P > 0.2$)

Figure 13-18.
Results from the Cardiovascular Health Study. In this study, among women with no clinical or subclinical cardiovascular disease (CVD) or CVD risk factors, there was a statistically significant 40% greater vasodilator response in hormone users compared with nonusers. In contrast, in women with established CVD, hormone therapy was not associated with vasodilator response. Thus, the coronary benefits of hormone use in this observational study appeared limited to healthier women. (*Adapted from* Herrington *et al.* [12].)

Hormones and Coronary Heart Disease in Women with Existing Vascular Disease: Nurses' Health Study

Analysis of those with prior report of:
  MI
  Revascularization surgery
  70% or greater occlusion of one or more coronary artery
Total = 2489 women, with 213 incident cases of recurrent nonfatal MI/coronary death

Figure 13-19.
Women with coronary disease history in the Nurses' Health Study. A separate analysis was conducted of women with a history of coronary disease—defined as myocardial infarction (MI), revascularization surgery, or > 70% occlusion of at least one coronary artery. In total, 2489 women in the cohort met these criteria; during the follow-up period, 213 of those women developed a recurrent coronary event (defined as nonfatal MI or coronary death). (*Adapted from* Grodstein *et al.* [13].)

Hormone Use and Risk of Recurrent Coronary Heart Disease in Women with Vascular Disease

Hormone duration and major CHD:
  < 1 year: RR = 1.25 (95% CI 0.78–2.00)
  2+ years: RR = 0.38 (95% CI 0.22–0.66)

Figure 13-20.
Effect of hormone use in women with vascular disease. In this study, there was a suggestion of an increase in recurrent coronary heart disease (CHD) in the first year of hormone use (similar to the findings in the Women's Health Initiative for hormone treatment and risk of new CHD), but over the long-term, there was a statistically significant inverse relation between current hormone therapy and recurrent CHD. These data indicate that hormone therapy may have different effects in women with existing vascular disease than had been reported in observational studies of healthier women, and especially that there may be short-term increases in risk of recurrent CHD for hormone users with existing vascular disease. RR—relative risk. (*Adapted from* Grodstein *et al.* [13].)

Hormones and Coronary Heart Disease in Women with Existing Vascular Disease: Coumadin/Aspirin Reinfarction Study

1857 Postmenopausal women post-MI in trial of
    aspirin/coumadin
28% (n = 524) never used hormones
6% (n = 111) new users
Composite endpoint: death, MI, angina

Figure 13-21.
The Coumadin/Aspirin Reinfarction Study (CARS). Other observational studies have also found results similar to those in Figure 13-20. CARS included 1857 postmenopausal women with a previous myocardial infarction (MI). Twenty-eight percent of the subjects currently used hormone therapy at the start of the study, or had used them in the past, whereas 6% of subjects initiated hormone therapy during the study follow-up. (*Adapted from* Alexander *et al.* [14].)

Hormones and Risk of Recurrent Coronary Heart Disease in Women with Existing Vascular Disease: Coumadin/Aspirin Reinfarction Study

	Cases, n	Relative risk (95% CI)
Never users	387	1.0
New users	46	1.44 (1.05–1.99)
Prior/current users	116	0.94 (0.75–1.18)

Figure 13-22.
Further data from the Coumadin/Aspirin Reinfarction Study: newly initiated hormone therapy. In this study, the women who had newly initiated hormone therapy after the study began had a statistically significant 44% increased risk of recurrent heart disease, compared with women who had never used hormone therapy. For women who were current or past hormone users when the study began, the rates of recurrent heart disease were similar to those of women who had never used hormone therapy. (*Adapted from* Alexander *et al.* [14].)

Estrogen Replacement and Atherosclerosis Trial

309 Women with established coronary disease
Mean age 65 years, mean follow-up 3.2 years
Randomized to estrogen alone, estrogen + progestin, placebo
Similar levels of atherosclerosis progression in all groups

Figure 13-23.
The Estrogen Replacement and Atherosclerosis ERA) trial.Clinical trials also have examined the effects of hormone therapy in women with existing vascular disease. The ERA included 309 women with established coronary disease assigned to one of three treatment arms: oral conjugated estrogen, oral conjugated estrogen with medroxyprogesterone acetate, and placebo. These were older women (mean age = 65 years), who were observed over 3.2 years with coronary angiograms to assess minimum coronary artery diameter. At the end of the trial, no difference was found in rates of progression of atherosclerosis between the three treatment groups. (*Adapted from* Herrington *et al.* [15].)

Heart and Estrogen/Progestin Replacement Study

2763 Women with established coronary disease
Mean age 66.7 years, mean follow-up 4.1 years
Randomized to 0.625 mg CEE + 2.5 mg MPA, or placebo
75% compliance after 3 years

Figure 13-24.
The Heart and Estrogen/progestin Replacement Trial (HERS). Finally, the largest randomized trial of hormone therapy and recurrent coronary events in women with existing coronary disease was HERS. This trial included 2763 women with established coronary disease (myocardial infarction, revascularization surgery, or at least 50% occlusion of at least one coronary artery). These were older women, with a mean age of approximately 67 years, and they were observed for a mean of 4.1 years. Women were randomly assigned to oral conjugated estrogen combined with medroxyprogesterone acetate (MPA) or placebo. CEE—conjugated equine estrogen. (*Adapted from* Hulley *et al.* [16].)

Heart and Estrogen/Progestin Replacement Study: Results for Recurrent Myocardial Infarction or Coronary Death

Overall RR = 0.99 (95% CI 0.80–1.22)
    Year 1: RR = 1.55
    Years 4 and 5: RR = 0.67
    P = 0.009

Figure 13-25.
Overall results from the Heart and Estrogen/Progestin Replacement Study. In this trial, overall, there were a similar number of cases of recurrent heart disease (myocardial infarction) or coronary death among the treated and the placebo groups. However, as in the observational data of women with established coronary disease, there was a suggestion of harm in the initial year of taking hormone therapy, with possible benefits after longer term use (P = 0.009). Thus, overall, studies may be suggesting that hormone therapy has harmful effects on coronary risk in specific situations—possibly in older women with existing coronary disease and especially in the initial years of treatment. RR—relative risk. (*Adapted from* Hulley *et al.* [16].)

Hormones and Risk of Coronary Heart Disease: Women's Health Initiative Combined Therapy Trial

Women < 10 years since menopause: RR = 0.89
Women 10–19 years since menopause: RR = 1.22
Women 20+ years since menopause: RR = 1.71

Figure 13-26.
Subgroup analyses from the Women's Health Initiative. These analyses also suggested that hormone therapy may have different effects in different women. In the trial of estrogen with progestin, subjects were separated according to the number of years between the onset of menopause and their enrollment in the trial. Although there was not a statistically significant interaction ($P = 0.33$), these data indicated that hormone therapy may slightly lower risk of heart disease compared with placebo in women who started treatment less than 10 years after the onset of menopause (relative risk [RR] = 0.89), while hormone therapy may slightly increase risk of heart disease compared with placebo in women who started treatment 10 to 19 or 20+ years after menopause (RR = 1.22 and RR = 1.71, respectively). (*Adapted from* Manson *et al.* [11].)

Hormones and Risk of Coronary Heart Disease: Women's Health Initiative Unopposed Estrogen Trial

Age 50–59 at trial enrollment: RR = 0.56
Age 60–69: RR = 0.92
Age 70–79: RR = 1.04

Figure 13-27.
The unopposed estrogen trial. Similarly, in the unopposed estrogen trial, subgroup analyses were conducted according to women's age at enrollment into the trial. Although the interaction was not statistically significant ($P = 0.14$), in subjects aged 50–59 years when they began the trial, there was a lower rate of development of heart disease for those assigned to treatment than placebo (relative risk [RR] = 0.56), whereas there was no effect of estrogen therapy on heart disease risk for women who began the trial at ages 60 to 69 or 70 to 79 years (RR = 0.92 and RR = 1.04, respectively).

Thus, although not conclusive, these data from the Women's Health Initiative also support the hypothesis that the apparent discrepancies in the results of the Women's Health Initiative compared with other studies of hormone therapy and primary prevention of heart disease might be explained by different effects of hormones on women at different stages of their life.

It is not completely clear why hormone therapy may have differing effects on coronary events. However, it is possible that in older women, at later stages of atherosclerosis, prothrombotic or plaque-destabilizing effects of hormone therapy may predominate. The increase in venous thromboembolism caused by hormones demonstrates its prothrombotic effects (*see* Figs. 13-8 and 13-9). In addition, hormone therapy increases levels of inflammatory markers (*see* Fig. 13-3), which may contribute to plaque destabilization. (*Adapted from* The Women's Health Initiative Steering Committee [6]).

Summary of Hormones and Risk of Coronary Heart Disease

HT increases risk of stroke and DVT
In observational studies and randomized trials of atherosclerosis, HT associated with reduced CHD risk and slower progression of carotid atherosclerosis in young, healthy women
Women's Health Initiative trials found increased CHD with E+P and similar CHD rates for E alone versus placebo
One explanation may be that HT is beneficial in younger or recently menopausal women and harmful in older women

Figure 13-28.
Summary of hormones and risk of coronary heart disease (CHD). To summarize, data from observational studies and randomized trials consistently show that hormone therapy (HT) increases risk of stroke and deep vein thrombosis (DVT) however, observational studies and randomized trials of atherosclerosis progression have reported lower rates of coronary heart disease and less progression of carotid atherosclerosis in women taking HT. In contrast, the Women's Health Initiative trial of estrogen with progestin found slightly higher rates of coronary disease for those assigned to therapy than placebo, and the unopposed estrogen trial found no difference in rates of coronary heart disease for the treatment and placebo groups. Currently, a plausible explanation for resolving these varying findings may be based on the populations who participated in the different studies; limited data suggest that HT may have coronary benefits if initiated in younger, healthier women but could cause harm when initiated in older women with subclinical or clinical vascular disease. E—estrogen; E+P—estrogen plus progestin.

Recommendations for Hormones and Risk of Coronary Heart Disease

Substantial controversy remains over the coronary benefits and risks of hormone therapy

Given established risks of hormone therapy (increase in stroke, deep vein thrombosis, and possibly breast cancer), hormone therapy should not be used for chronic disease prevention at any age

Alternate approaches to coronary health include:

Healthy lifestyle—exercise, weight maintenance, good diet, and avoidance of cigarette smoking

Nonhormonal pharmaceuticals (*eg*, statins)

Figure 13-29.
The data on hormone therapy and coronary heart disease remain controversial. National guidelines do not recommend the use of hormone therapy for heart disease prevention in primary or secondary prevention settings. Many other options exist for decreasing risk of heart disease, including nonpharmaceutical options such as exercise, a good diet, weight maintenance, and avoidance of cigarette smoking, as well as pharmaceutical options, such as statin medications, and antihypertensive drugs.

Future Challenges for Hormones and Risk of Coronary Heart Disease

More data are needed to identify possible subgroups that may receive benefits from hormone therapy

Information is needed on the variety of hormonal treatments, including lower-dose regimens and different routes of administration that may minimize the risks of hormone therapy, but provide chronic disease benefits

Figure 13-30.
Future research is needed to clarify the suggestive data regarding possibly different coronary effects of hormone therpay when initiated at different ages. In addition, the large majority of data on hormones and coronary heart disease regards the standard dose of 0.625 mg of oral conjugated estrogen and further research on lower doses, or alternate types of hormones (*eg*, transdermal estrogen) may also identify ways to minimize the risks while maintaining benefits.

References

1. The Writing Group for the PEPI Trial: Effects of estrogen or estrogen/progestin regimens on heart disease risk factors in post-menopausal women. The Postmenopausal Estrogen/Progestin Interventions (PEPI) Trial. *JAMA* 1995, 273:199–208.

2. Espeland MA, Hogan PE, Fineberg SE, *et al.*: Effect of postmenopausal hormone therapy on glucose and insulin concentrations. PEPI Investigators: Postmenopausal Estrogen/Progestin Interventions. *Diabetes Care* 1998, 21:1589–1595.

3. Cushman M, Legault C, Barrett-Connor E, *et al.*: Effect of post-menopausal hormones on inflammation-sensitive proteins: the Postmenopausal Estrogen/Progestin Interventions (PEPI) Study. *Circulation* 1999, 100:717–722.

4. Grodstein F, Manson JE, Colditz GA, *et al.*: A prospective, observational study of postmenopausal hormone therapy and primary prevention of cardiovascular disease. *Ann Intern Med* 2000, 133:933–941.

5. Writing Group for the Women's Health Initiative Investigators: Risks and benefits of estrogen plus progestin in healthy postmenopausal women: principal results from the Women's Health Initiative randomized controlled trial. *JAMA* 2002, 288:321–333.

6. The Women's Health Initiative Steering Committee: Effects of conjugated equine estrogen in postmenopausal women with hysterectomy: the Women's Health Initiative randomized controlled trial. *JAMA* 2004, 291:1701–1712.

7. Wassertheil-Smoller S, Hendrix SL, Limacher M, *et al.*: Effect of estrogen plus progestin on stroke in postmenopausal women: the Women's Health Initiative: a randomized trial. *JAMA* 2003, 289:2673–2684.

8. Grodstein F, Stampfer MJ, Goldhaber SZ, *et al.*: Prospective study of exogenous hormones and risk of pulmonary embolism in women. *Lancet* 1996, 348:983–987.

9. Cushman M, Kuller LH, Prentice R, *et al.*: Estrogen plus progestin and risk of venous thrombosis. *JAMA* 2004, 292:1573–1580.

10. Hodis HN, Mack WJ, Lobo RA, *et al.*: Estrogen in the prevention of atherosclerosis: a randomized, double-blind, placebo-controlled trial. *Ann Intern Med* 2001, 135:939–953.

11. Manson JE, Hsia J, Johnson KC, *et al.*: Estrogen plus progestin and the risk of coronary heart disease. *N Engl J Med* 2003, 349:523–534.

12. Herrington DM, Espeland MA, Crouse JR III, *et al.*: Estrogen replacement and brachial artery flow-mediated vasodilation in older women. *Arterioscler Thromb Vasc Biol* 2001, 21:1955–1961.

13. Grodstein F, Manson JE, Stampfer MJ: Postmenopausal hormone use and secondary prevention of coronary events in the Nurses' Health Study: a prospective, observational study. *Ann Intern Med* 2001, 135:1–8.

14. Alexander KP, Newby LK, Hellkamp AS, *et al.*: Initiation of hormone replacement therapy after acute myocardial infarction is associated with more cardiac events during follow-up. *J Am Coll Cardiol* 2001, 38:1–7.

15. Herrington DM, Reboussin DM, Brosnihan KB, *et al.*: Effects of estrogen replacement on the progression of coronary-artery atherosclerosis. *N Engl J Med* 2000, 343:522–529.

16. Hulley S, Grady D, Bush T, *et al.*: Randomized trial of estrogen plus progestin for secondary prevention of coronary heart disease in post-menopausal women. Heart and Estrogen/progestin Replacement Study (HERS) Research Group. *JAMA* 1998, 280:605–613.

Diet and Prevention of Coronary Heart Disease

Frank B. Hu

The relationship between diet and coronary heart disease (CHD) has been the subject of intense research for nearly a century. In the early 1900s, Russian scientists successfully developed an animal experimental model of atherosclerosis by feeding rabbits a diet high in cholesterol and saturated fat [1]. These observations led to the belief that dietary cholesterol was the primary agent for causing atherosclerosis. In the early 1950s, controlled feeding studies found that dietary fatty acids and cholesterol affected serum cholesterol concentration. Meanwhile, epidemiologic studies found that serum cholesterol predicted risk of CHD in healthy individuals. These discoveries led to the classical "diet-heart hypothesis," which postulated the primary role of dietary saturated fat and cholesterol in causing atherosclerosis and CHD in humans [2]. The further development of the diet-heart hypothesis was influenced heavily by ecologic correlations relating diet to rates of heart disease in different countries, along with findings from migration studies and special populations.

Until recently, most epidemiologic and clinical investigations of diet and CHD have been dominated by the classical diet-heart hypothesis. It is now recognized that dietary cholesterol is not the primary determinant of serum cholesterol or CHD in most populations and that the classical diet-heart hypothesis is overly simplistic [3]. In the past two decades, understanding of the nutrients and foods most likely to promote cardiac health has improved substantially, owing to the advances in several areas of research, including molecular mechanisms of atherosclerosis, metabolic effects of various nutrients and foods (beyond dietary fat and cholesterol), large and carefully conducted prospective cohort studies, and dietary intervention trials.

Although the search for the optimal diet for prevention of CHD is far from over, clearer and firmer evidence has now become available on the role of major types of fat and different classes of fatty acids and also other aspects of diet, including different types of carbohydrates, fiber, folate, antioxidant vitamins, phytochemicals, and overall eating patterns. This chapter reviews current evidence regarding the relationship between important dietary factors and risk of CHD.

Cumulative evidence from epidemiologic studies and clinical trials indicate that three dietary strategies are effective in preventing CHD: substitute nonhydrogenated unsaturated fats for saturated and trans-fats; increase consumption of omega-3 fatty acids from fish, fish oil supplements, or plant sources; and consume a diet high in fruits, vegetables, nuts, and whole grains and low in refined grain products [3]. Thus, diets including nonhydrogenated unsaturated fats as the predominate form of dietary fat, whole and minimally processed grains as the main form of carbohydrate, an abundance of fruits and vegetables, and adequate omega-3 fatty acids should offer significant protection against CHD. Such diets, together with avoidance of smoking and regular physical activity, can prevent the large majority of cardiovascular disease in Western populations.

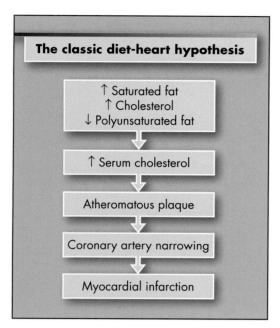

Figure 14-1.
The classic diet-heart hypothesis. According to this hypothesis, high intake of saturated fats and cholesterol and low intake of polyunsaturated fats increase serum cholesterol, leading to formation of atheromatous plaques. Accumulation of these plaques narrows the coronary arteries and reduces blood flow to the heart muscle, eventually leading to myocardial infarction [4].

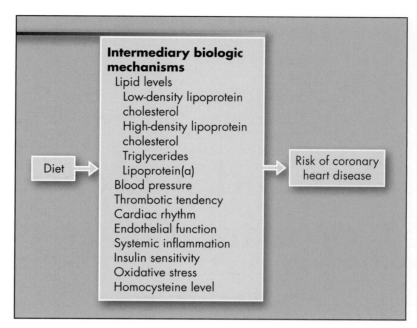

Figure 14-2.
Multiple mechanisms by which diet influences coronary heart disease (CHD). Besides blood lipid levels, dietary factors affect risk of CHD through several other biologic mechanisms [3]. For example, the source of dietary fat not only influences the level of low-density lipoprotein (LDL) and susceptibility to oxidative modification, but also is a primary determinant of vitamin E intake, the most important lipid-soluble dietary antioxidant. Most sources of animal fat tend to raise LDL levels and also contain few antioxidants. Liquid vegetable oils and nuts typically reduce LDL levels and also contain high amounts of antioxidant vitamins and phenolic compounds that protect essential fatty acids from oxidation. In addition, dietary factors have important influences on other major determinants of CHD, including blood pressure, thrombosis, arrhythmia, insulin resistance, and endothelial dysfunction. Because diet influences CHD through multiple complex pathways, it is important to consider all relevant intermediate biologic markers rather than just a single mechanism when evaluating the effects of a nutrient or food. (*Adapted from* Hu and Willett [3].)

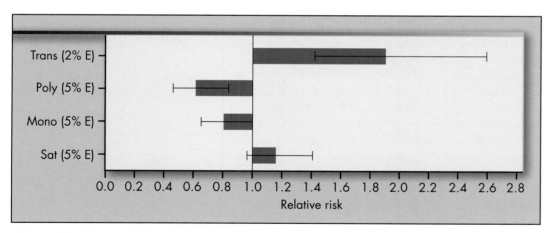

Figure 14-3.
Multivariate relative risks of coronary heart disease (CHD) associated with increase in major types of fat [5]. Ecologic studies showed a strong positive correlation between dietary intake of saturated fat and rates of CHD. In the Seven Countries Study [6], intake of saturated fat as a percentage of calories was strongly correlated with coronary death rates across 16 defined populations in seven countries ($r = 0.84$), although the correlation between the percentage of energy from total fat and CHD incidence was much weaker ($r = 0.39$). Hu *et al.* [5] conducted a prospective analysis of dietary fat and CHD among 80,082 women aged 34 to 59 in the Nurses' Health Study and found that type of fat was more important in predicting CHD risk than total amount of fat. In particular, higher intakes of trans-fat and saturated fat to less extent were associated with increased risk, whereas higher intakes of unhydrogenated mono- or polyunsaturated fats were associated with decreased risk. Because of opposing effects of different types of fat, total fat as percentage of energy was not appreciably associated with CHD risk. (*Adapted from* Hu *et al.* [5].)

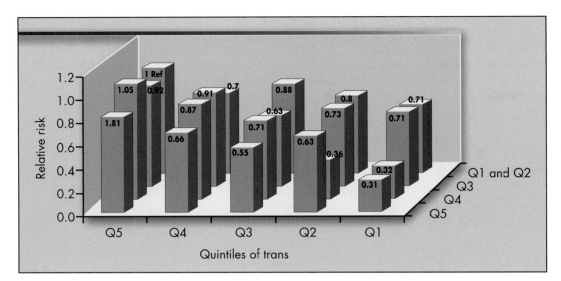

Figure 14-4.
Multivariate relative risk of coronary heart disease (CHD) according to dietary intake of trans- and polyunsaturated fats [5]. In the Nurses' Health Study, when intakes of polyunsaturated and trans-fat were considered together, the lowest risk of CHD was observed among those who had the highest intake of polyunsaturated and lowest intake of trans-fat (relative risk = 0.31 [95% CI 0.11–0.88]) [5], indicating a substantial benefit of substituting polyunsaturated fat (such as unhydrogenated vegetable oils) for trans-fat (such as hard margarine and vegetable shortenings) in the diet. (*Adapted from* Hu *et al.* [5].)

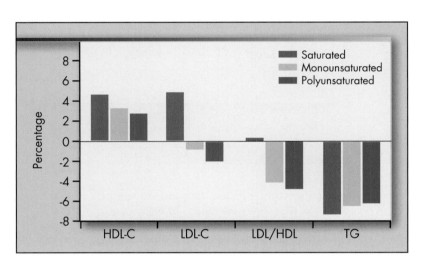

Figure 14-5.
Predicted changes in serum lipids and lipoproteins when 5% energy as carbohydrate is replaced by specific fatty acids under isocaloric conditions (assume baseline high-density lipoprotein [HDL] levels at 50 mg/dL, low-density lipoprotein [LDL] at 130 mg/dL, and triglycerides [TG] at 150 mg/dL) [7]. In controlled feeding studies, saturated fatty acids increase, and polyunsaturated fatty acids decrease total and LDL cholesterol (LDL-C). All three classes of fatty acids (saturated, monounsaturated, and polyunsaturated) elevate HDL cholesterol (HDL-C) when they replace carbohydrate in the diet, and this effect is slightly greater with saturated fatty acids. Also, TG levels increase when dietary fatty acids are replaced by carbohydrates. Because replacement of saturated fat with carbohydrate proportionally reduces LDL and HDL, and thus has little effect on the LDL/HDL ratio, and increases TG, this change in diet would be expected to have minimal benefit on coronary heart disease risk. However, when mono- or polyunsaturated fats replace saturated fat, LDL decreases and HDL changes only slightly. (*Adapted from* Hu and Willett [3].)

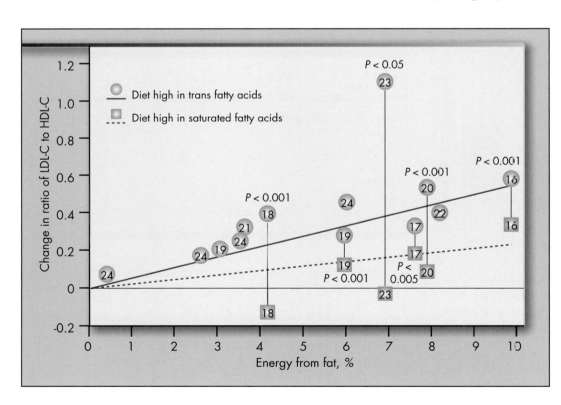

Figure 14-6.
Results of metabolic studies of the effects of a diet high in trans- or saturated fatty acids on the ratio of low- (LDL-C) and high-density lipoprotein cholesterol (HDL-C) [3]. In controlled metabolic studies, trans-fatty acids (found in stick margarine, vegetable shortenings, and commercial bakery and deep-fried foods) raise LDL-C levels and lower HDL-C relative to cis-unsaturated fatty acids, and the increase in the ratio of total to HDL-C for trans-fat is approximately double that for saturated fat. Also, high intake of trans-fat may promote insulin resistance [8] and increase risk of type 2 diabetes [9]. The unique adverse metabolic effects of trans-fatty acids may explain the strong positive association with coronary heart disease observed in epidemiologic studies. (*Adapted from* Hu and Willett [3].)

Diet and Prevention of Coronary Heart Disease

Traditional classification focuses on chemical structure
Mono-, di-, or polysaccharides or simple/complex
New classification emphasizes biologic effects of whole foods
    including physical forms, fiber contents, digestibility,
    metabolism, coexistence of fat and protein

Figure 14-7.

Types of carbohydrates. Prevailing dietary recommendations have emphasized high intake of complex carbohydrates, mainly starch, and avoidance of simple sugars. However, many complex carbohydrates, such as baked potatoes and white bread, are rapidly digested to glucose and produce even higher glycemic and insulinemic responses than sucrose (half glucose and half fructose). Thus, the new classification focuses on biologic effects of whole foods on blood glucose and insulin responses [10].

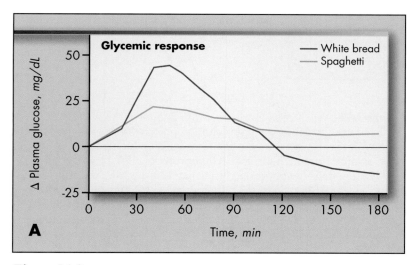

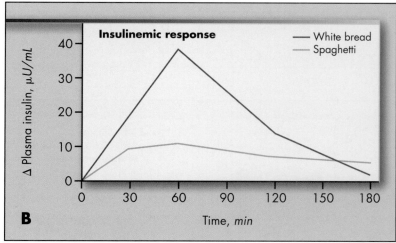

Figure 14-8.

Glycemic (**A**) and insulinemic (**B**) responses after ingestion of carbohydrates. Responses were measured after ingestion of 50 g of carbohydrate as white bread or spaghetti made from identical ingredients [10]. The glycemic index (GI) ranks foods based on rise in blood glucose (the incremental area under the curve for blood glucose levels) after ingestion compared with glucose or white bread, standardizing the carbohydrate content to 50 g [11,12]. Foods with a low degree of starch gelatinization (more compact granules), such as spaghetti and oatmeal, and a high level of viscose soluble fiber such as barley, oats, and rye tend to have a slower rate of digestion and thus lower GI values. In many controlled clinical studies [13], feeding low-GI meals to diabetic patients led to significant improvement in glycemic control and lipid profile. In addition, several large epidemiologic studies have found an inverse association between calculated overall dietary GI values and plasma high-density lipoprotein concentrations in free-living adults [14,15]. (*Adapted from* Ludwig [10].)

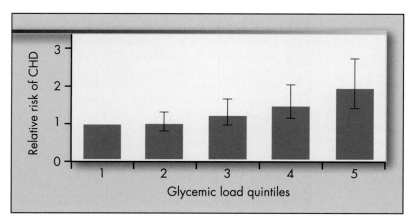

Figure 14-9.

Multivariate relative risk of coronary heart disease (CHD) according to quintiles of glycemic load in the Nurses' Health Study [16]. The overall blood glucose response to a food is determined not only by its glycemic index (GI) value, but also by the amount of carbohydrate. Thus, the glycemic load (GL; the product of the GI value of a food and its carbohydrate content) has been used to represent the quality *and* quantity of the carbohydrates consumed. A strong positive association between GL and risk of CHD (761 cases) was observed among 75,521 women during 10 years of follow-up (relative risk comparing the highest vs lowest quintiles was 1.98 [95% CI, 1.41–2.77]) [16]. The increased risk was more pronounced among overweight and obese women, consistent with metabolic studies that the adverse effects of a high-GL diet are exacerbated by underlying insulin resistance [17]. (*Adapted from* Liu *et al.* [16].)

Whole Grain Foods

Whole grain breakfast cereal
Wheat bread
Popcorn
Oatmeal
Brown rice
Bran, wheat germ, and other grains
    (*eg*, bulgar, kasha, or cous-cous)

Figure 14-10.

Types of whole grain foods. One way to classify dietary carbohydrate is to subdivide cereal grains—staple foods in most societies—into whole and refined grains. In traditional diets, grains were typically consumed in whole intact form or as coarse flours produced from stone grinding. In modern societies, however, most cereal grains are highly processed before they are consumed. Grinding or milling using modern technology produces fine flours with very small particle size. Milling also removes most of the bran and much of the germ. The resulting refined grain products contain more starch but substantially lower amount of dietary fiber, vitamins, minerals, essential fatty acids, and phytochemicals. In several epidemiologic studies, a higher consumption of whole grains was associated with a lower risk of coronary heart disease [2].

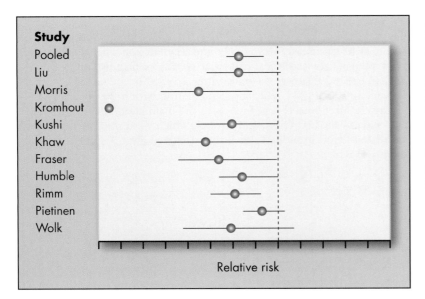

Figure 14-11.
Pooled analyses of prospective cohort studies on dietary fiber intake and risk of coronary heart disease [18]. Dietary fiber includes the cell walls of plants and other indigestible components of plants. Soluble fibers (pectins, gums, mucilages, and psyllium) lower total and low-density lipoprotein cholesterol through increased bile acid excretion and decreased hepatic synthesis of cholesterol and fatty acids, although the cholesterol-lowering effects are modest [19]. In addition, a high-fiber diet has been shown to improve glycemic control and insulin response. Several prospective cohort studies have consistently found an inverse association between fiber intake and risk of coronary heart disease. (*Adapted from* Liu *et al.* [18].)

A. Types of n-3 Fatty Acids

n-3 Fatty acid	Dietary source
α-Linolenic acid (C18:3n-3)	Some vegetable oils (canola, soybean), nuts (walnuts), seeds (flaxseed)
Eicosapentaenoic acid (C20:5n-3)	Fish and shellfish
Docosahexaenoic acid (C22:6n-3)	Fish and shellfish

ALA:	CH₃ ⟋⟍⟋⟍⟋⟍⟋⟍⟋⟍⟋⟍ COOH
EPA:	CH₃ ⟋⟍⟋⟍⟋⟍⟋⟍⟋⟍ COOH
DHA:	CH₃ ⟋⟍⟋⟍⟋⟍⟋⟍⟋⟍⟋ COOH

B

Figure 14-12.
A, Types of n-3 fatty acids. **B,** Formulas. There are two major classes of n-3 polyunsaturated fatty acids: eicosapentaenoic acid (20:5n-3; EPA) and docosahexaenoic acid (22:6n-3; DHA), found in high concentrations in fish oil, and α-linolenic acid (18:3n-3; ALA), found in vegetable oils (especially soybean and canola oil) and green leafy vegetables. ALA can be converted to EPA and DHA in humans, but with low efficiency. Fish n-3 fatty acids may reduce risk of coronary heart disease by lowering serum triglyceride levels, decreasing platelet aggregability, improving endothelial dysfunction, and preventing cardiac arrhythmia [20,21]. The antiarrhythmic effects of n-3 fatty acids, which are well established in cell-culture studies and animal experiments, may explain the protective effects of fish consumption at low levels (*ie*, one to two servings per week) against fatal coronary heart disease or sudden death.

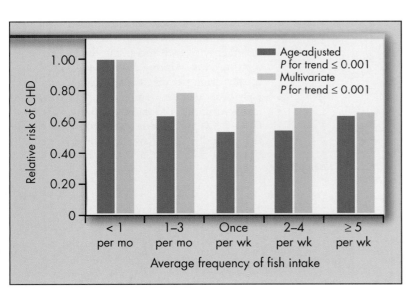

Figure 14-13.
Age- and multivariate-adjusted relative risks of coronary heart disease (CHD) according to categories of fish consumption. The Nurses' Health Study, including 1513 incident cases of CHD during 16 years of follow-up, found that fish consumption two to four times per week was associated with 30% lower risk of CHD, after adjustment for established CHD risk factors [22]. Intake of n-3 fatty acids was also associated with a lower risk of CHD, with multivariable relative risks of 1.0, 0.93, 0.78, 0.68, and 0.67 (*P* < 0.001 for trend) across quintiles of intake. These associations were stronger for fatal CHD than for nonfatal myocardial infarction. (*Adapted from* Hu *et al.* [22].)

Clinical Trials of Fish Oil after Myocardial Infarction

DART [23]
  1015 subjects using fish oil; 1015 control subjects
  Two fish meals per week or 0.3 g per day n-3 polyunsaturated
    fatty acids for 2 years
  Ischemic heart disease–related death reduced by 33%
GISSI [24]
  1 g per day n-3 polyunsaturated fatty acids for 3.5 years
  5666 subjects using fish oils; 5658 control subjects
  Cardiovascular disease–related death reduced by 30%

Figure 14-14.
Clinical trials of long-chain n-3 fatty acids and secondary prevention of coronary heart disease. In the Diet and Reinfarction Trial (DART) [23], patients advised to eat fish twice weekly or take fish oil (1.5 g/day) had a 29% lower mortality after 2 years. In the GISSI-Prevenzione trial [24], daily supplementation with n-3 fatty acids (1 g/day) resulted in a 15% reduction in the main endpoint (death, non-fatal myocardial infarction, and stroke), which was primarily because of a 45% reduction in sudden death that occurred after 3 months of treatment [25].

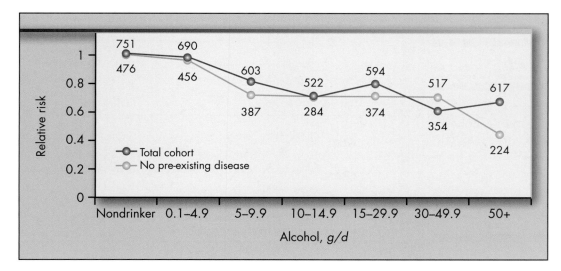

Figure 14-15.
Multivariate relative risks of coronary heart disease according to categories of alcohol consumption in the Health Professionals' Follow-up Study [26]. Alcohol consumption was strongly associated with lower risk of coronary heart disease in the total cohort. The results did not change after excluding 10,302 current nondrinkers or 16,342 men with disorders potentially related to coronary disease (*eg*, hypertension, diabetes, and gout), which may have led men to reduce their alcohol intake. Also, most epidemiologic studies suggest that wine, beer, and liquor confer similar benefits on coronary risk [27,28].

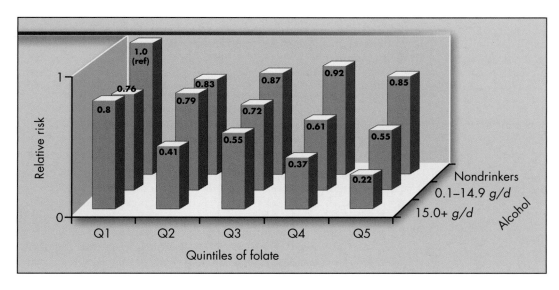

Figure 14-16.
Multivariate relative risk of coronary heart disease by quintiles of folate intake across levels of alcohol consumption among 80,082 women in the Nurses' Health Study. Women in the lowest quintile of folate who did not drink alcohol were the reference category [29]. The inverse association between folate intake and risk of coronary heart disease was stronger with each increasing level of alcohol consumption. Among women consuming up to one drink per day, the relative risk of coronary heart disease, comparing the highest with lowest quintiles of folate, was 0.69 (95% CI, 0.49–0.97) and among those consuming more than one drink per day, the comparable relative risk was 0.27 (95% CI, 0.13–0.58).

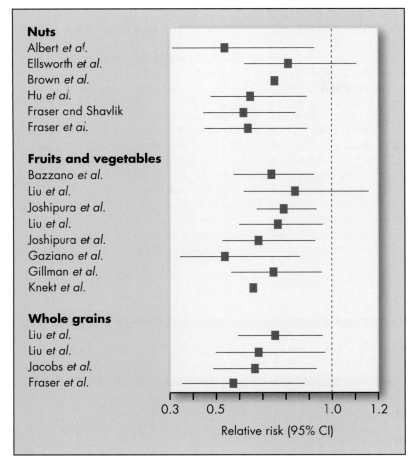

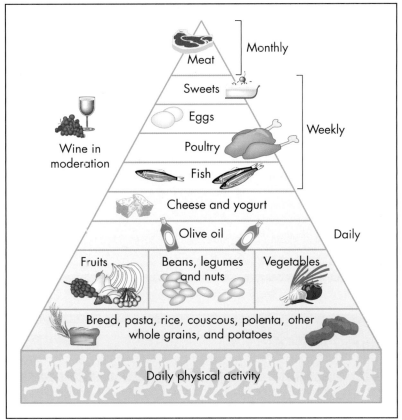

Figure 14-17.

Prospective cohort studies of consumption of nuts, fruits and vegetables, or whole grains and cardiovascular disease [3]. The relative risks (95% CI) were derived from the comparison of the incidence rates between the highest and lowest consumption groups (quintiles, quartiles, or specific intake categories) and adjusted for nondietary or dietary covariates. Substantial evidence from prospective cohort studies indicates that a higher consumption of plant-based foods, such as fruits and vegetables, nuts, and whole grains, is associated with significantly lower risk of coronary heart disease and stroke. The protective effects of these foods are probably mediated through multiple beneficial nutrients contained in these foods, including mono- and polyunsaturated fatty acids, omega-3 fatty acids, antioxidant vitamins, minerals, phytochemicals, fiber, and plant protein. (*Adapted from* Hu and Willett [3].)

Figure 14-18.

Food pyramid reflecting the traditional healthy Mediterranean diet [30]. The main characteristics of the Mediterranean diet include an abundance of plant food (fruits, vegetables, whole grain cereals, nuts, and legumes); olive oil as the principal source of fat; fish and poultry consumed in low to moderate amounts; lower consumption of red meat; and moderate consumption of wine, normally with meals. The concept of Mediterranean diet originated from the Seven Countries Study initiated by Ancel Keys in the 1950s. The study observed that, despite a high fat intake, the population of Crete Island in Greece enjoyed very low rates of coronary heart disease and of certain cancers and a long life expectancy [31]. (*Adapted from* Hu [30].)

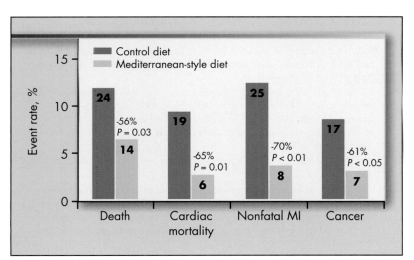

Figure 14-19.

Risk reductions in total mortality, cardiac mortality, recurrent myocardial infarction (MI), and cancer in the Mediterranean-type diet group compared with the control group during 4 years of follow-up in the Lyon Diet Heart Study [32,33]. The Lyon Diet Heart Study is a randomized secondary prevention trial testing whether a Mediterranean-type diet as opposed to an American Heart Association Step 1 diet may reduce the rate of recurrence after a first MI. The intervention diet is a Mediterranean-style diet supplemented with α-linolenic acid. This study showed a dramatic reduction in total and cardiac mortality, recurrent MIs, and cancer incidence in the intervention group compared with the control group. (*Adapted from* de Lorgeril *et al.* [32,33].)

Primary Prevention of Coronary Heart Disease: Five Attributes to Define Low-risk

1) Diet in upper 40% of cohort
   Good fat: low saturated and trans-fat, high polyunsaturated fat, high fish oil
   Good carbohydrates: low glycemic load, high fiber (whole grains)
   High folate (vegetables, fruit)
2) Not currently smoking
3) Moderate alcoholic beverage drinking
   One drink every other day or daily
4) Regular exercise
   One half-hour daily (*eg*, 2 miles per hour walking)
5) Body mass index < 25 kg/m^2 (optimal < 21 kg/m^2)

Figure 14-20.

Combined effects of diet and lifestyle on coronary heart disease (CHD) risk. The combination of multiple dietary factors is more powerful than a single factor alone. In the Nurses' Health Study cohort, a diet high in cereal fiber, marine n-3 fatty acids, and folate, with a high ratio of polyunsaturated to saturated fat, and low in trans-fat and glycemic load strongly predicted decreased risk of CHD (relative risk comparing highest with lowest quintiles of the composite score = 0.40 [95% CI, 0.31–0.53]) [34]. The analyses from the Nurses' Health Study estimated that 82% (95% CI, 58%–93%) of CHD events and 74% (95% CI, 55%–86%) of cardiovascular disease events (CHD or stroke) in the study cohort could be potentially prevented by moderate diet and lifestyle modifications. Among the nonsmokers, 74% (95% CI 39%–90%) of coronary events may have been prevented by eating a healthy diet, maintaining a healthy body weight, exercising regularly half an hour or more daily, and consuming a moderate amount of alcohol (5 g or more alcohol daily). (*Adapted from* Stampfer *et al.* [34].)

References

1. Anitschkow NN: A history of experimentation on arterial atherosclerosis in animals. In *Cowdry's Arteriosclerosis: A Survey of the Problem*, edn 2. Edited by Bleumenthal HT. Springfield: Charles C. Thomas; 1967:21–44.

2. Gordon T: The diet-heart idea: outline of a history. *Am J Epidemiol* 1988, 127:220–225.

3. Hu FB, Willett WC: Optimal diets for prevention of coronary heart disease. *JAMA* 2002, 288:2569–2578.

4. Willett WC: *Nutritional Epidemiology*, edn 2. New York: Oxford University Press; 1998.

5. Hu FB, Stampfer MJ, Manson JE, *et al.*: Dietary fat intake and the risk of coronary heart disease in women [see comments]. *N Engl J Med* 1997, 337:1491–1499.

6. Keys A: *Seven Countries: A Multivariate Analysis of Death and Coronary Heart Disease*. Cambridge: Harvard University Press; 1980.

7. Mensink RP, Katan MB: Effect of dietary fatty acids on serum lipids and lipoproteins: a meta-analysis of 27 trials. *Arterioscler Thromb* 1992, 12:911–919.

8. Lovejoy JC: Dietary fatty acids and insulin resistance. *Curr Atheroscler Rep* 1999, 1:215–220.

9. Salmeron J, Hu FB, Manson JE, *et al.*: Dietary fat intake and risk of type 2 diabetes in women. *Am J Clin Nutr* 2001, 73:1019–26.

10. Ludwig DS: The glycemic index: physiologic mechanisms relating to obesity, diabetes, and cardiovascular disease. *JAMA* 2002, 287:2414–2423.

11. Jenkins DJ, Wolever TM, Taylor RH, *et al.*: Glycemic index of foods: a physiological basis for carbohydrate exchange. *Am J Clin Nutr* 1981, 34:362–366.

12. Wolever TMS, Jenkins DJ, Jenkins AL, Josse RG: The glycemic index: methodology and clinical implications. *Am J Clin Nutr* 1991, 54:846–854.

13. Jenkins DJ, Kendall CW, Augustin LS, *et al.*: Glycemic index: overview of implications in health and disease. *Am J Clin Nutr* 2002, 76:266S–273S.

14. Frost G, Leeds AA, Dore CJ, *et al.*: Glycaemic index as a determinant of serum HDL-cholesterol concentration [see comments]. *Lancet* 1999, 353:1045–1048.

15. Ford E, Liu S: Glycemic index, glycemic load, and serum high-density lipoprotein (HDL) cholesterol concentration among United States adults. *Arch Intern Med* 2001, 161:572–576.

16. Liu S, Willett WC, Stampfer MJ, *et al.*: A prospective study of dietary glycemic load and risk of myocardial infarction in women. *Am J Clin Nutr* 2000, 71:1455–1461.

17. Jeppesen J, Schaaf P, Jones C, *et al.*: Effects of low-fat, high-carbohydrate diets on risk factors for ischemic heart disease in postmenopausal women. *Am J Clin Nutr* 1997, 65:1027–33.

18. Liu S, Buring JE, Sesso HD, *et al.*: A prospective study of dietary fiber intake and risk of cardiovascular disease among women. *J Am Coll Cardiol* 2002, 39:49–56.

19. Brown L, Rosner B, Willett WW, Sacks FM: Cholesterol-lowering effects of dietary fiber: a meta-analysis [see comments]. *Am J Clin Nutr* 1999, 69:30–42.

20. Harris WS: Fish oils and plasma lipid and lipoprotein metabolism in humans: a critical review. *J Lipid Res* 1989, 30:785–807.

21. Connor SL, Connor WE: Are fish oils beneficial in the prevention and treatment of coronary artery disease? *Am J Clin Nutr* 1997, 66:1020S–1031S.

22. Hu FB, Bronner L, Willett WC, *et al.*: Fish and omega-3 fatty acid and risk of coronary heart disease in women. *JAMA* 2002, 287:1815–1821.

23. Burr ML, Fehily AM, Gilbert JF, *et al.*: Effects of changes in fat, fish, and fiber intakes on death and myocardial reinfarction: diet and reinfarction trial (DART). *Lancet* 1989, 2:757–761.

24. GISSI-Prevenzione Investigators: Dietary supplementation with n-3 polyunsaturated fatty acids and vitamin E after myocardial infarction: results from the GISSI-Prevenzione trial. *Lancet* 1999, 354:447–455.

25. Marchioli R, Barzi F, Bomba E, *et al.*: Early protection against sudden death by n-3 polyunsaturated fatty acids after myocardial infarction: time-course analysis of the results of the Gruppo Italiano per lo Studio della Sopravvivenza nell'Infarto Miocardico (GISSI)-Prevenzione. *Circulation* 2002, 105:1897–1903.

26. Rimm EB, Giovannucci EL, Willett WC, *et al.*: A prospective study of alcohol consumption and the risk of coronary disease in men. *Lancet* 1991, 338:464–468.

27. Rimm EB, Katan MB, Ascherio A, *et al.*: Relation between intake of flavonoids and risk for coronary heart disease in male health professionals. *Ann Intern Med* 1996, 125:384–389.

28. Cleophas TJ: Wine, beer and spirits and the risk of myocardial infarction: a systematic review. *Biomed Pharmacother* 1999, 53:417–423.

29. Rimm EB, Willett WC, Hu FB, *et al.*: Folate and vitamin B6 from diet and supplements in relation to risk of coronary heart disease among women. *JAMA* 1998, 279:359–364.

30. Hu FB: The Mediterranean diet and mortality: olive oil and beyond. *N Engl J Med* 2003, 348:2595–2596.

31. Willett WC, Sacks F, Trichopoulou A, *et al.*: Mediterranean diet pyramid: a cultural model for healthy eating. *Am J Clin Nutr* 1995, 1(suppl):1403S–1406S.

32. de Lorgeril M, Salen P, Martin JL, *et al.*: Mediterranean dietary pattern in a randomized trial: prolonged survival and possible reduced cancer rate. *Arch Intern Med* 1998, 158:1181–1187.

33. de Lorgeril M, Salen P, Martin JL, *et al.*: Mediterranean diet, traditional risk factors, and the rate of cardiovascular complications after myocardial infarction: final report of the Lyon Diet Heart Study [see comments]. *Circulation* 1999, 99:779–785.

34. Stampfer MJ, Hu FB, Manson JE, *et al.*: Primary prevention of coronary heart disease in women through diet and lifestyle. *N Engl J Med* 2000, 343:16–22.

Cardiac Psychology/Behavioral Cardiology: Psychosocial Factors and Heart Disease

Robert Allan and Stephen Scheidt

Cardiac psychology and behavioral cardiology are two new closely related subspecialties in mental health and cardiology, respectively, informed by many hundreds of empiric studies conducted over nearly a half-century. The fields have evolved with the unifying hypothesis that psychologic and social variables, termed *psychosocial factors*, can affect the development of and outcome from coronary heart disease (CHD), the leading cause of death and disability in the Western World. In the late 1950s, some of the earliest research linked psychologic stress, such as the loss of a loved one or job, with increased risk of CHD. Since then, a number of psychosocial factors, including the type A behavior pattern, depression, social isolation, anger, anxiety, and job strain, among others, have attained some degree of empiric validity as CHD risk factors—some associated with development of CHD in healthy persons (potentially important in "primary prevention" of CHD), some associated with adverse outcomes in patients with known CHD (potentially important in "secondary prevention").

Of considerable interest are recent findings concerning "triggers" of clinical CHD events, particularly acute myocardial infarction (MI). Elegant research, particularly from the Myocardial Infarction Onset Study, has implicated major physical activity (especially in sedentary individuals), anger (but only of a very intense variety), sexual activity, cocaine and marijuana use (these last three perhaps statistically significant triggers, but clinically associated with small numbers of acute MIs in the real world); however, these same studies have not implicated other triggers that are widely prevalent in the popular mind (*eg*, "work stress").

Although improvement in psychosocial CHD risk factors has been considered a goal in and of itself, because of their generally negative impact on quality of life, the as yet unrealized "holy grail" of behavioral cardiology is a reduction in cardiac morbidity or mortality with intervention directed at presumed adverse psychosocial or behavioral characteristics.

Behavioral cardiology is evolving rapidly. A number of important studies have led to a changing emphasis in the relative importance ascribed to putative psychosocial CHD risk factors. Depression and social isolation have emerged from the literature as consistent and powerful risk factors. Type A behavior pattern seems of less importance than previously believed. Recent research on type A behavior has been quite limited, with the focus having shifted from the total behavior pattern to hostility, one of its major components.

Over the past few years, behavioral cardiology/cardiac psychology has attained considerable credibility in medicine, as evidenced by many recent studies published in cardiology and other medical journals in which they may be expected to have greater impact on patient care than in the past.

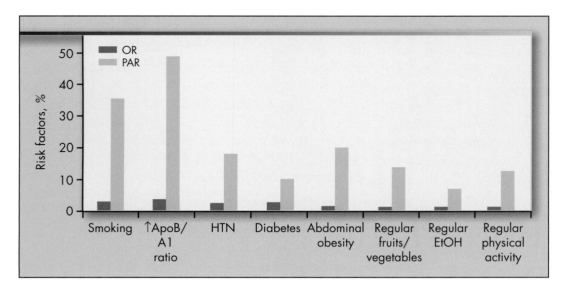

Figure 15-1.
"Traditional" risk factors for acute myocardial infarction and behavior. The recent case-control INTERHEART study of more than 15,152 cases admitted to hospital in 52 countries with a first myocardial infarction (MI) and 14,820 control subjects reported that the major risk factors around the world are the familiar ones stressed in preventive programs in developed countries. Most of the "traditional" CHD risk factors depicted as associated with acute MI are influenced by behavior, including cigarette smoking, regular physical activity, dietary lipids, abdominal obesity, daily consumption of fruits and vegetables, and hypertension [1]. EtOH—alcohol; HTN—hypertension; OR—odds ratio; PAR—population-attributable risk. (*Adapted from* Yusuf *et al.* [1].)

Psychosocial Risk Factors

The psychosocial risk factors consistently associated with coronary heart disease in many studies over the past several decades include depression, social isolation, intense anger, and perhaps hostility. "Stress" is difficult to define and less consistently a risk factor for coronary heart disease in studies published to date; there is no consensus as to the importance of other proposed psychosocial factors, including anxiety, Type A behavior pattern (including time pressure), "cardiac denial," and others. However, the INTERHEART study of patients admitted to hospital with a first myocardial infarction did find stress important. The INTERHEART study of psychosocial factors in 11,119 myocardial infarction patients and 13,648 controls from 262 centers around the world reported higher prevalence of four stress factors ($P < 0.0001$), including work stress, stress at home, general stress, and stress with finances in individuals with first myocardial infarction, compared with controls [2]. Stress was assessed with simple questions, rather than scientifically validated scales.

Depression

Depression is the strongest and most consistent psychosocial risk factor for coronary heart disease (CHD) in the literature. Figure 15-2, from the INTERHEART study, highlights the universality of depression as a risk factor for acute myocardial infarction, in all regions of the world and all ethnic groups [2]. Figure 15-3 presents results from studies assessing depression and the initial onset of CHD among *healthy* individuals; Figure 15-4 lists 20 studies on the adverse effects of depression in those with established CHD (over a twofold increase in death within 2 years in depressed subjects), and Figure 15-5 documents similar odds ratios for deaths and cardiovascular events in another meta-analysis of 22 studies of patients post myocardial infarction.

The mechanism(s) by which depression might be related to increased CHD events are surprisingly obscure, given the consistency and strength of the association of depression and increased CHD risk. One may postulate that depression affects behavior in ways that might be deleterious (*eg*, smoking, poor diet, medical noncompliance); or it may be that depression has physiologic effects that increase cardiovascular events. Figure 15-6 [3] is one schematic model of possible relationships between depression and CHD events.

Region	Number	Case, %	Control, %	Odds ratio (99%CI)
Overall	27,676	24.1	17.6	1.55 (1.42–1.69)
Western Europe	1375	28.4	22.9	1.20 (0.87–1.66)
Central and eastern Europe	3473	17.3	15.7	1.04 (0.82–1.33)
Middle East	2892	24.5	15.2	1.95 (1.51–2.52)
Africa	1259	30.3	19.7	1.69 (1.20–2.39)
South Asia	3300	30.0	19.0	1.62 (1.3–2.02)
China and Hong Kong	5894	20.4	9.7	2.38 (1.94–2.92)
Asia	1921	19.4	12.3	1.70 (1.21–2.39)
Australia and New Zealand	1255	25.6	22.1	1.18 (0.82–1.69)
South America and Mexico	2783	34.9	30.2	1.20 (0.96–1.50)
North America	615	23.7	19.3	1.37 (0.80–2.35)
Ethnic Group				
Overall	24,767	24.1	17.6	1.55 (1.42–1.69)
European	6737	22.1	18.6	1.16 (0.98–1.36)
Chinese	6034	20.2	9.6	2.38 (1.95–2.92)
South Asian	3825	29.5	18.4	1.64 (1.34–2.02)
Other Asian	1770	20.1	13.5	1.59 (1.13–2.25)
Arab	3538	25.5	15.7	2.03 (1.55–2.65)
Latin American	2632	34.5	29.8	1.21 (0.96–1.52)
Black African	471	35.2	21.9	1.63 (0.91–2.93)
Coloured African	601	26.9	17.8	1.72 (1.03–2.88)

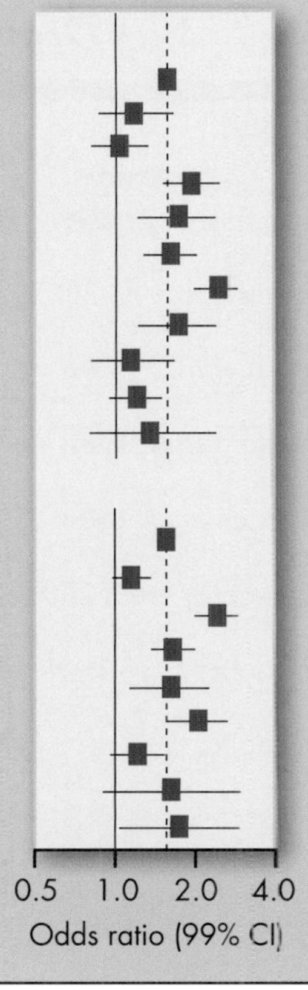

Odds ratio (99% CI)
0.5 1.0 2.0 4.0

Figure 15-2.
The INTERHEART study reported increased depression in myocardial infarction cases compared with control subjects in all areas of the world and in all ethnic groups. Overall, depression occurred in 24% of cases versus 17.6% of control subjects; odds ratio = 1.55 [1.42–1.69]).
(*Adapted from* Rosengren *et al.* [2].)

Onset of Coronary Heart Disease in Healthy Individuals

Study	Patients, *n*	Follow-up time, *y*	Endpoint(s)	Adjusted relative risk (RR)
Anda *et al.*	2832	Mean = 12.4	Fatal IHD; nonfatal IHD	RR = 1.5; 1.6
Barefoot *et al.*	730	27	MI	RR = 1.71
Ford *et al.*	1190	40	CHD events; MI	RR = 1.7; 2.12
Mendes de Leon *et al.*	2812	10	CHD deaths Diagnosis of CHD	Nonsignificant
Hippisley-Cox *et al.*	327 with IHD matched to 897 control subjects without IHD	Not specified	Diagnosis of IHD	Nonsignificant for women; Odds ratio = 2.75 for men
Ariyo *et al.*	4493	6	CHD	Hazard ratio = 1.15
Ferketich *et al.*	7893	10	Diagnosis of CHD; CHD mortality	Women: CHD RR = 1.73; CHD mortality not specified; Men: CHD RR = 1.71; CHD mortality 2.34
Pennix *et al.*	2397 ages 55–85 years	4	Cardiac mortality	RR = 3.9
Aromaa *et al.*	5355	6.6	CAD	Women: RR = 2.59; Men: RR = 2.45 (controlling for age only)

Figure 15-3.
Studies assessing depression and the initial onset of coronary heart disease (CHD) in healthy individuals. Most show the presence of depression increases the long-term risk of developing CHD 1.5 to three times over nondepressed healthy control subjects. CAD—coronary artery disease; IHD—ischemic heart disease; MI—myocardial infarction. (*Adapted from* Lett *et al.* [3].)

Depression as a Risk Factor for Mortality in Coronary Artery Disease

Study	Patients, *n* and type of CHD	Definition/assessment	Follow-up	Results
Barefoot *et al.* 1996, 2001	1250 post-PTCA	Depressive symptoms, Zung SDS	2–15 years	CV mortality HR 1.42 adjusted
Borowicz *et al.* 2002	172 post-CABG	Symptoms, CES-D	5 years	CV mortality OR 2.29 nonadjusted
Bush *et al.* 2001	258 post-MI	Symptoms, BDI	4 months	Total mortality OR 2.8 nonadjusted
Carney *et al.* 1988	52 post-MI, -CABG, -PTCA	Clinical depression, DSM-III-R	1 year	Total mortality OR 2.65 nonadjuester
Carney *et al.* 2003	766 post-MI	Major or minor depression, DSM-IV	30 months	Total mortality OR 2.4 adjusted
Connerey *et al.* 2001	309 post-CABG	Clinical depression, BDI	12 months	Cardiac mortality HR 2.31 adjusted
Denollet *et al.* 1998	303 post-MI, -PTCA	Symptoms, Million Behavioral Health Inventory	12 months	CV mortality OR 2.69 nonadjusted
Denollet *et al.*	87 post-MI	Symptoms, Million Behavioral Health Inventory	6–10 years	CV mortality OR 7.46 nonadjusted
Frasure-Smith *et al.* several	222 post-MI	Symptoms, BDI	6 months	CV mortality OR 6.24 nonadjusted
		Clinical depression (Diagnostic Interview Schedule; National Institutes of Health modified)	18 months	CV mortality OR 3.64 nonadjusted
Frasure-Smith *et al.* several	887–896 post-MI	Symptoms; BDI	5 years	CV mortality HR 3.16 adjusted
Hermann *et al.* 2000	2432 with CHD	Symptoms; Hospital Anxiety and Depression Scale	5–6 years	Total mortality HR 1.21 adjusted
Irvine *et al.* 1999	634 post-MI	Symptoms; BDI	2 years	Sudden cardiac death 2.45 adjusted
Jenkinson *et al.* 1993	1376 post-MI	Symptoms from three items of ASSET Study questionnaire	3 years	CV mortality OR 0.9
Kaufmann	331 post-MI	Clinical depression; Diagnostic Interview Schedule	1 year	Total mortality OR 2.34 nonadjusted
Ladwig *et al.* 1991, 1994	560 post-MI	Symptoms; Zerssen Self-rating Scale	1 year	CV mortality HR 4.9 adjusted
Lane *et al.* 2001, 2002	288 post-MI	Symptoms; BDI	3 years	CV mortality OR 0.84 nonadjusted
Mayou *et al.* 2000	344 post-MI	Symptoms; Hospital Anxiety and Depression Scale	18 months	Total mortality OR 1.64
Romanelli *et al.* 2002	153 post-MI	Clinical depression; BDI	4 months	CV mortality OR 4.71 nonadjusted
Schleifer *et al.* 1989	283 post-MI	Clinical depression; Schedule for Affective Disorders and Schizophrenia	3 months	CV mortality OR 0.59 nonadjusted
Welin *et al.* 2000	275 post-MI	Symptoms; BDI	10 years	CV mortality HR 3.16 adjusted

Figure 15-4.

Depression is a clear and powerful risk factor for mortality in patients with established coronary artery disease. A recent meta-analysis assessed outcome in 20 studies, with an overall odds ratio of 2.24 (1.37–3.60) for 2-year mortality in patients with symptoms of depression, compared with patients without such symptoms, at the time of assessment. BDI—Beck Depression Inventory; CABG—coronary artery bypass graft; CES-D—Center for Epidemiologic Studies Depression Scale; CHD—coronary heart disease; CV—cardiovascular; DSM—*Diagnostic and Statistical Manual of Mental Disorders*; HR—hazard ratio; MI—myocardial infarction; OR—odds ratio; SDS—Self-rating Depression Scale. (*Adapted from* Barth *et al.* [4].)

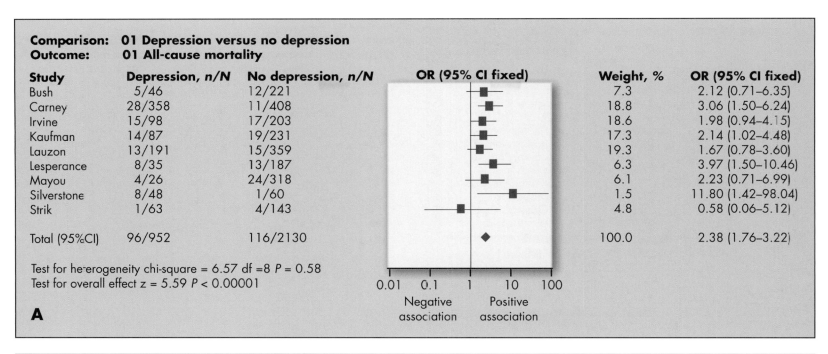

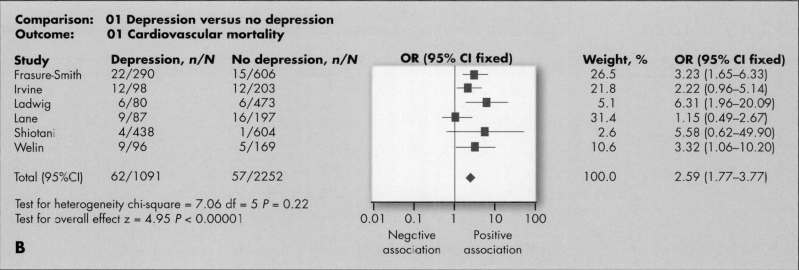

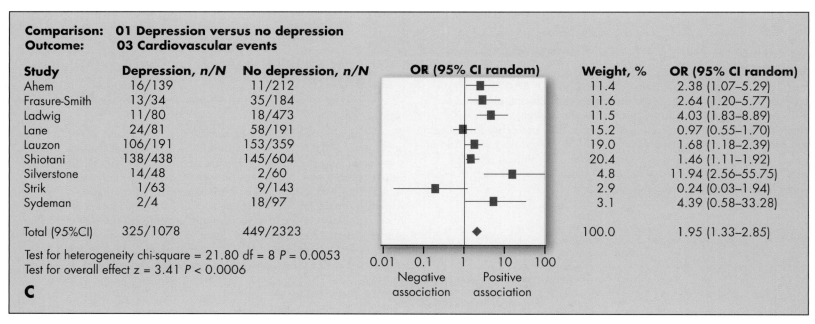

Figure 15-5.

A–C, Another recent meta-analysis by van Melle *et al.* [5] of 6367 patients in 16 studies with depression assessed within 3 months post-myocardial infarction, presented with odds ratios and confidence intervals; many of the studies are also listed in the Barth *et al.* [4] meta-analysis (Fig. 15-4).

van Melle *et al.* [5] reported an odds ratio of 2.38 (95 % CI; 1.76–3.22, *P* < 0.00001) for all-cause and 2.59 (95% CI; 1.77–3.77, *P* < 0.00001) for cardiac mortality in depressed patients, although the effect was more pronounced in studies done before 1992. (*Adapted from* van Melle *et al.* [5].)

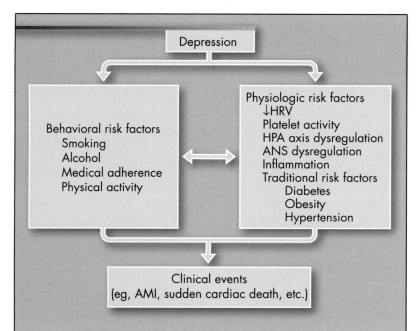

Figure 15-6.
Biobehavioral model for possible relationships between depression and coronary heart disease events. AMI—acute myocardial infarction; ANS—autonomic nervous system; HPA—hypothalamic pituitary adrenal; HRV—heart rate variability. (*Adapted from* Lett *et al.* [3].)

Social Isolation

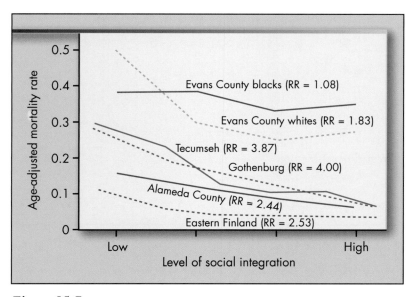

Figure 15-7.
A study by House *et al.* [6] reported on more than 37,000 people in five prospective studies in the United States and Europe observed for 8 to 13 years; categories of social ties included marriage, contact with extended family and friends, church membership, and other formal and informal affiliations. All-cause mortality was increased up to fourfold in initially healthy persons with the lowest versus the highest levels of social integration, with relative risk (RR) ratios higher for men than for women. (*Adapted from* House *et al.* [6].)

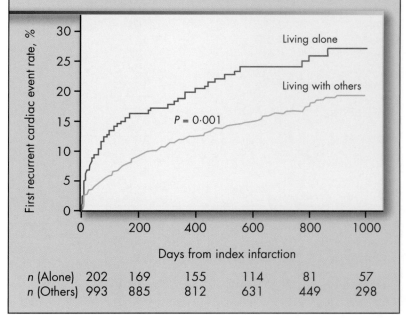

n (Alone)	202	169	155	114	81	57
n (Others)	993	885	812	631	449	298

Figure 15-8.
Case *et al.* [7] observed 1234 patients for 1 to 4 (mean 2.7) years after acute myocardial infarction. At 6 months post myocardial infarction, the rate of recurrent events (another nonfatal myocardial infarction or cardiac death) was 79% greater in those living alone compared with those living with others. This was independent of marital disruption (divorce, separation, or widowhood). Similarly, Williams *et al.* [8] observed 1368 consecutive patients undergoing cardiac catheterization and reported 3.34 times risk of death within 5 years in unmarried patients without a close confidant compared with those married or unmarried with a close confidant. (*Adapted from* Case *et al.* [7].)

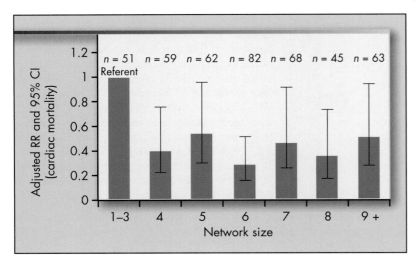

Figure 15-9.
More recently, Brummet *et al.* [9] reported that the most isolated coronary artery disease patients, those with three or fewer individuals in their social network, had the highest cardiac mortality over an approximately 4-year period after cardiac catheterization showing significant coronary artery disease (relative risk [RR] = 2.43). Socially isolated patients had less than half the number of social visits reported by the other patients, with more than one third averaging less than one network contact every 3 days. Isolated patients were less likely to be married or have a confidant, and they were pleased with a smaller proportion of the relationships that they did have. Once patients had social networks more than three individuals, there was no additional benefit for having larger networks. Apparently, once past a threshold, the adverse effect of social isolation is no longer a significant risk factor for cardiac death. (*Adapted from* Brummet *et al.* [9].)

Anger and Hostility

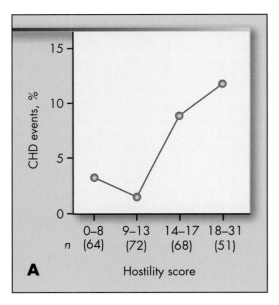

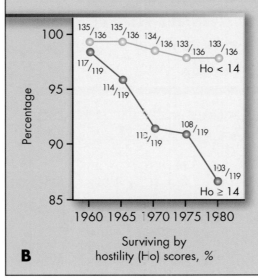

Figure 15-10.
In an early retrospective study, scores on the Cooke-Medley Hostility Scale (from a Minnesota Multiphasic Personality Inventory taken during medical school in 1954-59) were related to coronary heart disease incidence 25 years later among 255 graduates of the University of North Carolina Medical School (**A**) as well as to survival (**B**), showing worse survival for those above vs below the median hostility score. CHD—coronary heart disease. (*Adapted from* Barefoot *et al.* [10].)

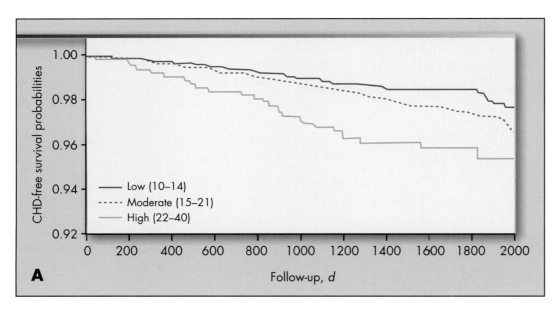

Figure 15-11.
In 2000, Williams *et al.* [11] reported on 12,986 Americans without known coronary heart disease at baseline, aged 45–64 at entry, who were observed for a median of 53 months in the Atherosclerosis Risk in Communities (ARIC) Study. Anger was assessed by the Spielberger Trait Anger Scale. There was a strong graded relationship between increasing "trait anger" and subsequent myocardial infarction (MI) and coronary heart disease mortality. The increased multivariate-adjusted hazard ratio (HR) of "hard events," (nonfatal and fatal MI) was 2.69 (95% CI, 1.48–4.90) for high versus low anger and 1.35 (95% CI, 0.87–2.10) for moderate versus low anger (**A**). Results were significant for only normotensive individuals, approximately two thirds of the population.

(*continued on next page*)

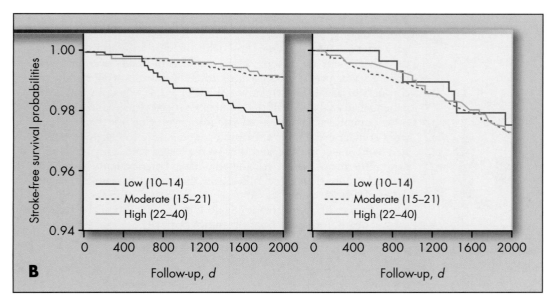

B

Figure 15-11. *continued*

A similar relationship between scores on the Spielberger Trait Anger Scale and increased risk of hemorrhagic and ischemic stroke was found in a sample of 13,851 men and women followed for a median of 77.3 months in the same study (**B**) [12]. After multivariate adjustment, results were significant for only those <60 years of age [high trait anger vs low trait anger relative risk = 2.82 (95% CI, 1.65–4.80)]. (In *right side panel* B, subjects are aged 60 or older; in *left side panel* B, subjects are aged younger than 60 years.) (*Adapted from* Williams *et al.* [11,12].)

Age-adjusted and Multivariate Relative Risk of Stroke and Cardiovascular Disease by Level of Anger Expression (95% CI)

	Level of Spielberger Anger-Out Expression Scale			
	8,9	10–12	13–32	Trend, *P*
Nonfatal stroke				
Cases	17	20	11	
Age-adjusted relative risk (RR)	1.00	0.66 (0.35–1.27)	0.46 (0.21–1.00)	0.09
Multivariate RR	1.00	0.64 (0.32–1.26)	0.44 (0.20–0.98)	0.09
Total stroke				
Cases	20	25	12	
Age-adjusted RR	1.00	0.71 (0.39–1.28)	0.43 (0.21–0.89)	0.04
Multivariate RR	1.00	0.68 (0.37–1.25)	0.42 (0.20–0.88)	0.04
Total CVD (includes total CHD and stroke)				
Cases	89	132	107	
Age-adjusted RR	1.00	0.81 (0.61–1.06)	0.81 (0.61–1.08)	0.40
Multivariate RR	1.00	0.78 (0.59–1.02)	0.76 (0.56–1.01)	0.21

Figure 15-12.
The largest study of anger failed to confirm the above results. Eng *et al.* [13] administered the Spielberger Anger-Out Expression Scale to 23,552 health professionals (primarily dentists, veterinarians, pharmacists, and other non-physicians), who were observed for 2 years. Moderate, compared with low, expressed anger conferred a *protective effect* on myocardial infarction (relative risk = 0.56; 95% CI, 0.32–0.97) and stroke (relative risk = 0.42; 95% CI, 0.20–0.88). CHD—coronary heart disease; CVD—cardiovascular disease. (*Adapted from* Eng *et al.* [13].)

Job Strain

Adjusted Hazard Ratio (95% CI) for Cardiovascular Mortality by Levels of Work Characteristics

Characteristic	Covariates in addition to age and gender			
	Occupational group	Behavioral risk factors (smoking and physical activity)	Biologic risk factors (SBP, cholesterol concentration, and BMI)	All aforementioned
Job strain				
Low	1.00	1.00	1.00	1.00
Intermediate	1.36 (0.72–2.57)	1.71 (0.92–3.17)	1.58 (0.84–2.95)	1.64 (0.85–3.19)
High	1.89 (0.93–3.81)	2.20 (1.12–4.32)	2.35 (1.22–4.52)	2.22 (1.04–4.73)
Job control (component of job strain)				
High	1.00	1.00	1.00	1.00
Intermediate	0.94 (0.48–1.82)	1.06 (0.57–1.98)	1.14 (0.62–2.11)	0.74 (0.39–1.50)
Low	1.55 (0.80–3.01)	1.79 (0.98–3.27)	1.89 (1.06–3.38)	1.42 (0.72–2.82)
Effort-reward imbalance				
Low	1.00	1.00	1.00	1.00
Intermediate	2.16 (1.04–4.49)	2.00 (1.06–3.78)	2.07 (1.09–3.91)	1.91 (0.90–4.05)
High	2.36 (1.06–5.46)	2.18 (1.15–4.13)	2.29 (1.21–4.35)	2.42 (1.02–5.73)

Figure 15-13.
This prospective cohort study of 812 employees at a metal company in Finland observed over a mean of 25.6 years reported a 2.2-fold increased risk (95% CI; 1.2–4.2) of cardiovascular mortality for those with high versus low strain [14]. BMI—body mass index; SBP—systolic blood pressure.

Triggers for Acute Cardiac Events

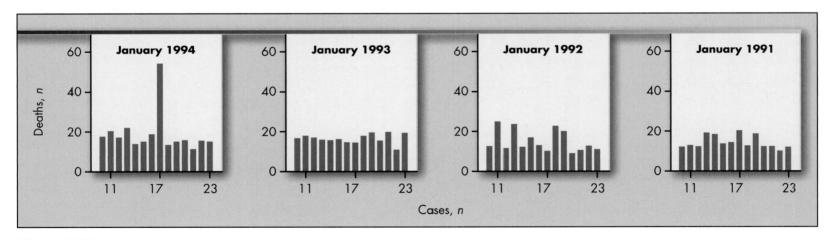

Figure 15-14.
The Northridge, California earthquake on January 17, 1994 was one of the largest earthquakes in the history of North America and caused widespread destruction. Although the absolute risk of increased sudden cardiac death is highly significant ($z = 4.41$, $P < 0.001$), the 24 cases should be compared with a daily average of 4.6 (SD ± 2.1) during the preceding week, as well as the 7000 injuries that were a direct result of the quake. (*Adapted from* Leor *et al.* [15].)

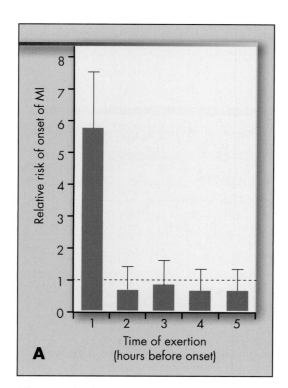

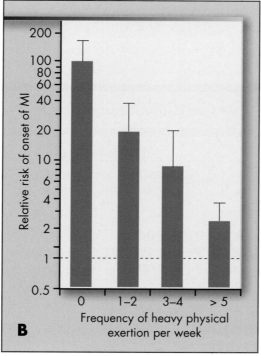

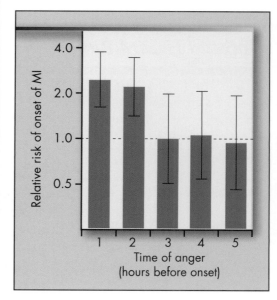

Figure 15-15.
A, Strenuous exertion is a trigger for myocardial infarction (MI) during exercise and for 1 hour afterwards [16]. **B,** The reduction in the relative risk for triggering MI in subjects with increasing levels of regular physical activity (although even the most habitually active individuals still have a significant [approximately twofold] relative risk during and for an hour after the activity— more than counterbalanced by a lower risk for these subjects during the many nonexercising hours of the week.) (*Adapted from* Mittleman *et al.* [16].)

Figure 15-16.
Intense anger is a trigger for myocardial infarction (MI) over a 2-hour hazard period [17], potentially useful information for individuals who are chronically angry. (*Adapted from* Mittleman *et al.* [17].)

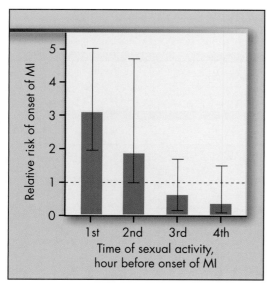

Figure 15-17.
The relative risk of triggering a cardiac event in the 2 hours after sexual activity is 2.5 (95% CI, 1.7–3.7) [1]. In counseling patients, it is important to point out the low absolute risk. Other notable triggers for acute cardiac events include use of marijuana (relative risk = 4.8; 95% CI, 2.4–9.5) [18] and cocaine (relative risk = 23.7; 95% CI, 8.5–66.3) [19]. Regular exercise and aspirin reduce the risk of triggering a cardiac event with most of the above factors. MI—myocardial infarction. (*Adapted from* Muller *et al.* [20].)

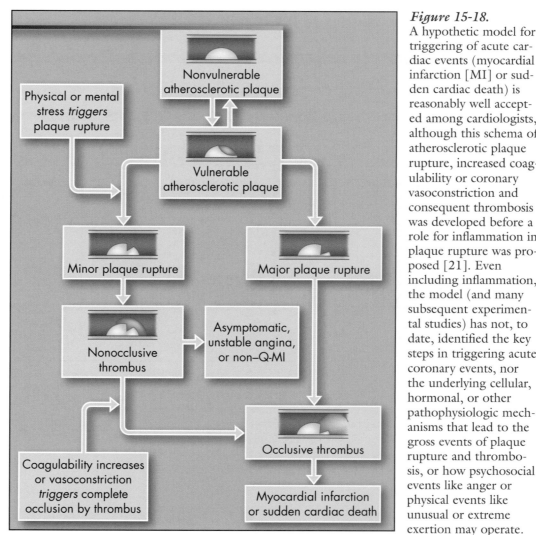

Figure 15-18.
A hypothetic model for triggering of acute cardiac events (myocardial infarction [MI] or sudden cardiac death) is reasonably well accepted among cardiologists, although this schema of atherosclerotic plaque rupture, increased coagulability or coronary vasoconstriction and consequent thrombosis was developed before a role for inflammation in plaque rupture was proposed [21]. Even including inflammation, the model (and many subsequent experimental studies) has not, to date, identified the key steps in triggering acute coronary events, nor the underlying cellular, hormonal, or other pathophysiologic mechanisms that lead to the gross events of plaque rupture and thrombosis, or how psychosocial events like anger or physical events like unusual or extreme exertion may operate.

Psychosocial Intervention Trials

Study	Year published	Patients, n	Intervention	Follow-up duration	Psychologic outcome	Cardiac outcome
Psychologic interventions						
Recurrent Coronary Prevention Project	1986	862; 270 controls, 592 experimental	Group therapy for type A behavior	4.5 years	Reductions in type A behavior	44% reduction in second MI; reductions in SCD
ENRICHD	2003	2481; 1238 controls; 1243 experimental	Cognitive behavioral group plus individual psychotherapy and sertraline (as needed)	41 months	Improvement in depression and social isolations at 6 months	No differences in morbidity or mortality
Jones and West	1996	2328; 1155 controls, 1159 experimental	Seven 2-hour group sessions	1 year	No improvement	No improvement
Blumenthal *et al.*	1997 2002	107; 40 controls, 34 exercise, 33 stress management	4 month group and two sessions of biofeedback	38 months and 5 years, respectively	Reduction in depression and hostility	0.26 ($P = 0.04$); risk of adverse cardiac events in stress management group compared with controls
Denollet and Brutsaert	2001	150; 72 controls, 78 experimental	6 weekly group sessions plus selected patient individual therapy	9 years	43% improvement, 15% worsening of mood	17% vs 4% mortality ($P = 0.009$)
Hamlainen	1995	375; 187 controls, 188 experimental	Multiple risk factor rehabilitation, including discussion of psychologic problems, for 3 months plus close contact for 3 years	15 years	Not reported	Lower incidence SCD (16.5% vs 28.9%; $P = 0.006$); cardiac mortality (47.9% vs 58.5%; $P = 0.04$) in treated group
Project New Life	1996	268; 133 controls, 128 experimental	17 3-hour group sessions plus 5–6 booster sessions	4.5 years	Not reported	Significant difference in total (7 vs 16; $P = 0.02$) deaths; fewer cardiac events ($P = 0.04$)
Pharmacologic intervention						
SADHART	2002	369; 183 controls, 186 experimental	Sertraline—safety		Modest improvement, more effective if one prior episode of major depression	No significant difference in morbidity; not powered for mortality
Lifestyle trials with a psychologic or behavioral component						
LIFESTYLE	1990 1993 1998	48; 20 controls, 28 experimental	Major life change: diet plus yoga plus exercise plus group therapy	1, 4, and 5 years, respectively	Not reported	Regression of atherosclerotic plaques on quantitative angiogram; improved myocardial perfusion on PET
Multicenter LIFESTYLE	1998	333; 139 controls, 194 experimental	Same as LIFESTYLE	3 years	Not reported	No difference in MI, stroke, or mortality; cost savings $29,528 per patient

Figure 15-19.

Noteworthy psychosocial interventional trials [22–26]. ENRICHD—Enhancing Recovery in Coronary Heart Disease; MI—myocardial infarction; PET—positron emission tomography; SADHART— Sertraline Antidepressant Heart Attack Randomized Trial; SCD—sudden cardiac death. (*Adapted from* Allan and Scheidt [27].)

Cardiac Psychology/Behavioral Cardiology: Psychosocial Factors and Heart Disease

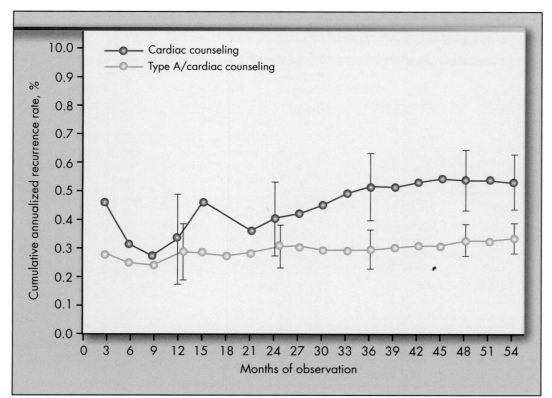

Figure 15-20.
The Recurrent Coronary Risk Reduction
Program (RCPP) was the first large-scale clinical trial and was completed in 1986. The study
was designed to reduce type A behavior. The
RCPP demonstrated a 44% reduction in second myocardial infarction for patients who
received group type A counseling plus cardiac
education compared with control subjects who
received only cardiac education [23].
Ironically, since the RCPP, three studies have
reported that type A behavior is protective for
future cardiac events [24–26]. (*Adapted from*
Friedman *et al.* [23].)

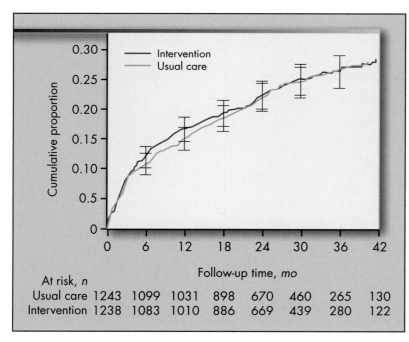

At risk, *n*							
Usual care	1243	1099	1031	898	670	460	265	130
Intervention	1238	1083	1010	886	669	439	280	122

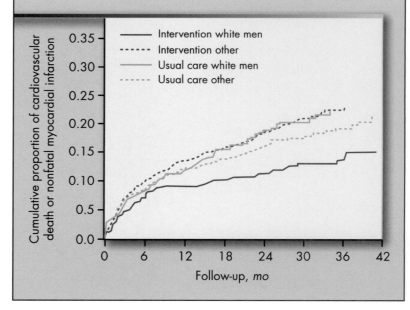

Figure 15-21.
The Enhancing Recovery in Coronary Heart Disease study provided
individual or group cognitive-behavioral group psychotherapy plus
sertraline (as needed) for 6 months or routine care to 2481 (1084
women) randomized post-myocardial infarction patients with major or
minor depression and/or low perceived social support. Patients were
observed for a minimum of 18 months (average 29 months). After 30
months of follow-up, there were no significant differences in psychologic or cardiac outcome (death or nonfatal myocardial infarction in
Fig. 15-20; also no difference in secondary endpoints including total
mortality). (*Adapted from* Writing Committee for the ENRICHD
Investigators [27].)

Figure 15-22.
A post hoc analysis of Enhancing Recovery in Coronary Heart Disease
study reported that treated white men (*n* = 973), but not the three
other subgroups (424 minority men, 674 white women, and 410
minority women), had improved cardiac mortality and recurrent nonfatal myocardial infarction. (*Adapted from* Schneiderman *et al.* [28].)

Relative Risk of Death and Urgent Cardiovascular Rehospitalizations

Endpoint*	Patients, *n*		Relative risk (95% CI)
	Sertraline	**Placebo**	
Death	2	5	0.39 (0.08–1.39)
Myocardial infarctions	5	7	0.70 (0.23–2.16)
Congestive heart failure	5	7	0.70 (0.23–2.16)
Stroke	2	2	0.98 (0.14–6.93)
Angina	26	30	0.85 (0.53–1.38)
Composite endpoint	32	41	0.77 (0.51–1.16)

*If a patient is hospitalized more than once for the same endpoint, that patient is counted only once. A patient may be included for more than one endpoint. In the composite endpoint, a patient is counted only once.

Figure 15-23.

The Sertraline Antidepressant Heart Attack Randomized Trial was a drug trial, with *no psychotherapy*, for depression in 369 post-myocardial infarction and unstable angina patients, conducted to establish the safety and efficacy of sertraline in the cardiac population. Sertraline was found to be safe, with no reductions in ejection fraction. The incidence of major cardiovascular events was 14.5% in the sertraline treated group compared with 22.4% in the placebo group, a non-significant difference. The study was not powered to detect differences in mortality or cardiovascular events. Sertraline-treated patients showed significantly greater improvement than controls on the Clinical Global Impression Improvement Scale, supporting a potential benefit of psychotropic intervention for depressed post-MI patients [29]. Of note, the Enhancing Recovery in Coronary Heart Disease study and Sertraline Antidepressant Heart Attack Randomized Trial found unexpectedly high rates of improvement in depression in the control group, confounding both study designs. (*Adapted from* Glassman *et al.* [29].)

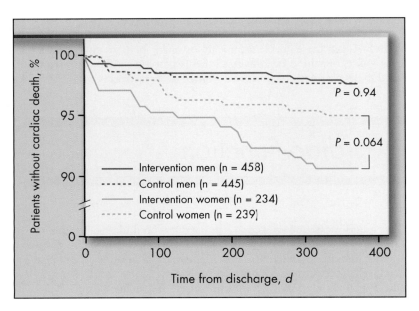

Figure 15-24.

After an encouraging pilot study with men, the Montreal Heart Attack Readjustment Trial [30] provided home visits by psychiatrically supervised nurses to 1376 male and female post-myocardial infarction patients whenever their stress scores exceeded a threshold. Intervention did not improve outcome for men in the study. Notably, there was a trend for increased cardiac mortality among women in the intervention compared with control subjects. A post hoc analysis reported that successful, compared with unsuccessful, home visits resulted in improved psychosocial and cardiac outcome at 1 year [31]. (*Adapted from* Frasure-Smith *et al.* [30].)

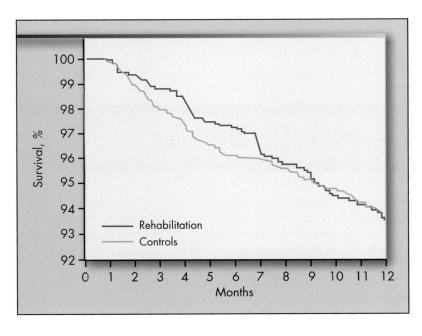

Figure 15-25.

In Wales, UK, Jones and West [32] randomized 2328 post-myocardial infarction patients to seven 2-hour psychologic interventions or routine medical care. At the end of 1 year, there were no differences in psychologic or cardiac outcome. The negative results of this study suggest that such intervention is too brief to have a significant impact. All patients were included in the study, rather than those reporting some level of psychologic distress, likely limiting the power of the study design.

There are a number of other intervention trials, most summarized here, with methodologic problems that limit their importance.

Burrell *et al.* [33] in Sweden reported on a modified replication of the Recurrent Coronary Risk Reduction Program, Project New Life, in 265 nonsmoking postcoronary artery bypass graft patients. During the first year post-bypass, intervention patients met for 17 3-hour group sessions with five to six "booster sessions" in years 2 and 3. Cardiac events and mortality were reduced over 5 years. This study was published in a psychology textbook, rather than a peer reviewed journal.

Hamalainen *et al.* [34] studied a group of 375 acute myocardial infarction patients (74 women) younger than 65 years of age at entry in Finland. Patients were given a comprehensive rehabilitation program that included exercise, smoking cessation, dietary advice, and psychologic discussion. Intervention was most intensive during the first 3 months, but there was close contact with the health care team for 3 years. Patients were

(*continued on next page*)

Figure 15-25. *continued*

observed for 15 years, with a significantly lower incidence of sudden death (16.5% vs 28.9%; *P* = 0.006) and cardiac mortality (47.9% vs 58.5%; *P* = 0.04) in the intervention compared with the control group. Total mortality, however, was similar between groups because of excess deaths from cancer in the intervention group.

In the Netherlands, Denollet and Brutsaert [35] studied 150 men with coronary heart disease (*n* = 78 experimental and 72 control subjects; nonrandomized) who received six weekly 2-hour group therapy sessions with a significant other plus exercise or routine care. In an effort to tailor treatment to patients' particular needs, 49% (38 of 78) patients also received weekly individual cognitive-behavioral psychotherapy with one of the study authors. The intervention lasted 3 months, with 43% of patients (*n* = 64) reporting improvement and 15% (*n* = 22) worsening of distress on the Global Mood Scale. At 9-year follow-up, death rate was 17% (12 of 72) for control patients compared with 4% (3 of 78) for intervention patients (*P* = 0.009).

Blumenthal *et al.* [36,37] provided a 4-month program of "stress management," exercise, or usual care to a group of 107 post-myocard-ial infarction patients with evidence of ambulatory or mental stressed myocardial ischemia. The psychosocial intervention consisted of sixteen 1.5-hour sessions of group cognitive-behavioral therapy; it made use of a number of the treatment components of the Recurrent Coronary Risk Reduction Program as well as biofeedback. There was improved cardiac outcome compared to exercise and routine care control subjects, as well as reduction in depression and hostility, after 3 to 5 years of follow-up.

Nortriptyline, compared with paroxetine, resulted in significantly higher rates of adverse cardiac events in 81 patients with major depressive disorder (*Diagnostic and Statistical Manual of Mental Disorders,*

Fourth Edition) and documented coronary heart disease randomized to 6 weeks therapy with either drug [38]. Both drugs improved depression in substantial numbers of patients but there were more "adverse effects" with nortriptyline (even though most of these effects were asymptomatic sinus tachycardia or asymptomatic increase in ventricular premature contraction frequency). Selective serotonin reuptake inhibitors, compared with tricyclic antidepressants, are probably the drugs of choice for treating depression in coronary heart disease patients, especially given the larger Sertraline Antidepressant Heart Attack Randomized Trial study that demonstrated safety of sertraline in post-myocardial infarction patients.

Finally, Ornish *et al.* [39] has had considerable impact on the American psyche after reporting reversal of coronary atherosclerosis with intensive lifestyle changes, including a very low fat vegetarian diet, daily meditation for a minimum of 1 hour, thrice-weekly exercise, and twice-weekly support groups. The intervention required 14 hours per week and the study was based on 28 patients and 20 control subjects. Regression of atherosclerotic lesions was associated with overall adherence to the program.

All of these trials suffer from inadequate numbers of patients, and in some, a much more fundamental problem, lack of randomization and blinding. In addition, several include multiple interventions, for example, physical exercise or diet counseling, in addition to the psychologic intervention. It is impossible to be sure how much of the benefit in the intervention groups is because of prior selection, perhaps self-selection, of subjects likely to be more compliant or diligent in many areas of care, and how much is related to the particular intervention espoused in the reported study. Given these problems, it is unfortunate, perhaps unfair, but most cardiologists remain to be convinced that psychologic interventions are useful in patients with established coronary heart disease.

Psychologic Stress and Abnormal Cardiac Function

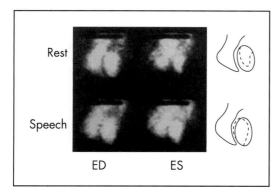

Figure 15-26.
Comparative still-frames of left anterior oblique scintigrams in patient who underwent radionuclide ventriculography at rest and then during a mental stress task involving a speech task given in imaging laboratory. Patient had worsening of left ventricular segmental wall motion while speaking about feelings of personal distress concerning his problems in caring for his family. Images shown for rest are on top and those for the speaking task on bottom. Shown are end-diastolic (ED) images (*left*), end-systolic (ES) images (*middle*), and superimposed ED and ES edges (*right*). During speech, frank dyskinesis (abnormal outward motion during systole) developed in septum. (*Adapted from* Rozanski *et al.* [40].)

Patients with an Implantable Cardioverter Defibrillator

An area of emerging importance is psychosocial adjustment in implantable cardioverter defibrillator (ICD) patients. Many ICD patients are sudden death survivors and a significant percentage suffer from depression, anxiety, and posttraumatic stress disorder [41]. Additionally, two small studies have reported that physical and psy-

chological stress, as well as anger, can serve as "triggers" for ICD discharge [42,43]. A recent pilot study in England reported reduced anxiety with psychological intervention, with benefits extending to the waiting list control group after they received the treatment [44].

Cardiac Denial and Prehospital Delay in Seeking Treatment of Acute Myocardial Infarction

With widespread availability of thrombolytic therapy and emergent percutaneous transluminal angioplasty (PTCA), myocardial necrosis often can be limited and sometimes eliminated, if individuals obtain prompt medical attention. Ironically, in one study, those with a history of coronary heart disease actually arrived at the hospital later than those without a history [45].

A number of community interventions have attempted to educate the public about the importance of early intervention. One of the largest, the Rapid Early Action for Coronary Treatment (REACT), was conducted in 20 pair-matched communities in the United States [46,47]. After intervention, there was a 34% increase in the use of Emergency Medical Services to provide transportation to the hospital. However, the community intervention did not improve the time from symptom onset to hospital arrival. Similarly disappointing results occurred after an intensive multimedia campaign undertaken in Goteborg, Sweden [48]. The "HJARTA-SMARTA" program provided newspaper articles, ads on radio and public transportation, and leaflets distributed twice to all 200,000 households. Median delay time was reduced from 3 hours to 2 hours and 20 minutes. However, neither in-hospital nor 1 year mortality were improved. The lack of success of REACT and HJARTA-SMARTA suggests that some factor(s) other than lack of information may play a crucial role in preventing individuals from seeking prompt medical attention for symptoms of myocardial infarction.

"Cardiac denial" is the tendency to minimize or deny the significance of cardiac symptoms. A 1992 review reported on 21 studies and concluded that cardiac denial has a long-term negative effect on health outcome [49]. Additionally, a scale has been developed for assessment [50]. This is an area worthy of future research, in light of the enormous potential health benefits as well as the failure of past ambitious public education trials.

The Current State of Behavioral Cardiology/Cardiac Psychology

Over the past several decades, the database linking psychosocial factors with the onset and outcome from coronary heart disease has been greatly expanded, with depression and social isolation strongly linked with worsened outcome. The intervention literature, however, has produced mixed results. Most daunting have been the disappointing results of Enhancing Recovery in Coronary Heart Disease, the largest and most costly clinical trial in behavioral medicine to date.

In spite of encouraging results in the Recurrent Coronary Prevention Project, Project New Life, and the intervention of Blumenthal et al. [36,37], several large studies did not corroborate type A behavior as a risk factor. Research on type A behavior pattern has been largely abandoned in favor of a more specific focus on hostility, one of its core components.

A major issue confronting cardiac psychology is the rapid progress of clinical cardiology. To detect differences in treatment effects on hard endpoints, such as myocardial infarction and sudden cardiac death, intervention studies will now have to be quite large and costly. Many cardiologists are now keenly aware of the importance of treating depression; hence, "routine care" control groups will now contain many patients who have been prescribed antidepressants or referred for psychotherapy, making it even more difficult to detect differences between groups.

Measurement of psychosocial variables is still a major issue. Most recent studies have relied on self-report questionnaires, which bias responses by limitations in subjects' self-awareness, as well as their (un)willingness to acknowledge socially undesirable personality characteristics. At present, there are no agreed-on standards for assessment of any of the psychosocial risk factors, although some questionnaires, such as the Beck Depression Inventory, the Cook-Medley Hostility Scale, and the Spielberger anger scales, have been used extensively.

A critical issue for intervention is its breadth and intensity. At one extreme, the Ornish et al. [39] program requires a great effort— a minimum of 14 hours a week—whereas Jones and West [32] provided only seven 2-hour sessions over a year. The Recurrent Coronary Prevention Project required 28 sessions, then monthly sessions for 2 additional years before achieving a reduction in recurrent myocardial infarction; Project New Life provided 15 to 16 3-hour sessions in the first year followed by "booster sessions" in years 2 and 3 to demonstrate reduced morbidity and mortality. We find that it is difficult for most cardiac patients to maintain heart-healthy habits and after a "honeymoon" of several months, most revert back to their former unhealthy habits, A substantial "dose" and response to lifestyle change intervention is likely needed for improved outcome.

Although the "holy grail" of cardiac psychology/behavioral cardiology is the reduction of morbidity and morality, this has not yet been achieved. It should be pointed out, however, that most psychosocial interventions have reported improvements in quality of life, a worthy goal in its own right; it's not just how long one lives, but how well. It may be added that many of the interventions in clinical cardiology, such as coronary artery bypass graft (other than for left main coronary artery and triple vessel disease) and percutanous transluminal coronary angioplasty, do not necessarily lead to reductions in morbidity and mortality. Modern trials of new medical therapies increasingly include assessments of quality of life and cost effectiveness. Although psychologic or behavioral interventions have yet to definitely increase survival or decrease future cardiac events, the recent increased emphasis on psychologic issues in cardiac patients probably yields improved quality of life, and is likely cost effective.

References

1. Yusuf S, Hawken S, Ounpuu S, for the INTERHEART Investigators: Effect of potentially modifiable risk factors associated with myocardial infarction in 52 countries (the INTERHEART study): case-control study. *Lancet* 2004, 364:937–952.

2. Rosengren A, Hawken S, Ounpuu S, for the INTERHEART Investigators: Association of psychosocial risk factors with risk of acute myocardial infarction in 11 119 cases and 13 648 controls from 52 countries (the INTERHEART study): case-control study. *Lancet* 2004, 364:953–962.

3. Lett HS, Blumenthal JA, Babyak MA, *et al.*: Depression as a risk factor for coronary artery disease, mechanisms, and treatment. *Psychosom Med* 2004, 66:305–315.

4. Barth J, Schumacher M, Herrmann-Lingen C: Depression as a risk factor for mortality in patients with coronary heart disease. *Psychosom Med* 2004, 66:802–813.

5. van Melle JP, de Jonge P, Spijkerman TA, *et al.*: Prognostic association of depression following myocardial infarction with mortality and cardiovascular events: a meta-analysis. *Psychosom Med* 2004, 66:814–822.

6. House JS, Landis KR, Umberson D: Social relationships and health. *Science* 1988, 241:540–545.

7. Case RB, Moss AJ, Case N, *et al.*: Living alone after myocardial infarction: impact on prognosis. *JAMA* 1992, 267:515–519.

8. Williams RB, Barefoot JC, Califf RM: Prognostic importance of social and economic resources among medically treated patients with angiographically documented coronary artery disease. *JAMA* 1992, 267:520–524.

9. Brummett BH, Barefoot JC, Siegler IC, et al.: Characteristics of socially isolated patients with coronary artery disease who are at elevated risk for mortality. *Psychosom Med* 2001, 63:267–272.

10. Barefoot JC, Dahlstrom WG, Williams RB: Hostility, CHD incidence, and total mortality: a 25-year follow-up study of 255 physicians. *Psychosom Med* 1984, 45:59–63.

11. Williams JE, Paton CC, Siegler IC, *et al.*: Anger proneness predicts coronary heart disease risk: prospective analysis from the Atherosclerosis Risk in Communities (ARIC) Study. *Circulation* 2000, 101:2034–2039.

12. Williams JE, Nieto FJ, Sanford CO, *et al.*: The association between trait anger and incident stroke risk: The Atherosclerosis Risk in Communities (ARIC) Study. *Stroke* 2002, 33:13–20.

13. Eng PM, Fitzmaurice G, Kubzansky LD, *et al.*: Anger expression and risk of stroke and coronary heart disease among male health professionals. *Psychosom Med* 2003, 65:100–110.

14. Kawachi I, Colditz GA, Ascherio A, *et al.*: Prospective study of phobic anxiety and risk of coronary heart disease in men. *Circulation* 1994, 89:1992–1997.

15. Leor J, Poole WK, Kloner RA: Sudden cardiac death triggered by an earthquake. *N Engl J Med* 1996, 334:413–419.

16. Meisel SR, Kutz I, Davan KI, *et al.*: Effect of the Iraqi missile war on incidence of acute myocardial infarction and sudden death in Israeli citizens. *Lancet* 1991, 338; 660–661.

16. Mittleman MA, Maclure M, Tofler GH, *et al.*: Triggering of acute myocardial infarction by heavy physical exertion. *N Engl J Med* 1993, 329:1677–1683.

17. Mittleman MA, Maclure M, Sherwood JB, for the Determinants of Myocardial Infarction Onset Study Investigators: Triggering of acute myocardial infarction onset by episodes of anger. *Circulation* 1995, 92:1720–1725.

18. Willich SN, Lowel H, Lewis M, *et al.*: Increased Monday risk of acute myocardial infarction in the working population. *Circulation* 1992, 86(suppl):61.

18. Mittleman MA, Lewis RA, Maclure M, *et al.*: Triggering myocardial infarction by marijuana. *Circulation* 2001, 103:2805–2809.

19. Mittleman MA, Mintzer D, Maclure M, *et al.*: Triggering of myocardial infarction by cocaine. *Circulation* 1999, 99:2737–2741.

20. Muller JE, Mittleman MA, Maclure M, *et al.*: Triggering myocardial infarction by sexual activity: low absolute risk and prevention by regular physical exertion. Determinants of Myocardial Infarction Onset Study Investigators. *JAMA* 1996, 275:1405–1409.

21. Muller JE, Tofler GH, Stone PH: Circadian variations and triggers of onset of acute cardiovascular disease. *Circulation* 1989, 79:733–741.

22. Allan R, Scheidt S: Cardiac psychology: psychosocial factors. In *Clinical Trials in Heart Disease: A Companion to Braunwald's Heart Disease*, edn 2. Edited by Manson JE, Ridker PM, Gaziano JM. Philadelphia: Elsevier Saunders; 2004:386-398.

23. Friedman M, Thoresen CE, Gill JJ, *et al.*: Alteration of type-A behavior and its effect on cardiac recurrences in post myocardial infarction patients: summary results of the Recurrent Coronary Prevention Project. *Am Heart J* l986, ll2:653–665.

24. Case RB, Heller SS, Case NB, Moss AJ: Type A behavior and survival after acute myocardial infarction. *N Eng J Med* 1985, 312:737–741.

25. Ragland DR, Brand RJ: Type A behavior and mortality from coronary heart disease. *N Engl J Med* 1988, 318:65–69.

26. Ahern DK, Gorkin L, Anderson J, *et al.*: Biobehavioral variables and mortality in the Cardiac Arrhythmic Pilot Study (CAPS). *Am J Cardiol* 1990, 66:59–62.

27. Writing Committee for the ENRICHD investigators: Effects of treating depression and low perceived social support on clinical events after myocardial infarction: the enhancing recovery in coronary heart disease patients (ENRICHD) randomized trial. *JAMA* 2003, 289:3106–3116.

28. Schneiderman N, Saab PG, Catellier DJ, for the ENRICHD Investigators: Psychosocial treatment within sex by ethnicity subgroups in the Enhancing Recovery in Coronary Heart Disease Clinical Trial. *Psychosom Med* 2004, 66:475–483.

29. Glassman AH, O'Connor CM, Califf RM, for the Sertraline Antidepressant Heart Attack Randomized Trial (SADHART) Group: Sertraline treatment of major depression in patients with acute MI or unstable angina. *JAMA* 2002, 288:701–709.

30. Frasure-Smith N, Lesperance F, Prince R, *et al.*: Randomized trial of home-based psychosocial nursing intervention for patients recovering from myocardial infarction. *Lancet* 1997, 350:473–479.

31. Cosette S, Frasure-Smith N, Lesperance F: Clinical implications of a reduction in psychological distress on cardiac prognosis in a psychosocial intervention program. *Psychosom Med* 2001, 63:257–266.

32. Jones DA, West RR: Psychological rehabilitation after myocardial infarction: multicentre randomized controlled trial. *BMJ* 1996, 313:1517–1521.

33. Burell G: Group psychotherapy in Project New Life: treatment of coronary-prone behavior for post coronary artery bypass patients. In *Heart and Mind: The Practice of Cardiac Psychology*. Edited by Allan R, Scheidt S. Washington, DC: American Psychological Association; 1996.

34. Hamalainen H, Luurila OJ, Kallio V, Knuts L-R: Reduction in sudden deaths and coronary mortality in myocardial infarction patients after rehabilitation: 15-year follow-up study. *Eur Heart J* 1995, 16:1839–1844.

35. Denollet J, Brutsaert DL: Reducing emotional distress improves prognosis in coronary heart disease. *Circulation* 2001, 104:2018–2023.

36. Blumenthal JA, Jiang W, Babyak M, *et al.*: Stress management and exercise training in patients with myocardial ischemia. *Arch Intern Med* 1997, 157:2213–2223.

37. Blumenthal JA, Babyak M, Wei J, *et al.*: Usefulness of psychosocial treatment of mental stress-induced myocardial ischemia in men. *Am J Cardiol* 2002, 89:164–168.

38. Roose SP, Laghrissi-Thode F, Kennedy JS, *et al.*: Comparison of paroxetine and nortriptyline in depressed patients with ischemic heart disease. *JAMA* 1998, 279:287–291.

39. Ornish D, Scherwitz LW, Billings JH, *et al.*: Intensive lifestyle changes for reversal of coronary heart disease. *JAMA* 1998, 280:2001–2007.

40. Rozanski A, Blumenthal JA, Kaplan J: Impact of psychological factors on the pathogenesis of cardiovascular disease and implications for therapy. *Circulation* 1999, 99:2192–2217.

41. Sears SF, Todaro JF, Lewis TS, *et al.*: Examining the psychosocial impact of implantable cardioverter defibrillators: a literature review. *Clin Cardiol* 1999, 22:481–489.

42. Fries R, Konig J, Schafers HJ, Bohm M: Triggering effect of physical and mental stress on spontaneous ventricular tachyarrhythmias in patients with implantable cardioverter-defibrillators. *Clin Cardiol* 2002, 25:474–478.

43. Lampert R, Joska T, Burg MM, et al.: Emotional and physical precipitants of ventricular arrhythmia. *Circulation* 2002, 106:1800–1805.

44. Frizelle DJ, Lewin RJP, Kaye G, *et al.*: Cognitive-behavioral rehabilitation programme for patients with an implantable cardioverter defibrillator: a pilot study. *Br J Health Psychol* 2004, 9:381–392.

45. Mumford AD, Warr KV, Owen SJ, Fraser AG: Delays by patients in seeking treatment for acute chest pain: implications for achieving earlier thrombolysis. *Postgrad Med J* 1999, 75:90–95.

46. Luepker RV, Raczynski JM, Osganian S, *et al.*: Effect of a community intervention on patient delay and medical service use in acute coronary heart disease: the Rapid Early Action for Coronary Treatment (REACT) Trial. *JAMA* 2000, 284:60–67.

47. Osganian SK, Zapka JG, Feldman HA, *et al.*: Use of emergency medical services for suspected acute cardiac ischemia among demographic and clinical patient subgroups: the REACT trial. *Prehosp Emerg Care* 2002, 6:175–185.

48. Blohm M, Herlitz J, Hartford M, *et al.*: Consequences of a media campaign focusing on delay in acute myocardial infarction. *Am J Cardiol* 1992, 69:411–413.

49. Sirous F Le: Deni dans la maladie coronarienne. [Denial in coronary disease.] *Can Med J* 1992, 147:315–321.

50. Fowers BJ: The cardiac denial of impact scale: a brief, self-report research measure. *J Psychosom Res* 1992, 36:469–475.

Novel Risk Factors: Focus on High-sensitivity C-reactive Protein

Paul M Ridker

Half of all heart attacks and strokes occur among apparently healthy men and women with normal or even low levels of cholesterol, and 20% of all acute vascular events occur among individuals without any major risk factor for heart disease. In an effort to better identify high-risk patients, several risk factors, including homocysteine, lipoprotein(a), lipid-subfractions, and measures of fibrinolysis and inflammation, have been explored. However, of available biomarkers, only high-sensitivity C-reactive protein (CRP) has been shown to predict risk of heart disease independent of traditional risk factors included in global prediction scores. Broadly, levels of high-sensitivity CRP less than 1, 1 to 3, and greater than 3 mg/L correspond to lower, moderate, and higher risk of cardiovascular disease at all levels of low-density lipoprotein (LDL) cholesterol, at all levels of metabolic syndrome, and at all levels of the Framingham Risk Score. Laboratory evidence further indicates that CRP is not only a marker of disease risk, but likely is a direct participant in the atherothrombotic process. In secondary prevention, patients taking statin agents who achieve lower levels of CRP appear to have reduced atherosclerotic progression and improved survival at all levels of LDL cholesterol. These observations suggest that "dual goals" may need to be considered for statin therapy that include target levels for LDL cholesterol (< 70 mg/dL) and target levels for CRP (< 2 mg/L). Trials in primary prevention are ongoing to determine whether statin therapy has clinical benefits among those with low levels of cholesterol who nonetheless are at elevated risk because of the presence of increased high-sensitivity CRP levels.

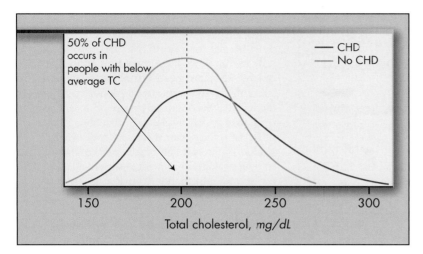

Figure 16-1.
Total cholesterol distribution: coronary heart disease (CHD) versus non-CHD population. Although elevated total and low-density cholesterol levels are major risk factors for myocardial infarction, 50% of those with CHD have below-average cholesterol levels. Thus, although measuring and managing cholesterol is crucial for heart disease prevention, cholesterol evaluation alone cannot be relied on for full risk prediction. TC—total cholesterol. (*Adapted from* Castelli [1].)

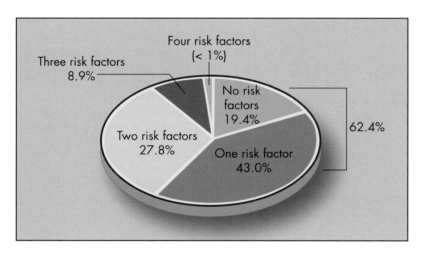

Figure 16-2.
Prevalence of conventional risk factors in patients with coronary heart disease ($n = 87{,}869$). Many studies indicate that a large proportion of heart attacks occur in the absence of any major risk factor, defined as smoking, hypertension, hyperlipidemia, or diabetes. As shown here in an analysis of over 87,000 women, one event in five had no major risk factor at all, and more than half (62%) had only one risk factor. (*Adapted from* Khot *et al.* [2].)

Evaluating Novel Cardiovascular Risk Factors

Does/is the biomarker/risk factor:
Add independent information on risk or prognosis?
Account for a clinically significant proportion of disease?
Reliable and accurate?
Provide good sensitivity, specificity, and predictive value?
Available and practical for widespread use?

Figure 16-3.
Evaluating novel cardiovascular risk factors. In evaluating any novel risk factor or biomarker for disease, several important issues must be addressed. These include evidence that the biomarker of interest provides independent information on risk, that it accounts for a clinically significant proportion of disease, that the test itself is reliable and has adequate predictive value, and is available for widespread use. Because cardiovascular screening must be done on broad populations, it is desirable for the test of interest to be inexpensive and capable of being used in the outpatient primary care setting. It is for this reason that most novel risk factors have relied on simple blood tests that can be run along with cholesterol evaluation. It is also for this reason that imaging modalities that require radiologic interpretation have been less desirable. (*Adapted from* Manolio [3].)

Clinical Epidemiology of Proposed Plasma-based Biomarkers for the Prediction of Future Cardiovascular Events

Biomarker	Prospective studies convincing?	Standardized commercial assay?	Additive to lipid screening?	Additive to Framingham Risk Score?
Inflammation				
hsCRP	++++	+++	+++	+++
sICAM-1	++	+/-	+	-
SAA	++	-	+	-
IL-6/IL-18	++	-	+	-
Myeloperoxidase	+	-	+/-	-
sCD40L	+	-	-	-
Altered thrombosis				
t-PA/PAI-1	++	+/-	-	-
Fibrinogen	+++	+/-	++	-
Homocysteine	++++	+++	+/-	-
D-dimer	++	+	-	-
Oxidative stress				
Oxidized LDL	+/-	-	-	-
Altered lipids				
Lipoprotein(a)	+++	+/-	+/-	-
LDL particle size	++	+/-	+/-	-

Figure 16-4.
Criteria to assess novel biomarkers. Four criteria must be met for a novel risk marker to be clinically useful. First, there must be a consistent set of large-scale prospective studies that demonstrate the factor of interest to consistently predict events. Second, there must be a standardized assay widely available so that clinicians in different settings can accurately measure the marker of interest. Third, the marker should add to lipid evaluation. Finally, it should add to prognostic information to that available from global risk prediction models such as the Framingham Risk Score. As shown, many blood-based markers have been evaluated including multiple markers of inflammation, markers of altered thrombosis, oxidative stress, and lipid subfractions. However, with the exception of high sensitivity C-reactive protein (hsCRP), none of these have been found to add to the predictive value of the Framingham Risk Score. For this reason, only hsCRP has been recommended by the American Heart Association and the Centers for Disease Control and Prevention as a new method to assist clinicians in predicting cardiovascular risk. IL—interleukin; LDL—low-density lipoprotein; PAI-1—plaminogen activator inhibitor-1; SAA—serum amyloid A; sICAM—soluble intercellular adhesion molecule; t-PA—tissue-type plasminogen activator. (*Adapted from* Ridker *et al.* [4].)

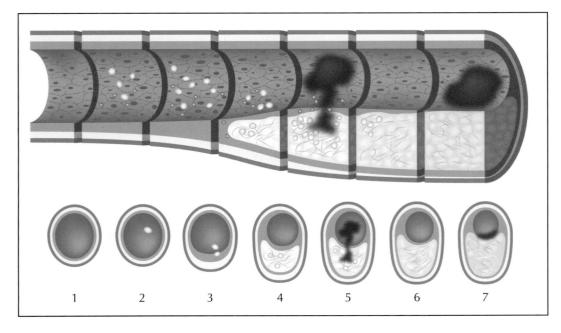

Figure 16-5.
The atherothrombotic process. It is now understood that, in addition to being a process of lipid accumulation, atherothrombosis and acute plaque rupture are fundamentally inflammatory processes characterized by infiltration of leukocytes and heightened cytokine activity. C-reactive protein is a systemic marker of that inflammatory process [5].

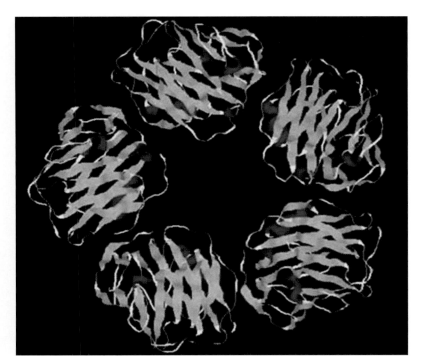

Figure 16-6.
Illustration of high-sensitivity C-reactive protein (hsCRP). In clinical practice, the easiest marker of inflammation to measure for risk prediction is hsCRP. CRP is a pentraxin and functions as a pattern recognition molecule for innate immunity. There is no circadian variation in hsCRP levels, the plasma half-life is long, and the protein is highly stable, making it easy to measure in outpatient settings.

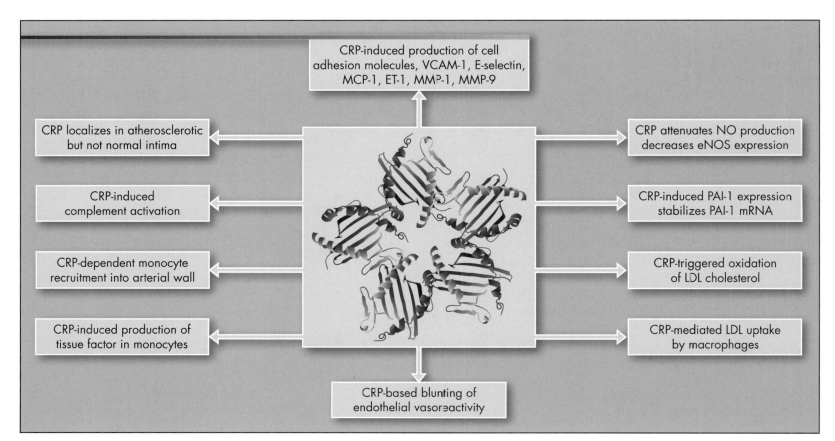

Figure 16-7.
More than a marker: does C-reactive protein (CRP) play a direct role in atherothrombosis? Current data indicate that CRP may be more than a marker of disease—it may also play a direct role in the atherothrombotic process. Potential mechanisms of this effect include complement activation, tissue factor production, changes in fibrinolytic potential, attenuated nitric oxide (NO) production, and enhanced production of cell adhesion molecules. eNOS—endothelial nitric oxide synthase; ET-1—endothelin-1; LDL—low-density lipoprotein; MCP-1—monocyte chemoattractant protein; MMP—matrix metalloproteinase; PAI-1—plasminogen activator inhibitor-1; VCAM-1—vascular cellular adhesion molecule. (*Adapted from* Ridker [6].)

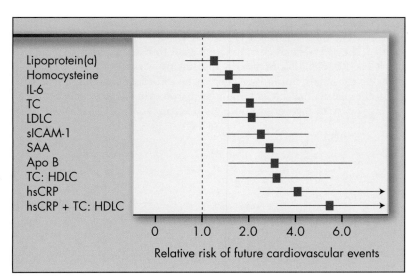

Figure 16-8.
Risk factors for future cardiovascular events. In a head-to-head comparison of multiple "novel" risk factors, high-sensitivity C-reactive protein (hsCRP) performed better than lipoprotein(a), homocysteine, total cholesterol, low-density lipoprotein cholesterol (LDLC), and apolipoprotein B (Apo B) in predicting future vascular events. hsCRP was also a superior predictor of risk as compared with other markers of inflammation, including interleukin-6 (IL-6), soluble intercellular adhesion molecule type 1 (sICAM-1), and serum amyloid A (SAA). It is important to recognize that hsCRP levels minimally correlate with cholesterol measures. Thus, adding hsCRP to lipid measures such as the total cholesterol to high-density lipoprotein cholesterol (TC: HDLC) ratio is the best way to use these data. (*Adapted from* Ridker *et al.* [7].)

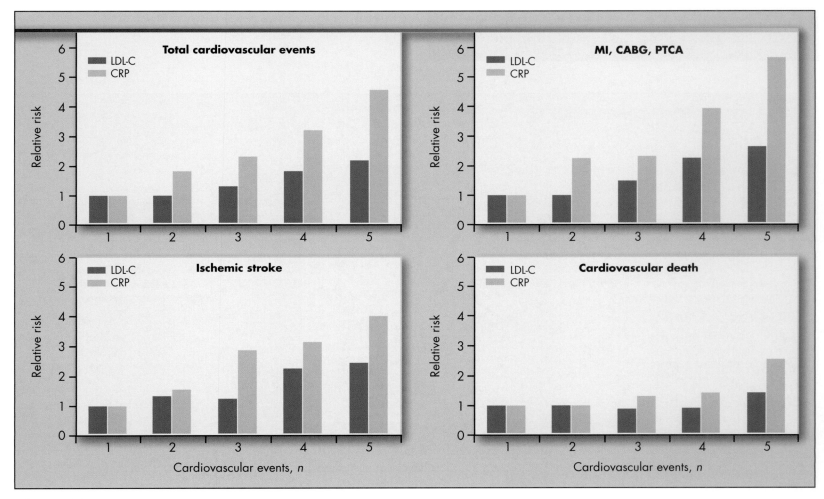

Figure 16-9.
A direct comparison of low-density lipoprotein cholesterol (LDL-C) and C-reactive protein (CRP) in the prediction of first-ever cardiovascular events among 17,939 women. In a direct comparison, high-sensitivity CRP levels were a better predictor of total cardiovascular events, coronary events, stroke events, and cardiovascular death than was LDL-C. CABG—coronary artery bypass graft; MI—myocardial infarction; PTCA—percutaneous transluminal coronary angioplasty. (*Adapted from* Ridker *et al.* [7].)

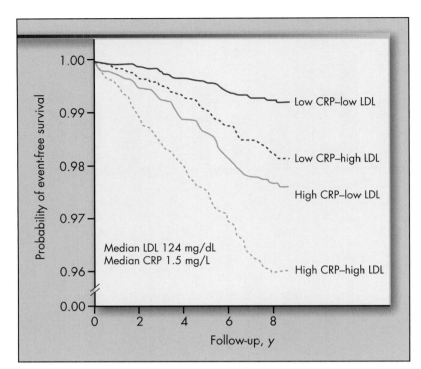

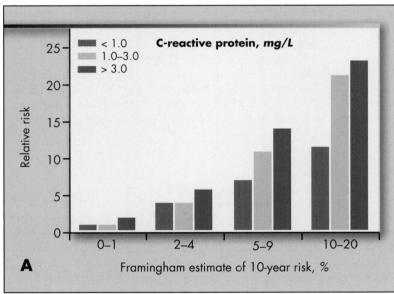

A

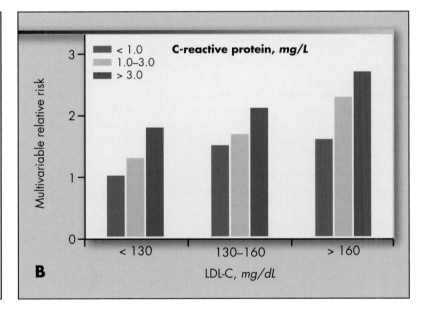

B

Figure 16-10.
Cardiovascular event-free survival using combined high-sensitivity C-reactive protein (CRP) and low-density lipoprotein cholesterol (LDL-C). Cardiovascular event-free survival in the general population can be divided into four groups on the basis of LDL and CRP values greater than or less than median levels. As shown, those with high levels of LDL-C and CRP are at highest risk. However, as also shown, those with elevated levels of CRP and low levels of LDL are at higher absolute risk than those with elevated levels of LDL and low CRP levels. Such individuals are largely outside current risk algorithms. (*Adapted from* Ridker *et al.* [7].)

Figure 16-11.
C-reactive protein (CRP) adds prognostic information at all levels of Framingham Risk Score (**A**) and at all levels of low-density lipoprotein cholesterol ([**B**] LDL-C). In the Women's Health Study, high-sensitivity CRP values were coded as less than 1 mg/L for lower risk, 1 to 3mg/L for moderate risk, and greater than 3 mg/L for higher risk.

These levels of high-sensitivity CRP added important prognostic information on risk at all levels of LDL-C after adjusting for usual risk factors (*panel B*) and across the full spectrum of the Framingham Risk Score (*panel A*). (*Adapted from* Ridker *et al.* [7].)

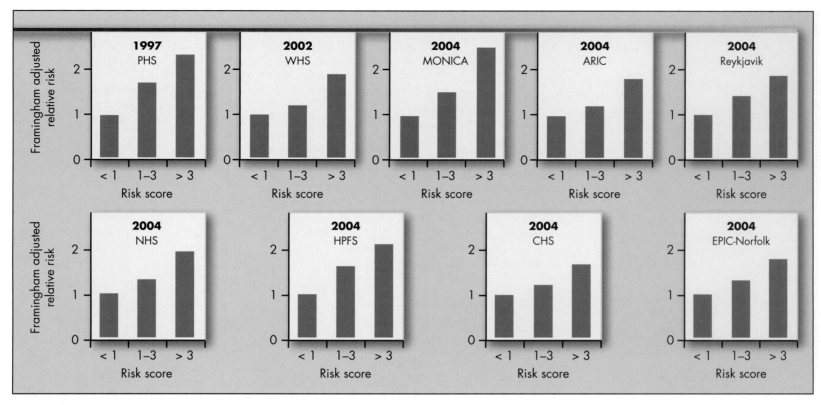

Figure 16-12.
High-sensitivity C-reactive protein (hsCRP) adds prognostic information beyond the Framingham Risk Score in *all* major cohorts evaluated. There are now over 30 prospective studies evaluating hsCRP, and all have found positive relationships with incident cardiovascular disease. The nine largest have also consistently found that hsCRP levels add information on risk even after adjusting for the Framingham covariates. These studies include the Physicians' Health Study (PHS), the Women's Health Study (WHS), the Monitoring Trends and Determinants in Cardiovascular Disease (MONICA) study, the Atherosclerosis Risk in Communities study (ARIC), the Reykjavik Heart Study (Reykjavik), the Nurses Health Study (NHS), the Health Professional follow-Up Study (HPFS), the Coronary Heart Study (CHS), and the European-Norfolk (EPIC) study. (*Adapted from* Ridker *et al.* [7].)

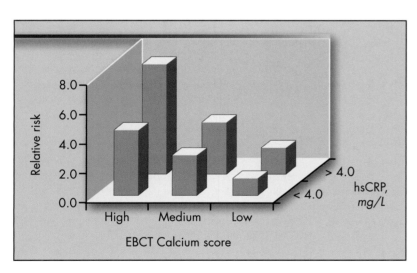

Figure 16-13.
Combined use of CT calcium scores and C-reactive protein (CRP) in the prediction of cardiovascular events: South Bay Heart Watch. Imaging techniques such as electron beam CT (EBCT) scanning reflect atherosclerotic burden and are used by some prevention groups to assist in risk detection. High-sensitivity CRP (hsCRP) levels do not strongly correlate with coronary calcium, and at all levels of coronary calcification, knowledge of hsCRP levels increases risk. This suggests that hsCRP is not a marker of disease burden but rather a marker for plaque instability. (*Adapted from* Park *et al.* [8].)

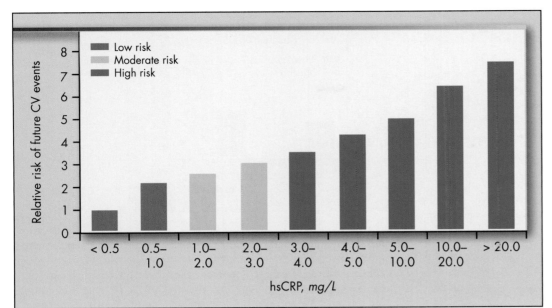

Figure 16-14.
Clinical predictive value of very low as well as very high levels of high-sensitivity C-reactive protein (hsCRP). The relationship of hsCRP to future cardiac risk is linear across a full range of values. Thus, those with very high levels of hsCRP are at very high risk, whereas those with very low levels are at very low risk. CV—cardiovascular. (*Adapted from* Ridker and Cook [9].)

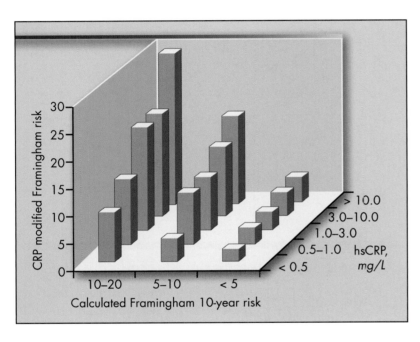

Figure 16-15.
Moving toward a high-sensitivity C-reactive protein (hsCRP) modified Framingham Risk Score. On the basis of these data, algorithms have been proposed that add information from hsCRP measurement to traditional global risk factors such as those shown here from the Framingham Risk Score. (*Adapted from* Ridker *et al.* [10].)

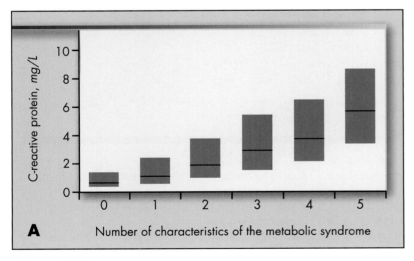

B. Adult Treatment Panel III Definition of Metabolic Syndrome

Three of the following five characteristics:
Midline obesity
Elevated triglycerides
Low high-density lipoprotein
Hypertension
Glucose intolerance

Figure 16-16.
A and **B**, C-reactive protein (CRP) levels correlate with the Adult Treatment Program III definition of the metabolic syndrome (*n* = 14,719 apparently healthy American women). Levels of high-sensitivity CRP also predict the onset of type 2 diabetes and are related to the metabolic syndrome. As shown here, high-sensitivity CRP levels increase on a population basis as the number of metabolic syndrome characteristics increase. (*Adapted from* Ridker *et al.* [11].)

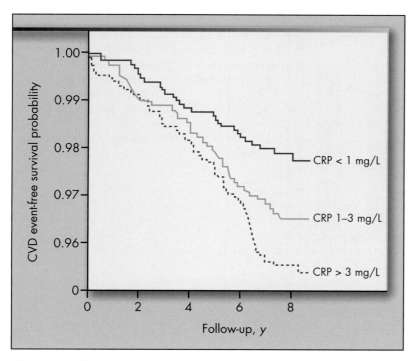

Figure 16-17.
C-reactive protein (CRP) adds to the Adult Treatment Program III (ATP-III) definition of the metabolic syndrome (*n* = 3097 patients with ATP-III metabolic syndrome). Knowledge of high-sensitivity CRP levels increases the ability to predict high and low vascular risk, even among those already defined as having metabolic syndrome. As shown here in a prospective study of over 3000 individuals with ATP-III–defined metabolic syndrome, vascular survival was much worse for those who also had high-sensitivity CRP levels greater than 3 mg/L. This indicates that inflammation also is a critical part of the metabolic syndrome. Newer definitions of metabolic syndrome are thus likely to include high-sensitivity CRP evaluation. CVD—cardiovascular disease. (*Adapted from* Ridker *et al.* [11].)

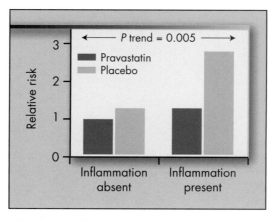

Figure 16-18.
Inflammation, statin therapy, and relative risk of coronary events. Statin therapy has been found more effective among those with increased systemic inflammation. In these data from the Cholesterol and Recurrent Events trial of secondary prevention, the magnitude of benefit of statin therapy was greatest among those with increased levels of inflammation as assessed by high-sensitivity C-reactive protein. (*Adapted from* Ridker *et al.* [12].)

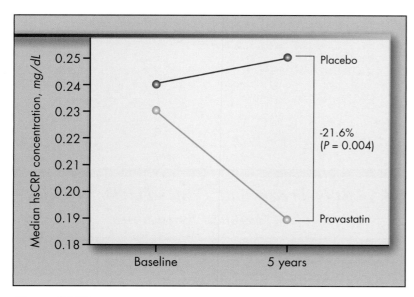

Figure 16-19.
Long-term effect of pravastatin on high-sensitivity C-reactive protein (hsCRP): placebo and pravastatin groups. In addition to lowering cholesterol levels, statins also lower hsCRP levels. This was first shown in the Cholesterol and Recurrent Events trial and is now known to be a class effect of these agents. However, for all statins, the magnitude of low-density lipoprotein reduction is a very poor predictor of the magnitude of hsCRP reduction. These data support basic laboratory evidence of direct anti-inflammatory effects of statin therapy. (*Adapted from* Ridker *et al.* [13].)

C-reactive Protein as a Method to Target Statin Therapy in Primary Prevention: AFCAPS/TexCAPS

Study Group	Statin	Placebo	NNT
Low LDL-C/low CRP	0.025	0.022	—
Low LDL-C/high CRP	0.029	0.051	48
High LDL-C/low CRP	0.020	0.050	33
High LDL-C/high CRP	0.038	0.055	58

Median LDL-C = 149 mg/dL.
Median CRP = 0.16 mg/dL.

Figure 16-20.
In primary prevention, it has been hypothesized that high-sensitivity C-reactive protein (hsCRP) levels may provide a method to better target statin therapy. For example, within the Air Force/Texas Coronary Atherosclerosis Prevention Study (AFCAPS/TexCAPS) trial of lovastatin, it was observed that the number needed to treat (NNT) with statin therapy for individuals with low levels of low-density lipoprotein cholesterol (LDL-C) but high levels of hsCRP was 48, well within the range observed for those who had overt hyperlipidemia (NNT = 33–58). However, such individuals are not currently considered candidates for statin therapy because their LDL-C cholesterol levels are too low. The ongoing Justification for the Use of statins in Primary prevention; an Intervention Trial Evaluating Rosuvastatin (JUPITER) trial is directly evaluating this hypothesis. (*Adapted from* Ridker *et al.* [14].)

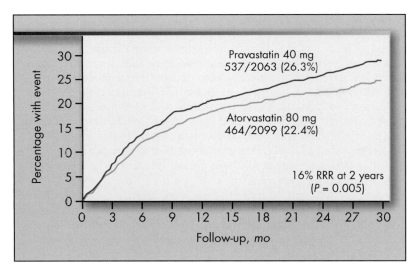

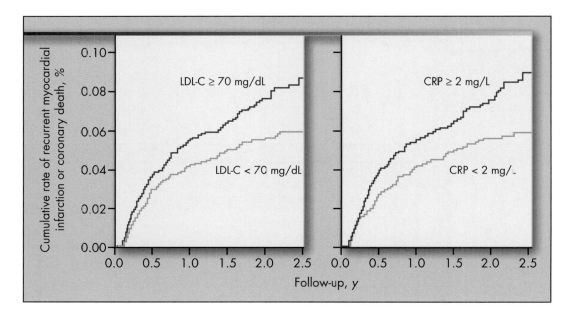

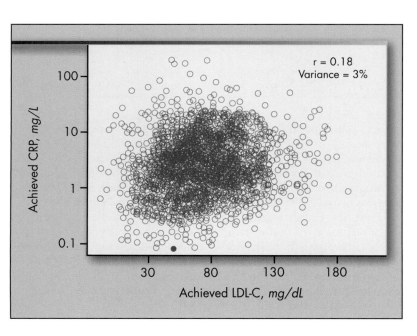

Figure 16-21.
Pravastatin or Atorvastatin Evaluation and Infection Therapy trial (PROVE-IT/TIMI-22) results: all-cause death or major cardiovascular events in all randomized subjects. In high-risk secondary prevention, recent data from the PROVE-IT/TIMI-22 clinical trial have been instructive in understanding the role of inflammation and statin therapy in heart disease. The primary findings of the PROVE-IT/TIMI-22 trial conducted among very high-risk acute coronary syndrome (ACS) patients were that a more aggressive statin regimen resulted in fewer vascular events compared with a modest statin regimen. RRR—relative risk reduction. (*Adapted from* Cannon *et al.* [15].)

Figure 16-22.
Clinical relevance of achieved low-density lipoprotein (LDL) and achieved C-reactive protein (CRP) after treatment with statin therapy. Within the Pravastatin or Atorvastatin Evaluation and Infection Therapy trial, achieving LDL cholesterol (LDL-C) of less than 70 mg/dL was associated with significantly lower rates of recurrent myocardial infarction or vascular death as compared with those who did not lower LDL-C levels below this cut-off point (*left panel*). However, an almost identical set of survival curves was observed in the Pravastatin or Atorvastatin Evaluation and Infection Therapy trial according to whether or not the study participants also achieved high-sensitivity CRP levels less than 2 mg/L. These data were not changed after adjustment for all available baseline characteristics. Thus, LDL-C reduction and high-sensitivity CRP reduction are highly predictive of statin efficacy. (*Adapted from* Ridker *et al.* [16].)

Figure 16-23.
Minimal relationship between achieved low-density lipoprotein (LDL) and achieved C-reactive protein (CRP) after initiation of statin therapy. It is important to recognize that the relationship between the achieved level of LDL cholesterol (LDL-C) after statin therapy is minimally related to the achieved levels of high-sensitivity CRP after initiating statin therapy. (*Adapted from* Ridker *et al.* [16].)

Novel Risk Factors: Focus on High-sensitivity C-reactive Protein

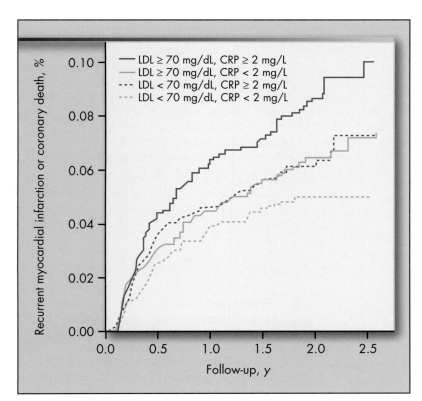

Figure 16-24.
Clinical relevance of achieved low-density lipoprotein (LDL) and achieved
C-reactive protein (CRP) after treatment with statin therapy. Because
achieved high-sensitivity CRP levels and achieved LDL levels after statin
therapy are unrelated, and because each of these is independently associated with outcome, it is possible to classify Pravastatin or Atorvastatin
Evaluation and Infection Therapy trial subjects into four groups on the
basis of achieved LDL and achieved high-sensitivity CRP levels. As shown
here, the worst outcomes were observed among those statin-treated
patients in whom LDL cholesterol after 30 days was greater than 70
mg/dL and high-sensitivity CRP was greater than 2 mg/L. However, for
those who reduced high-sensitivity CRP less than 2 mg/L or who
reduced LDL less than 70 mg/dL, there were substantial benefits. These
effects were almost identical in magnitude suggesting that high-sensitivity
CRP reduction alone has a magnitude of benefit almost exactly the same
as that of LDL reduction alone. Clinically, those who not only lowered
LDL cholesterol to less than 70 mg/dL but who also lowered high-sensitivity CRP levels to less than 2 mg/L enjoyed by far the greatest benefit
of statin therapy. On this basis, it has been suggested that physicians must
meet the "dual goals" of lowering high-sensitivity CRP and LDL cholesterol when treating with statins. (*Adapted from* Ridker *et al.* [16].)

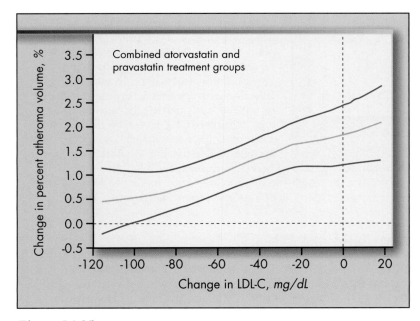

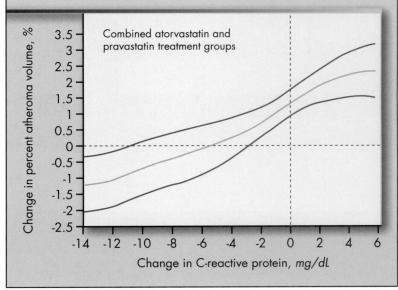

Figure 16-25.
Low-density lipoprotein cholesterol (LDL-C) change versus atherosclerosis progression. Evidence that reduction in LDL-C and high-sensitivity C-reactive protein is crucial for patient survival also comes from the
Reversal of Atherosclerosis with Lipitor (REVERSAL) study in which
statin therapy was given over an 18-month period, and the amount of
coronary atheroma was evaluated using intravascular ultrasound. In that
study, the change in percent atheroma volume declined with larger
levels of LDL reduction. These data are consistent with the hypothesis
that LDL reduction can lead to a slowing of atherosclerotic progression
(*Adapted from* Nissen *et al.* [17].)

Figure 16-26.
C-reactive protein (CRP) change versus atherosclerosis progression. Of
great interest, however, was the simultaneous observation in the Reversal
of Atherosclerosis with Lipitor (REVERSAL) trial that there was also a
direct relationship between the change in percent of atheroma volume and
the magnitude of high-sensitivity CRP reduction achieved. Specifically, as
high-sensitivity CRP levels came down, there was less atheroma observed
and those who had the largest high-sensitivity CRP reductions enjoyed
plaque regression. As in the Pravastatin or Atorvastatin Evaluation and
Infection Therapy trial, these effects were fully independent, and thus low-
density lipoprotein reduction and CRP reduction appear critical for best
patient outcomes. Within the REVERSAL study, only those who had CRP
reductions saw actual regression of disease as measured by intravascular
ultrasound. (*Adapted from* Nissen *et al.* [17].)

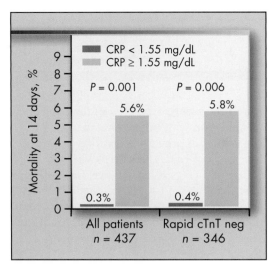

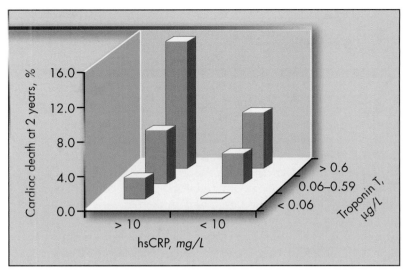

Figure 16-27.
Baseline C-reactive protein (CRP) and mortality. Many physicians measure high-sensitivity CRP during acute ischemia as a method of improving risk prediction in acute coronary syndrome settings. As shown here in data from the Thrombolysis in Myocardial Infarction-11A trial, those with elevated high-sensitivity CRP levels during acute coronary syndrome had substantially increased short-term risks of death, even when troponin (cTnT) levels were normal. These data demonstrate that presence of inflammation is highly associated with recurrent plaque rupture. (*Adapted from* Morrow *et al.* [18].)

Figure 16-28.
Incidence of cardiac death at 2 years according to high-sensitivity C-reactive protein (hsCRP) and maximal 24-hour troponin T levels. High-sensitivity CRP levels at the time of hospital admission are strongly related to long-term cardiac survival. As shown in these data from the Fragmin during Instability in Coronary Artery Disease Study (FRISC), levels of hsCRP were highly predictive of cardiac death at 2 years, again fully additive to troponin levels. (*Adapted from* Lindahl *et al.* [19].)

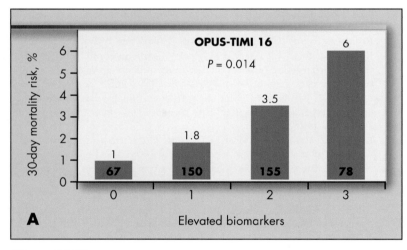

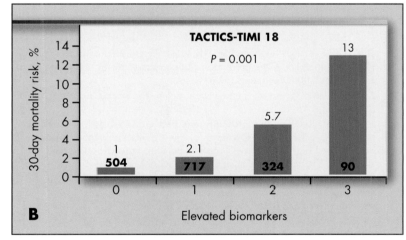

Figure 16-29.
Troponin-1, C-reactive protein, and β-type natriuretic peptide (BNP) as determinants of 30-day mortality in acute coronary ischemia: a multimarker approach. The combined use of troponin, BNP, and high-sensitivity C-reactive protein has been proposed as a "multimarker" approach

to the diagnosis of acute coronary ischemia. As shown here for the Thrombolysis in Myocardial Infarction (TIMI)-16 (**A**) and TIMI-18 trials (**B**), the number of elevated biomarkers was closely related to subsequent 30-day mortality. (*Adapted from* Sabatine *et al.* [20].)

Figure 16-30.
Interrelation of C-reactive protein (CRP), myeloperoxidase (MPO), and recurrent clinical events after unstable angina. Recent data have found high-sensitivity CRP to add prognostic information beyond that attributed to other markers being considered in unstable angina, in particular MPO. (*Adapted from* Baldus *et al.* [21].)

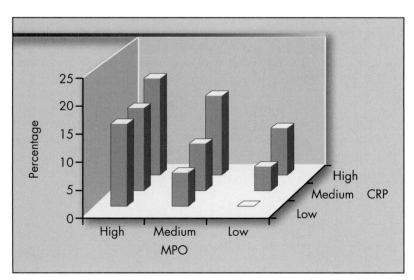

Novel Risk Factors: Focus on High-sensitivity C-reactive Protein

Summary

In summary, high-sensitivity C-reactive protein (hsCRP) levels have been found to predict risk at all levels of low-density lipoprotein (LDL) cholesterol, at all levels of the metabolic syndrome, and all levels of the Framingham Risk Score, and the use of hsCRP has been advocated by the American Heart Association and the Centers for Disease Control for those at "intermediate risk" by conventional screening. hsCRP levels also have utility in the targeting of statin therapy in primary prevention, and in high-risk secondary prevention the use of a "dual goal" strategy to lower LDL and lower CRP has been advocated. Finally, in acute ischemia, elevated levels of hsCRP are associated with markedly increased vascular risk, even in the absence of a troponin leak, and in conjunction with other novel markers of acute ischemic risk. Ongoing studies in primary prevention will determine whether those with low levels of LDL cholesterol who are nonetheless at high risk because of increased hsCRP may benefit from statin therapy. In the meantime, the use of hsCRP in primary prevention has proven highly effective as an adjunct to global risk prediction. In secondary prevention, measurement and management of hsCRP in a manner analogous to that of LDL cholesterol provides a new method to optimize the efficacy of statin therapy.

References

1. Castelli WP: Lipids, risk factors and ischemic heart disease. *Atherosclerosis* 1996, 124(suppl):S1–S9.

2. Khot UN, Khot MB, Bajzer CT, *et al.*: Prevalence of conventional risk factors in patients with coronary heart disease. *JAMA* 2003, 290:898–904.

3. Manolio T: Novel risk markers and clinical practice. *N Engl J Med* 2003, 349:1587–1589.

4. Ridker PM, Brown NJ, Vaughan DE, *et al.*: Established and emerging plasma biomarkers in the prediction of first atherothrombotic events. *Circulation* 2004, 109(suppl):IV6–IV19.

5. Libby P: Atherosclerosis: the new view. *Scientific American* 2002, 286:46–55.

6. Ridker PM: Rosuvastatin in the primary prevention of cardiovascular disease among patients with low levels of low-density lipoprotein cholesterol and elevated high-sensitivity C-reactive protein: rationale and design of the JUPITER trial. *Circulation* 2003, 108:2292–2297.

7. Ridker PM, Hennekens CH, Buring JE, Rifai N: C-reactive protein and other markers of inflammation in the prediction of cardiovascular disease in women. *N Engl J Med* 2000, 342:836–843.

8. Park R, Detrano R, Xiang M, *et al.*: Combined use of computed tomography coronary calcium scores and C-reactive protein levels in predicting cardiovascular events in nondiabetic individuals. *Circulation* 2002, 106:2073–2077.

9. Ridker PM, Cook N: Clinical usefulness of very high and very low levels of C-reactive protein across the full range of Framingham Risk Scores. *Circulation* 2004, 109:1955–1999.

10. Ridker PM, Wilson PW, Grundy SM: Should C-reactive protein be added to metabolic syndrome and to assessment of global cardiovascular risk? *Circulation* 2004, 109:2818–2825.

11. Ridker PM, Buring JE, Cook NR, Rifai N: C-reactive protein, the metabolic syndrome, and risk of incident cardiovascular events: an 8-year follow-up of 14,719 initially healthy American women. *Circulation* 2003, 107:391–397.

12. Ridker PM, Rifai N, Pfeffer MA, *et al.*: Inflammation, pravastatin, and the risk of coronary events after myocardial infarction in patients with average cholesterol levels. Cholesterol and Recurrent Events (CARE) Investigators. *Circulation* 1998, 98:839–844.

13. Ridker PM, Rifai N, Pfeffer MA, *et al.*: Long-term effects of pravastatin on plasma concentration of C-reactive protein. The Cholesterol and Recurrent Events (CARE) Investigators. *Circulation* 1999, 100:230–235.

14. Ridker PM, Rifai N, Clearfield M, *et al.*: Measurement of C-reactive protein for the targeting of statin therapy in the primary prevention of acute coronary events. *N Engl J Med* 2001, 344:1959–1965.

15. Cannon CP, Braunwald E, McCabe CH, *et al.*: Intensive versus moderate lipid lowering with statins after acute coronary syndromes. *N Engl J Med* 2004, 350:1495–1504.

16. Ridker PM, Cannon CP, Morrow D, *et al.*: C-reactive protein levels and outcomes after statin therapy. *N Engl J Med* 2005, 352:20–28.

17. Nissen SE, Tuzcu EM, Schoenhagen P, *et al.*: Statin therapy, LDL cholesterol, C-reactive protein, and coronary artery disease. *N Engl J Med* 2005, 352:29–38.

18. Morrow DA, Rifai N, Antman EM, *et al.*: C-reactive protein is a potent predictor of mortality independently of and in combination with troponin T in acute coronary syndromes: a TIMI 11A substudy. Thrombolysis in Myocardial Infarction. *J Am Coll Cardiol* 1998, 31:1460–1465.

19. Lindahl B, Toss H, Siegbahn A, *et al.*: Markers of myocardial damage and inflammation in relation to long-term mortality in unstable coronary artery disease. FRISC Study Group. Fragmin during Instability in Coronary Artery Disease. *N Engl J Med* 2000, 343:1139–1147.

20. Sabatine MS, Morrow DA, de Lemos JA, *et al.*: Multimarker approach to risk stratification in non-ST elevation acute coronary syndromes: simultaneous assessment of troponin I, C-reactive protein, and B-type natriuretic peptide. *Circulation* 2002, 105:1760–1763.

21. Baldus S, Heeschen C, Meinertz T, *et al.*: Myeloperoxidase serum levels predict risk in patients with acute coronary syndromes. *Circulation* 2003, 108:1440–1445.

Genetic Markers

Sekar Kathiresan and Christopher J. O'Donnell

Many diseases of the heart have a substantial genetic component. Over the past 25 years, the genetic basis for a number of heart diseases has been identified. Initial successes in gene discovery have occurred primarily for rare, mendelian conditions such as familial hypercholesterolemia and familial long QT syndrome. With completion of the sequencing of the human genome, the sequence of nearly the entire 2.85 billion base pairs and the approximately 20,000 to 25,000 human genes is now available, and the pace of discovery in genetics is sure to accelerate. Much of the focus has turned now to the genetic determinants of more common, complex cardiovascular diseases that comprise the leading cause of death in men and women, such as myocardial infarction and heart failure. Genetic markers (or *genotypes*) can be broadly defined as variations in the human genome sequence that are associated with a specific disease parameter or treatment response (also termed a *phenotype*).

This chapter discusses the concepts and methods involved in the search for genes contributing to cardiovascular disease.

Use of Genetic Markers

Disease phenotype identified by marker	Utility
Prevalent disease	Pathophysiology
Incident disease	Risk assessment
Disease subtype	Diagnosis
Treatment response, disease progression	Optimal therapy

Figure 17-1.

Uses of genetic markers. A specific sequence variant in the human genome may be related to a number of disease parameters (phenotypes). A genetic marker may be related to the prevalence of a disease, incidence of a disease, specific subtypes of a disorder, response to treatment or disease progression. Thus, genetic markers may allow us to dissect the pathophysiology of a disease, assess risk for incident disease, aid in the diagnosis, or better predict response to a therapy.

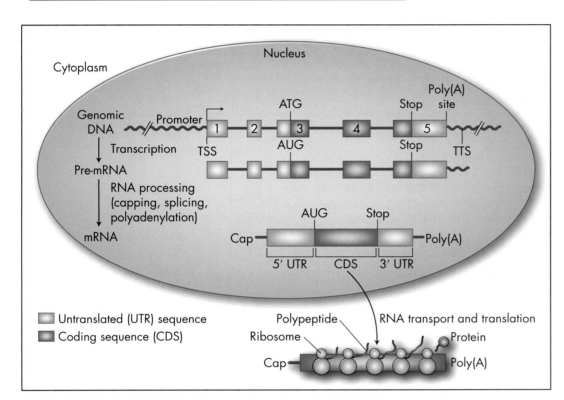

Figure 17-2.

The central dogma of genetics. DNA is the molecular building block for genes. DNA is packaged in human cells into chromosomes (46 in total). Genes are encoded by DNA. Premessenger RNA (pre-mRNA) is transcribed from the DNA in the nucleus. After transcription, the pre-mRNA undergoes modifications including splicing of intronic DNA, capping, and polyadenylation to produce a mature mRNA. The mature mRNA is transported from the nucleus to the cytoplasm where it is translated into a protein polypeptide chain, mediated by the cellular apparatus called ribosomes. In a departure from the central dogma, splicing of mRNA may occur and lead to more than one mRNA molecule and/or more than one protein polypeptide chain. TSS—transcription start site; TTS—transcription termination site. (*Adapted from* Zhang [1].)

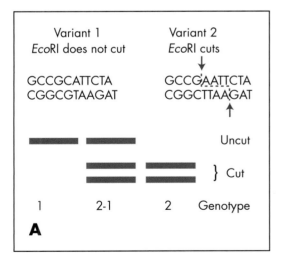

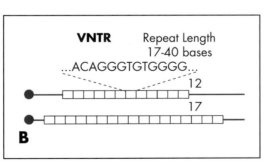

Figure 17-3.

Types of sequence variants in the human genome. **A,** A restriction fragment length polymorphism (RFLP) is a single base-pair change that creates or removes a cleavage site for a DNA restriction enzyme. Restriction enzymes such as the *Escherichia coli* enzyme (*Eco*RI) identify and cut DNA only at very specific DNA sequences. Digesting DNA with the specific restriction enzyme creates DNA fragments of differing lengths. **B,** Variable number tandem repeats (VNTR) are repetitive sequences ranging from 14 to 100 base-pairs in length. The number of times that a sequence is repeated varies in the population. **C,** Short tandem repeats or microsatellites are sequences two to four bases in length that repeat a variable number of times. Short tandem repeats occur throughout the human genome and provide easily measured markers spaced along the genome.

(*continued on next page*)

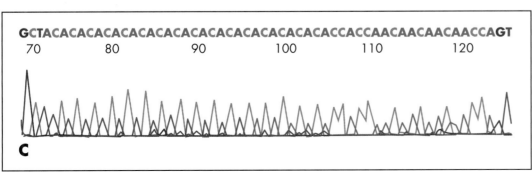

Atlas of Cardiovascular Risk Factors

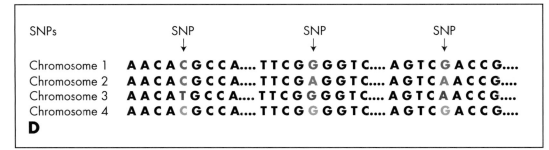

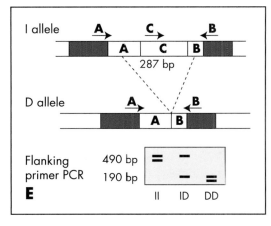

Figure 17-3. continued

D, A single nucleotide polymorphism (SNP) is a common (*ie*, present in > 1% of the population) base change that occurs in a specific site in the human genome. It is estimated that at least 10,000,000 SNPs are present in the human genome. **E**, Insertion-deletion polymorphisms represent the insertion (I) or deletion (D) of a specific sequence in the human genome. Shown here is the angiotensin-converting enzyme D/I polymorphism. bp—base-pair; PCR—polymerase chain reaction.

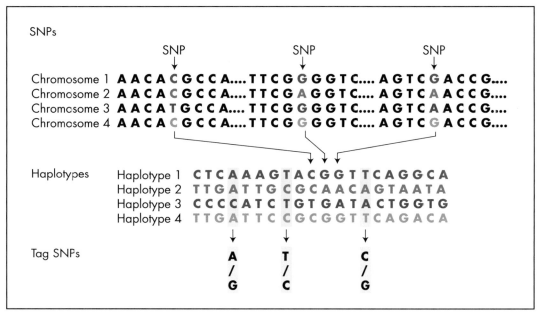

Figure 17-4.

Single nucleotide polymorphisms (SNPs), haplotypes, linkage disequilibrium, and tag SNPs. Three SNPs across are shown in the *upper portion* of the figure. SNPs occur approximately every 300 base-pairs in the population and in any given individual, approximately every 1000 base-pairs, so any two individuals are identical at essentially 99.9% of all bases in the human genome sequence. At the first SNP, most versions of this hypothetical chromosome carry the C allele, and one version of this hypothetic chromosome carries the T allele. Haplotypes (*middle portion* of the figure) are specific combinations of SNP alleles along a chromosome. Twenty SNP variant sites are shown along a sequence consisting of approximately 6000 bases. Only the SNP sites are shown. Although the number of possible combinations of haplotypes for X SNPs is 2^X, it has been empirically observed that only a limited number of common (*ie*, present in > 1%) haplotypes are observed for long stretches of the human sequence. In this case, although as many as 2^{20} possible haplotype combinations could occur, only four common haplotypes are reported. This correlation between nearby SNPs is known as *linkage disequilibrium*. A few SNPs, termed *tag SNPs* (*bottom portion* of the figure), may mark specific haplotypes. Thus, to identify all four haplotypes uniquely, only three of the 20 SNP variants need to be studied. (*Adapted from* the International HapMap Consortium [2].)

Completed Human Genome Sequence Overview

Human genome overview

Number of bases	2.85 billion base-pairs
Estimated number of genes	20,000–25,000
Average gene size	27,000 bases
Gene with the most exons	Titin (234 exons)
Most gene-rich chromosome	19
Estimated rate of SNP variation	One SNP every 300 bases

Figure 17-5.

Completed human genome sequence. The Human Genome Project, an open collaboration involving 20 centers in six countries [3], and Celera Genomics [4] reported their completed draft sequence in 2001, and the Human Genome Project reported its finished genome sequence in 2004 [5]. Non-sex chromosomes are numbered roughly according to size, with chromosome 1 being the largest and chromosome 22 the smallest. The Y chromosome is the smallest of both sex chromosomes and of the rest of the human chromosomes. Interestingly, the largest gene in the genome, titin, plays an important role in cardiovascular physiology. Titin is involved in the regulation of filament length and assembly in cardiomyocytes as well as skeletal muscle cells. SNP—single nucleotide polymorphism.

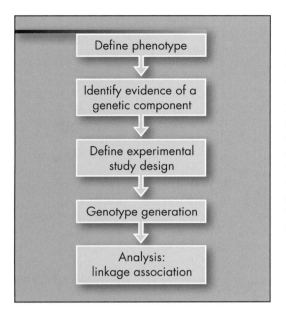

Figure 17-6.
Genetic dissection of traits. Understanding the genetic contribution to a medical trait involves a number of steps. Defining the phenotype, or measurable manifestations or characteristics of the disease, is the first step. Establishing that the phenotype of interest has a genetic component will ensure that a search for genetic markers is warranted. The genetic component is also known as "heritability," the extent to which variation in the disease phenotype is determined by genes. Experimental study designs for identifying a genetic component include studies of families and studies of unrelated individuals. Common forms of family study designs include studies of affected sibling pairs, studies of trios of parents and a single offspring, and linkage studies comprised of multiple extended multigenerational families. One of the most common study designs of unrelated individuals is the "case-control" study. A number of technologies are available to define genotypes with almost all methods depending on amplification of the genomic region that spans the single nucleotide polymorphism before the actual genotyping reaction. Finally, analytic tools to identify genetic markers related to the phenotype include genetic linkage and genetic association approaches.

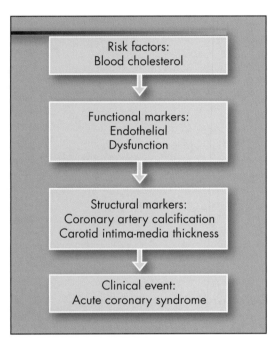

Figure 17-7.
Defining the phenotype in genetic studies. For heart diseases such as atherosclerotic cardiovascular disease, possible phenotypes for genetic studies range from risk factors (*eg*, blood cholesterol) to subclinical disease functional (*eg*, endothelial dysfunction) and structural measures (*eg*, coronary artery calcification or carotid intima-media thickness) to clinical events (acute coronary syndrome).

Heritability of Cardiovascular Phenotypes

Phenotype	Heritability, %
High-density lipoprotein cholesterol [6]	55
Low-density lipoprotein cholesterol [7]	50
Systolic blood pressure [8]	42
Maximum body mass index [9]	40
Coronary artery calcification [10]	38
Abdominal aortic calcification [11]	38

Figure 17-8.
Heritability of cardiovascular phenotypes. For quantitative traits such as blood cholesterol levels, heritability estimates the proportion of phenotypic variance caused by the additive effects of many genes. The remaining proportion of variance is related to environmental or unmeasured factors. Thus, 55% of the measured variability in high-density lipoprotein cholesterol may be attributable to genes. There is evidence for a substantial genetic component to many quantitative cardiovascular traits.

Premature Parental History of Cardiovascular Disease as a Risk Factor for Offspring Cardiovascular Disease

Model adjustment	Risk for offspring CVD, OR (95% CI)				
	None	Paternal CVD	Maternal CVD	Both	One or both parents
Offspring men					
Unadjusted	1.0	3.0 (1.7–5.0)	3.4 (2.1–5.6)	3.3 (1.2–9.0)	3.2 (2.1–5.0)
Age-adjusted	1.0	2.7 (1.6–4.7)	2.4 (1.5–4.0)	3.1 (1.1–8.3)	2.6 (1.7–4.1)
Age and SBP and antihypertensive therapy	1.0	2.5 (1.4–4.3)	2.2 (1.3–3.7)	2.7 (1.0–7.6)	2.4 (1.5–3.8)
Age and total/HDL cholesterol ratio	1.0	2.8 (1.6–4.9)	2.1 (1.2–3.4)	2.9 (1.1–8.1)	2.3 (1.5–3.7)
Age and smoking	1.0	2.4 (1 4–4.1)	2.2 (1.4–3.7)	2.8 (1.0–7.8)	2.4 (1.5–3.8)
Age and diabetes and BMI	1.0	2.5 (1 4–4.3)	2.2 (1.3–3.7)	2.7 (1.0–7.5)	2.4 (1.5–3.8)
Multivariable-adjusted*	1.0	2.2 (1.2–3.9)	1.7 (1.0–2.9)	2.4 (0.9–6.8)	2.0 (1.2–3.1)
Offspring women					
Unadjusted	1.0	2.7 (1.3–5.8)	3.2 (1.7–6.0)	4.3 (1.2–15)	2.9 (1.6–5.3)
Age-adjusted	1.0	2.8 (1.3–6.1)	2.3 (1.2–4.5)	4.1 (1.1–15)	2.3 (1.3–4.3)
Age and SBP and antihypertensive therapy	1.0	2.3 (1.1–5.1)	1.9 (0.9–3.7)	3.1 (0.8–12)	1.9 (1.0–3.6)
Age and total/HDL cholesterol ratio	1.0	1.9 (0.8–4.3)	2.0 (1.0–3.9)	3.8 (1.1–14)	1.9 (1.0–3.6)
Age and smoking	1.0	2.8 (1.3–6.0)	2.3 (1.2–4.4)	4.5 (1.2–17)	2.3 (1.2–4.2)
Age and diabetes and BMI	1.0	2.4 (1.1–5.3)	2.2 (1.1–4.3)	3.5 (1.0–13)	2.2 (1.2–4.1)
Multivariable-adjusted*	1.0	1.7 (0.7–3.9)	1.7 (0.8–3.4)	2.8 (0.7–11)	1.7 (0.9–3.1)

*Adjusted for age, total/HDL cholesterol ratio, SBP, antihypertensive therapy, diabetes, BMI, and current smoking.

Figure 17-9.

Premature parental history of cardiovascular disease (CVD) is a risk factor for offspring CVD. In the Framingham Heart Study, the occurrence of premature (men < 55 years, women < 65 years) onset of CVD in one or both parents led to twofold increase in the offspring's risk of CVD twofold [12]. This risk imparted by family history is independent of other CVD risk factors. The totality of evidence suggests that the parental history of myocardial infarction or other CVDs, particularly at an early age, is an independent risk factor. Thus, there appears to be a significant genetic contribution to the phenotype of CVD. BMI—body mass index; HDL—high-density lipoprotein; OR—odds ratio; SBP—systolic blood pressure. (*Adapted from* Lloyd-Jones *et al.* [12].)

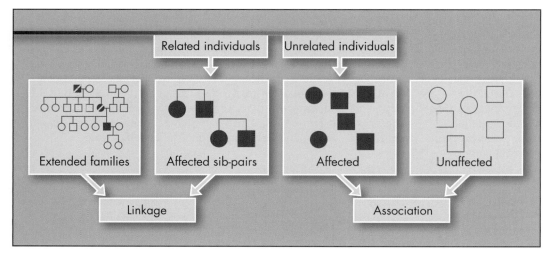

Figure 17-10.

Experimental study design. Sets of related or unrelated individuals may be studied to identify the genetic component of a disease [13]. For related individuals, linkage analysis is the main analytic approach. For a study of unrelated individuals, association analysis may be used to isolate genetic markers associated with disease.

Monogenic Versus Complex Traits

Mendelian or monogenic disorders	Complex traits
Genotype-phenotype correlation nearly perfect	Genotype-phenotype correlation imperfect
Simple inheritance pattern (autosomal dominant, autosomal recessive, X-linked)	No clear simple inheritance pattern
Single causative gene	Multiple susceptibility genes
Large effect of the gene	Each gene with modest effect
Rare in the population	Common in population
	Environmental mimics (phenocopy)

Figure 17-11.

Monogenic versus complex traits. Monogenic (also termed *Mendelian*) disorders often result from one or a few defects in a single gene. For over a 1000 apparently monogenic conditions, the causative gene(s) has been identified. In contrast, most common cardiovascular diseases, such as hypertension or myocardial infarction, are complex in origin and are the result of interplay between multiple susceptibility genes and environmental factors. The search for genetic markers related to complex traits has been underway in earnest during only the past 5 years since completion of the human genome sequence. To date, there have not been a large number of reliably replicated genetic associations with complex traits.

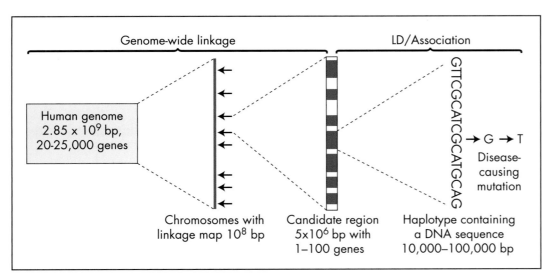

Figure 17-12.

Isolating cardiovascular disease genes. Two complimentary methods, linkage analysis and association (also known as linkage disequilibrium [LD]) studies, have been available to isolate disease genes. In linkage analyses, members of families with evidence of aggregation of a disease are genotyped using a set of highly polymorphic markers (typically microsatellites), evenly spaced across the genome. Markers close to a disease-causing genetic variant will tend to be less commonly separated from the causal variant by recombinations within a family, whereas those further away will be more likely to have observable recombinations.

Linkage analysis leads to less evidence of linkage to disease for the more distant markers and greater evidence for linkage to disease for the nearby markers. Summation of the evidence across multiple families allows the estimation for each marker using the "LOD score," the log of the ratio of the likelihood of marker linkage to a disease to the likelihood of no linkage. Once a segment of DNA that is shared by affected individuals is identified, association studies may help refine the region of interest and identify the specific disease causing mutation. bp—base-pairs.

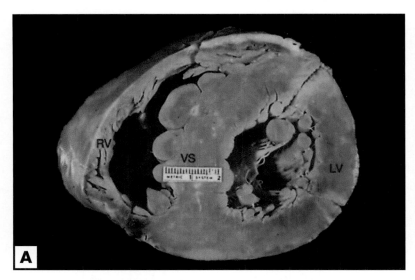

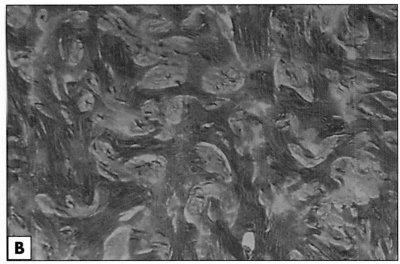

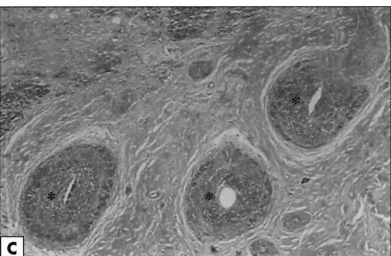

Figure 17-13.

Hypertrophic cardiomyopathy. Hypertrophic cardiomyopathy is a mendelian genetic disorder that occurs in approximately one in 500 individuals. Gene mutations in one of at least 10 sarcomere proteins have been shown to cause hypertrophic cardiomyopathy. The three most common genes affected are β-myosin heavy chain, cardiac troponin T, and myosin-binding protein C. The morphologic features on pathology are displayed here. **A,** In this autopsy heart specimen, there is thickening of the ventricular septum (VS) compared with the right ventricular (RV) and left ventricular (LV) free walls. **B,** There is disarray of myocardial cells; and (**C**) abnormally thickened intramural coronary arteries (marked with an *asterisk*) on hematoxylin and eosin–stained sections of the myocardium. (*From* Maron [14]; with permission.)

A. Diagnostic Criteria for Long QT Syndrome

Features	Points
ECG findings*	
QTc	
0.48 s or greater	3
0.46–0.47 s	2
0.45 s	1
Torsade de pointes[†]	2
T wave alternans	1
Notched T wave in three leads	1
Low heart rate for age[‡]	0.5
Clinical history	
Syncope[†]	
With stress	2
Without stress	1
Congenital deafness	0.5
Family history	
Family members with LQTS[§]	1
Unexplained sudden cardiac death before age 30 among immediate family members[§]	0.5

*Findings in the absence of medications or disorders known to affect ECG findings. QTc calculated by Bazett's formula, in which QTc = QT/RR.
[†]Mutually exclusive.
[‡]Resting heart rate below the second percentile for age.
[§]The same family member cannot be counted for each of these criteria.
Scoring: 1 point or less=low probability of LQTS; 2–3 points=intermediate probability of LQTS; 4 points or higher=high probability of LQTS.

B. Causal Genes Implicated in Long QT Syndrome

Disease	Gene (alternate name)	Protein
LQT-1	KVLQT (KNCQ1)	l_{Ks} K+ channel α subunit
LQT-2	HERG (KCNH2)	l_{Kr} K+ channel α subunit
LQT-3	SCN5A	i_{Na} K+ channel α subunit
LQT-4	ANKB	ANKRIN-β
LQT-5	mink (KCNE1)	l_{Ks} K+ channel β subunit
LQT-6	MiRP1 (KCNE2)	l_{Kr} K+ channel β subunit
LQT-7	KCNJ2	i_{Kr} K+ channel α subunit

Figure 17-14.
A and **B**, Congenital long QT syndrome (LQTS). LQTS is a rare monogenic condition caused by mutations in one of several ion channel genes. Mutation carriers are at increased risk for polymorphic ventricular tachycardia or sudden cardiac death. Diagnostic criteria for the LQTS are presented in *panel A* and the genes implicated as causal are listed in *panel B*. (*Adapted from* Schwartz *et al.* [15] and Kass and Moss [16].)

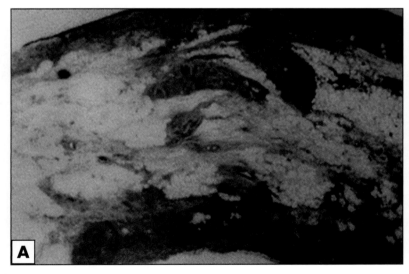

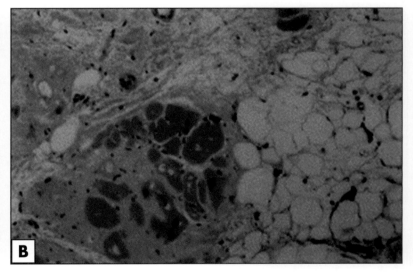

Figure 17-15.
Arrythmogenic right ventricular cardiomyopathy (ARVC). ARVC, also called *right ventricular dysplasia*, is a genetic disorder of heart muscle characterized by increased risk of sudden death and heart failure. Hemotoxylin and eosin stain under low (**A**) and high (**B**) power magnification reveals extensive replacement of the right ventricular myocardium by fibrofatty tissue. Mutations in cell adhesion protein genes, including desmoplakin and plakoglobin, have been linked to the etiology of ARVC. (*From* McKoy *et al.* [17]; with permission.)

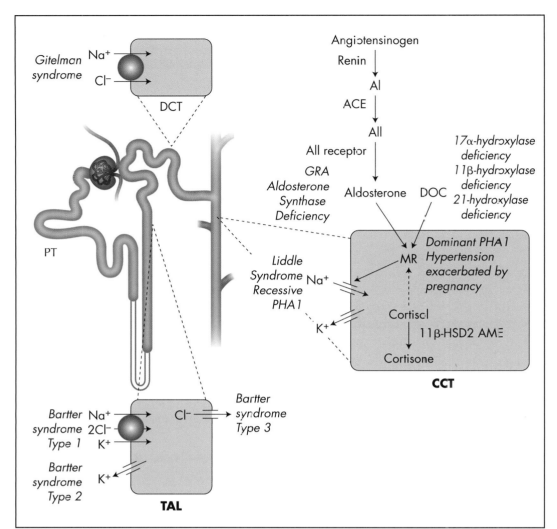

Figure 17-16.
Mendelian forms of hypertension. Multiple genes for monogenic forms of hypertension and hypotension have been identified. Almost all of the genes identified to date play a role in salt handling in the kidney. ACE—angiotensin-converting enzyme; AI—angiotensin I; AII—angiotensin II; AME—apparent mineralocorticoid excess; CCT—cortical collecting tubule; DCT—distal converting tubule; DOC—deoxycorticosterone; GRA—glucocorticoid-remediable aldosteronism; MR—mineralocorticoid receptor; PHA1—pseudohypoaldosteronism type-1; PT—proximal tubule; TAL—thick ascending limb of the loop of Henle. (*Adapted from* Lifton *et al.* [18].)

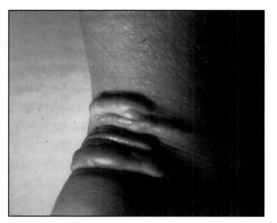

Figure 17-17.
Tendon xanthoma in familial hypercholesterolemia. Familial hypercholesterolemia is an autosomal dominant disorder of lipid metabolism. Mutations in the low-density lipoprotein receptor lead to marked elevations in blood serum cholesterol. Lipid deposits are localized to the tendons, skin, and eyelids. Lipid infiltration of the Achilles tendon is shown here.

Complex Cardiovascular Trait Genetics

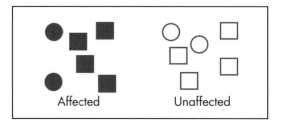

Figure 17-18.
Genetic association study. Genetic association studies seek to relate variation in human DNA sequence with a disease or trait. Compared with linkage analysis, the association study design provides greater power to detect common genetic variants conferring susceptibility to complex phenotypes such as atherosclerosis and myocardial infarction. In a case-control study, a common and convenient association study design, the frequency of a harmful genetic variant is expected to be greater among cases than controls (a protective variant is less frequent in cases). (*Adapted from* Lander and Schork [13].)

Candidate Gene Association Studies of Myocardial Infarction

Genetic variant	Variant type	Gene	Alleles	Risk allele or genotype	Phenotype	Summary odds ratio (95% CI)	Study
Glu298Asp	SNP	Endothelial nitric oxide synthase	Glu, Asp	Asp	Ischemic heart disease	1.31 (1.13–1.51)	Casas et al. [19]
ApoE	Two SNPs	Apolipoprotein E	ε2, ε3, ε4	ε4	Coronary heart disease	1.42 (1.26–1.61)	Song et al. [20]
PAI-1 4G/5G	Indel	Plaminogen activa-tor inhibitor-1	4G, 5G	4G/4G	Myocardial infarction	1.20 (1.04–1.39)	Boekholdt et al. [21]
ACE D/I	Indel	Angiotensin-convert-ing enzyme	D, I	D/D	Myocardial infarction	1.10 (1.00–1.21)	Keavney et al. [22]
Q192R	SNP	Paraoxonase-1	Q, R	R	Coronary heart disease	1.12 (1.07–1.16)	Wheeler et al. [23]
PIA2	SNP	Glyocprotein IIIa	A1, A2	A2	Coronary heart disease	1.10 (1.03–1.18)	Di Castelnuovo et al. [24]

Figure 17-19.

Candidate gene association studies of myocardial infarction. Thousands of studies have been performed relating one or a few genetic markers in a candidate gene, usually a single nucleotide polymorphism (SNP), with complex cardiovascular traits, such as myocardial infarction. Often, the frequency of the alleles is compared between cases with the trait and controls without the trait. Summarized here are results from several published meta-analyses or large overviews of specific genetic variants and the risk of cardiovascular disease. The results to date suggest that multiple gene variants with low to moderate relative risk effects are likely to underlie complex traits like myocardial infarction.

Assessing If A Genetic Association Is Real

Reasons for apparent significant association
  True-positive
    Variant is causal
    Variant is in linkage disequilibrium with causal variant
  False-positive
    False-positive related to multiple testing
    False-positive related to systematic genotyping error
    False-positive related to population stratification or other confounder
Reasons for lack of replication
  False-positive
    Original report is a false-positive
  False-negative
    Phenotypes differ across studies
    Study populations differ in genetic or environmental background
    Replication study is underpowered

Figure 17-20.

Assessing whether a reported genetic association is real. A central issue in the genetic association study literature has been the general lack of replication of associations reported to date [25]. A recent examination of 301 published studies of 25 different reported associations found that less than half of all the reported associations had strong evidence of replication [26]. False-positive reports, false-negative replication studies, or true variability in association among different populations may explain the inconsistency in the literature. However, in pooled analyses of all follow-up studies, eight of the associations yielded a significant replication of the initial report, with modest genetic effect sizes (with odds ratios generally between 1.1 and 2.0). Thus, despite the abundant false positive associations in the literature, many real associations lurk among the data.

Genome-wide Association Study

Screening cohort	Replication cohort
94 Japanese with MI	1133 Japanese with MI
658 control subjects free of MI	1006 control subjects free of MI
65,671 SNPs across the genome	849 SNPs tested
849 SNPs with $P < 0.01$	2 SNPs in lymphotoxin-α gene associated with MI

Figure 17-21.

Genome-wide association study design. A genome-wide association seeks to sift through single nucleotide polymorphism (SNP) variants throughout the genome in search of evidence for associations of specific SNPs to a phenotype. Of the approximately 10,000,000 SNPs in the genome, it is estimated that, in populations of European ancestry, 300,000 to 500,000 SNPs will capture the majority of the relevant information. This study by Ozaki et al. [27] exemplifies a pilot study of this more dense genome-wide SNP approach. Relevant study design components include a screening cohort, a large number of SNPs, cases with trait, controls without trait, and a replication cohort. MI—myocardial infarction. (Adapted from Ozaki et al. [27].)

Pharmacogenetics: Daily Dose of Warfarin in Relation to Cytochrome P 2C9 Genotype

	Genotype					
	*1/*1	*1/*2	*1/*3	*2/*2	*2/*3	*3/*3
Patients, *n* Daily maintenance dose of warfarin, *mg*	127	28	18	4	3	5
Mean (SD)	5.63 (2.56)	4.88 (2.57)	3.32 (0.94)	4.07 (1.48)	2.34 (0.35)	1.60 (0.81)
Median (IQR)	5.27 (3.93–7.14)	4.64 (3.61–5.29)	2.92 (2.50–3.93)	3.86 (2.50–4.00)	2.32 (2.00–2.70)	1.61 (1.14–1.96)

Figure 17-22.

Pharmacogenetics. Pharmacogenetics is the study of genetic variations and their relations to drug metabolism, drug safety, and drug efficacy. Warfarin is a commonly used drug in heart disease treatment and is metabolized by the liver enzyme cytochrome P2C9 (CYP2C9). Two genetic variants in the enzyme (*2 and *3) are related to decreased activity of the CYP2C9 enzyme. Because of the decreased CYP2C9 activity associated with the *2 and *3 alleles, individuals carrying the *2 and *3 alleles may be expected to metabolize warfarin slowly and,

consequently, need lower maintenance doses of warfarin. Higashi *et al.* [28] demonstrated this phenomenon in a study of 185 individuals treated in an anticoagulation clinic. Patients with two copies of the *3 allele had a mean prescribed daily warfarin dose of 1.60 mg compared with a maintenance dose of 5.63 mg in patients with two copies of the *1 allele. IQR—interquartile range; SD—standard deviation. (*Adapted from* Higashi *et al.* [28].)

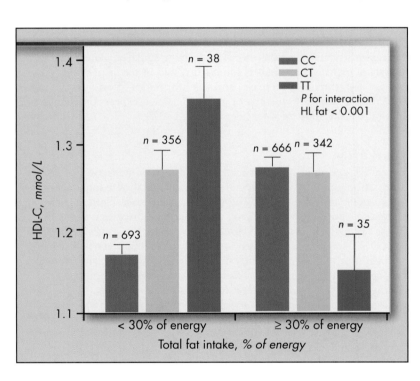

Figure 17-23.

Gene-environment interaction. Complex traits are related to the effects of multiple genes and environment. Gene-environment interaction studies seek to untangle the relationship between genetic variants and environmental exposures in influencing a phenotype. Illustrated here is an example of such an interaction involving cardiovascular risk factors. Ordovas *et al.* [29] studied the role of dietary fat in influencing the relations between a gene variant in the hepatic lipase gene and high-density lipoprotein cholesterol (HDL-C). They observed that the TT genotype was associated with higher HDL-C in the setting of low dietary fat intake (< 30% of energy), whereas the converse was true in the setting of high fat intake. Thus, genotyping this single nucleotide polymorphisms in populations with different fat intakes may yield diametrically opposite association study results. (*Adapted from* Ordovas *et al.* [29].)

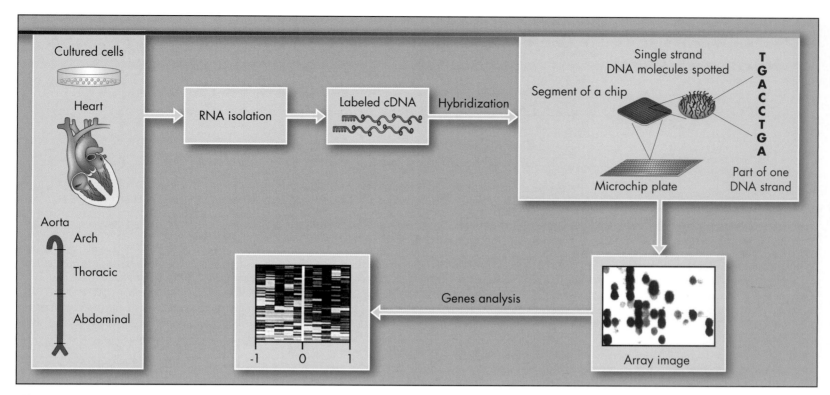

Figure 17-24.

Transcriptomics. Transcriptomics (also referred to as *gene expression profiling*) is the study of all cellular messenger RNA (mRNA) transcripts of an organism. This figure depicts the several stages involved in such experiments, including 1) preparation of relevant tissues; 2) isolation of mRNA; 3) reverse transcription of mRNA into complementary DNA (cDNA); 4) hybridization of cDNA onto a microchip; 5) detection of genes expressed by hybridization; and 6) software analysis of these expression signals into a list of up- and downregulated genes. The analysis of expression signals is often expressed in terms of "fold-change" (*eg*, threefold increase) and bioinformatics techniques are used to identify groups, or clusters, of genes for which expression change is simultaneous. (*Adapted from* Napoli *et al.* [30].)

Integrative Genomics and Bioinformatics

DNA	mRNA	Protein
Known and predicted genes in the LSFC candidate region	Mitochondria neighborhood analysis in four, large-scale expression sets	Tandem mass spectra from mitochondria proteomics

Figure 17-25.

Integrative genomics. Integrative genomics is the integration of global information about DNA, RNA, and protein/metabolite information for disease-gene identification. Using bioinformatics tools, large experimental data sets are jointly considered to aid in gene discovery. Recently, Mootha *et al.* [31] integrated three different types of genomic information (DNA sequences of known and predicted human genes, mRNA expression profiles from a wide range of cells and tissues, and tandem mass spectrometry data from a mitochondria proteomics project) to identify a specific candidate gene for a mendelian disorder, Leigh Syndrome French-Canadian variant (LSFC). They proceeded to experimentally show that the isolated candidate gene was responsible for the disorder. (*Adapted from* Mootha *et al.* [31].)

References

1. Zhang MQ: Computational prediction of eukaryotic protein-coding genes. *Nat Rev Genet* 2002, 3:698–709.

2. The International HapMap Consortium: The International HapMap Project. *Nature* 2003, 426:789–796.

3. Lander ES, Linton LM, Birren B, *et al.*: Initial sequencing and analysis of the human genome. *Nature* 2001, 409:860–921.

4. Venter JC, Adams MD, Myers EW, *et al.*: The sequence of the human genome. *Science* 2001, 291:1304–1351.

5. International Human Genome Sequencing Consortium: Finishing the euchromatic sequence of the human genome. *Nature* 2004, 431:931–945.

6. Mahaney MC, Blangero J, Comuzzie AG, *et al.*: Plasma HDL cholesterol, triglycerides, and adiposity. A quantitative genetic test of the conjoint trait hypothesis in the San Antonio Family Heart Study. *Circulation* 1995, 92:3240–3248.

7. Perusse L, Rice T, Despres JP, *et al.*: Familial resemblance of plasma lipids, lipoproteins and postheparin lipoprotein and hepatic lipases in the HERITAGE Family Study. *Arterioscler Thromb Vasc Biol* 1997, 17:3263–3269.

8. Levy D, DeStefano AL, Larson MG, *et al.*: Evidence for a gene influencing blood pressure on chromosome 17. Genome scan linkage results for longitudinal blood pressure phenotypes in subjects from the Framingham Heart Study. *Hypertension* 2000, 36:477–483.

9. Atwood LD, Heard-Costa NL, Cupples LA, *et al.*: Genomewide linkage analysis of body mass index across 28 years of the Framingham Heart Study. *Am J Hum Genet* 2002, 71:1044–1050.

10. Peyser PA, Bielak LF, Chu JS, *et al.*: Heritability of coronary artery calcium quantity measured by electron beam computed tomography in asymptomatic adults. *Circulation* 2002, 106:304–308.

11. O'Donnell CJ, Chazaro I, Wilson PW, *et al.*: Evidence for heritability of abdominal aortic calcific deposits in the Framingham Heart Study. *Circulation* 2002, 106:337–341.

12. Lloyd-Jones DM, Nam BH, D'Agostino RB Sr, *et al.*: Parental cardiovascular disease as a risk factor for cardiovascular disease in middle-aged adults: a prospective study of parents and offspring. *JAMA* 2004, 291:2204–2211.

13. Lander ES, Schork NJ: Genetic dissection of complex traits. *Science* 1994, 265:2037–2048.

14. Maron BJ: Hypertrophic cardiomyopathy: a systematic review. *JAMA* 2002, 287:1308–1320.

15. Schwartz PJ, Moss AJ, Vincent GM, *et al.*: Diagnostic criteria for the long QT syndrome: an update. *Circulation* 1993, 88:782–784.

16. Kass RS, Moss AJ: Long QT syndrome: novel insights into the mechanisms of cardiac arrhythmias. *J Clin Invest* 2003, 112:810–815.

17. McKoy G, Protonotarios N, Crosby A, *et al.*: Identification of a deletion in plakoglobin in arrhythmogenic right ventricular cardiomyopathy with palmoplantar keratoderma and woolly hair (Naxos disease). *Lancet* 2000, 355:2119–2124.

18. Lifton RP, Gharavi AG, Geller DS: Molecular mechanisms of human hypertension. *Cell* 2001, 104:545–556.

19. Casas JP, Bautista LE, Humphries SE, *et al.*: Endothelial nitric oxide synthase genotype and ischemic heart disease: meta-analysis of 26 studies involving 23028 subjects. *Circulation* 2004, 109:1359–1365.

20. Song Y, Stampfer MJ, Liu S: Meta-analysis: apolipoprotein E genotypes and risk for coronary heart disease. *Ann Intern Med* 2004, 141:137–147.

21. Boekholdt SM, Bijsterveld NR, Moons AH, *et al.*: Genetic variation in coagulation and fibrinolytic proteins and their relation with acute myocardial infarction: a systematic review. *Circulation* 2001, 104:3063–3068.

22. Keavney B, McKenzie C, Parish S, *et al.*: Large-scale test of hypothesised associations between the angiotensin-converting-enzyme insertion/deletion polymorphism and myocardial infarction in about 5000 cases and 6000 controls. International Studies of Infarct Survival (ISIS) Collaborators. *Lancet* 2000, 355:434–442.

23. Wheeler JG, Keavney BD, Watkins H, *et al.*: Four paraoxonase gene polymorphisms in 11212 cases of coronary heart disease and 12786 controls: meta-analysis of 43 studies. *Lancet* 2004, 363:689–695.

24. Di Castelnuovo A, de Gaetano G, Donati MB, *et al.*: Platelet glycoprotein receptor IIIa polymorphism PLA1/PLA2 and coronary risk: a meta-analysis. *Thromb Haemost* 2001, 85:626–633.

25. Kathiresan S, Newton-Cheh C, Gerszten RE: On the interpretation of genetic association studies. *Eur Heart J* 2004, 25:1378–1381.

26. Lohmueller KE, Pearce CL, Pike M, *et al.*: Meta-analysis of genetic association studies supports a contribution of common variants to susceptibility to common disease. *Nat Genet* 2003, 33:177–182.

27. Ozaki K, Ohnishi Y, Iida A, *et al.*: Functional SNPs in the lymphotoxin-alpha gene that are associated with susceptibility to myocardial infarction. *Nat Genet* 2002, 32:650–654.

28. Higashi MK, Veenstra DL, Kondo LM, *et al.*: Association between CYP2C9 genetic variants and anticoagulation-related outcomes during warfarin therapy. *JAMA* 2002, 287:1690–1698.

29. Ordovas JM, Corella D, Demissie S, *et al.*: Dietary fat intake determines the effect of a common polymorphism in the hepatic lipase gene promoter on high-density lipoprotein metabolism: evidence of a strong dose effect in this gene-nutrient interaction in the Framingham Study. *Circulation* 2002, 106:2315–2321.

30. Napoli C, Lerman LO, Sica V, *et al.*: Microarray analysis: a novel research tool for cardiovascular scientists and physicians. *Heart* 2003, 89:597–604.

31. Mootha VK, Lepage P, Miller K, *et al.*: Identification of a gene causing human cytochrome c oxidase deficiency by integrative genomics. *Proc Natl Acad Sci U S A* 2003, 100:605–610.

Aspirin in the Prevention of Heart Disease

Tobias Kurth, Julie E. Buring, and J. Michael Gaziano

Aspirin was first synthesized in the late 19th century and became the most widely used drug in the world in the 20th century. However, its potential to decrease risk of cardiovascular disease (CVD) has only been demonstrated during the past few decades [1].

In 1971 the Nobel Prize winning research of Sir John Vane [2] demonstrated that, in platelets, small amounts of aspirin (*ie*, 50–80 mg/day) irreversibly acetylate the active site of the isoenzyme cyclo-oxygenase (COX)-1, which is required for the production of thromboxane A2, a powerful promoter of platelet aggregation. This effect persists for the entire life of the platelet and is so pronounced that higher dosages of aspirin appear to yield no additional benefit.

The beneficial effects of aspirin in the secondary prevention of CVD and primary prevention of myocardial infarction (MI) have been conclusively demonstrated in numerous randomized trials and their meta-analyses [3–6]. The Antithrombotic Trialists' Collaboration reviewed, in their third meta-analyses, 287 trials including 194 that randomized 135,000 patients to antiplatelet therapy, particularly aspirin at various doses versus control, and 93 trials that randomized 77,000 patients to different antiplatelet regimens [5]. Overall, among high-risk patients for CVD, there was a highly significant reduction of approximately a quarter in the combined outcome of any serious vascular event among those assigned to antiplatelet therapy, particularly aspirin. This effect persisted in a wide range of patients at increased risk of occlusive vascular events, including those with previous MI, stroke or transient cerebral ischemia, unstable or stable angina, peripheral artery disease, or atrial fibrillation, as well as during acute MI or acute occlusive stroke.

In primary prevention, a meta-analysis included the six published primary prevention trials of aspirin, which randomized over 95,000 apparently healthy individuals [6]. Overall, aspirin was associated with a statistically significant reduction of 24% in the risk of first MI. However, there were no significant effects on nonfatal stroke or vascular death. In the randomized trials of secondary and primary prevention, the absolute access risk of hemorrhagic stroke is about 0.3 per 1000 [5].

The current recommendation from the United States Preventive Services Task Force (USP-STF) [7] states that aspirin is likely to have net benefits for apparently healthy individuals whose risk of a first coronary heart disease event is sufficiently high (6% or greater risk over 10 years). The American Heart Association recommends aspirin for all apparently healthy individuals with a 10% or greater risk of a first coronary heart disease event [8].

Milestones for Aspirin	
Date	**Milestone**
5th Century BC	Hippocrates
1897	Felix Hoffmann/Friedrich Bayer
1970	Sir John Vane
2000	Most widely used drug in the world

Figure 18-1.
Milestones for aspirin. The history of aspirin dates to the fifth century BC, when Hippocrates discovered that an extract of white willow bark had analgesic properties. The painkilling effect was the result of salicin, a naturally occurring chemical in willow bark, which is closely related to acetylsalicylic acid, the synthetic aspirin available today. Aspirin was synthesized in 1897, but it is only over the past few decades that attention has focused on the potential role of aspirin in reducing the risks of occlusive vascular disease.

Aspirin Daily Dose	
Dose	**Type**
40–150 mg	Antiplatelet
> 325 mg	Antipyretic; analgesic
> 3000 mg	Anti-inflammatory

Figure 18-2.
Aspirin daily dose. The dose of aspirin seems to determine its physiologic effects. At doses as low as 30–40 mg, platelet function is affected. To achieve an analgesic or antipyretic effect, doses of 325 mg or more are required. Much higher daily doses are necessary to achieve a sustained anti-inflammatory effect.

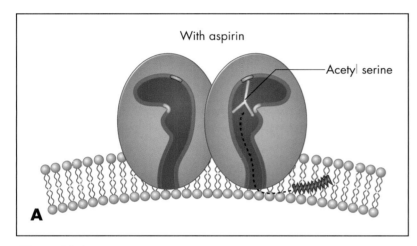

Figure 18-3.
A and **B**, Findings from basic research demonstrate that, in platelets, small amounts of aspirin (*ie*, 50–80 mg/day) irreversibly acetylate the active site of the isoenzyme cyclo-oxygenase-1 (COX-1) [9], which is required for the production of thromboxane A_2 [10], a powerful promoter of aggregation [2]. This effect persists for the entire life of the platelet (approximately 10–12 days) and is so pronounced that higher dosages of aspirin appear to yield no additional benefit. The basic research findings raise the possibility that less than daily frequency of administration (*eg*, alternate-day dosing) may be as effective as a daily regimen, whereas more frequent dosing may, in theory, compromise the favorable effects of aspirin by activating reversible vessel wall enzymes.

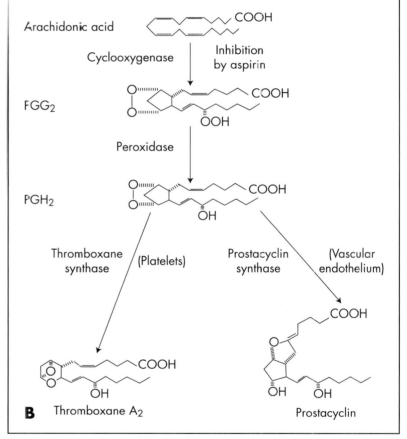

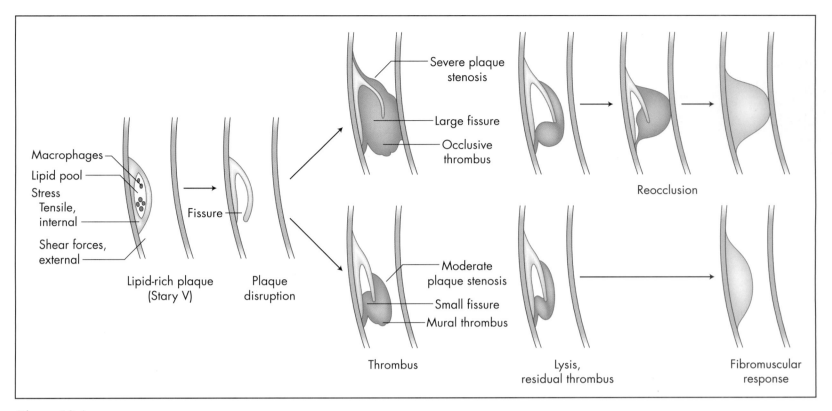

Figure 18-4.

Mechanisms of coronary thrombosis. The hypothesized mechanism for aspirin's benefit derives from its ability to decrease platelet aggregation and thereby reduce the risk of thrombotic vascular events. The disruption of platelet- and fibrin-rich atherosclerotic plaque may lead to aggressive platelet deposition and, ultimately, to the formation of a thrombus, which can precipitate an acute clinical event. (*Adapted from* Fuster *et al.* [11].)

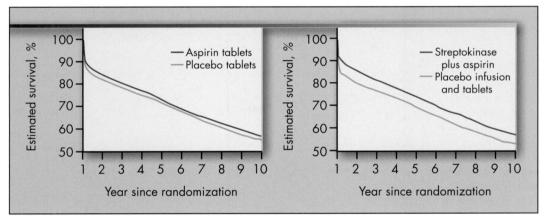

Figure 18-5.

Estimate of 10-year survival with aspirin. The second International Study of Infarct Survival (ISIS-2) was a two-by-two randomized, double-blind trial of aspirin versus placebo and streptokinase versus placebo in patients with acute myocardial infarction (AMI) [12]. Aspirin was given in a dose of 162.5 mg immediately (with the first tablet crushed or chewed), followed by 162.5 mg daily for approximately 1 month. Overall, 17,187 patients with suspected AMI presenting within 24 hours of symptom onset were randomized. There was a 23% reduction in vascular mortality at 1 month with aspirin versus placebo (804/8587 [9.4%] vs 1016/8600 [11.8%], relative risk 0.77, $P < 0.00001$). This reduction represents the avoidance of about 25 early deaths for every 1000 patients with AMI who are treated with aspirin for 1 month. The benefits at 1 month were maintained through 10 years of follow-up [13]. Further, there were additional reductions with aspirin reinfarction.

These reductions translate into the avoidance of about 25 deaths and 10 to 15 nonfatal reinfarctions and strokes. The benefits of aspirin in ISIS-2 were similar irrespective of the delay from symptom onset to the start of treatment, indicating that aspirin should be given to all patients with acute MI, even if they present late after the onset of symptoms. The benefits of aspirin were additive to the benefit of fibrinolysis with streptokinase, which itself reduced mortality by one quarter (9.2% vs 12.0%, relative risk 0.75, $P < 0.00001$). Thus in patients receiving aspirin and streptokinase versus neither agent, there was an impressive 42% reduction in vascular death ($P < 0.0001$). In ISIS-2, the incidence of major bleeding (*ie*, bleeds requiring transfusion) occurred with a similar frequency in the aspirin and placebo groups (0.4% vs 0.4%), and there was no significant excess in cerebral hemorrhage with aspirin. (*Adapted from* Baigent *et al.* [13].)

Antithrombotic Trialists' Collaborations

Publication year	Trials, n	Total subjects, n
1988	25	29,000
1994	145	51,000 subjects with prior disease; 28,000 low-risk subjects
2002	287	136,000 aspirin vs placebo

Figure 18-6.
Antithrombotic Trialists' Collaborations. Over the past three decades, several hundred trials of antiplatelet agents in secondary prevention have been conducted. These included trials of aspirin and other antiplatelet agents (alone or in combination) versus placebo and trials of antiplatelet agents (alone or in combination) versus other agents. The trials were conducted among a wide range of patients at high risk of occlusive vascular events. To this end, the Antiplatelet Trialists' Collaboration, whose investigators have directed randomized trials of antiplatelet therapy worldwide, conducted meta-analyses in 1988, 1994, and 2002.

Antithrombotic Trialists' Collaborative: 1988

25% reduction in vascular events
32% reduction in nonfatal MI
27% reduction in nonfatal stroke
15% reduction in vascular mortality

Figure 18-7.
Antithrombotic Trialists' Collaborative: 1988. In 1988, the first meta-analysis was conducted on 25 completed trials of antiplatelet therapy among individuals with a history of cardiovascular disease [3]. This overview included the results of the 10 completed trials among approximately 18,000 post–myocardial infarction (MI) patients [13], completed trials among approximately 9000 patients with prior cerebrovascular disease (stroke or transient ischemic attack [TIA]), and two trials among approximately 2000 patients with unstable angina.

When all 25 secondary prevention trials were considered together, antiplatelet therapy was associated with statistically significant reductions of 32% in nonfatal MI (standard deviation [SD] = 5%), 27% in nonfatal stroke (SD = 6%), 15% in total vascular mortality (SD = 4%), and 25% (SD = 3%) in the combined endpoint of important vascular events (a composite outcome that comprised nonfatal MI, nonfatal stroke, and vascular mortality). There was no apparent effect of antiplatelet treatment on nonvascular death. Therefore, the statistically significant ($P = 0.0003$) benefit observed on total mortality was largely explained by the significant reduction in vascular death.

Antithrombotic Trialists' Collaboration: 1994

Gender*	Subjects, n	Vascular events prevented/1000 patients treated for 1 year
Men	40,000	37
Women	10,000	33

*29 trials provided data separated by gender

Figure 18-8.
Antithrombotic Trialists' Collaborative: 1994. In 1994, an updated meta-analysis was published that included subsequently completed trials among a broader range of patients with prior manifestations of vascular disease (eg, prior coronary revascularization, peripheral vascular disease, atrial fibrillation) [4]. This overview included a total of 145 trials of antiplatelet therapy among 51,144 patients with prior vascular disease and about 28,000 low-risk subjects in primary prevention trials.

The findings among patients with prior myocardial infarction, stroke, transient ischemic attack, and unstable angina were similar to the 1988 overview. The 1994 meta-analysis also provided reliable data that antiplatelet treatment in high-risk patients produces vascular event reductions of similar size in various patient subgroups. Specifically, separate data for men and women were available from 29 trials conducted among approximately 40,000 men and 10,000 women. There were comparable benefits on vascular events, with reductions per 1000 patients treated of 37 events for men (standard deviation = 4; $P < 0.00001$) and 33 events for women (standard deviation = 7; $P < 0.0001$). The data from these 29 trials also demonstrate similar reductions in vascular events for middle-aged and older patients, for hypertensive and normotensive groups, and for diabetic and nondiabetic persons.

Antithrombotic Trialists' Collaboration: 2002

Objective:
 To determine the effects of antiplatelet therapy among patients at high risk of occlusive vascular events
Data reviewed:
 287 studies involving:
  135,000 patients in comparisons of antiplatelet therapy vs control
  77,000 patients in comparisons of different antiplatelet regimens
Main outcome measure:
 Serious vascular event; nonfatal myocardial infarction, nonfatal stroke, or vascular death

Figure 18-9.
Antithrombotic Trialists' Collaborative: 2002. In 2002, the Antithrombotic Trialists' Collaboration published its third major meta-analysis [5]. This meta-analysis included all new trials through September 1997 among high-risk patients, which included additional trials of aspirin at various doses, other antiplatelet drugs, the combination of aspirin with other antiplatelet drugs with a different mechanism of action, and the addition of anticoagulants to antiplatelet drugs. This meta-analysis included data from 287 studies involving 135,640 patients at high risk of occlusive arterial disease of antiplatelet therapy, and 77,000 patients in comparison of different antiplatelet regimes.

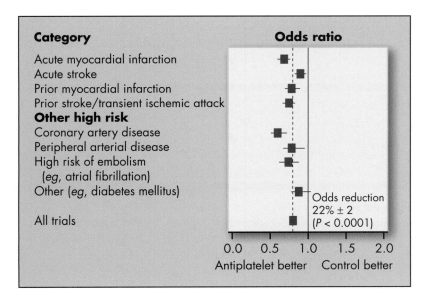

Category	Odds ratio
Acute myocardial infarction	
Acute stroke	
Prior myocardial infarction	
Prior stroke/transient ischemic attack	
Other high risk	
Coronary artery disease	
Peripheral arterial disease	
High risk of embolism (eg, atrial fibrillation)	
Other (eg, diabetes mellitus)	
All trials	Odds reduction 22% ± 2 (P < 0.0001)

0.0   0.5   1.0   1.5   2.0
Antiplatelet better   Control better

Figure 18-10.
Antithrombotic Trialists' Collaborative 2002: effect of antiplatelet therapy on vascular events. Overall, among these high-risk patients, there was a highly significant reduction in the proportion of the combined outcome of any serious vascular event among patients assigned to antiplatelet therapy compared with those assigned to the control group (10.7% vs 13.2%, P < 0.0001). Antiplatelet therapy was protective in most types of patients at increased risk of occlusive vascular events, including those with an acute myocardial infarction or ischemic stroke, unstable or stable angina, previous myocardial infarction, stroke or cerebral ischemia, peripheral artery disease, or atrial fibrillation. (*Adapted from* Antithrombotic Trialists' Collaboration [5].)

Antithrombotic Trialists' Collaboration: 2002

Event	Percentage	Result	P Value
Nonfatal MI	34	Reduction	< 0.0001
Total CHD	26	Reduction	< 0.0001
Nonfatal stroke	25	Reduction	< 0.0001
Total ischemic stroke	30	Reduction	< 0.0001
Total hemorrhagic stroke	22	Increase	< 0.01
Fatal or nonfatal pulmonary embolism	25	Reduction	< 0.01
Vascular death	15	Reduction	< 0.0001

Figure 18-11.
Antithrombotic Trialists' Collaborative: 2002. With respect to specific outcomes, antiplatelet therapy was associated with a 34% proportional reduction in nonfatal myocardial infarction ([MI] P < 0.0001), a 26% reduction in nonfatal MI or fatal coronary heart disease (P < 0.0001), and a 25% reduction in nonfatal stroke (P < 0.0001). When strokes were classified by type, antiplatelet treatment was associated with a 30% decrease in total ischemic stroke (P < 0.0001) and a 22% increase in total hemorrhagic stroke (P < 0.01). Antiplatelet therapy also reduced the risk of fatal or nonfatal pulmonary embolism by 25% (P < 0.01). In addition, there was a highly significant 15% proportional reduction in vascular death. CHD—coronary heart disease. (*Adapted from* Antithrombotic Trialists' Collaboration [5].)

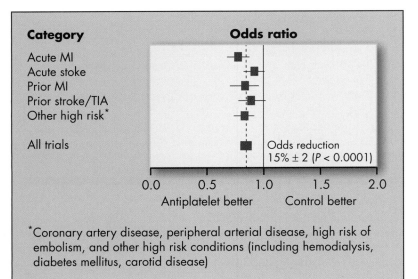

Category	Odds ratio
Acute MI	
Acute stoke	
Prior MI	
Prior stroke/TIA	
Other high risk*	
All trials	Odds reduction 15% ± 2 (P < 0.0001)

0.0   0.5   1.0   1.5   2.0
Antiplatelet better   Control better

*Coronary artery disease, peripheral arterial disease, high risk of embolism, and other high risk conditions (including hemodialysis, diabetes mellitus, carotid disease)

Figure 18-12.
Antithrombotic Trialists' Collaborative 2002: reduction of risk in vascular events. The magnitude of the overall treatment effect on serious vascular events varied across the five categories of high-risk patients studied (previous myocardial infarction [MI], acute MI, previous stroke/transient ischemic attack, acute stroke, and other high risk) and ranged from a proportional reduction of 11% (standard error [SE] = 4%) for patients with acute stroke to 30% (SE = 4%) in patients with acute MI. Overall, there was a 22% reduction (SE = 2%). The heterogeneity was related primarily to the somewhat smaller (but still significant) reduction in risk of serious vascular events among patients treated for acute stroke. TIA—transient ischemic attack. (*Adapted from* Antithrombotic Trialists' Collaboration [5].)

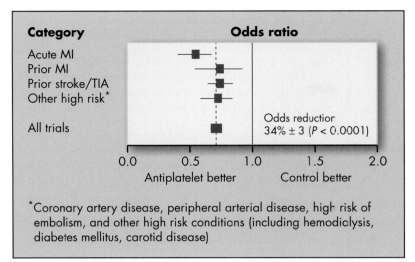

Figure 18-13.

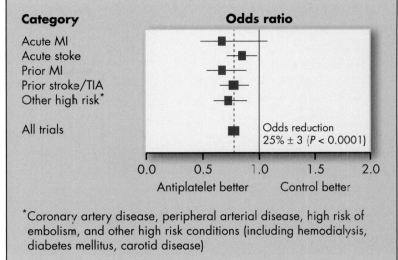

Figure 18-14.

Figure 18-13.
Antithrombotic Trialists' Collaborative 2002: reduction of risk in nonfatal myocardial infarction. The overall reductions in myocardial infarction were apparent in all groups. There was a suggestion of a strong effect among those in the throws of an acute myocardial infarction. MI—myocardial infarction; TIA—transient ischemic attack. (*Adapted from* Antithrombotic Trialists' Collaboration [5].)

Figure 18-14.
Antithrombotic Trialists' Collaborative 2002: reduction of risk in nonfatal stroke. Nonfatal stroke rates were also reduced in all groups treated with aspirin compared with placebo. (*Adapted from* Antithrombotic Trialists' Collaboration [5].)

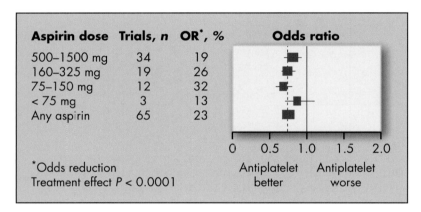

Figure 18-15.
Efficacy of aspirin doses on vascular events in high-risk patients. With respect to dose, daily aspirin doses of 75 to 150 mg appeared to confer the same level of cardioprotective benefit as did larger doses. Indirect comparisons using data from trials testing a particular aspirin dose versus no aspirin estimated a proportional reduction in serious vascular events of 19% (standard error [SE] = 3%) for dosages of 500 to 1500 mg/day, 26% (SE = 3%) for dosages of 160 to 325 mg/day, and 32% (SE = 6%) for dosages of 75 to 150 mg/day. Dosages below 75 mg/day had a somewhat smaller effect (13% [SE = 8%]). However, a combined analysis of the three trials that directly compared doses of 75 mg/day or greater with dosages less than 75 mg/day found no significant difference in efficacy. Therefore, more data are needed to determine conclusively whether doses of less than 75 mg/day offer as comparable a protection against vascular events as dosages exceeding that amount. OR—odds ratio. (*Adapted from* Antithrombotic Trialists' Collaboration [5].)

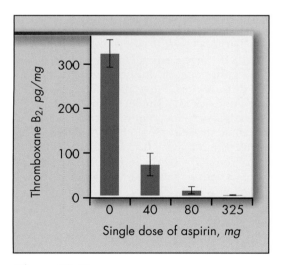

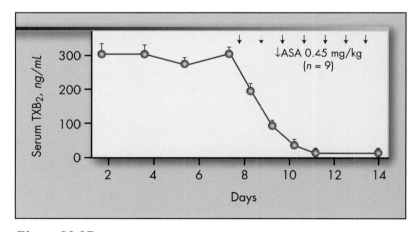

Figure 18-16.
Effect of aspirin on thromboxane A_2 biosynthesis on platelets. When given as a single dose, maximal inhibition of thromboxane A_2 is achieved at a dose of 325 mg.

Figure 18-17.
Accumulation of effect of low-dose aspirin on platelet cyclo-oxygenase. When given as a daily dose, much smaller doses of aspirin are required to achieve maximal platelet inhibition, but this was not achieved for several days. For this reason, in a patient with acute myocardial infarction in whom the effect is needed in a short time, a full dose of 325 mg should be given. However, among those who are taking aspirin daily, the Antithrombotic Trialists' Collaborations together with this physiologic data suggest that doses of 75 to 150 mg per day will result in maximal benefit.

Aspirin in the Prevention of Heart Disease

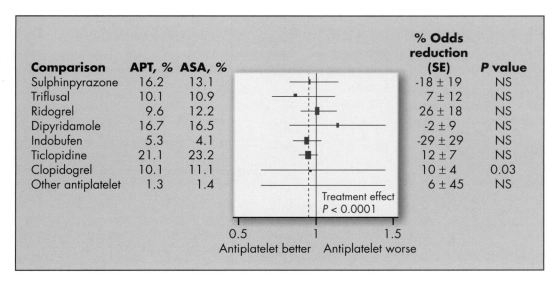

Comparison	APT, %	ASA, %	% Odds reduction (SE)	P value
Sulphinpyrazone	16.2	13.1	-18 ± 19	NS
Triflusal	10.1	10.9	7 ± 12	NS
Ridogrel	9.6	12.2	26 ± 18	NS
Dipyridamole	16.7	16.5	-2 ± 9	NS
Indobufen	5.3	4.1	-29 ± 29	NS
Ticlopidine	21.1	23.2	12 ± 7	NS
Clopidogrel	10.1	11.1	10 ± 4	0.03
Other antiplatelet	1.3	1.4	6 ± 45	NS

Treatment effect P < 0.0001

0.5   1   1.5

Antiplatelet better   Antiplatelet worse

Figure 18-18.
Antithrombotic Trialists' Collaborative: other antiplatelet (APT) drugs versus aspirin (ASA). The 2002 Antithrombotic Trialists' Collaboration directly compared data from three trials of dipyridamole and ASA and found no difference between the two agents with respect to vascular events. An indirect comparison yielded similar proportional reductions of dipyridamole and 75 mg aspirin when compared with placebo [5]. NS—not significant. (*Adapted from* Antithrombotic Trialists' Collaboration [5].)

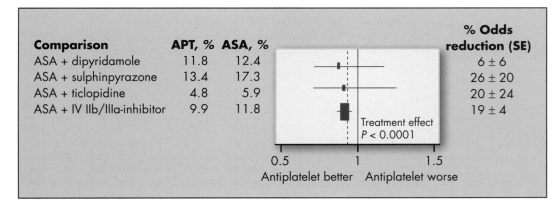

Comparison	APT, %	ASA, %	% Odds reduction (SE)
ASA + dipyridamole	11.8	12.4	6 ± 6
ASA + sulphinpyrazone	13.4	17.3	26 ± 20
ASA + ticlopidine	4.8	5.9	20 ± 24
ASA + IV IIb/IIIa-inhibitor	9.9	11.8	19 ± 4

Treatment effect P < 0.0001

0.5   1   1.5

Antiplatelet better   Antiplatelet worse

Figure 18-19.
Antithrombotic Trialists' Collaborative: aspirin (ASA) plus another antiplatelet therapy (APT) versus ASA alone. The addition of dipyridamole to ASA has not been clearly shown to produce additional reductions in serious vascular events. With respect to ticlopidine versus ASA, the 2002 Antithrombotic Trialists' Collaboration meta-analysis found a nonsignificant proportional reduction in serious vascular events of 12% (standard error = 7%) [5]. (*Adapted from* Antithrombotic Trialists' Collaboration [5].)

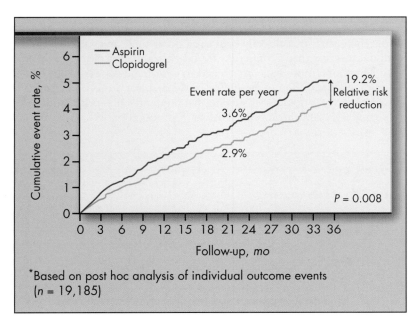

*Based on post hoc analysis of individual outcome events (n = 19,185)

Figure 18-20.
Primary endpoint: myocardial infarction, stroke, or cardiovascular death. The thienopyridine derivatives clopidogrel and ticlopidine are antiplatelet agents that inhibit the platelet aggregation induced by adenosine diphosphate—dependent activation of the platelet glycoprotein IIb/IIIa complex. Thus, these agents have a different action on platelets than aspirin (ASA), and combining one of these agents with ASA, which blocks the thromboxane-mediated pathway, may have an additive effect. However, initial trials examined the thienopyridines against ASA, not in combination. Most importantly, a large-scale randomized secondary prevention trial comparing clopidogrel versus ASA alone has been reported by the Clopidogrel Versus Aspirin in Patients at Risk of Ischemic Events (CAPRIE) investigators [14]. A total of 19,185 patients with atherosclerotic vascular disease were randomized to clopidogrel (75 mg/day) or to ASA (325 mg/day). As compared with ASA alone, clopidogrel alone was associated with an 8.7% reduction in the annual risk of the composite endpoint of vascular death, myocardial infarction, or ischemic stroke (5.3 vs 5.8%; *P* = 0.043). The reduction of events in patients with MI was 5.03% in the clopidogrel group and 4.84% in the ASA group (*P* = 0.66). In CAPRIE, the benefit was most prominent for patients with peripheral arterial disease. (*Adapted from* CAPRIE [14].)

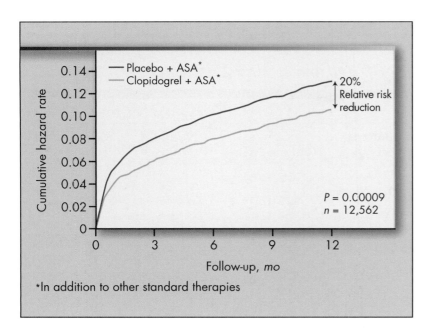

*In addition to other standard therapies

Figure 18-21.

Risk reduction in myocardial infarction outcome events: fatal and nonfatal. The effect of clopidogrel plus aspirin versus placebo plus aspirin was tested in the Clopidogrel in Unstable Angina to Prevent Recurrent Events (CURE I) trial [15]. In this multicenter trial, 12,562 patients with acute coronary syndrome without ST-segment elevation were randomized to receive clopidogrel (300 mg immediately, followed by 75 mg once daily) or placebo in addition to aspirin (daily recommended dose of 75–300 mg) for 3 to 12 months. Compared with the combination of aspirin and placebo, the combination of active clopidogrel and aspirin was associated with a statistically significant 20% reduction (relative risk [RR] = 0.80; 95% CI 0.72–0.90; $P < 0.001$) of death from cardiovascular causes, nonfatal myocardial infarction, or stroke. However, major bleeding complications were significantly more common in the clopidogrel plus aspirin group as compared with the aspirin and placebo group (RR = 1.38; 95% CI 1.13–1.67; $P < 0.001$). (*Adapted from* CURE I [15].)

Any Important Vascular Event and Vascular Death from Five Randomized Trials of Aspirin in Primary Prevention of Cardiovascular Disease

	Aspirin			Control		
Trial	Any important vascular event, *n*	Vascular death, *n*	Subjects, *n*	Any important vascular event, *n*	Vascular death, *n*	Subjects, *n*
PHS	307	81	11,037	370	83	11,034
BDT	289	148	3429	147	79	1710
TPT	228	101	2545	260	81	2540
HOT	315	133	9399	368	140	9391
PPP	47	17	2226	71	31	2269
Total	1186	480	28,636	1216	414	26,944
Statistical analysis						
Relative risk	0.85	0.98				
95% CI	0.79–0.93	0.85–1.12				

Figure 18-22.

Aspirin for the primary prevention of cardiovascular events: meta-analysis. The data discussed in the previous sections do not address the role of aspirin in the primary prevention of cardiovascular disease (CVD) among individuals at usual risk. In primary prevention, the benefit-risk ratio for aspirin must be even more carefully weighed than in secondary prevention settings. Any agent that inhibits platelet aggregation may pose a risk of increased bleeding. Although these risks may be deemed acceptable for those at high risk of a CVD event because of acute myocardial infarction or other CVD history, they must be carefully weighed against the likely benefits for those at lower baseline risk of occlusive vascular events. The dosage of aspirin must also be carefully considered; although the benefits on CVD appear comparable over the wide dose range tested in trials to date, the major side effects of the drug are dose-dependent [15]. The goal for primary prevention is to choose the lowest dosage of aspirin that has a cardioprotective effect while minimizing side effects.

Aspirin has been evaluated in five completed primary prevention trials. The British Doctors' Trial (BDT) trial was conducted among 5139 apparently healthy male physicians aged 50 to 78 years in Great Britain [16]. The Physicians' Health Study (PHS) was a randomized, double-blind, placebo-controlled trial of 325 mg of aspirin on alternate days (as well as 50 mg of beta-carotene on alternate days) conducted among 22,071 apparently healthy US male physicians, 40 to 84 years of age [17].

The Thrombosis Prevention Trial (TPT) used a factorial design to randomize 5085 men aged 45 to 69 years who were at elevated risk for ischemic heart disease based on a risk score that included family history, smoking history, body mass index, blood pressure, cholesterol, plasma fibrinogen, and plasma factor VII activity, to low-dose aspirin (75 mg/day), warfarin (target International Normalized Ratio = 1.5), both agents, or placebo [18].

In the 26-country Hypertension Optimal Treatment (HOT) trial, 18,790 persons (47% of whom were women) with elevated diastolic blood pressure (between 100 and 115 mm Hg) were randomly assigned to one of three target diastolic blood pressure ranges (80, 85, and 90 mm Hg or less) and to controlled-release aspirin (75 mg/day) or placebo [19].

The Primary Prevention Project (PPP) trial was a randomized, open-label two-by-two factorial trial of enteric-coated, low-dose aspirin (100 mg/day) and vitamin E in 4495 individuals (58% women) 50 years or older who had one or more cardiovascular risk factors [20].

Despite design differences between the primary prevention trials, five of the six trials have been generally consistent in showing that aspirin therapy reduces the incidence of first coronary heart disease. (*Adapted from* Eidelman *et al.* [21].)

Nonfatal Myocardial Infarction and Nonfatal Stroke: Five Randomized Trials of Aspirin in Primary Prevention of Cardiovascular Disease

	Aspirin			Control		
Trial	Nonfatal MI, n	Nonfatal stroke, n	Randomized subjects, n	Nonfatal MI, n	Nonfatal stroke, n	Randomized subjects, n
PHS	129	110	11,037	213	92	11,034
BDT	80	61	3429*	41	27	1710*
TPT	94	33	2545	137	42	2540
HOT	NA	NA	NA	NA	NA	NA
PPP	15	15	2226	22	18	2269
Total	318	219	19,237	413	179	17,553
Statistical analysis						
Relative risk	0.68	1.06				
95% CI	0.59–0.79	0.87–1.29				

*A two-to-one randomization of aspirin to control was used

Figure 18-23.

Nonfatal myocardial infarction (MI) and stroke in trials of aspirin for primary prevention. A recent update on the role of aspirin in primary prevention of cardiovascular disease took all five primary prevention trials into account [21]. Among the 55,580 randomized participants, aspirin was associated with a statistically significant 32% (relative risk = 0.68, 95% CI 0.59–0.79) reduction in the risk of first MI and a significant 15% (relative risk = 0.85, 95% CI 0.79–0.93) reduction in the risk of all important vascular events. BDT—British Doctors' Trial; HOT—Hypertension Optimal Treatment trial; NA—no data available; PHS—Physicians' Health Study; PPP—Primary Prevention Project; TPT—Thrombosis Prevention Trial. (*Adapted from* Eidelman *et al.* [21].)

Ischemic Versus Hemorrhagic Stroke (Fatal and Nonfatal): Five Randomized Trials of Aspirin in Primary Prevention of Cardiovascular Disease

	Aspirin			Control		
Trial	Ischemic stroke, n	Hemorrhagic stroke, n	Randomized subjects, n	Ischemic stroke, n	Hemorrhagic stroke, n	Randomized subjects, n
PHS	91	23	11,037	82	12	11,034
BDT	21	13	3429*	7	6	1710*
TPT	21	12	2545	33	6	2540
HOT	NA	NA	NA	NA	NA	NA
PPP	14	2	2226	21	3	2269
Total	147	50	19,237	141	27	17,553
Statistical analysis						
Relative risk	0.97	1.56				
95% CI	0.77–1.22	0.99–2.46				

*A two-to-one randomization of aspirin to control was used

Figure 18-24.

Ischemic and hemorrhagic stroke in trials of aspirin in primary prevention. However, there were no significant effects on nonfatal stroke or vascular death. With respect to hemorrhagic stroke, although based on small numbers of events, there was a 56% increase, which was of borderline statistical significance (relative risk = 1.56, 95% CI 0.99–2.46).

Additional data from primary prevention trials are needed for the complete assessment of aspirin's benefit-risk ratio in apparently healthy persons. None of these trials had an adequate number of women to evaluate the role of aspirin in this group. The primary concern in extrapolating findings to women from trial data in men is that the benefit-risk ratio for prophylactic aspirin use in women may differ from that in men. Women's risk of myocardial infarction, the principal outcome that aspirin may prevent, is lower at almost all ages than men's risk, whereas women and men have roughly comparable rates of stroke, the hemorrhagic forms of which may be increased by aspirin. Gender-specific subgroup analyses of data from the Hypertension Optimal Treatment trial among hypertensive individuals suggested that women may not benefit from aspirin therapy to the same degree as their male counterparts [22]. In women, aspirin was associated with a non-significant 19% reduction in myocardial infarction incidence (relative risk = 0.81, 95% CI 0.49–1.31; 1.7 vs 2.1 events per 1000 person-years of observation), whereas in men, a highly significant 42% reduction was achieved (relative risk = 0.58, 95% CI 0.41–0.81; 2.9 vs 5.0 events per 1000 person-years of observation). Gender differences in the effect of aspirin were not found for stroke or total mortality, however. Gender-stratified analyses were not provided in the Primary Prevention Project trial, the only other completed primary prevention trial that included women. BDT—British Doctors' Trial; HOT—Hypertension Optimal Treatment trial; NA—no data available; PHS—Physicians' Health Study; PPP—Primary Prevention Project; TPT—Thrombosis Prevention Trial. (*Adapted from* Eidelman *et al.* [21].)

Incidence and Relative Risk of Confirmed Cardiovascular Endpoints in the WHS

Endpoint	Events, n		Relative risk (95% CI)	P value
	Aspirin (n = 19,934)	Placebo (n = 19,942)		
Major cardiovascular event*	477	522	0.91 (0.80–1.03)	0.13
Stroke	221	266	0.83 (0.69–0.99)	0.04
Ischemic	170	221	0.76 (0.63–0.93)	0.009
Hemorrhagic	51	41	1.24 (0.82–1.87)	0.31
Fatal	23	22	1.04 (0.58–1.86)	0.90
Nonfatal	198	244	0.81 (0.67–0.97)	0.02
Myocardial infarction	198	193	1.02 (0.84–1.25)	0.83
Fatal	14	12	1.16 (0.54–2.51)	0.70
Nonfatal	184	181	1.01 (0.83–1.24)	0.90
Death from cardiovascular causes	120	126	0.95 (0.74–1.22)	0.68
Transient ischemic attack	186	238	0.78 (0.64–0.94)	0.01
Coronary revascularization	389	374	1.04 (0.90–1.20)	0.61
Death from any cause	609	642	0.95 (0.85–1.06)	0.32

*A major cardiovascular event was defined as a nonfatal myocardial infarction, a nonfatal stroke, or death from cardiovascular causes

Figure 18-25.
Findings from the Women's Health Study (WHS). The WHS is a recently completed two-by-two factorial, randomized placebo-controlled trial testing the balance of risks and benefits of low-dose aspirin (100 mg every other day) and vitamin E (600 IU every other day) in the primary prevention of cardiovascular disease and cancer. The trial included a total of 39,876 apparently healthy female health professionals without history of cardiovascular disease or cancer. After a mean follow-up of 10.1 years, 477 major cardiovascular events were confirmed in the aspirin group, as compared with 522 in the placebo group, a nonsignificant 9% reduction [6]. With regard to the individual cardiovascular endpoints, there was a statistically significant 17% reduction in the risk of total stroke, a 24% reduction of ischemic stroke, but no effect on myocardial infarction or vascular death. There was a nonsignificant increase in the risk of hemorrhagic stroke of 24%, but the absolute numbers were small. In subgroup analyses, women aged 65 years or older had statistically significant reductions in major cardiovascular events, stroke, ischemic stroke, and myocardial infarction. With regard to severe side effects, there were significantly more gastrointestinal bleeds that required transfusion (127 in the aspirin and 91 in the placebo group; P = 0.02). Reports of hematuria, easy bruising, and epistaxis were also more frequent in the aspirin than the placebo group.

When the results of the WHS were added to the meta-analysis by Eidelman et al. [21], there was a 24% reduction in the risk of myocardial infarction (relative risk = 0.76; 95% CI, 0.62–0.95; P = 0.01), but no significant effect on the risk of stroke among the 95,456 randomized participants [6]. In analyses stratified by gender, combined data on women from the WHS, Hypertension Optimal Treatment trial [22], and Primary Prevention Project indicated that aspirin therapy was associated with a significant 19% reduction in the risk of stroke with no reduction in the risk of myocardial infarction. The combined data for men from the Physicians' Health Study, British Doctors' Trial, Thrombosis Prevention Trial, Hypertension Optimal Treatment trial, and Primary Prevention Project indicated a 32% reduction in the risk of myocardial infarction but no significant effect on stroke [6].

Nonsteroidal Anti-inflammatory Drugs

Nonselective NSAIDs, like aspirin, inhibit cyclo-oxygenase-1 (COX-1), but they bind reversibly, leading to impaired platelet function only during their dosing interval

Aspirin and other NSAIDs share a common docking site on COX-1

This raises the possibility of a competitive interaction between aspirin and other NSAIDs afforded by these structural relations

A crossover study in healthy subjects by Catella-Lawson et al. [34], reported that concomitant administration of aspirin and ibuprofen (an NSAID) antagonizes the irreversible platelet inhibition induced by aspirin

Figure 18-26.
Nonselective, nonaspirin, nonsteroidal anti-inflammatory drugs (NSAIDs), such as ibuprofen or naproxen, as well as other drugs, such as sulfinpyrazone, also inhibit the cyclo-oxygenase (COX)-1 isoenzyme [23]. Unlike aspirin, however, these agents bind reversibly at the active site of the isoenzyme, leading to impaired platelet function for only a portion of the dosing interval [24]. Although it has been suggested that the effect of the nonselective NSAID naproxen on COX-1 persists throughout the dosing interval [25], its cardioprotective effect remains controversial. Results from a subgroup analysis of a randomized trial [26] and from case-control studies [27–29] found a reduced risk of cardiovascular events among naproxen users, whereas other studies found no association [30,31].

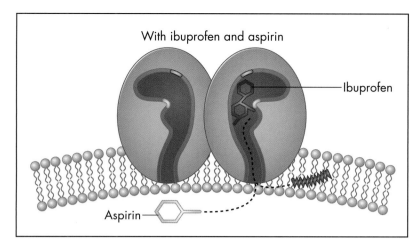

With ibuprofen and aspirin

Ibuprofen

Aspirin

Figure 18-27.

Mechanisms of interaction. There is recent evidence that aspirin and other nonaspirin nonsteroidal anti-inflammatory drugs may interact because these medications share a common docking site on cyclo-oxygenase (COX)-1 [32,33]. Basic research findings [34,35], a crossover study in healthy subjects [36], and one observational study in secondary prevention [37] support this hypothesis. In the crossover study by Catella-Lawson *et al.* [36], concomitant administration of 400 mg ibuprofen every morning antagonized the irreversible platelet inhibition of COX-1 induced by 81 mg aspirin (*see* Fig. 18-3). This inhibition could be bypassed, such as when aspirin was given before a single dose of ibuprofen. Intake of enteric-coated ibuprofen three times per day inhibited the effect of aspirin on platelets, even when the aspirin was taken before the ibuprofen. No interaction was found between concomitant intake of aspirin and rofecoxib, acetaminophen, or diclofenac.

Effect of Ibuprofen on the Cardioprotective Effect of Aspirin

		Mortality	
Drug	Patients, *n*	All causes	CVD
Aspirin	6285	1.00	1.00
Aspirin + ibuprofen	187	1.93 (1.30–2.87)	1.73 (1.05–2.84)
Aspirin + diclofenac	206	0.82 (0.54–1.25)	0.80 (0.49–1.31)
Aspirin + other NSAIDs	429	1.10 (0.87–1.40)	1.03 (0.77–1.37)

Figure 18-28.

Effect of ibuprofen on the cardioprotective effect of aspirin. The recent observational study of secondary prevention by MacDonald and Wei [37] identified 7107 patients from Scotland who were discharged after first admission for cardiovascular disease and observed for 8 years. Four discharge groups were compared: low-dose (< 325 mg/day) aspirin alone, aspirin plus ibuprofen, aspirin plus diclofenac, and aspirin plus another nonsteroidal anti-inflammatory drug. Compared with aspirin-only users, ibuprofen users had a relative risk of 1.73 (95% CI 1.05–2.84) for cardiovascular mortality. Combined use of aspirin and diclofenac or other nonsteroidal anti-inflammatory drugs did not increase the risk. Although the authors could control for several potential confounding factors, the nature of their data did not allow them to control for lifestyle factors, such as smoking and exercise. CVD—cardiovascular disease; NSAIDs—nonsteroidal anti-inflammatory drugs. (*Adapted from* MacDonald and Wei [37].)

Relative Hazard of Myocardial Infarction According to Randomized Aspirin or Placebo Group and Nonsteroidal Anti-inflammatory Drug Use Categories

NSAIDs	Age-adjusted HR (95% CI)	Model* HR (95% CI)
Placebo	1.00	1.00
+ NSAIDs: 1–59 days/year	1.14 (0.82–1.59)	1.13 (0.80–1.58)
+ NSAIDs: 60 or more days/year	0.22 (0.03–1.55)	0.21 (0.03–1.50)
Aspirin	0.55 (0.43–0.70)	0.56 (0.44–0.72)
+ NSAIDs: 1–59 days/year	0.67 (0.44–1.01)	0.69 (0.46–1.05)
+ NSAIDs: 60 or more days/year	1.49 (0.66–3.37)	1.57 (0.70–3.56)

*Model: Age, body mass index, exercise, arthritis, and smoking; plus hypertension, diabetes, and family history of MI

Figure 18-29.

Relative hazard of myocardial infarction (MI) according to randomized aspirin or placebo group and nonsteroidal anti-inflammatory drug (NSAID) use categories. A recent study from the randomized aspirin arm of the Physicians' Health Study [17] suggested that the clinical benefit of aspirin in the primary prevention of MI is inhibited by regular but not intermittent use of NSAIDs [38]. In this trial, randomized aspirin assignment was associated with a 44% reduction in risk of MI (relative risk [RR] = 0.56; 95% CI 0.44–0.72). Among participants randomized to aspirin, use of NSAIDs 1 to 59 days per year was still associated with a suggested reduction in risk of MI (RR = 0.69; 95% CI 0.46–1.05), whereas the use of NSAIDs on 60 days or more per year was associated no apparent benefit of aspirin on MI (RR = 1.57; 95% CI 0.70–3.56). In the placebo group, the RRs for MI across the same categories of NSAID use were 1.13 (95% CI 0.80–1.58), and 0.21 (95% CI 0.03–1.50), respectively. A limitation of the study was that no information could be provided about dosing and brand of NSAIDs. However, ibuprofen was one of the most often used NSAIDs during the period of the study (1982–1988). Although the information from the secondary prevention study on NSAIDs was observational, the most plausible interpretation of the available data is that the regular use of the NSAID ibuprofen may inhibit the clinical benefit of aspirin in secondary prevention of cardiovascular disease and in the primary prevention of MI. HR—hazard ratio. (*Adapted from* Kurth *et al.* [38].)

Estimates of Benefit and Harm of Aspirin Given for 5 Years per 1000 Individuals

Benefits and harms	Baseline risk for CHD over 5 years		
	1%	3%	5%
Total mortality	No effect	No effect	No effect
CHD events	1–4 avoided	4–12 avoided	6–20 avoided
Hemorrhagic stroke	0–2 caused	0–2 caused	0–2 caused
Major GI bleeding events	2–4 caused	2–4 caused	2–4 caused

Figure 18-30.

Estimates of benefit and harm of aspirin given for 5 years per 1000 individuals: US Preventive Services Task Force. In 2002, the US Preventive Services Task Force (USPSTF) [7] reviewed the available data from primary prevention trials and found "good" evidence that aspirin decreases the incidence of coronary heart disease (CHD) in adults at high risk for heart disease, "good" evidence that aspirin increases the incidence of gastrointestinal (GI) bleeding, and "fair" evidence that aspirin increases the incidence of hemorrhagic strokes. For primary prevention, the USPSTF concluded that aspirin may be beneficial for those whose risk of CHD is sufficiently high (*ie*, 5-year risk = 3% or greater and 10-year risk = 6% or greater) to warrant exposure to any risks of long-term administration of the drug. Thus, clinicians should discuss aspirin therapy with patients at increased risk for CHD, including men older than 40 years of age; postmenopausal women; and younger persons with CHD risk factors, such as hypertension, diabetes, or smoking. (The USPSTF reported that statistical prediction tools, such as that provided at http://www.med-decisions.com [39], are likely to produce a more accurate estimate of CHD risk than is a simple count of coronary risk factors.) Discussions with patients should focus on benefit and harm of aspirin, and should consider individual preferences and risk aversions with respect to myocardial infarction, stroke, and GI bleeding. Although the benefit-risk balance is most favorable in individuals whose 5-year CHD risk exceeds 3%, some lower-risk individuals may want to consider the potential benefits to outweigh the potential harm.

In 2002, the American Heart Association also updated its Guidelines for Primary Prevention of Cardiovascular Disease and Stroke [8]. The American Heart Association recommended the use of low-dose aspirin, 75 to 160 mg/day, in men and women with a 10-year risk of CHD of 10% or greater who are not at increased risk for GI bleeding or hemorrhagic stroke. On the basis of these guidelines, a middle-aged man who is a current smoker and has a strong family history of premature CHD would be a strong candidate for prophylactic aspirin use. Similarly, aspirin may be warranted for a 60-year-old woman with a cholesterol level of 250 mg/dL and a recent diagnosis of type 2 diabetes. However, aspirin would not be indicated—and may even be contraindicated—in a 44-year-old premenopausal woman whose only cardiovascular risk factor is poorly controlled hypertension (average readings of 160/100 mm Hg), because she is at greater risk of hemorrhagic stroke than myocardial infarction.

References

1. Williams A, Hennekens CH: The role of aspirin in cardiovascular diseases: forgotten benefits? *Expert Opin Pharmacother* 2004, 5:109–115.

2. Vane JR: Inhibition of prostaglandin synthesis as a mechanism of action for aspirin-like drugs. *Nat N Biol* 1971, 231:232–235.

3. Antiplatelet Trialists' Collaboration: Secondary prevention of vascular disease by prolonged antiplatelet therapy. *BMJ* 1988, 296:320–332.

4. Antiplatelet Trialists' Collaboration: Collaborative overview of randomised trials of antiplatelet treatment: I. Prevention of death, myocardial infarction, and stroke by prolonged antiplatelet therapy in various categories of patients. *BMJ* 1994, 308:81–106.

5. Antithrombotic Trialists' Collaboration: Collaborative meta-analysis of randomised trials of antiplatelet therapy for prevention of death, myocardial infarction, and stroke in high risk patients. *BMJ* 2002, 324:71–86.

6. Ridker PM, Cook NR, Lee IM, *et al.*: A randomized trial of low-dose aspirin in the primary prevention of cardiovascular disease in women. *N Engl J Med* 2005, 352:1293–1304.

7. US Preventive Services Task Force: Aspirin for the primary prevention of cardiovascular events: recommendation and rationale. *Ann Intern Med* 2002, 136:157–160.

8. Pearson TA, Blair SN, Daniels SR, *et al.*: AHA guidelines for primary prevention of cardiovascular disease and stroke: 2002 update. *Circulation* 2002, 106:388–391.

9. Funk CD, Funk LB, Kennedy ME, *et al.*: Human platelet/erythroleukemia cell prostaglandin G/H synthase: cDNA cloning, expression, and gene chromosomal assignment. *FASEB J* 1991, 5:2304–2312.

10. FitzGerald GA: Mechanisms of platelet activation: thromboxane A_2 as an amplifying signal for other agonists. *Am J Cardiol* 1991, 68:11B–15B.

11. Fuster V, Dyken ML, Vokonas PS, *et al.*: Aspirin as a therapeutic agent in cardiovascular disease: AHA scientific statement. *N Engl J Med* 1993, 87:659

12. Randomised trial of intravenous streptokinase, oral aspirin, both, or neither among 17,187 cases of suspected acute myocardial infarction: ISIS-2. ISIS-2 (Second International Study of Infarct Survival) Collaborative Group. *Lancet* 1988, 2:349–360.

13. Baigent C, Collins R, Appleby P, *et al.*: ISIS-2: 10 year survival among patients with suspected acute myocardial infarction in randomised comparison of intravenous streptokinase, oral aspirin, both, or neither. The ISIS-2 (Second International Study of Infarct Survival) Collaborative Group. *BMJ* 1998, 316:1337–1343.

14. CAPRIE Steering Committee: A randomised, blinded, trial of clopidogrel versus aspirin in patients at risk of ischaemic events (CAPRIE). *Lancet* 1996, 348:1329–1339.

15. CURE I: Effects of clopidogrel in addition to aspirin in patients with acute coronary syndromes without ST-segment elevation. *N Engl J Med* 2001, 345:494–502.

16. UK-TIA Study Group: United Kingdom Transient Ischemic Attack (UK-TIA) aspirin trial: final results. *J Neurol Neurosurg Psychiatry* 1991, 54:1044–1054.

17. Steering Committee of the Physicians' Health Study Research Group: Final report on the aspirin component of the ongoing Physicians' Health Study. *N Engl J Med* 1989, 321:129–135.

18. Medical Research Council's General Practice Research Framework: Thrombosis prevention trial: randomised trial of low-intensity oral anticoagulation with warfarin and low-dose aspirin in the primary prevention of ischaemic heart disease in men at increased risk. *Lancet* 1998, 351:233–241.

19. Hansson L, Zanchetti A, Carruthers SG, *et al.*: Effects of intensive blood-pressure lowering and low-dose aspirin in patients with hypertension: principal results of the Hypertension Optimal Treatment (HOT) randomised trial. *Lancet* 1998, 351:1755–1762.

20. deGaetano G, for the Collaborative Group of the Primary Prevention Project (PPP): Low-dose aspirin and vitamin E in people at cardiovascular risk: a randomised trial in general practice. *Lancet* 2001, 357:89–95.

21. Eidelman RS, Hebert PR, Weisman SM, Hennekens CH: An update on aspirin in the primary prevention of cardiovascular disease. *Arch Intern Med* 2003, 163:2006–2010.

22. Kjeldsen SE, Kolloch RE, Leonetti G, *et al.*: Influence of gender and age on preventing cardiovascular disease by antihypertensive treatment and acetylsalicylic acid: the HOT Study. *J Hypertens* 2000, 18:629–642.

23. Schafer AI: Effects of nonsteroidal antiinflammatory drugs on platelet function and systemic hemostasis. *J Clin Pharmacol* 1995, 35:209–219.

24. Pedersen AK, FitzGerald GA: Cyclooxygenase inhibition, platelet function, and metabolite formation during chronic sulfinpyrazone dosing. *Clin Pharmacol Ther* 1985, 37:36–42.

25. Van Hecken A, Schwartz JI, Depre M, *et al.*: Comparative inhibitory activity of rofecoxib, meloxicam, diclofenac, ibuprofen, and naproxen on COX-2 versus COX-1 in healthy volunteers. *J Clin Pharmacol* 2000, 40:1109–1120.

26. Bombardier C, Laine L, Reicin A, *et al.*: Comparison of upper gastrointestinal toxicity of rofecoxib and naproxen in patients with rheumatoid arthritis. VIGOR Study Group. *N Engl J Med* 2000, 343:1520–1528.

27. Solomon DH, Glynn RJ, Levin R, Avorn J: Nonsteroidal anti-inflammatory drug use and acute myocardial infarction. *Arch Intern Med* 2002, 162:1099–1104.

28. Rahme E, Pilote L, LeLorier J: Association between naproxen use and protection against acute myocardial infarction. *Arch Intern Med* 2002, 162:1111–1115.

29. Watson DJ, Rhodes T, Cai B, Guess HA: Lower risk of thromboembolic cardiovascular events with naproxen among patients with rheumatoid arthritis. *Arch Intern Med* 2002, 162:1105–1110.

30. Ray WA, Stein CM, Hall K, *et al.*: Non-steroidal anti-inflammatory drugs and risk of serious coronary heart disease: an observational cohort study. *Lancet* 2002, 359:118–123.

31. Garcia Rodriguez LA, Varas C, Patrono C: Differential effects of aspirin and non-aspirin nonsteroidal antiinflammatory drugs in the primary prevention of myocardial infarction in postmenopausal women. *Epidemiology* 2000, 11:382–387.

32. Loll PJ, Picot D, Ekabo O, Garavito RM: Synthesis and use of iodinated nonsteroidal antiinflammatory drug analogs as crystallographic probes of the prostaglandin H2 synthase cyclooxygenase active site. *Biochemistry* 1996, 35:7330–7340.

33. Loll PJ, Picot D, Garavito RM: The structural basis of aspirin activity inferred from the crystal structure of inactivated prostaglandin H2 synthase. *Nat Struct Biol* 1995, 2:637–643.

34. Livio M, Del Maschio A, Cerletti C, de Gaetano G: Indomethacin prevents the long-lasting inhibitory effect of aspirin on human platelet cyclooxygenase activity. *Prostaglandins* 1982, 23:787–796.

35. Rao GH, Johnson GG, Reddy KR, White JG: Ibuprofen protects platelet cyclooxygenase from irreversible inhibition by aspirin. *Arteriosclerosis* 1983, 3:383–388.

36. Catella-Lawson F, Reilly MP, Kapoor SC, *et al.*: Cyclooxygenase inhibitors and the antiplatelet effects of aspirin. *N Engl J Med* 2001, 345:1809–1817.

37. MacDonald TM, Wei L: Effect of ibuprofen on cardioprotective effect of aspirin. *Lancet* 2003, 361:573–574.

38. Kurth T, Glynn RG, Walker AM, *et al.*: Inhibition of clinical benefits of aspirin on first myocardial infarction by nonsteroidal antiinflammatory drugs. *Circulation* 2003, 108:1191–1195.

39. Wilson PW, D'Agostino RB, Levy D, *et al.*: Prediction of coronary heart disease using risk factor categories. *Circulation* 1998, 97:1837–1847.

Secondary Prevention

Akshay S. Desai and Peter H. Stone

The latter part of the 20th century witnessed dramatic progress in the care of patients with coronary heart disease and associated steep declines in cardiovascular morbidity and mortality. The development of coronary care units in the 1960s enabled rapid identification and treatment of arrhythmias after myocardial infarction, dramatically reducing the incidence of peri-infarct sudden cardiac death. Subsequent development and refinement of early reperfusion strategies in the 1980s and 1990s using thrombolytic therapy and primary percutaneous transluminal coronary angioplasty allowed further reductions in mortality by limiting infarct size and better preserving left ventricular function. Simultaneously, progressive understanding of the pathophysiology of atherosclerosis and ventricular remodeling has contributed to the development of a burgeoning array of pharmacologic and nonpharmacologic therapies for reducing the incidence of recurrent myocardial infarction, congestive heart failure, and cardiac death after an index event.

Recent evidence, however, suggests that this steady rate of decline in cardiovascular mortality among Western nations has slowed. Age-adjusted death rates from coronary heart disease have plateaued, while morbidity and mortality related to congestive heart failure have steadily risen [1]. Moreover, the mortality gap between certain population subgroups (defined by race/ethnicity, socioeconomic status, and geography) and the rest of the US population continues to increase. Although the prevalence of many risk factors, such as smoking, dietary saturated fat and cholesterol intake, serum cholesterol, and hypertension, fell until 1990, there has been little or no progress since then. Along with notable increases in the prevalence of obesity and type 2 diabetes, these trends forecast a possible resurgence in the cardiovascular morbidity and mortality in the near future.

Because nearly 70% of deaths from coronary heart disease and 50% of myocardial infarctions occur in patients who have previously established atherosclerosis, the first presentation with myocardial infarction represents a major opportunity to reduce the burden of recurrent cardiovascular complications. Key strategies for secondary prevention include the control of traditional cardiovascular risk factors and the institution of pharmacologic therapies with demonstrated benefit in reducing mortality and cardiovascular disease progression. Lifestyle modifications, including regular physical exercise, weight reduction, cessation of cigarette smoking, and stress reduction, all of which have a favorable impact on blood coagulation, fibrinolysis, and platelet reactivity are also critical in reducing the vulnerability to atherothrombotic events. Structured programs of cardiac rehabilitation can be particularly helpful in attaining these goals.

A growing number of randomized, blinded, placebo-controlled studies highlight smoking cessation, aggressive lipid lowering, control of hypertension and diabetes, and prophylactic use of antiplatelet agents, β-blockers, and angiotensin-converting enzyme inhibitors, as the cornerstones of secondary prevention in survivors of myocardial infarction. Further, newer guidelines emphasize that atherosclerosis is a systemic process, and that aggressive secondary prevention strategies may be appropriate in other high-risk patient subsets, including those with cerebrovascular disease, peripheral arterial disease, and diabetes [2]. Nonetheless, recent data suggest that these strategies remain grossly underutilized [3].

This chapter reviews the evidence base supporting the various secondary prevention strategies, with a specific emphasis on data from prospective, randomized trials.

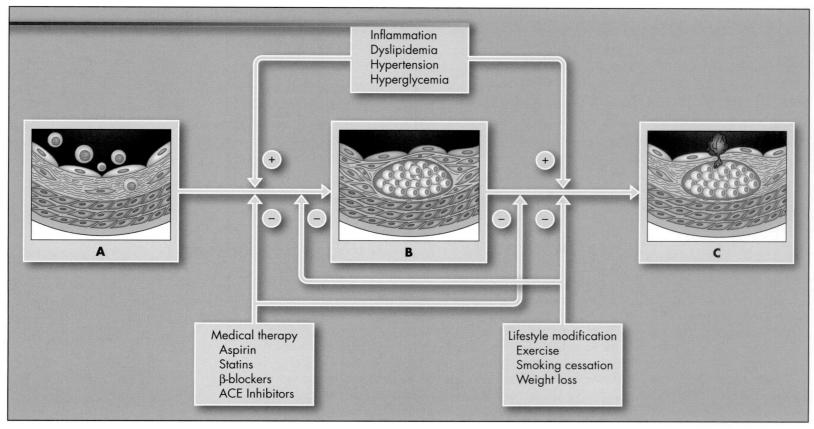

Figure 19-1.

Progression of atherosclerosis and targets for secondary prevention. The atherosclerotic plaque begins with inflammation of the vascular endothelium, which induces expression of cellular adhesion molecules that promote leukocyte adhesion (A). Activation of proinflammatory cytokines promotes migration of leukocytes to the intima, where they participate in and perpetuate a local inflammatory response. Activated macrophages express scavenger receptors for modified lipoproteins, allowing them to ingest lipid and become foam cells. Activated T lymphocytes secrete cytokines and growth factors that promote proliferation and migration of smooth muscle cells from the media to the intima, in which they proliferate and help to generate a dense, collagen-rich extracellular matrix (the fibrous cap) that insulates the prothrombotic contents of the plaque from the flow of blood within the vessel (B). Over time, ongoing inflammation inhibits collagen synthesis in the fibrous cap and evokes expression of collagenases from foam cells within the lesion that actively degrade the fibrous cap and render it susceptible to rupture. Within the plaque core, macrophages produce procoagulant tissue factor, which is released into the circulation as the plaque fissures, generating local platelet activation, adherence, and vascular thrombosis (C).

Inflammatory processes not only promote initiation of atheroma, but also contribute decisively to the precipitating acute thrombotic complications of atheroma. Traditional cardiovascular risk factors, such as dyslipidemia, high blood pressure, cigarette smoking, and diabetes contribute to plaque inflammation and instability. Low-density lipoprotein (LDL) retained in the intima undergoes oxidative modification, enhancing expression of proinflammatory cytokines by macrophages and vascular wall cells. Angiotensin II, a key mediator in hypertension, also promotes inflammation within the intima. Hyperglycemia associated with diabetes can lead to formation of advanced glycation end products that further augment the production of inflammatory mediators and activate inflammatory pathways in endothelial cells. Obesity not only predisposes to insulin resistance and diabetes, but also contributes to atherogenic dyslipidemia.

Retarding plaque progression and preventing plaque rupture by reducing vascular inflammation are therefore key goals of secondary prevention. As a result, strategies for secondary prevention must take into account aggressive control of traditional risk factors through lifestyle modification and pharmacologic therapy. Antiplatelet drugs (especially aspirin), lipid-lowering medications, β-blockers, and angiotensin-converting enzyme (ACE) inhibitors are the cornerstones of therapy, with proven benefits in reducing the complications of atherosclerotic vascular disease, especially among those at highest risk for complications. (*Adapted from* Libby *et al.* [4].)

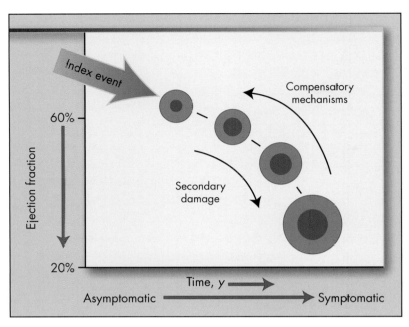

Figure 19-2.
Progressive ventricular remodeling and the development of heart failure. Left ventricular (LV) dysfunction begins with initial injury to the myocardium and subsequently progresses, often in the absence of any identifiable new insult. The index event may take any of several forms:

In the vast majority of patients in the United States (> 70%), the inciting event is myocyte damage as a result of coronary artery disease and resultant myocardial infarction that directly interferes with myocardial force generation. After the initial decline in LV function, a variety of compensatory homeostatic mechanisms (adrenergic nervous system, renin-angiotensin-aldosterone axis, natriuretic peptides, prostaglandins, and nitric oxide) are activated to restore cardiac function to the normal range. As a result, many patients may remain asymptomatic or minimally symptomatic for years after the initial insult. Over time, however, the sustained activation of these compensatory neurohormonal systems leads to ventricular remodeling and alteration in myocyte function that further impair LV contraction, promote salt and water retention, and ultimately lead to cardiac decompensation and symptomatic heart failure. Increasingly, then, heart failure is understood as the pathologic consequence of sustained neurohormonal activation that ensues as a result of LV dysfunction [5]. The overexpression of biologically active molecules such as norepinephrine, angiotensin II, endothelin, aldosterone, and tumor necrosis factor is sufficient to contribute to disease progression in the failing heart independent of the hemodynamic status of the patient, by virtue of the direct toxic effects that these molecules exert on the heart and circulation. Antagonism of these molecules (with β-blockers, angiotensin-converting enzyme inhibitors, and aldosterone receptor antagonists) in an attempt to limit the impact of neurohormonal activation, arrest progression, and ventricular remodeling has therefore been the cornerstone of pharmacologic therapy following myocardial infarction. (*Adapted from* Mann [6].)

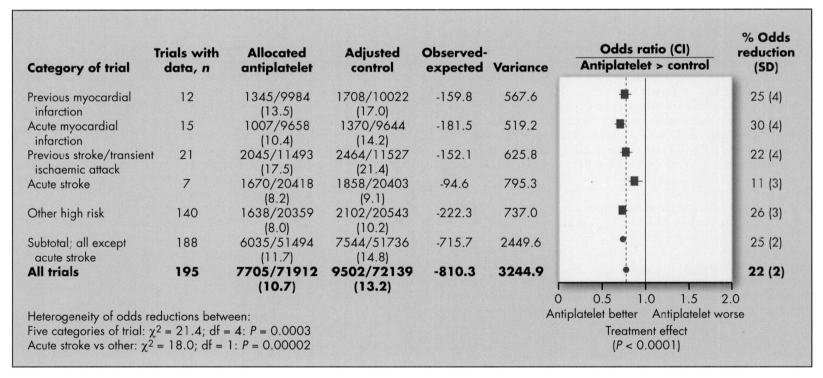

Category of trial	Trials with data, *n*	Allocated antiplatelet	Adjusted control	Observed-expected	Variance	Odds ratio (CI) Antiplatelet > control	% Odds reduction (SD)
Previous myocardial infarction	12	1345/9984 (13.5)	1708/10022 (17.0)	-159.8	567.6		25 (4)
Acute myocardial infarction	15	1007/9658 (10.4)	1370/9644 (14.2)	-181.5	519.2		30 (4)
Previous stroke/transient ischaemic attack	21	2045/11493 (17.5)	2464/11527 (21.4)	-152.1	625.8		22 (4)
Acute stroke	7	1670/20418 (8.2)	1858/20403 (9.1)	-94.6	795.3		11 (3)
Other high risk	140	1638/20359 (8.0)	2102/20543 (10.2)	-222.3	737.0		26 (3)
Subtotal; all except acute stroke	188	6035/51494 (11.7)	7544/51736 (14.8)	-715.7	2449.6		25 (2)
All trials	**195**	**7705/71912 (10.7)**	**9502/72139 (13.2)**	**-810.3**	**3244.9**		**22 (2)**

Heterogeneity of odds reductions between:
Five categories of trial: $\chi^2 = 21.4$; df = 4: $P = 0.0003$
Acute stroke vs other: $\chi^2 = 18.0$; df = 1: $P = 0.00002$

0   0.5   1.0   1.5   2.0
Antiplatelet better   Antiplatelet worse
Treatment effect
($P < 0.0001$)

Figure 19-3.
Antithrombotic Trialists' Collaboration. Impact of antiplatelet therapy on vascular events in high-risk patient subsets [7]. Data presented are from a meta-analysis of 287 studies, involving 135,640 patients in trials of various antiplatelet regimens versus control and 77,000 patients in comparison of different antiplatelet regimens. Included patients were considered to be at high risk of occlusive arterial events related to prior myocardial infarction, stroke, transient ischemic attack, peripheral arterial disease, chronic stable angina, atrial fibrillation, or coronary artery revascularization. Overall, among these high-risk patients, there was a highly significant reduction in the combined outcome of any serious vascular event among patients assigned to antiplatelet therapy compared with those assigned to the control group (10.7% vs 13.2%, $P < 0.0001$). More specifically, antiplatelet therapy was associated with a 25% reduction in serious vascular events among patients with prior myocardial infarction (13.5% vs 17.0%, $P < 0.0001$). Aspirin was the most widely studied antiplatelet drug, with comparable effects observed among lower (75–150 mg daily) and higher daily doses. The effects of doses lower than 75 mg daily were less certain. Clopidogrel reduced serious vascular events by 10% compared with aspirin, which was similar to the 12% reduction observed with its analogue ticlopidine. Addition of dipyridamole to aspirin produced no significant further reduction in vascular events compared with aspirin alone.

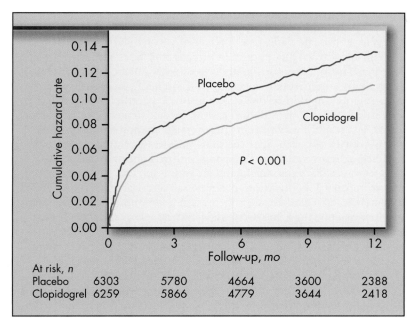

At risk, n

Placebo	6303	5780	4664	3600	2388
Clopidogrel	6259	5866	4779	3644	2418

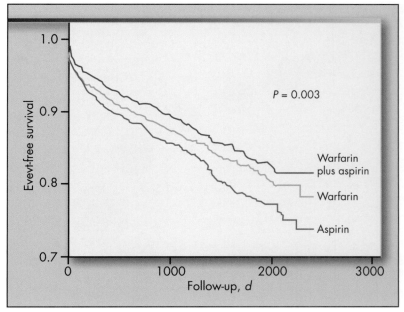

Figure 19-4.

The Clopidogrel in Unstable Angina to Prevent Recurrent Events (CURE) trial [8]; aspirin, clopidogrel, or combination of the two for secondary prevention of coronary artery disease. The thienopyridines ticlopidine and clopidogrel inhibit adenosine diphosphate (ADP) receptor–mediated platelet activation; they are more potent platelet inhibitors than aspirin. Maximal inhibition of ADP-induced platelet aggregation occurs 3 to 5 days after the initiation of a standard dose (75 mg daily), but within 4 to 6 hours after the administration of a larger loading dose (300–600 mg) [9]. The CURE trial randomized 12,562 patients within 24 hours of presentation with an acute coronary syndrome to therapy with clopidogrel (300 mg immediately, followed by 75 mg once daily) or placebo in addition to aspirin over a mean treatment duration of 9 months. The administration of aspirin and clopidogrel in combination was more effective than aspirin alone in reducing the combined incidence of death from cardiovascular causes, myocardial infarction, or stroke (event rate 9.3% vs 11.4%, relative risk for clopidogrel as compared with placebo 0.80, 95% CI 0.72–0.91, $P < 0.001$). This figure presents the cumulative hazard rates for the primary endpoint over the first 12 months of the study.

There was significantly more major bleeding in clopidogrel-treated patients relative to placebo (3.7% vs 2.7%; relative risk, 1.38; $P = 0.001$), but no excess of life-threatening bleeds or hemorrhagic strokes. Those who received aspirin and clopidogrel during the 5 days before coronary-artery bypass grafting were more likely than those receiving aspirin alone to have major bleeding and to require transfusions, reoperation, or both. This observation has led some physicians to delay clopidogrel therapy until the results of coronary angiography are known and confirm that bypass grafting is not necessary. Routine utilization of clopidogrel in addition to aspirin for secondary prevention benefit is not cost-effective [10]; however, in aspirin-intolerant patients, clopidogrel is a viable alternative.

Figure 19-5.

The Warfarin-Aspirin Reinfarction Study II (WARIS II) [11]; warfarin, aspirin or a combination of the two after myocardial infarction. WARIS II was a randomized trial of warfarin (in a dose intended to achieve an international normalized ratio [INR] of 2.8–4.2), aspirin (160 mg daily), or low-dose aspirin (75 mg daily) combined with warfarin (in a dose intended to achieve an INR of 2.0–2.5) in 3630 patients after myocardial infarction. Over 4 years of follow-up, the primary endpoint of death, nonfatal reinfarction, or thromboembolic cerebral stroke occurred in 20% of patients receiving aspirin alone, 16.7% of patients receiving warfarin (rate ratio as compared with aspirin, 0.81; 95% CI, 0.69–0.95; $P = 0.03$), and 15% of patients receiving warfarin and aspirin (rate ratio as compared with aspirin, 0.71; 95% CI, 0.60–0.83; $P = 0.001$). There was no difference in mortality between the three arms, and the observed benefit to warfarin therapy was driven by a reduction in the rates of nonfatal myocardial infarction and stroke. Event-free survival curves for the primary endpoint are displayed in this figure. The benefit to warfarin therapy, alone or in combination with aspirin, was balanced by a higher risk of major, nonfatal bleeding. As well, 35% of patients in the trial discontinued warfarin therapy. Other trials of combination therapy with aspirin and oral anticoagulants confirm that the rates of major bleeding with oral anticoagulants are increased, even if the intensity of anticoagulation is adjusted downwards. Poor compliance with warfarin therapy and the increased risk of bleeding are justifiable concerns in using oral anticoagulants for secondary prevention benefits [12].

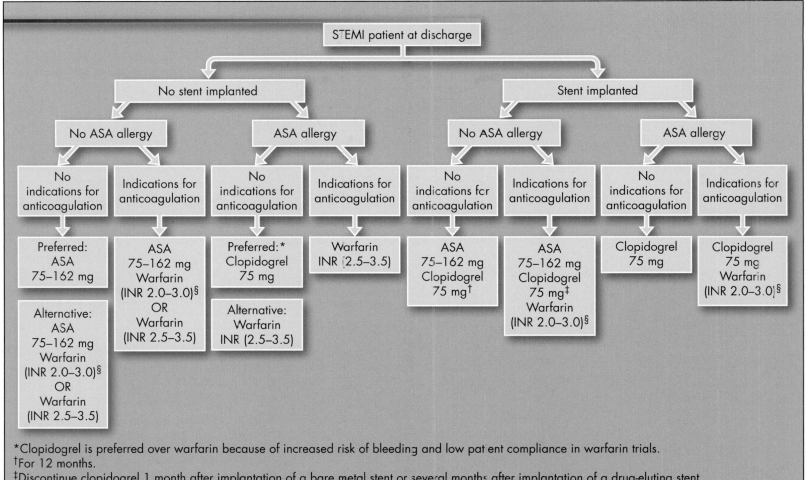

*Clopidogrel is preferred over warfarin because of increased risk of bleeding and low patient compliance in warfarin trials.
†For 12 months.
‡Discontinue clopidogrel 1 month after implantation of a bare metal stent or several months after implantation of a drug-eluting stent
    (3 months after sirolimus and 6 months after paclitaxel) because of the potential increased risk of bleeding with warfarin and two antiplatelet agents.
    Continue aspirin and warfarin long term if warfarin is indicated for other reasons such as atrial fibrillation, LV thrombus, cerebral emboli,
    or extensive regional wall-motion abnormality.
§An INR of 2.0 to 3.0 is acceptable with tight control, but the lower end of this range is preferable. The combination of antiplatelet therapy and
    warfarin may be considered in patients aged less than 75 years with low bleeding risk who can be monitored reliably.

Figure 19-6.

American College of Cardiology/American Heart Association algorithm for management of long-term antithrombotic therapy at hospital discharge after myocardial infarction. Level of evidence is reported according to the American College of Cardiology/American Heart Association format, and reflects the strength of published data supporting the recommendations. Although the recommendations are designed for patients presenting with ST-elevation myocardial infarction (STEMI), they are equally applicable to those presenting with acute coronary syndromes and non-STEMI. Few patients under the age of 75 have been studied in clinical trials. Given the increased risks of bleeding complications in this subset, additional caution should be exercised in prescribing oral anticoagulant medications, particularly in combination with antiplatelet therapy. ASA—aspirin; INR—international normalized ratio; LV—left ventricular. (*Adapted from* Antman *et al.* [13].)

Effect of β-adrenergic Receptor Antagonists on Morbidity and Mortality after Myocardial Infarction

Study	Drug and dose	Study design	Randomized, *n*	Timing of therapy after MI	Mean follow-up	Total mortality	Reinfarction
Norwegian Multicenter Study 1981 [15]	Timolol 10 mg orally twice daily	RCT	1884	7 to 28 days	17 months	16.2% placebo (152/939); 10.4% timolol (98/945); RR = 0.64 ($P < 0.001$)	15.0% placebo (141/939); 9.3% timolol (88/945); RR = 0.62 ($P < 0.001$)
BHAT 1982 [16]	Propranolol 80 mg orally three times daily or 60 mg orally three times daily; dose based on serum drug levels	RCT	3837	5 to 21 days	25 months (early termination)	9.8% placebo (188/1921); 7.2% propranolol (138/1916); RR = 0.74 ($P < 0.005$)	13.0% placebo (249/1921); 10.0% propranolol (192/1926); RR = 0.77 ($P < 0.01$)
APSI 1990 [17]	Acebutolol 200 mg orally twice daily	RCT	607	3 to 21 days	10.5 months	11.0% placebo (34/309); 5.7% acebutolol (17/298); RR = 0.52 ($P = 0.019$)	Not studied
CAPRICORN 2001 [18]	Carvedilol titrated to 25 mg orally twice daily	RCT	1959	3 to 21 days	15.6 months	15.3% placebo (151/984); 11.9% carvedilol (116/975); RR = 0.78 ($P = 0.031$)	5.8% placebo (57/984); 3.5% carvedilol (34/975); RR = 0.60 ($P = 0.014$)

Figure 19-7.

Effect of β-adrenergic receptor antagonists on morbidity and mortality after myocardial infarction (MI) [14]. Multiple clinical trials have demonstrated the efficacy of β-adrenergic receptor antagonists in the secondary prevention of death or recurrent infarction in survivors of MI. Summary data are presented in this figure for four of the largest trials of chronic β-blocker therapy after MI: the Norwegian Multicenter Study Group [15], the Beta-blocker Heart Attack Trial (BHAT) [16], the Acebutolol et Prevention Secondaire de L'Infarctus (APSI) [17], and the Carvedilol Post-Infarct Survival Control in Left Ventricular Dysfunction (CAPRICORN) [18] trial. Consistently, prolonged use of β-blockers after MI is associated with significant reductions in total mortality, sudden death, and reinfarction. RCT—randomized controlled trial; RR—relative risk. (*Adapted from* Gornik and O'Gara [14].)

Adjusted Risk and Relative Risk of Death in Patients Who Received or Did Not Receive β-blockers at Hospital Discharge

Characteristic	Risk of death at 2 years			Relative risk (95% CI)
	Receiving β-blocker, %	Not receiving β-blocker, %	Difference in risk, %[†]	
Patient without complications*	14.4	23.9	-9.5	0.60 (0.57–0.63)
Age, y				
< 70	11.3	18.7	-7.4	0.60 (0.57–0.63)
70–79	15.3	24.0	-8.7	0.64 (0.58–0.70)
80 or older	22.6	33.1	-10.5	0.68 (0.63–0.75)
Black race	16.5	23.0	-6.4	0.72 (0.66–0.79)
Previous COPD	16.8	27.8	-11.1	0.60 (0.57–0.63)
Asthma	11.9	19.7	-7.8	0.60 (0.57–0.63)
Diabetes mellitus	17.0	26.6	-9.6	0.64 (0.60–0.69)
Q-wave MI	14.2	23.6	-9.4	0.60 (0.57–0.63)
Non–Q-wave MI	14.4	23.9	-9.5	0.60 (0.57–0.63)
Previous CHF	17.4	28.9	-11.5	0.60 (0.57–0.63)
Previous MI	16.8	25.1	-8.4	0.67 (0.62–0.72)
Systolic blood pressure				
< 100 mm Hg	16.9	28.1	-11.2	0.60 (0.57–0.63)
100–139 mm Hg	10.4	17.2	-6.8	0.60 (0.57–0.63)
140 mm Hg or greater	9.8	14.8	-5.0	0.66 (0.61–0.71)
Ejection fraction				
< 20%	23.5	34.5	-11.0	0.68 (0.58–0.80)
20%–49%	15.3	25.4	-10.1	0.60 (0.57–0.63)
50% or greater	11.6	19.3	-7.7	0.60 (0.57–0.63)
Missing data	12.3	20.4	-8.1	0.60 (0.57–0.63)
Serum creatinine				
< 0.8 mg/dL	12.9	21.4	-8.5	0.60 (0.57–0.63)
0.8–1.4 mg/dL	13.9	23.1	-9.2	0.60 (0.57–0.63)
> 1.4 mg/dL	19.4	29.9	-10.5	0.65 (0.61–0.69)
Heart rate, bpm				
< 70	13.1	21.7	-8.6	0.60 (0.57–0.63)
70–99	14.9	24.8	-9.9	0.60 (0.57–0.63)
100 or more	16.9	26.2	-9.3	0.65 (0.60–0.69)
Treatment during current hospitalization				
CABG	6.1	10.2	-4.0	0.60 (0.57–0.63)
PTCA	9.2	15.2	-6.0	0.60 (0.57–0.63)
Thrombolytic agents	11.8	19.6	-7.8	0.60 (0.57–0.63)
Calcium-channel blockers	16.4	23.6	-7.1	0.70 (0.65–0.75)
ACE inhibitors	14.4	23.9	-9.5	0.60 (0.57–0.63)
Aspirin	13.8	22.9	-9.1	0.60 (0.57–0.63)

*For patients without complications, all risk factors were set at the Cooperative Cardiovascular Project population mean, with none of the factors that alter the effect of β-blockers.

†Because of rounding, the difference in risk does not always equal the difference between the risks shown for patients receiving a β-blocker and those not receiving a β-blocker.

Figure 19-8.
Benefits of β-adrenergic receptor antagonists among high-risk and low-risk patients after myocardial infarction (MI). The Cooperative Cardiovascular Project abstracted medical records from 201,752 patients with myocardial infarction and compared mortality among β-blocker–treated patients with that among untreated patients during 2-year follow-up. In their analysis, only 34% of patients admitted with a diagnosis of MI were treated with β-blockers. Those less likely to receive β-blockers included patients who were elderly or black, and patients with the lowest ejection fractions, congestive heart failure (CHF), chronic obstructive pulmonary disease (COPD), elevated serum creatinine concentrations, or type 1 diabetes mellitus. As shown in this figure, however, the mortality reduction associated with β-blocker therapy is robust across all patient subgroups, including those presumed to be at high risk for complications (such as those with heart failure, pulmonary disease, or older age). Patients at the highest risk for post-MI complications (such as those with ventricular arrhythmias or left ventricular dysfunction) derive the greatest benefit from β-blocker therapy. β-blockers are a cornerstone of secondary prevention after acute MI, though they remain underutilized in practice. ACE—angiotensin-converting enzyme; bpm—beats per minute; CABG—coronary artery bypass graft; PTCA—percutaneous transluminal coronary angioplasty. (*Adapted from* Gottlieb *et al.* [19].)

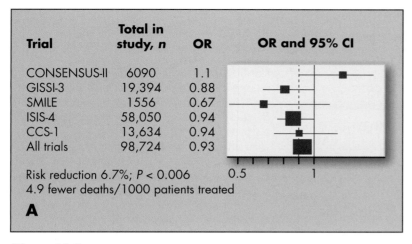

Trial	Total in study, n	OR	OR and 95% CI
CONSENSUS-II	6090	1.1	
GISSI-3	19,394	0.88	
SMILE	1556	0.67	
ISIS-4	58,050	0.94	
CCS-1	13,634	0.94	
All trials	98,724	0.93	

Risk reduction 6.7%; P < 0.006
4.9 fewer deaths/1000 patients treated

A

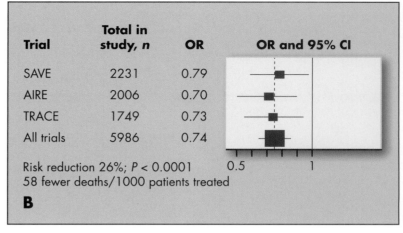

Trial	Total in study, n	OR	OR and 95% CI
SAVE	2231	0.79	
AIRE	2006	0.70	
TRACE	1749	0.73	
All trials	5986	0.74	

Risk reduction 26%; P < 0.0001
58 fewer deaths/1000 patients treated

B

Figure 19-9.
A and **B**, Impact of angiotensin-converting enzyme (ACE) inhibition on mortality after myocardial infarction. ACE inhibitors block the conversion of angiotensin I to angiotensin II and potentiate the activity of bradykinin. Through their ability to reduce myocardial afterload, limit progressive ventricular remodeling, and attenuate ventricular dilation over time, ACE inhibitors improve clinical outcomes among patients with left ventricular dysfunction (ejection fraction < 0.40) after myocardial infarction. In patients with prior myocardial infarction but no clinical heart failure, ACE inhibitors have also been shown to reduce cardiovascular mortality, reinfarction, and sudden death. This figure summarizes the data from randomized, controlled, clinical trials [20–29] enrolling over 100,000 patients supporting the use of ACE inhibition in the short-term and long-term after myocardial infarction. In the peri-infarct setting, the use of ACE inhibitors is associated with a 6.7% reduction in mortality at 30 days, with the greatest benefit seen among patients with anterior myocardial infarction and low ejection fraction. Over the long-term, ACE inhibitors are associated with a highly significant 26% reduction in mortality. Comparable benefits seen across

multiple trials of different agents suggest a class effect to these medications, with higher doses potentially associated with greater protection. The American College of Cardiology/American Heart Association guidelines currently recommend initiation of oral ACE inhibitors within 24 hours of myocardial infarction in patients without contraindications. Titration to doses achieved in large-scale clinical trials is particularly important for the subgroup of patients with large, anterior myocardial infarction, clinical heart failure, or left ventricular ejection fraction less than 0.40, in whom the long-term benefits are most pronounced. AIRE—Acute Infarction Ramipril Efficacy; CCS—Chinese Cardiac Study; CONSENSUS—Cooperative New Scandinavian Enalapril Survival Study; GISSI—Gruppo Italiano per lo Studio della Sopravivenza nell'Infarto; ISIS—International Study of Infarct Survival; OR—odds ratio; SAVE—Survival and Ventricular Enlargement trial; SMILE—Survival of Myocardial Infarction Long-Term Evaluation trial; TRACE—Trandolapril Cardiac Evaluation study group. (*Adapted from* Flather and Pfeffer [20].)

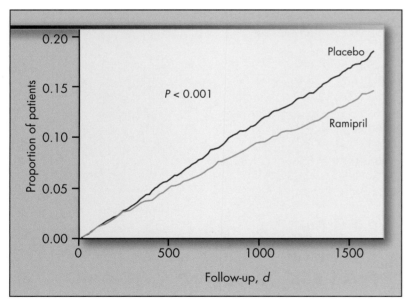

Figure 19-10.
Impact of angiotensin-converting enzyme (ACE) inhibitors in high-risk patients with vascular disease: the results of the Heart Outcomes Prevention Evaluation (HOPE) trial [30]. In the HOPE trial, 9297 high-risk patients (52% with prior evidence of myocardial infarction, the remainder with history of stroke, peripheral arterial disease, or diabetes with one additional cardiovascular risk factor) were randomized to therapy with ramipril 10 mg or vitamin E in a two-by-two factorial design. At mean follow-up of 5 years, use of ramipril was associated with a highly significant 22% reduction in the primary endpoint of myocardial infarction, stroke, or cardiovascular death relative to placebo (*P* < 0.001). The Kaplan-Meier survival curves for ramipril and placebo with regard to this composite endpoint are presented.

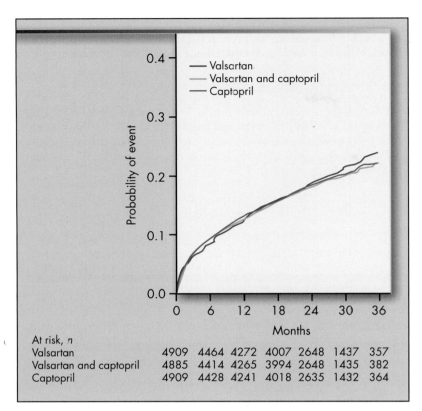

At risk, n

Valsartan	4909	4464	4272	4007	2648	1437	357
Valsartan and captopril	4885	4414	4265	3994	2648	1435	382
Captopril	4909	4428	4241	4018	2635	1432	364

Figure 19-11.
Relative benefits of angiotensin-receptor blockade and angiotensin converting enzyme (ACE) inhibition after myocardial infarction: the Valsartan In Acute Myocardial Infarction (VALIANT) Study [31]. The VALIANT trial compared the effects of captopril (target dose 50 mg three times daily), valsartan (target dose 160 mg twice daily), and the combination (captopril target dose 50 mg three times daily; and valsartan target dose 80 mg twice daily) on mortality with left ventricular dysfunction after myocardial infarction. During a median follow-up of 24.7 months, death occurred in 19.9% of the valsartan group, 19.5% of the captopril group, and 19.3% of the combined-treatment group. The hazard ratio for death in the valsartan group compared with the captopril group was 1.00 (97.5% CI, 0.90–1.11; $P = 0.98$), and the hazard ratio for death in the combination therapy group versus the captopril group was 0.98 (97.5% CI, 0.8–1.09; $P = 0.73$). The Kaplan-Meier estimates for the rate of death from any cause according to treatment group are superimposable. The results of VALIANT suggest that the valsartan is as effective as captopril in patients who are at high risk for cardiovascular events after myocardial infarction. Combining valsartan and captopril was associated with an increase in drug-related adverse events, but no improvement in survival. Because of the more extensive randomized trial and routine clinical experience with ACE inhibitors, they remain the logical first agent for inhibition of the renin-angiotensin-aldosterone system in post-MI patients. However, valsartan may be administered to patients with myocardial infarction who are intolerant of ACE inhibitors and have evidence of left ventricular dysfunction.

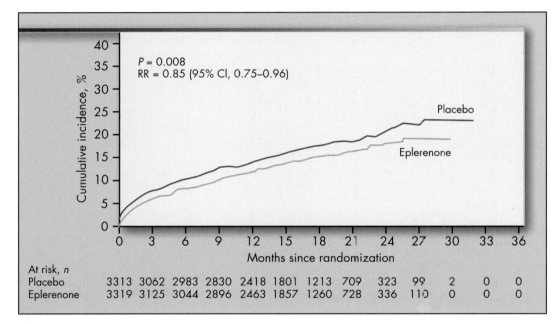

At risk, n

Placebo	3313	3062	2983	2830	2418	1801	1213	709	323	99	2	0	0
Eplerenone	3319	3125	3044	2896	2463	1857	1260	728	336	110	0	0	0

Figure 19-12.
Incremental benefit of adding aldosterone antagonists to optimal medical therapy in patients with left ventricular dysfunction after myocardial infarction. The Eplerenone Post-Acute Myocardial Infarction Heart Failure Efficacy and Survival (EPHESUS) Study [32].

Activation of the renin-angiotensin system generates high levels of circulating aldosterone that promote fluid retention, myocardial fibrosis, and progressive clinical deterioration in patients with heart failure. The EPHESUS study randomized 6632 post–myocardial infarction patients with left ventricular ejection fraction 0.40 or greater and clinical evidence of heart failure to receive the aldosterone blocker eplerenone (target dose 50 mg daily) or placebo in addition to optimal medical therapy. In this population managed aggressively with reperfusion, aspirin, angiotensin-converting enzyme inhibitors, β-blockers, and 3-hydroxy-3-methylglutaryl coenzyme A reductase inhibitors (statins), eplerenone therapy was associated with a highly significant 15% reduction in all-cause mortality relative to placebo (relative risk [RR] 0.85; 95% CI, 0.75–0.96, $P = 0.008$). As well, there was a statistically

significant reduction in the rate of sudden death from cardiac causes in eplerenone-treated patients (RR 0.79; 95% CI, 0.64–0.97, $P = 0.03$). Serious hyperkalemia occurred in 5.5% of patients treated with eplerenone and 3.9% of patients treated with placebo ($P = 0.002$). These results are comparable to those reported in the Randomized Aldactone Evaluation Study [33] trial of spironolactone in patients with New York Heart Association Class III-IV heart failure (55% related to ischemic heart disease). On the basis of these studies, therapy with an aldosterone receptor blocker (in addition to angiotensin-converting enzyme inhibitors and/or angiotensin-receptor blockers) should be considered in patients with ST-elevation myocardial infarction, heart failure, and an ejection fraction of 0.40 or less, in the absence of contraindications (creatinine clearance < 50 cc/min or hyperkalemia at baseline). Although the greater specificity of eplerenone for the mineralocorticoid receptor implies a more favorable side effect profile, it has not demonstrated clinical benefits over generic spironolactone.

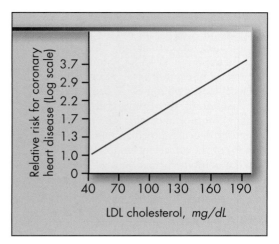

Figure 19-13.

Log-linear relationship between serum low-density lipoprotein (LDL) and relative risk for coronary heart disease. Report of the National Cholesterol Education Panel, Adult Treatment Program III [34].

Epidemiologic evidence and evidence from several randomized clinical trials suggests that serum total cholesterol levels are continuously correlated with cardiovascular risk over a broad range of cholesterol values. Although the association between LDL cholesterol levels and the risk of cardiovascular events is continuous, it is not linear; the risk rises more steeply with increasing LDL cholesterol concentrations. This results in a curvilinear, or log-linear, relationship. These data suggest that for every 30 mg/dL change in LDL cholesterol, the relative risk for coronary heart disease is changed in proportion by approximately 30%.

Modified Guidelines for Lipid-lowering Therapy Based on the Results of Randomized Controlled Trials: The Adult Treatment Panel III

Risk category	LDL-C Goal	Initiate therapeutic lifestyle change	Consider drug therapy§§
High risk: CHD* or CHD risk equivalents (10-year risk > 20%)†	< 100 mg/dL (optional: < 70 mg/dL)**	100 mg/dL or greater‡‡	100 mg/dL or greater¶¶ (< 100 mg/dL: consider drug options§§)
Moderately high risk: two or more risk factors‡ (10-year risk 10%–20%§)	< 130 mg/dL††	130 mg/dL or greater‡‡	130 mg/dL or greater (100–129 mg/dL: consider drug options***)
Moderate risk: two or more risk factors‡ (10-year risk < 10%§)	< 130 mg/dL	130 mg/dL or greater	160 mg/dL or greater
Lower risk: Zero to one risk factor¶	< 160 mg/dL	106 mg/dL or greater	190 mg/dL or greater (160–189 mg/dL: LDL-lowering drug is optional)

*Includes history of myocardial infarction, unstable angina, stable angina, coronary artery procedures (angioplasty or bypass surgery), or evidence of clinically significant myocardial ischemia.

†Risk equivalents include clinical manifestations of noncoronary forms of atherosclerotic disease (peripheral artery disease, abdominal aortic aneurysm, and carotid artery disease [transient ischemic attack or stroke of carotid origin or > 50% obstruction of carotid artery]), diabetes, and two or more risk factors with 10-year risk for hard CHD > 20%.

‡Include cigarette smoking, hypertension (blood pressure 140/90 mm Hg or greater or antihypertensive medication), low HDL-C (< 40 mg/dL), family history of premature CHD (male first-degree relative < 55 years of age; female first-degree relative < 65 years of age), and age (men 45 or older; women 55 or older).

§A 10-year risk calculator is available at http://www.nhlbi.nhi.gov/guidelines/cholesterol.

¶Almost all people with 0 or one risk factor have a 10-year risk < 10%, and 10-year risk assessment in people with zero or one risk factor is not necessary.

**Very high risk favors the optional LDL-C goal of < 70 mg/dL, and in patients with high triglycerides, non-HDL-C < 100 mg/dL.

††Optional LDL-C goal < 100 mg/dL.

‡‡Any person at high risk or moderately high risk who has lifestyle-related risk factors (*eg*, obesity, physical inactivity, elevated triglyceride, low HDL-C, or metabolic syndrome) is a candidate for therapeutic lifestyle changes to modify these risk factors regardless of LDL-C level.

§§When LDL-lowering drug therapy is used, it is advised that intensity of therapy be sufficient to achieve at least a 30% to 40% reduction in LDL-C levels.

¶¶If baseline LDL-C is < 100 mg/dL, institution of LDL-lowering drug is a therapeutic option on the basis of available clinical trial data. If a high-risk individual has high triglyceride levels or low HDL-C, combining a fibrate or nicotinic acid with a LDL-lowering therapy can be taken under consideration.

***For moderately high-risk individuals, when LDL-C is 100–129 mg/dL, baseline or on lifestyle therapy, initiation of LDL-lowering drug to achieve LDL-C level < 100 mg/dL is an option on the basis of available clinical trial data.

Figure 19-14.

Modified guidelines for lipid-lowering therapy based on the results of randomized controlled trials. Report of the National Cholesterol Education Panel, Adult Treatment Program III [34]. Recent clinical trial data (in particular, data from the Heart Protection Study [35] and the Pravastatin or Atorvastatin Evaluation and Infection Therapy/Thrombolysis in Myocardial Infarction–22 Study [36]) suggest that that the relationship between low-density lipoprotein cholesterol (LDL-C) levels and risk of cardiovascular disease persists even at low serum cholesterol levels, such that incremental reduction in cardiovascular risk may be achieved by further reducing already low LDL-C levels. The most recent iteration of the guidelines on cholesterol reduction therefore suggest that for high-risk patients (including those with established coronary artery disease or prior myocardial infarction), and LDL target of < 70 mg/dL may be appropriate. CHD—coronary heart disease; HDL-C—high-density lipoprotein cholesterol. (*Adapted from* Grundy *et al.* [34].)

Large-scale Randomized Trials of HMG CoA Reductase Inhibitors for Cholesterol Lowering in the Secondary Prevention of Cardiovascular Disease

Study	Baseline LDL-C, *mg/dL*	Study population, *n*	Intervention	Duration, *y*	LDL reduction	CVD event reduction: relative risk (95% CI)	Overall mortality: relative risk (95% CI)
4S 1999 [38]	187	4444 men and women (mean age 59 years)	Simvastatin, titration	5.4	35	0.58 (0.46–0.73)	0.70 (0.58–0.85)
CARE 1996 [39]	139	4159 men and women (mean age 59 years)	Pravastatin 40 mg	5.0	28	0.76 (0.64–0.91)	0.91 (0.74–1.12)
LIPID 1998 [40]	150	9014 men and women (age 31–75 years)	Pravastatin 40 mg	6.1	25	0.76 (0.65–0.88)	0.78 (0.69–0.87)
HPS 2002 [35]	132	20,526 men and women (age 40–80 years)	Simvastatin 40 mg	5.5	29	0.83 (0.75–0.91)	0.87 (0.81–0.94)
PROSPER 2002 [41]	147	5804 men and women (age 70–82 years)	Pravastatin 40 mg	3.2	34	0.85 (0.74–0.97)	—
GREACE 2002 [42]	180	1600 men and women (mean age 58 years)	Atorvastatin 10–80 mg	3.0	46	0.49 (0.27–0.73)	0.57 (0.39–0.78)
ASCOT-LLA 2003 [43]	133	19,342 men and women (age 40–79 years)	Atorvastatin 10 mg	3.3	29	0.64 (0.50–0.83)	0.87 (0.71–1.06)

Figure 19-15.

Large-scale randomized trials of 3-hydroxy-3-methylglutaryl coenzyme A (HMG CoA) reductase inhibitors for cholesterol lowering in the secondary prevention of cardiovascular disease (CVD) [37]. Trials presented include the Scandinavian Simvastatin Survival Study (4S) [38], the Cholesterol and Recurrent Events (CARE) Trial [39], the Long-term Intervention with Pravastatin in Ischemic Disease (LIPID) Trial [40], the Heart Protection Study (HPS) [35], The Pravastatin in Elderly Individuals at Risk of Vascular Disease (PROSPER) [41] study, the Greek Atorvastatin and Coronary Heart Disease Evaluation Study (GREACE) [42], and the Anglo-Scandinavian Cardiac Outcomes Trial (ASCOT-LLA) [43]. Serial randomized controlled trials in post–myocardial infarction patients and in high-risk patients with established vascular disease demonstrate consistent and irrefutable benefit from lipid-lowering therapy with HMG CoA reductase inhibitors (statins) relative to placebo with regard to recurrent cardiovascular events and all-cause mortality. Subgroup analyses of the HPS, as noted previously, suggest that the benefits to statin therapy are independent of baseline low-density lipoprotein-cholesterol (LDL-C) levels, and persist even for even those patients with baseline LDL less than 100 mg/dL. In a meta-analysis of over 30,000 patients enrolled in randomized trials [44], statin therapy in secondary prevention was associated with a 21% reduction in all-cause mortality and a 31% reduction in major coronary events. The benefits to lipid lowering with statins appear to accrue equally to younger and older patients and to men and women. (*Adapted from* Scranton and Gaziano [37].)

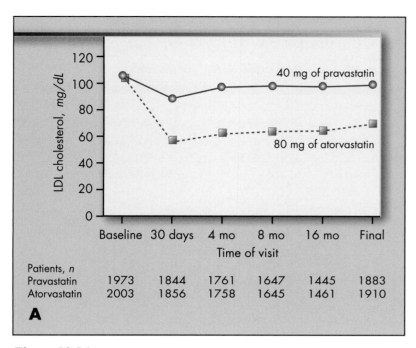

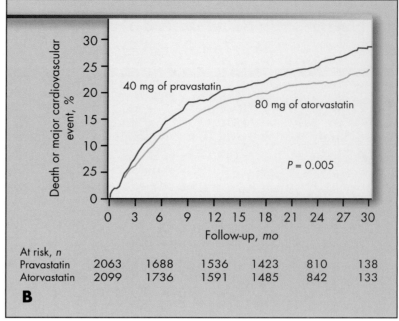

A	Patients, n					
	Baseline	30 days	4 mo	8 mo	16 mo	Final
Pravastatin	1973	1844	1761	1647	1445	1883
Atorvastatin	2003	1856	1758	1645	1461	1910

B	At risk, n					
Pravastatin	2063	1688	1536	1423	810	138
Atorvastatin	2099	1736	1591	1485	842	133

Figure 19-16.

The Pravastatin or Atorvastatin Evaluation and Infection Therapy/Thrombolysis in Myocardial Infarction–22 (PROVE IT/TIMI-22) trial. Benefits of intensive over moderate lipid lowering in patients with acute coronary syndromes. To investigate the relative benefits of intensive versus moderate lipid lowering using statins in patients with acute coronary syndromes, the PROVE-IT investigators randomized 4162 patients within 10 days of hospitalization for an acute coronary syndrome to therapy with pravastatin 40 mg or atorvastatin 80 mg. The primary endpoint was a composite of death from any cause, myocardial infarction, documented unstable angina requiring revascularization, and stroke. Over a mean 2-year follow up, the median low-density lipoprotein (LDL) cholesterol achieved was 95 mg/dL in the standard-dose pravastatin group and 62 mg/dL in the high-dose atorvastatin group (**A**; *P* < 0.001). The incremental LDL reduction with high-dose atorvastatin was associated with a 16% reduction at 2 years in the hazard ratio for the primary endpoint relative to pravastatin-treated patients (95% CI, 5%–26%; *P* = 0.005). **B**, Kaplan Meier estimates. The relative benefits to more aggressive statin therapy in this trial support early and intensive lowering of serum LDL cholesterol with high-dose statins to less than 70 mg/dL in patients presenting with acute coronary syndromes. (*Adapted from* Cannon *et al.* [36].)

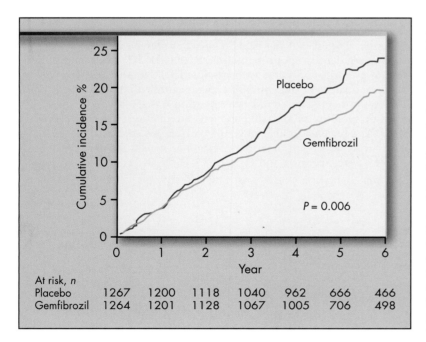

At risk, n						
Placebo	1267	1200	1118	1040	962	666	466
Gemfibrozil	1264	1201	1128	1067	1005	706	498

Figure 19-17.

High-density lipoprotein (HDL)-cholesterol as a therapeutic target. The Veterans Affairs High-Density Lipoprotein Cholesterol Intervention Trial (VA-HIT) Study Group [45]. Patients with low serum HDL cholesterol are at substantial risk for cardiovascular events, even in the setting of normal serum low-density lipoprotein (LDL)-cholesterol. Though ample data support the use of pharmacologic therapy to lower LDL-cholesterol in patients with coronary artery disease, there is less guidance for pharmacologic management of patients with isolated low HDL cholesterol. The VA-HIT trial enrolled 2531 men with coronary artery disease, HDL cholesterol less than 40 mg/dL, and LDL cholesterol less than 140 mg/dL and randomized them to therapy with gemfibrozil 1200 mg daily or placebo. Over median follow-up of 5.1 years, gemfibrozil treatment was associated with a 6% increase in serum HDL and 31% reduction in serum triglycerides, but no change in serum LDL. This modulation of the lipid profile was associated with a 4.4% absolute reduction in cardiovascular events and 22% reduction in relative risk of the primary outcome of nonfatal myocardial infarction or cardiovascular death (95% CI, 7%–35%, *P* = 0.006). Kaplan-Meier estimates of the hazard for the primary endpoint according to treatment group are displayed. The results of the VA-HIT trial support therapy with gemfibrozil in the secondary prevention of cardiovascular events among patients whose primary lipid abnormality is a low serum HDL cholesterol. Raising serum HDL and decreasing serum triglycerides alone were sufficient to achieve cardiovascular risk reduction, supporting the use of these parameters as secondary targets of anti-lipid therapy. Of note, because no patients in the VA-HIT trial were treated with statins, the incremental or additive benefit of fibrate derivatives in statin-treated patients remains unknown.

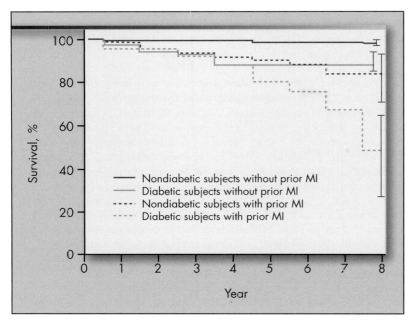

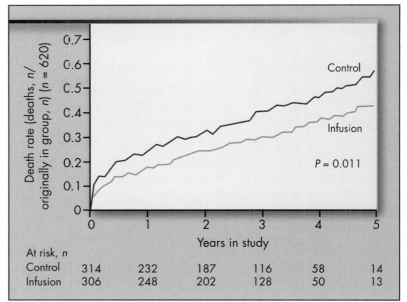

Figure 19-18.
Diabetes mellitus substantially enhances cardiovascular risk in patients
with and without prior myocardial infarction (MI). These data from
1373 nondiabetic and 1059 diabetic subjects in a Finnish-based cohort
represent the Kaplan-Meier estimates of the probability of death from
coronary heart disease, stratified according to the presence of diabetes
and the presence of prior MI. Notably, the 7-year incidence rates of de
novo MI in nondiabetic subjects with and without history of MI were
18.8% and 3.5%, respectively. By contrast, the 7-year incidence rates of
MI in diabetic subjects with and without history of MI were 45.0% and
20.2%, respectively. Further, the hazard ratio for death from coronary
heart disease among diabetic subjects without prior MI relative to nondiabetic subjects with prior MI was 1.4 (95% CI, 0.7–2.6, P value was
not significant). The suggestion is that patients with diabetes and no
history of MI have as high a risk of cardiovascular events as nondiabetic
patients with a history of MI. Patients with diabetes and prior MI
represent an extremely high-risk group, and warrant aggressive therapy
for secondary prevention. (*Adapted from* Haffner *et al.* [46].)

Figure 19-19.
Intensive glycemic control reduces mortality in patients with myocardial
infarction. The Diabetes Mellitus Insulin Glucose Infusion in Acute
Myocardial Infarction (DIGAMI) trial. The DIGAMI study sought to
test the hypothesis that intensive glycemic control in diabetic patients
with acute myocardial infarction would improve mortality relative to
standard hypoglycemic therapy. The investigators randomized 620
patients (mean hemoglobin A1c 8.0%) with diabetes and acute myocardial infarction to intensive therapy with insulin and glucose infusion for
at least 24 hours followed by four times daily subcutaneous insulin
injections for at least 3 months or standard diabetic control (using
insulin only as necessary). At 1 year, glycemic control as measured by
the hemoglobin A1c was significantly improved in the insulin infusion
arm relative to control. Over a mean follow-up of 3.4 years, there were
102 (33%) deaths in the treatment group compared with 138 (44%)
deaths in the control group (relative risk 0.72; 95% CI, 0.55–0.92;
P = 0.011). Kaplan-Meier estimates of survival according to treatment
assignment are displayed. The results of this trial are buttressed by the
results of the United Kingdom Prospective Diabetes Study (UKPDS)
[47,48], which found a marked reduction in the incidence of microvascular disease and diabetes-related complications (including myocardial
infarction) among patients managed with tight glucose control (defined
as hemoglobin A1c < 7.0%). Aggressive management of hyperglycemia
is likely important, therefore, to prevention of cardiovascular complications in patients with diabetes. (*Adapted from* Malmberg [47].)

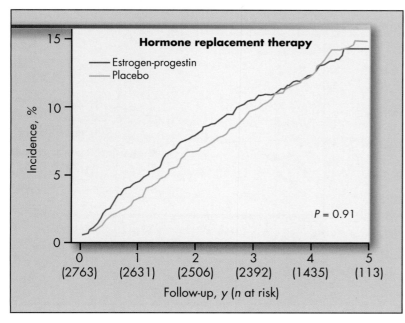

Figure 19-20.
Hormone replacement therapy (HRT) provides no benefit in secondary prevention of cardiovascular events: the Heart Estrogen/progestin Replacement Study (HERS). Estrogen replacement therapy is associated with beneficial effects on serum lipoprotein levels, vasomotor tone, and atherogenesis. Limited epidemiologic evidence initially suggested a ben-

efit to estrogen replacement in secondary prevention of cardiovascular events. However, to date, no prospective, randomized controlled trials of hormone replacement have confirmed evidence of reduction in death or myocardial infarction. HERS was the first large-scale trial to address the role of HRT in the secondary prevention of coronary heart disease. In this trial, 2763 postmenopausal women with pre-existing coronary artery disease and an intact uterus, were randomized to therapy with placebo or 0.625 mg of conjugated equine estrogens plus 2.5 mg of medroxyprogesterone acetate. Over a median follow-up of 4.1 years, there were significant differences between the two groups with regard to the primary outcome of nonfatal myocardial infarction or cardiovascular death (hazard ratio for hormone therapy relative to placebo = 0.99, 95% CI, 0.80–1.22, $P = 0.91$; Kaplan-Meier estimates for survival by treatment group are displayed). A time-trend analysis of the data, however, suggested a possible increase in the risk of cardiovascular events in the first year, with a decrease in risk in subsequent years. However, extended, unblinded follow-up of participants who continued hormone replacement therapy after the conclusion of HERS did not suggest a late benefit with longer duration of therapy [49]. Extensive post hoc subgroup analyses of HERS failed to identify any subgroup of participants in whom HRT was clearly beneficial. More women in the hormone group than in the placebo group experienced venous thromboembolic events. The lack of benefit (and potential harm) associated with HRT in postmenopausal women have led the American College of Cardiology and the American Heart Association to recommend that HRT not be initiated for secondary prevention of coronary heart disease. (*Adapted from* Hulley *et al.* [50].)

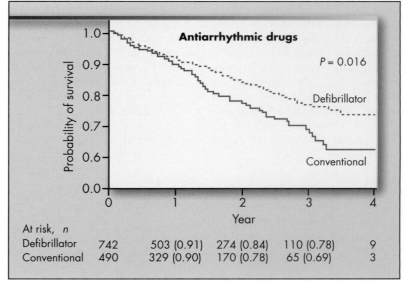

Figure 19-21.
Suppression of premature ventricular contractions with antiarrhythmic drugs after myocardial infarction is associated with increased mortality: the Cardiac Arrhythmia Suppression Trial. The Cardiac Arrhythmia Suppression Trial investigated the potential benefit of arrhythmia suppression utilizing class IC antiarrhythmic drugs. The investigators enrolled 1498 patients within 6 days to 2 years of myocardial infarction with frequent premature ventricular contractions or nonsustained ventricular tachycardia and randomized them to therapy with encainide, flecainide, or placebo. The trial was terminated prematurely at a mean follow up of 10 months because of a more than twofold increase in the risk of all-cause mortality in patients treated with either encainide or flecainide (relative risk = 2.38, $P = 0.0001$; Kaplan-Meier survival estimates by treatment group are shown). Suppression of ventricular ectopy using antiarrhythmic drugs, in particular class I antiarrhythmic agents, is therefore contraindicated after myocardial infarction. (*Adapted from* Echt *et al.* [51].)

Figure 19-22.
Prophylactic implantation of an implantable cardioverter-defibrillator (ICD) is associated with improved survival in patients with prior myocardial infarction and reduced ejection fraction: the Multicenter Automatic Defibrillator Implantation Trial II. Although suppression of ventricular ectopy after myocardial infarction with antiarrhythmic drugs is associated with no benefit and possible harm, implantation of an ICD in high-risk patients after myocardial infarction is associated with improved survival. The Multicenter Automatic Defibrillator Implantation Trail II randomly assigned 1232 patients with a prior myocardial infarction and a left ventricular ejection fraction of 0.30 or greater to receive an ICD or conventional medical therapy. During an average follow-up of 20 months, 14.2% of patients in the ICD arm and 19.8% of patients in the medical arm died. The hazard ratio for ICD relative to medical therapy with regard to all-cause mortality was 0.69 (95% CI, 0.51–0.93; $P = 0.016$; Kaplan-Meier estimates of survival stratified by treatment assignment are presented). Based on the results of this trial, the American College of Cardiology/American Heart Association guidelines support prophylactic implantation of an ICD in patients with prior myocardial infarction and a left ventricular ejection fraction 0.30 or greater (measured > 1 month after myocardial infarction).

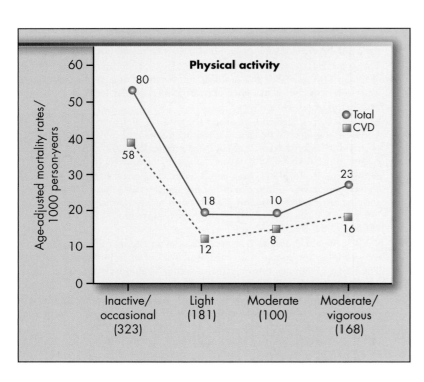

Study	Year	Patients, n
Mulcahy et al. [53]	1977	190
Sparrow et al. [54]	1978	195
Salonen [55]	1980	523
Rodda [56]	1983	918
Aberg et al. [57]	1983	983
Perkins and Dick [58]	1985	119
Johannson et al. [59]	1985	156
Burr et al. [60]	1992	1186
Hedback et al. [61]	1993	157
Tofler et al. [62]	1993	702
Herlitz et al. [63]	1995	217
Greenwood et al. [64]	1995	532
Overall		5878

Smoking cessation

0.02 0.05 0.10 0.20 0.50 1 2 5 10 20 50

Favors smoking cessation   Favors continued smoking

Odds ratio (95% CI)

Figure 19-23.
Favorable effect of smoking cessation on mortality after myocardial infarction. A meta-analysis of cohort studies demonstrated a substantial reduction in mortality with smoking cessation after myocardial infarction across several trials. In random effects models, the pooled odds ratio for death was 0.54 for smoking cessation relative to placebo (95% CI, 0.46–0.62; individual trial data is displayed) Benefit to smoking cessation was seen in every study included in the meta-analysis, with consistent benefits seen in men and women. These data are substantiated by subgroup analyses of prospective, randomized trials of therapeutic interventions for heart failure. The increased risk associated with smoking dissipates rapidly over the first 1 to 3 years after smoking cessation, such that the risk among former smokers approaches that of never-smokers after 10 to 15 years of abstinence. Smoking cessation is therefore essential after myocardial infarction. (*Adapted from* Wilson *et al.* [52].)

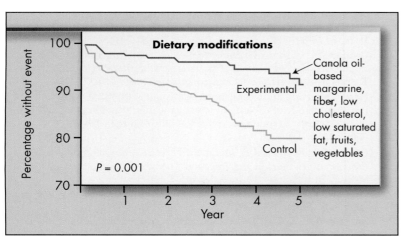

Figure 19-24.
Light-to-moderate activity is associated with a significantly lower risk of all-cause mortality in patients with established coronary artery disease [65]. Abundant epidemiologic data suggest that physical activity is strongly and inversely related to the risk of death from coronary heart disease. Increasing body mass index (BMI) is also associated with an increased risk of cardiovascular death and nonfatal myocardial infarction, with overweight (BMI 25–29.9 kg/m^2) and obese (BMI 30 kg/m^2 or greater) experiencing a high risk of cardiovascular events relative to those with BMI in the normal range [66]. This figure presents data for total and cardiovascular mortality for a cohort of 772 men with established coronary artery disease, according to level of reported physical activity. Those who pursued at least light physical activity on a regular basis experienced significantly lower mortality rates. Specifically, activities such as moderate or heavy gardening or regular walking (> 40 minutes per day) were associated with a significant reduction in all-cause mortality. Because of facilitation of weight loss, risk factor modification, and early resumption of physical activity, enrollment in a structured program of exercise-based cardiac rehabilitation significantly reduces mortality rates after myocardial infarction [67]. (*Adapted from* Wannamethee *et al.* [65].)

Figure 19-25.
Consumption of a Mediterranean-style diet is associated with a lower rate of cardiovascular complications following myocardial infarction. Dietary modification is a cornerstone of secondary prevention after myocardial infarction. Key features of the American Heart Association Step I diet include decreased intake of saturated fat and cholesterol and greater intake of fruits, vegetables, and whole grain products. Increasing data support the benefits of a Mediterranean-style diet, high in monounsaturated fat, for reducing cardiovascular risk. In the Lyon Heart Study, patients with previous myocardial infarction were randomized to a standard, Western-type diet or a Mediterranean style diet. Patients in the intervention group were instructed to consume fruit every day; eat more bread, fish, and root and green vegetables; eat less red meat; and replace butter and cream with canola oil–based margarine. At 46-month follow-up, patients on the Mediterranean diet experienced a significant reduction in the composite endpoint of death or nonfatal myocardial infarction. This figure contains the survival curves according to treatment assignment for the composite endpoint (relative risk, 0.28 for Mediterranean diet vs control; 95% CI, 0.15–0.53; P = 0.0001). (*Adapted from* De Lorgeril *et al.* [68].)

Secondary Prevention

References

1. Cooper R, Cutler J, Desvigne-Nickens P, *et al.*: Trends and disparities in coronary heart disease, stroke, and other cardiovascular diseases in the United States: findings of the National Conference on Cardiovascular Disease Prevention. *Circulation* 2000, 102:3137.

2. Third Report of the National Cholesterol Education Program (NCEP) Expert Panel on Detection, Evaluation, and Treatment of High Blood Cholesterol in Adults (Adult Treatment Panel III) final report. *Circulation* 2002, 106:3143–3421.

3. Qureshi AI, Suri MF, Guterman LR, Hopkins LN: Ineffective secondary prevention in survivors of cardiovascular events in the US population: report from the Third National Health and Nutrition Examination Survey. *Arch Int Med* 2001, 161:1621–1628.

4. Libby PL, Ridker PM, Maseri A: Inflammation and atherosclerosis. *Circulation* 2002, 105:1135–1143.

5. Packer M: The neurohormonal hypothesis: a theory to explain the mechanism of disease progression in heart failure. *J Am Coll Cardiol* 1992, 20:248–254.

6. Mann DL: Mechanisms and models in heart failure: a combinatorial approach. *Circulation* 1999, 100:999–1008.

7. Antithrombotic Trialists' Collaboration: Collaborative meta-analysis of randomised trials of antiplatelet therapy for prevention of death, myocardial infarction, and stroke in high risk patients. *BMJ* 2002, 324:71–86.

8. The Clopidogrel in Unstable Angina to Prevent Recurrent Events Investigators: Effects of clopidogrel in addition to aspirin in patients with acute coronary syndromes without ST-segment elevation. *N Engl J Med* 2001, 345:494–502.

9. Helft G, Osende JI, Worthley SG, *et al.*: Acute antithrombotic effect of a front-loaded regimen of clopidogrel in patients with atherosclerosis on aspirin. *Arterioscler Thromb Vasc Biol* 2000, 20:2316–2321.

10. Gaspoz JM, Coxson PG, Goldman PA, *et al.*: Cost effectiveness of aspirin, clopidogrel, or both for secondary prevention of coronary heart disease. *N Engl J Med* 2002, 346:1800–1806.

11. Hurlen M, Abdelnoor M, Smith P, *et al.*: Warfarin, aspirin, or both after myocardial infarction. *N Engl J Med* 2002, 347:969–974.

12. Anand S, Yusuf S: Oral anticoagulant therapy in patients with coronary artery disease: a meta-analysis. *JAMA* 1999, 282:2058–2067.

13. Antman EM, Anbe DT, Armstrong PW, *et al.*: ACC/AHA guidelines for management of patients with ST-elevation myocardial infarction: executive summary. *J Am Coll Cardiol* 2004, 44:671–719.

14. Gornik HL, O'Gara PT: Adjunctive medical therapy. In *Clinical Trials in Heart Disease*, edn 2. Edited by Manson JE, Buring JE, Ridker PM, Gaziano JM. Philadelphia: Elsevier Saunders; 2004:109–129.

15. The Norwegian Multicenter Study Group: Timolol-induced reduction in mortality and reinfarction in patients surviving acute myocardial infarction. *N Engl J Med* 1981, 301:801–807.

16. Beta-blocker Heart Attack Trial Research Group: A randomized trial of propranolol in patients with acute myocardial infarction: I. Mortality results. *JAMA* 1982, 247:1707–1714.

17. Boissel JP, Leizorovicz A, Picolet H, *et al.*: Secondary prevention after high-risk acute myocardial infarction with low dose acebutolol. *Am J Cardiol* 1990, 66:251–260.

18. Carvedilol Post-Infarct Survival Control in LV dysfunction Investigators: Effect of carvedilol on outcome after myocardial infarction in patients with left-ventricular dysfunction: the CAPRICORN randomized trial. *Lancet* 2001, 357:1385–1390.

19. Gottlieb SS, McCarter RJ, Vogel RA: Effect of beta-blockade on mortality among high-risk and low-risk patients after myocardial infarction. *N Engl J Med* 1998, 339:489–497.

20. Flather MD, Pfeffer MA: Angiotensin-converting enzyme inhibitors. In *Clinical Trials in Cardiovascular Disease: A Companion to Braunwald's Heart Disease*. Edited by Hennekens CH. Philadelphia: WB Saunders; 1999:97.

21. Swedberg K, Held P, Kjekshus J, *et al.*: Effects of the early administration of enalapril on mortality in patients with aute myocardial infarction. Results of the Cooperative New Scandinavian Enalapril Survival Study II (CONSENSUS II). *N Engl J Med* 1992, 327:678–684.

22. Gruppo Italiano per lo Studio della Sopravivenza nell'Infarto Miocardiaco (GISSI-3): Effects of lisinopril and transdermal glyceryl trinitrate singly and together on 6-week mortality and ventricular function after acute myocardial infarction. Gruppo Italiano per lo Studio della Sopravivenza nell'Infarto Miocardiaco. *Lancet* 1994, 343:1115–1122.

23. Chinese Cardiac Study Collaborative Group (CCS-1): Oral captopril versus placebo among 14,962 patients with suspected acute myocardial infarction: a multicenter, randomized, double-blind, placebo-controlled clinical trial. *Chinese Med J* 1997, 110:834–838.

24. Chinese Cardiac Study Collaborative Group: Oral captopril versus placebo among 13,634 patients with suspected acute myocardial infarction: interim report from the Chinese Cardiac Study (CCS-1). *Lancet* 1995, 345:686–687.

25. Fourth International Study of Infarct Survival (ISIS-4) Collaborative Group (ISIS-4): A randomized factorial trial assessing early captopril, oral mononitrate, and intravenous magnesium sulphate in 58,050 patients with suspected acute myocardial infarction. *Lancet* 1995, 345:669–685.

26. Pfeffer MA, Braunwald E, Moye LA, *et al.*: Effect of captopril on mortality and morbidity in patients with left ventricular dysfunction after myocardial infarction. Results of the survival and ventricular enlargement trial. The SAVE Investigators. *N Engl J Med* 1992, 327:669–677.

27. The Acute Infarction Ramipril Efficacy (AIRE) Study Investigators: Effect of ramipril on mortality and morbidity of survivors of acute myocardial infarction with clinical evidence of heart failure. *Lancet* 1993, 342:821–828.

28. Kober L, Torp-Pedersen C, Carlsen JE, *et al.*: A clinical trial of the angiotensin converting enzyme-inhibitor trandolapril in patients with left ventricular dysfunction after myocardial infarction. Trandolapril Cardiac Evaluation (TRACE) Study Group. *N Engl J Med* 1995, 333:1670–1676.

29. Ambrosioni E, Borghi C, Magnani B, *et al.*: The effect of the angiotensin converting enzyme-inhibitor zofrenopril on mortality and morbidity after anterior myocardial infarction. The Survival of Myocardial Infarction Long-Term Evaluation (SMILE) Study Investigators. *N Engl J Med* 1995, 332:80–85.

30. Yusuf S, Sleight P, Pogue J, *et al.*: Effects of an angiotensin-converting-enzyme inhibitor, ramipril, on cardiovascular events in high-risk patients. The Heart Outcomes Prevention Evaluation Study Investigators. *N Engl J Med* 2000, 342:145–153.

31. Pfeffer MA, McMurray JJV, Velazquez EJ, *et al.*: Valsartan, captopril, or both in myocardial infarction complicated by heart failure, left ventricular dysfunction, or both. *N Engl J Med* 2003, 349:1893–1906.

32. Pitt B, Remme W, Zannad F, *et al.*: Eplerenone, a selective aldosterone blocker, in patients with left ventricular dysfunction after myocardial infarction. *N Engl J Med* 2003, 348:1309–1321.

33. Pitt B, Zannad F, Remme W, *et al.*: The effect of spironolactone on morbidity and mortality in patients with severe heart failure. The Randomized Aldactone Evaluation Study Investigators. *N Engl J Med* 1999, 341:709–717.

34. Grundy SM, Cleeman JI, Bairey Merz CN, *et al.*: Implications of recent clinical trials for the National Cholesterol Education Program Adult Treatment Panel III Guidelines. *Circulation* 2004, 110:227–239.

35. Heart Protection Study Collaborative Group: MRC/BHF Heart Protection Study of cholesterol lowering with simvastatin in 20,536 high-risk individuals: a randomised placebo-controlled trial. *Lancet* 2002, 360:7–22.

36. Cannon CP, Braunwald E, McCabe CH, *et al.*: Pravastatin or Atorvastatin Evaluation and Infection Therapy-Thrombolysis in Myocardial Infarction 22 Investigators. Intensive versus moderate lipid lowering with statins after acute coronary syndromes. *N Engl J Med* 2004, 350:1495–1504.

37. Scranton RE, Gaziano JM: Cholesterol reduction. In *Clinical Trials in Heart Disease*, edn 2. Edited by Manson JE, Buring JE, Ridker PM, Gaziano JM. Philadelphia: Elsevier Saunders; 2004:267–277.

38. Randomised trial of cholesterol lowering in 4444 patients with coronary heart disease: the Scandinavian Simvastatin Survival Study (4S). *Lancet* 1994, 344:1383–1389.

39. Sacks FM, Pfeffer MA, Moye LA, *et al.*: The effect of pravastatin on coronary events after myocardial infarction in patients with average cholesterol levels: Cholesterol and Recurrent Events Trial investigators. *N Engl J Med* 1996, 335:1001–1009.

40. The Long-Term Intervention with Pravastatin in Ischaemic Disease (LIPID) Study Group: Prevention of cardiovascular events and death with pravastatin in patients with coronary heart disease and a broad range of initial cholesterol levels. *N Engl J Med* 1998, 339:1349–1357

41. Shepherd J, Blauw GJ, Murphy MB, *et al.*: PROSPER study group. Pravastatin in elderly individuals at risk of vascular disease (PROSPER): a randomized controlled trial. Prospective Study of Pravastatin in the Elderly at Risk. *Lancet* 2002, 360:1623–1630.

42. Mikhailidis DP, Wierzbicki AS: The Greek Atorvastatin and Coronary-heart-disease Evaluation (GREACE) study. *Curr Med Res Opin* 2002, 18:215–219.

43. Sever PS, Dahlof B, Poulter NR, *et al.*: Prevention of coronary and stroke events with atorvastatin in hypertensive patients who have average or lower-than-average cholesterol concentrations, in the Anglo-Scandinavian Cardiac Outcomes Trial–Lipid Lowering Arm (ASCOT-LLA): a multi-centre randomised controlled trial. *Lancet* 2003, 361:1149–1158.

44. LaRosa JC, He J, Vupputuri S: Effect of statins on risk of coronary disease: a meta-analysis of randomized controlled trials. *JAMA* 1999, 282:2340–2346.

45. Rubins HB, Robins SJ, Collins D, *et al.*: Gemfibrozil for the secondary prevention of coronary heart disease in men with low levels of high-density lipoprotein cholesterol: Veterans Affairs High Density Lipoprotein Cholesterol Intervention Trial Study Group. *N Engl J Med* 1999, 341:410–418.

46. Haffner SM, Lehto S, Ronnemaa T, *et al.*: Mortality from coronary heart disease in subjects with type 2 diabetes and in nondiabetic subjects with and without prior myocardial infarction. *N Engl J Med* 1998, 339:229–234.

47. Malmberg K, for the Diabetes Mellitus Insulin Glucose Infusion in Acute Myocardial Infarction (DIGAMI) Study Group: Prospective randomised study of intensive insulin treatment on long term survival after acute myocardial infarction in patients with diabetes mellitus. *BMJ* 1997, 314:1512–1515.

48. UK Prospective Diabetes Study (UKPDS) Group: Intensive blood-glucose control with sulphonylureas or insulin compared with conventional treatment and risk of complications in patients with type 2 diabetes (UKPDS 33). *Lancet* 1998, 352:837–853.

49. Grady D, Herrington D, Bittner V, *et al.*: Cardiovascular disease outcomes during 6.8 years of hormone therapy. Heart and Estrogen/progestin Replacement Study follow-up (HERS II). *JAMA* 2002, 288:49–57.

50. Hulley S, Grady D, Bush T, *et al.*: Randomized trial of estrogen plus progestin for secondary prevention of coronary heart disease in postmenopausal women. *JAMA* 1998, 280:605–613.

51. Echt DS, Liebson PR, Mitchell LB, *et al.*: Mortality and morbidity in patients receiving encainide, flecainide, or placebo. The Cardiac Arrhythmia Suppression Trial. *N Engl J Med* 1991, 324:781–788.

52. Wilson K, Gibson N, Willan A, *et al.*: Effect of smoking cessation on mortality after myocardial infarction: meta-analysis of cohort studies. *Arch Int Med* 2000, 160:939–944.

53. Mulcahy R, Hicker N, Graham IM, *et al.*: Factors affecting the 5 year survival rate of men following acute coronary heart disease. *Am Heart J* 1977, 93:556–559.

54. Sparrow D, Dawber TR: The influence of cigarette smoking on prognosis after a first myocardial infarction: a report from the Framingham study. *J Chronic Dis* 1978, 31:425–432.

55. Salonen JT: Stopping smoking and long-term mortality after acute myocardial infarction. *Br Heart J* 1980, 430:463–469.

56. Rodda BE: The Timolol Myocardial Infarction Study: an evaluation of selected variables. *Circulation* 1983, 67:I101–I106.

57. Aberg A, Bergstrand R, Johansson S, *et al.*: Cessation of smoking after myocardial infarction: effects on mortality after 10 years. *Br Heart J* 1983, 49:416–422.

58. Perkins J, Dick TB: Smoking and myocardial infarction: secondary prevention. *Postgrad Med J* 1985, 61:295–300.

59. Johansson S, Bergstrand R, Pennert K, *et al.*: Cessation of smoking in myocardial infarction in women: effects on mortality and reinfarction. *Am J Epidemiol* 1985, 121:823–831.

60. Burr ML, Holliday RM, Rehily AM, *et al.*: Haematological prognostic indices after myocardial infarction: evidence from the Diet and Reinfarction Trial (DART). *Eur Heart J* 1992, 13:166–170.

61. Hedback B, Perk J, Wodlin P: Long-term reduction of cardiac mortality after myocardial infarction: 10-year results of a comprehensive rehabilitation program. *Eur Heart J* 1993, 14:831–835.

62. Tofler GH, Muller JE, Stone PH, *et al.*: Comparison of long-term outcome after acute myocardial infarction in patients never graduated from high school with that in more educated patients. Multicenter Investigation of the Limitation of Infarct Size (MILIS). *Am J Cardiol* 1993, 71:1031–1035.

63. Herlitz J, Bengston A, Hjalmarson A, *et al.*: Smoking habits in consecutive patients with myocardial infarction: prognosis in relation to other risk indicators and to whether or not they quit smoking. *Cardiology* 2005, 86:496–502.

64. Greenwood DC, Muir KR, Packham CJ, *et al.*: Stress social support and stopping smoking after myocardial infarction in England. *J Epidemiol Community Health* 1995, 49:583–587.

65. Wannamethee SG, Shaper AG, Walker M: Physical activity and mortality in older men with diagnosed coronary heart disease. *Circulation* 2000, 102:1358–1363.

66. National Institutes of Health and National Heart, Lung, and Blood Institute: Clinical guidelines on the identification, evaluation, and treatment of overweight and obesity in adults. The Evidence Report. *Obes Res* 1998, 6:51S–209S.

67. Oldrige NB, Guyatt GH, Fischer ME, *et al.*: Cardiac rehabilitation after myocardial infarction: combined experience of randomized clinical trials. *JAMA* 1988, 260:945–950.

68. De Lorgeril M, Salen P, Martin JL, *et al.*: Mediterranean diet, traditional risk factors, and the rate of cardiovascular complications after myocardial infarction: Final Report of the Lyon Diet Heart Study. *Circulation* 1999, 99:779–785.

Childhood Risk Factors Predict Adult Cardiovascular Risk and Strategies for Prevention: The Bogalusa Heart Study

Gerald S. Berenson for the Bogalusa Heart Study Group

Cardiovascular (CV) risk factors can be identified in childhood and are predictive of CV disease later in life. Observations in the Bogalusa Heart Study have shown an important correlation of clinical risk factors in early life, with anatomic changes at autopsy in the aorta and coronary vessels with atherosclerosis and cardiac and renal changes related to hypertension. These observations have been extended by echocardiographic Doppler studies of carotid arteries and intima media thickness (IMT). A close association of risk factors in young adults, 20 to 38 years of age, occurs with IMT, and a marked increase in IMT is observed as the numbers of risk factors increase. Obesity and low-density lipoprotein cholesterol are strong predictors of subclinical disease; even childhood levels predict adult CV changes. Observations of risk factors in young individuals and noninvasive studies of structure and function changes of the CV system have strong implications for prevention by cardiologists. Health education of children as a population approach for prevention is a practical strategy that needs encouragement from the medical profession.

Cardiovascular risk factors in childhood are predictive of future CV risk in adulthood [1,2]. Although clinical events occur in middle aged and older individuals, the diseases of atherosclerosis, hypertension, and diabetes mellitus clearly begin in childhood. Studies of environmental and genetic factors related to CV disease, although continuingly being investigated as the earliest determinants of CV risk, indicate a great deal has been achieved in understanding susceptibility (risk) in early life [1–4]. Risk factors as measured clinically are governed by genes and environment; the genetic-environmental interaction is what is perceived when measured clinically. This interaction is expressed as a long-term burden on the CV system. Many studies now show that risk factor levels at an early age are associated with anatomic changes in the CV-renal system. Lifestyles and behaviors developing in early childhood contribute considerably to this long-term burden and ultimately result in overt clinical CV disease. Unhealthy lifestyles, such as high-fat high-calorie diet, physical inactivity leading to obesity, and tobacco use represent strong environmental conditions that relate to latent or "silent" CV lesions and disease in the CV system.

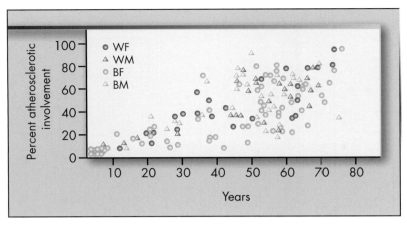

Figure 20-1.
Atherosclerotic involvement in sampling of human aortas of varying ages. This figure illustrates increasing occurrence of atherosclerotic lesions by age and race. Pathologists long ago determined that atherosclerosis occurred at a young age [5]. Cardiologists, who understand the clinical aspects of the endstage process of heart disease, have the opportunity to study cardiovascular risk, the subtle underlying cardiac and vascular changes in young individuals at the beginning stages of disease, and to implement prevention strategies. BF—black female; BM—black male; WF—white female; WM—white male.

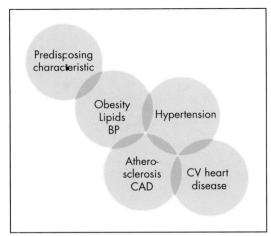

Figure 20-2.
Natural history of cardiovascular (CV) heart disease. The Bogalusa Heart Study is a comprehensive study of the early natural history of CV disease in a population of children and young adults from a biracial (65% white, 35% black), semi-rural community [1,2]. The study began in 1973 as an effort to understand the evolution of adult heart disease beginning in early life. This figure shows conceptually the natural history of CV disease beginning in early life with predisposing characteristics, the lifelong burden of CV risk factors, and clinical expression of heart disease at an older age. The study has continued with multiple cross-sectional surveys in childhood and longitudinal studies extending from young adult age into the middle age to overlap with observations from the Framingham Study [6]. BP—blood pressure; CAD—coronary artery disease.

Enigmas of the Early Natural History of Coronary Artery Disease and Essential Hypertension

Is it possible to diagnose coronary atherosclerosis in early life?
Is it possible to diagnose type 2 diabetes in childhood?
What is the evidence that essential hypertension begins in childhood?
    High blood pressure: hypertensions
    Hypertensive cardiovascular end-stage disease

Figure 20-3.
Major questions that form the basis for the Bolagusa Heart Study. The Bolagusa Heart Study provides observations of secular trends, long-term observations, and predictors of adult risk from childhood. Extensive cardiovascular risk factor data on approximately 16,000 individuals compose a database from birth to 45 years of age. Many subjects have had multiple observations, from one to 12 repeated studies with an average of seven examinations. These have provided data on secular trends over time, tracking of risk factors and longitudinal changes, and observations on the interrelation of risk factors. As children aged, these studies extended into the adult years. With certain limitations we can answer all of these questions in a positive manner.

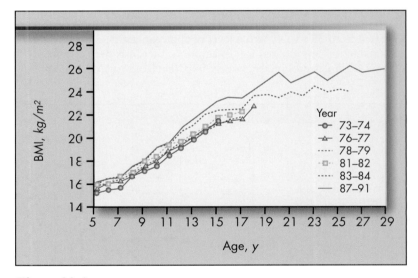

Figure 20-4.
Body mass index (BMI) in children and young adults. Repeated surveys have shown secular trends by repeated examinations of subjects years apart but following a common protocol. Figure 20-4 illustrates the dramatic increase of obesity as body mass index, *without* an increase in height. Although the increase of obesity has occurred in the population generally, it is especially great in black females and in the children at the higher percentiles of the distribution.

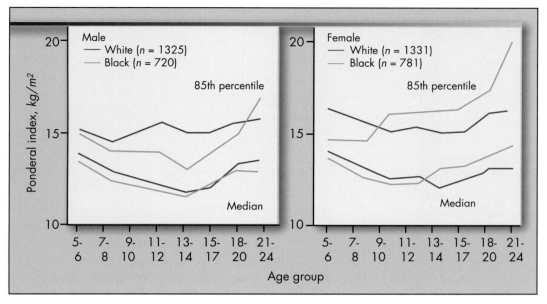

Figure 20-5.

Race and gender distribution of the Ponderal index in 5- to 24-year-old subjects. This figure shows the marked increase of body fatness in black females at puberty. Since 1973, children on average gained 5 kilograms of body weight without comparable increase in height [7,8]. This upward secular trend in childhood obesity reflects the national trend seen in children and in adults [9].

With this increasing obesity, there is a notable increase in the incidence of type 2 diabetes mellitus in adults and an increase in an early onset of diabetes during adolescence [9]. In addition, a secular trend in dietary intake has also occurred. An increase of P/S ratio from 0.30 to approximately 0.45 occurred in the mid-1970s with the industrial introduction of liquid oils for cooking. The total fat consumption has decreased from 38% to 40% to a level of approximately 33% of the diet and a reduction in saturated fat. In addition, there has been a marked decrease of cholesterol intake, largely in part related to a decreased consumption of eggs [10]. Although increased body weight has occurred, little detectable change of caloric intake has been reported. However, the limitations in the methods of quantitating diet limits accurately documenting slight caloric increases. Yet, the availability of food and its composition have changed. Dietary caloric imbalance with decreasing physical inactivity have contributed to and account for the dramatic increase of body weight and body fatness [11]. The dietary patterns show a large increase of high-carbohydrate soft drinks, high intake of corn starch and snacks, and diet composition has been associated with risk factors related to the metabolic syndrome [12].

Although dietary characteristics have changed, physical inactivity has also changed. There has been a considerable increase of computer activities and computer games. Television watching is documented to occur 2 to 4 hours per day. Consequently, decreased physical activity has become a major contributor to increasing obesity.

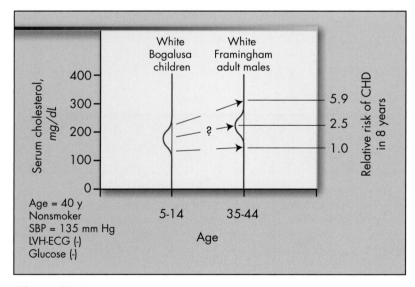

Figure 20-6.

Do risk factor variables in children become risk factors in adults? This figure shows the importance of tracking risk factors. Levels of risk factor variables for an individual "track" and tend to remain over time in a given rank for an individual relative to peers. "Tracking," based on findings beginning in early life, is important because childhood risk factors predict adult cardiovascular risk factors and underlying clinical disease. Although risk factors track to varying degrees, the measures of obesity track at a very high level and relate to adult cardiovascular risk [13,14]. CHD—coronary heart disease; LVH-ECG—electrocardiographic left ventricular hypertrophy; SBP—systolic blood pressure.

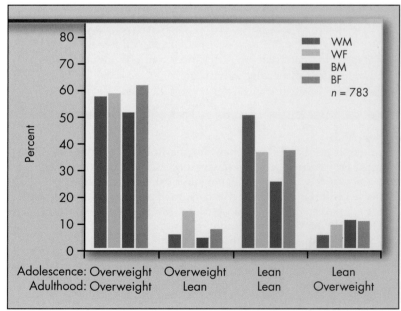

Figure 20-7.

Persistence of obese or lean adolescents over 12 to14 years at 25 to 31 years of age. Obesity, which begins in infancy and childhood, persists into adulthood, and body mass index levels in childhood are strongly predictive of adult body mass index. Serum total cholesterol and low-density lipoprotein cholesterol track almost as well. The magnitude of tracking of triglycerides, high-density lipoprotein cholesterol, and blood pressure is somewhat lower, likely because of biologic and measurement variability. BF—black female; BM—black male; WF—white female; WM—white male.

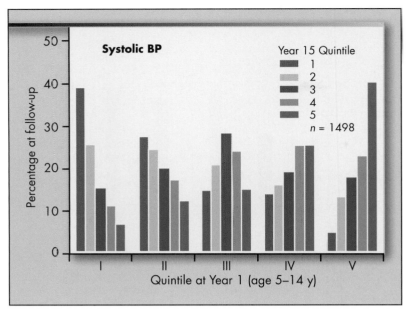

Figure 20-8.
Tracking of blood pressure from childhood to young adulthood: individuals remaining at respective quintiles of systolic blood pressure over a 15-year period [15].

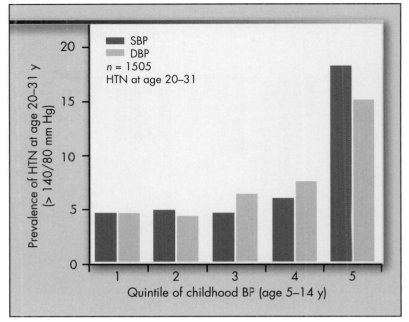

Figure 20-9.
Association between childhood blood pressure and adult hypertension (HTN) over 15 years. Childhood measurements are predictable of adult HTN [15]. DBP—diastolic blood pressure; SBP—systolic blood pressure.

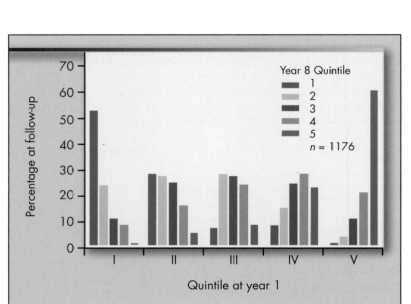

Figure 20-10.
Persistence of multiple cardiovascular risk clustering from childhood to young adulthood: individuals remaining at respective quintiles of multiple risk index (rank sum of systolic blood pressure, insulin, and total and high-density lipoprotein cholesterol) over an 8-year period [16]. The adverse impact of obesity on individual cardiovascular risk variables has been found in children and adults. Although obesity strongly relates to adverse changes of other risk factors, obesity correlates with higher insulin levels [17–19]. Analyses from childhood to adulthood show adiposity in childhood precedes the hyperinsulinemia at older age periods, independently of race, gender, and baseline fasting insulin levels [20]. Developing adiposity becomes an independent predictor of the evolving cluster of risk variables consistent with the metabolic or insulin resistance syndrome. Risk factors are additive and interactive in these constellations. The occurrence of multiple risk factors produces a burden on the cardiovascular (CV) system over time, and accelerates the development of systemic atherosclerosis and hypertensive CV disease [21].

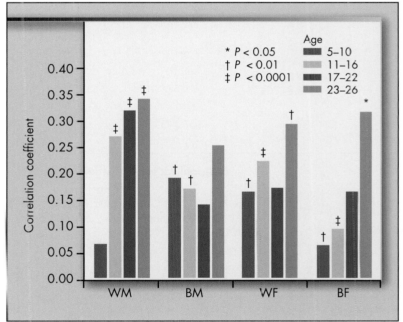

Figure 20-11.
Relationship of very low-density lipoprotein cholesterol with Wt/Ht^3 by age group, race, and gender. This figure (as well as Fig. 20-15) shows a strong association of ponderal index (Wt/Ht^3), equivalent to body mass index, with adverse changes of lipoproteins. Very low density lipoprotein cholesterol increases markedly with obesity and the association increases with age in white males, and particularly high-density lipoprotein cholesterol decreases with obesity. BF—black female; BM—black male; WF—white female; WM—white male.

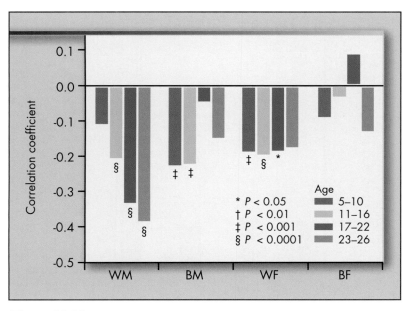

Figure 20-12.
Relationship of high-density lipoprotein cholesterol with Wt/Ht³ by age group, race, and gender. BF—black female; BM—black male; WF—white female; WM—white male.

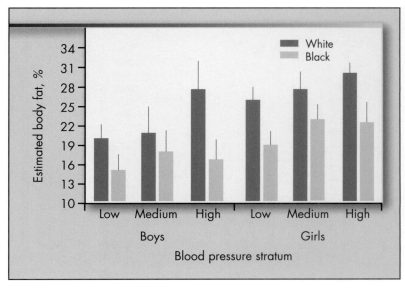

Figure 20-13.
Estimated percent of body fat by race, gender, and blood pressure stratum in children aged 7 to 15 years. Even though obesity is clearly shown to relate to higher blood pressure levels in children [22], this figure shows obesity in white children is associated more with higher blood pressure levels than in young blacks [23,24]. Although individual risk factors correlate with other risk factors in childhood and adulthood alike, obesity potentially relates to higher blood pressure levels through multiple mechanisms. Risk factors are interactive and tend to occur in constellations. Based on these observations, the metabolic or insulin resistance syndrome, which includes dyslipidemia, hypertension, hyperinsulinemia/insulin resistance, and central obesity, is evident in childhood, but seems to increase with age. Ultimately, abnormal clinical levels occur according to criteria of the Adult Treatment Panel III and World Health Organization [25,26]. Because childhood levels differ from adult levels, childhood criteria, such as the 75th percentile, are used to designate abnormal levels. Age-related changes of abdominal obesity and the attendant insulin resistance are central to the degree of clustering.

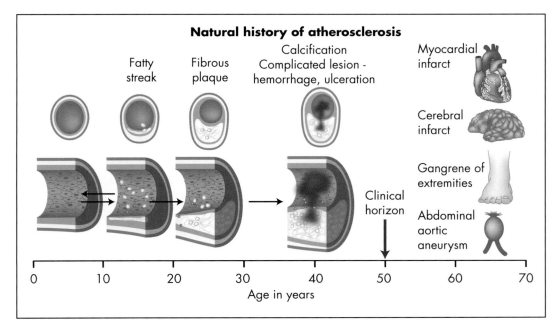

Figure 20-14.
The natural history of cardiovascular disease at an anatomic level. Autopsy studies in young individuals in the Bogalusa Heart Study provide the most compelling data to show that an unusually high prevalence of coronary atherosclerosis occurs at an early age in the general population [27–29]. By the third decade of life perhaps 90% of individuals in the United States show coronary atherosclerosis. The occurrence of atherosclerosis at an early age was found in autopsy studies in the International Atherosclerosis Study, and emphasized by McGill [30] and in studies soldiers dying in the Korean and Vietnamese wars [31,32].

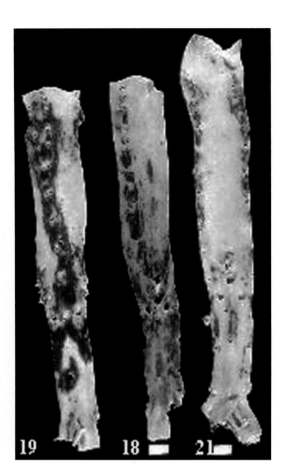

Figure 20-15.
Subjects of adolescent and young adult age with atherosclerotic involvement are shown for individuals who participated in the Bogalusa Heart Study and died from accidental causes. Fatty streaks begin to appear in the aorta even earlier than 3 years of age, and it has been recently reported that anatomic changes in the fetal arterial wall are conditioned by maternal hypercholesterolemia during pregnancy [33]. These early lesions adversely influence the rate of progression of lesions throughout childhood. Lesions also appear in other vascular beds early and show a predilection for different vascular sites [34]. In adolescence, progressive lesions involve the coronary arteries. Coronary vessels demonstrate fatty streaks and the fibrous plaques of raised, collagen-capped disease, and these become the precursors of more advanced lesions that occlude vessels by thrombosis.

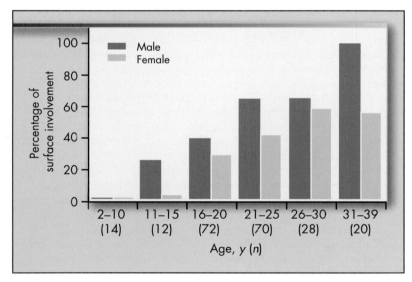

Figure 20-16.
Prevalence of coronary artery fibrous plaque by gender and age in children and young adults. This figure demonstrates gender differences and definite lag in the development of lesions in females versus males at a young age. Blacks also show more aorta fatty streaks [35], whereas white males show more coronary artery fibrous plaques [27,28]. Of importance is the strong relationship of antemortem cardiovascular risk factors to the extent of lesions.

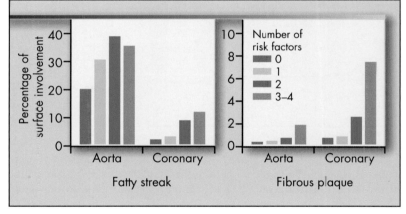

Figure 20-17.
Atherosclerotic surface involvement in children and young adults by risk factor status. The severity of atherosclerosis increases as a curvilinear increase in lesions in the aorta and coronaries with the increase in number of the multiple risk factors [28]. The Pathobiologic Determinants of Atherosclerosis in Youth (PDAY) study has confirmed the extent of these autopsy findings and has shown the importance of multiple risk factors in a young population [29]. These observations support the multiple risk factor concept of the Framingham Risk Score for predicting morbidity and mortality and emphasize the burden of multiple risk factors on the cardiovascular system. In addition to aorta and coronary vessels, involvement at various vascular sites, including carotid, cerebral, and renal vessels, indicates the systemic distribution of atherosclerosis. Other lesions, nonatherosclerotic, also are related to the effect of risk factors. For example, small renal artery changes occur with remodeling and are associated with higher levels of blood pressure [27]. Histologic studies of the kidney arteriolar bed also indicate the early effects of hypertension [36].

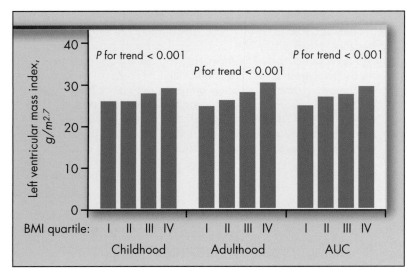

Figure 20-18.

Mean levels of left ventricular mass index in young adults by body mass index (BMI) quartile. The increase of left ventricular mass is associated with higher levels of blood pressure in young individuals. This is important because increased left ventricular mass in adults is an independent risk factor for cardiac events as shown in the Framingham Study [37]. Obesity and insulin resistance in children are also predictive of left ventricular hypertrophy [38]. Echocardiographic studies in children indicate that although linear growth is a major determinant of cardiac growth, overweight is equal to that of blood pressure as an important determinant of the acquisition of increased left ventricular mass in adulthood. AUC—area under the curve. (*Adapted from* Li *et al.* [39].)

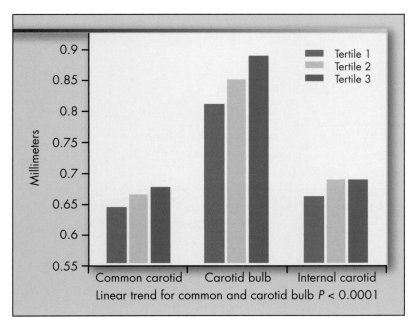

Figure 20-19.

Effect of Framingham Risk Score on the intima-media thickness in young adults. This figure shows the relation of the Framingham Risk Score with carotid intima-media thickness. Data from the Bogalusa Heart Study also reported increases in intima-media thickness with increasing numbers of risk factors (0, 1, 2, 3 or more) similar to the Framingham multivariate risk score at different segments. Changes especially for the common carotid and the carotid bulb segments are observed.

Although a profile of cardiovascular (CV) risk factors is useful in predicting CV events, inclusion of measurements of subclinical atherosclerosis by noninvasive imaging techniques are helpful in determining the extensiveness and severity of asymptomatic disease and potential future risk—evidence of "silent" disease. Imaging for calcification of coronary arteries indicates advanced coronary disease, but these observations do not determine the extensiveness of coronary atherosclerosis of noncalcified lesions, even in individuals with known coronary artery disease and risk factors. The Muscatine Study [40] has shown a relation of obesity from childhood with coronary calcification. Of the methods, such as coronary arteriography and intravascular coronary ultrasound studies (IVUS), that can confirm atherosclerotic disease at a young age, some are not applicable for large population studies, and they cannot be recommended for asymptomatic individuals. In contrast, the noninvasive ultrasonography studies of the carotid arteries, for example, are readily available and can be adapted for large numbers of asymptomatic individuals.

Intima media thickness (IMT) of carotid arteries by B-mode duplex ultrasonography in black and white subjects, aged 20 to 38 years, is shown in Figure 20-19 related to a Framingham score. Risk factor variables including age, gender, parental history, blood pressure, obesity measures, lipoproteins, insulin, glucose, and cigarette smoking all have a deleterious effect on carotid changes as has been shown for coronary vessel lesions. The means of three values, each for right and left farwall have been used for the common, the bulb or bifurcation, and internal carotid segments, and these show differences as illustrated in the figure. IMT in the common carotid and the bulb segments were significantly greater in blacks, males, and older individuals. Lumen narrowing by encroaching atherosclerotic plaques is unusual at a young age, except in familial hypercholesterolemia and in individuals with diabetes. However, changes of IMT do occur that can reveal increased CV risk.

The association of carotid IMT with multiple risk factor variables is likely a predictor of the severity of systemic atherosclerosis. Systolic blood pressure, race, age, low-density lipoprotein cholesterol and high-density lipoprotein cholesterol explain 16% variance in the common carotid IMT; age, systolic blood pressure, high-density lipoprotein cholesterol, low-density lipoprotein cholesterol, race, and, importantly, insulin explain 19.4% variance in the carotid bulb IMT; and gender and body mass index explain 4.7% variance in the internal carotid IMT.

Locations of the carotid vessels reflect variations in severity at different sites. These observations are consistent with the notion that the carotid bulb or bifurcation is more susceptible for atherosclerotic damage than the common carotid or internal carotid segments. Ku *et al.* [41] showed the importance of pulsatile hemodynamic forces on arterial wall structure, which led Glagov [41] to the concept of remodeling. Even earlier, Fry [42] showed the effect of hemodynamic forces on lipoprotein influx in the arterial wall. The thicker IMT at the bulb segment and stronger association of risk factors similar to that observed for coronary arteries suggest that sites of musculoelastic vessels in structural composition are more susceptible to the multiple risk factor influences on atherosclerosis. The common carotid site seems to reflect a more diffuse effect of hypertension. More elaborate investigations are needed to show the complexity and even genetic effects on vascular disease and different locations for progression of atherothrombotic disease.

Marked individual differences occur in IMT to reflect severity and advancement of disease in asymptomatic individuals in the general population. The top 5% of carotid artery at the common segment showed a range of 0.83 to 1.1 mm IMT, with a mean of 0.89 mm, and for the carotid bulb 0.90 to 2.57 mm, with a mean of 1.36 mm. These were significantly greater than for those at the low 5% of the population: range of 0.44 to 0.54 mm with a mean of 0.52 mm for the common carotid and 0.52 to 0.64 mm with a mean of 0.61 for the bulb.

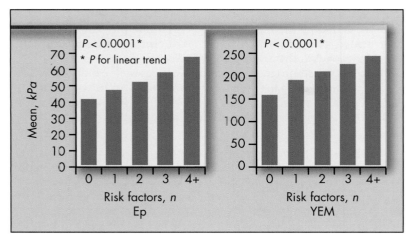

Figure 20-20.
The effect of multiple risk factors on measures of artery elasticity in young adults. Earlier, in a related study regarding vascular carotid artery distensibility in 10- to 17-year old subjects, an association of increased stiffness in terms of pressure-strain elastic modulus (Peterson's elastic modulus [Ep]) was reported, with elevated levels of serum total cholesterol and systolic blood pressure and a positive parental history of myocardial infarction [43]. This observation indicated that cardio-vascular (CV) risk factors already had a detectable effect on vascular changes at a young age. It is possible that studies of compliance and distensibility could show that functional changes occur prior to detectable structural disease of the arterial wall with evidence of seg-mental atherosclerotic lesions. In this figure, Peterson's Ep and Young's elastic modulus (YEM) related to increasing numbers of risk factors similar to atherosclerotic changes of coronary and carotid vessels [44].

The subclinical underlying structure/function changes in the carotid arteries, especially at the bulb site, by relating to multiple CV risk factors in young individuals are a predictor of future CV events. Carotid ultra-sound measurements are relatively easy to obtain and reflect the intensity of the long-term burden of CV risk factors. Studies of such changes of "vascular age" compared with "chronologic age," as determined by a Framingham score, may advance the capability of disease prediction. Understanding risk factors at a young age and observing their effects on the CV system are useful to guide early prevention modalities.

Guidelines for Prevention of Adult Heart Disease in Early Life

A family at risk = a member with:
Myocardial infarction before age of 60
Hypertension and/or cerebrovascular accident
High level of LDL-C (> 75th percentile for age, gender)
Low level of HDL-C (< 25th percentile for age, gender)
Obesity (> 85th percentile for age, gender)
Adult-onset diabetes
Smoking habit

Figure 20-22.
The High Risk Model: Heart Smart Family Health Promotion. This model is an approach to improve healthy lifestyles of an entire family [45,46]. The program uses lectures, counseling, demonstrations and hands-on activities, and behavioral training strategies. The program increases knowledge of heart-healthy behavior and is directed toward improving eating and exercise habits in families with known increased risk for coronary artery disease. Although the program was initially developed in a school setting and for a military base [47], it is a clinical program to be adapted by hospitals or in clinical-office based settings in which a detailed program of preventive care

Practical Concepts for Prevention in Children of Adult Heart Disease "Heart Smart" Program

Intervention methods:
Population strategy
Cardiovascular health education for school children
High-risk strategy
Family health promotion

Figure 20-21.
There are two epidemiologic approaches to preventive cardiology devoted to adoption of healthy lifestyles that can potentially influence and delay the development of heart disease. These are the "High Risk Approach" and a more general "Public Health Model." Although the former address individuals and families with known high risk, the latter addresses the entire population. Both approaches are important, because of the need for prevention and because of the persuasiveness of heart disease in the total population. There are numerous clinical trials and available medications indicating the utility and effectiveness of pharmacologic management of risk factors in patients with documented heart disease. However, based on the discussed message of silent under-lying cardiovascular changes, these clinical trials address, for the most part, manifestations of endstage disease. The rest of the figures in this chapter will focus primarily on strategies to change behaviors and achieve healthy lifestyles. Obviously, subtleties in understanding the role of components of dietary intake and physical activity will change over time, but learning behavioral skills and decision-making are important for both approaches. Education and skills will aid decision-making in which choices based on new information can influence achieving healthy lifestyles. It is difficult to overestimate the importance of healthy eating and exercise habits for disease prevention, easy to under-stand the detrimental effects of poor lifestyles, for example, tobacco use and excess alcohol or drug use, but achieving healthy lifestyles requires a concerted effort to balance environmental and social forces.

can be developed by a multidisciplinary team. Ideally, the program is imple-mented with a multidisciplinary team consisting of 1) a preventive cardiolo-gist, 2) a nurse specialist, 3) a nutritionist, 4) exercise physiologist, and 5) a psychologist. The multiple talents of such a team are needed to train families and individuals to achieve healthy lifestyles over a period of time for training. The Heart Smart Family Health Promotion programs recommends training be taught to all family members for a period of 10 to 12 weeks [48].

Individuals with known coronary heart disease and high-risk factors, for example, individuals with hypertension, dyslipidemia or diabetes, or clinical coronary heart disease, provide a basis for involving their fami-lies along with their own personal care. Patients with coronary heart disease bypass surgery stents usually are treated and guided for lifestyle changes, but they and their families, including children, also should be enrolled in family health promotion as shown in this figure.

The Family Health Promotion Program is a useful collaboration of cardiologists, pediatricians, and primary care physicians who can help guide individuals to enter a preventive program and guide the multidis-ciplinary team. This figure helps target families including children at markedly increased risk for coronary heart disease. Elevated risks through heritability and shared household effects run in families. Behavior is notoriously difficult to change, and patients are more likely to adopt healthy lifestyles in which there is family support. When necessary changes are expected from everyone, not just the family member with apparent illness, it is likely that lifestyles can be improved.

Children and parents are recruited into a 2- to 3-month program to gradually train family members on lifestyles to reduce risk factors. Weekly sessions are followed by monthly visits.

(*continued on next page*)

Figure 20-22. *continued*
The goal of the program is to encourage all family members to adopt healthy lifestyles, which, understandably, takes time. All members of the family, children and parents, undergo cardiovascular risk factor profiling. This examination consists of blood pressure, anthropometric measurements, evaluation, serum lipids and lipoproteins, urinalysis, and self-reported personal and family medical history. Information on dieting and exercise habits and use of tobacco and alcohol are obtained. Although the Family Health Promotion program is ideally implemented with a multidisciplinary team, primary care physicians can adapt this model to their own setting with trained personnel. Components of the program, behavioral strategies, nutritional and exercise training, and a maintenance phase are all part of the Family Health Promotion program. HDL-C—high-density lipoprotein cholesterol; LDL-C—low-density lipoprotein cholesterol.

Cardiovascular Health Promotion for Families and Children

Behavioral concepts	
Behavioral	**Social/cognitive**
Self-monitoring	Social support
Feedback	Modeling
Stimulus control	Self-efficacy
Shaping/skills building	Positive self-statements
Positive reinforcement	
Goal setting/contracting	
Relaxation skills	

Figure 20-23.
Cardiovascular health promotion for families and children. Behavioral contracts can be made with children and parents, between participants and caregivers, or between adult members of a family. They include a specific behavior to be performed within a time frame with some kind of reward for performance. Awards are combined with the mastery experiences, and the satisfaction of having accomplished a task. For each desired behavior change, the staff implementing the program can use incentives or social reinforcement by congratulations or other forms of approval. The ultimate goal of the program is to achieve a feeling of intrinsic satisfaction to encourage the person to maintain new behavior over a long period. The dietary component includes modules that provide families with ways to develop and practice skills to observe healthy eating close to that recommended by the American Heart Association. Specific lesson plans should include menu planning, label reading, snacking, and eating out. Activities help motivate and adopt better habits of food intake. Role-playing games, food demonstrations, and food intake monitoring are part of the training. In addition, activities for improving eating at fast food outlets and restaurants are provided. Heart-healthy food coupons, food samples, and recipe booklets are part of the program. Tasting of several food products take place while families participate in brief discussions on nutrition concepts. Potluck picnics and exchange of modified family recipes are encouraged with discussions by staff on the dietary composition.

The exercise component involves counseling on specific exercises and instructions during at each session being devoted to an aerobic exercise led by the exercise trainer. Families are asked to design a program of outside physical activity with recommendations to achieve physical activity conducted over 45 minutes to 1 hour daily. Physical activity encourages aerobic and isometric exercise or cross-training, and the benefit of each are to be discussed. Families may choose a form of exercise similar to what children do in school, or they may select an activity such as walking or bicycling that can be done together. Specific goals are set and contracts negotiated with an award built in for meeting activity goals.

A maintenance phase is intended to help families continue changes once they have completed the program. Group strategies, for example, Weight Watchers and Alcoholics Anonymous, are important to gain peer support. Suggestions and information from various members with problems of high cardiovascular risks common to several members participating in the heart-healthy programs become valuable reinforcement. An overlap of family members completing the Heart Smart Family Health Promotion program will spill over to new members joining the group for the series of sessions. By repeated sessions over time, the members become more aware of their lifestyles, which are likely to be achieved by repeating the message of achieving healthy lifestyles over time.

Cardiac patients need preventive cardiology programs, such as the Family Health Promotion/Heart Smart program, for moral support. Children of cardiac patients carry the genetic risk for coronary artery disease and risk factor screening in early life can detect abnormal levels early. The multidisciplinary model can be adapted according to facilities available and modified by a setting for implementing the program. It is important that a primary care physician or cardiologist with interest in prevention oversee the program, particularly for coordinating medical management and pharmacologic treatment for specific risk factors, such as uncontrolled hypertension or dyslipidemia. Although there are controversies for screening children for cardiovascular risk factors, the pathologic and epidemiologic findings from Bogalusa research argue for universal evaluation and appropriate intervention beginning for all school-age children. Certainly, a positive family history is important in this regard as recommended in guidelines, but it is important for individuals to realize that the same risk factors found in adults also affect their offspring. Physicians in general, especially cardiologists, concern themselves with endstage heart disease with preventive medicine playing a secondary role. A trained and developed multidisciplinary team will require little time from physicians to help implement a prevention program for their patients and families.

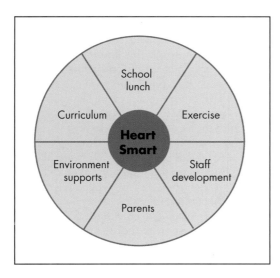

Figure 20-24.
Public health strategy and population model. The prevention of heart diseases through the development of healthy lifestyles in the general population involves understanding of the high prevalence of heart disease and a change of attitudes and personal involvement to make a change in lifestyles [49]. For children, prevention entails adoption and learning healthy lifestyles. Equally necessary is the need for socioeconomic changes in the population structure. Recognizing the development of heart disease at a young age to be so widespread in our population, the public health approach addressing the entire population of youth becomes paramount.

This figure shows an effective and comprehensive health education program (Health Ahead/Heart Smart) for elementary school children [50]. The program addresses the entire school environment including the students, the teachers, the parents, the cafeteria facilities, and the community [51]. The program includes classroom guides, a cafeteria and nutrition protocol, physical education curriculum and activities, lifestyles of teachers, and efforts to involve parents in the education process [52].

Cardiovascular Health Promotion for School Children

An interactive program

Multiple targeted areas	Multiple approaches
Nutrition	School
Exercise	Family
Cognitive/behavior (skills)	Community
	Media

Figure 20-25.
Cardiovascular health promotion for school children. As an interactive program, the targeted areas to approach are shown this figure. Lifestyles and behaviors that influence cardiovascular risk factors are learned in childhood. Therefore, healthy lifestyles need to be adopted early because they are critical to modulating risk factors in adult life. The observations of tracking show the difficulty and importance of being able to change or prevent risk factors begun earlier. However, cardiologists, pediatricians, and primary care family physicians have a tremendous opportunity to guide and help propagate prevention programs for the young [53]. If not, these children will be destined to be the next generation of cardiac patients.

Practical Problems Addressed by Health Education

Dropouts
Tobacco use
Alcohol abuse
Drug abuse
Teenage pregnancies
Suicides
Violent behavior

Figure 20-26.
Practical problems addressed by health educators. Although much emphasis is placed on improving nutrition and physical activity for children, it is equally important to address social problems, as listed in this figure. Drugs, alcohol, tobacco use, teenage pregnancy, sexually transmitted diseases, and even violent behavior accompanying poor lifestyles of students leading to dropouts. Health education needs to broadly address such problems and health in general. Without adoption of appropriate lifestyles, including healthy attitudes and morals, children cannot achieve lifestyles that will avoid the long-term burden of cardiovascular risk and, ultimately, chronic diseases as adults. Parents and teachers, as role models, are critical to this process and a health education program needs to be internalized to them as role models.

Although school activities help to implement a health education program, broad curriculum on general health, nutrition, physical activity and skills, and stress release should be internalized by teachers. Students are encouraged to have respect for their own bodies and respect for teachers and their parents by teaching self-esteem beginning in kindergarten. An adoption of good attitudes toward health starts as early as the age the education program addresses. The Health Ahead/Heart Smart materials are kindergarten through sixth grade, but preschool programs are important. Physical activity depends on facilities and available personnel. With a lack of physical educators. the classroom teacher should be able to implement physical activity for their students. The "Feeling Good" program emphasizes these aspects [54]. It is also important to include noncompetitive exercises so that all students, not just athletes, can participate. The Super Kids/Super Fit program emphasizes physical activity for all children. Physical education should be introduced as a lifestyle for fun for all children to be engaged in individually and with family and others [55]. Competitive exercises and team sports are important, but individual activities are most needed for a total population approach.

School nurses, if available, can obtain weight and height, body mass index, and blood pressures, and they can ensure adequate vaccination programs. A Wellness Committee at each school can help implement various health activities related to the health education program, and assist teachers and students in participating in health activities. Health fairs and a week devoted to health, a Heart Smart Week, involving English compositions on health and ethics and a demonstration of exercise programs, are activities that a wellness committee can oversee. A parent seeing these types of programs spills over to the family and community.

Acknowledgments

Supported by grants HL38844 from the National Heart, Lung, and Blood Institute, AG16592 from the National Institute on Aging, and HD43820 from the National Institute of Child Health and Human Development.

The Bogalusa Heart Study is a joint effort of many individuals whose cooperation is gratefully acknowledged. We are especially grateful for the children who grew up contributing to this research.

References

1. Berenson GS, McMahan CA, Voors AW, *et al.*: *Cardiovascular Risk Factors in Children: The Early Natural History of Atherosclerosis and Essential Hypertension*. Edited by Andrews C, Hester HE. New York: Oxford University Press; 1980.

2. Berenson GS: *Causation of Cardiovascular Risk Factors in Children: Perspectives on Cardiovascular Risk in Early Life*. New York: Raven Press; 1986.

3. Lauer RM, Shekelle RB: *Childhood Prevention of Atherosclerosis and Hypertension*. New York: Raven Press; 1980.

4. Raitakari OT, Porkka KV, Viikari JS, *et al.*: Clustering of risk factors for coronary heart disease in children and adolescents. The Cardiovascular Risk in Young Finns Study. *Acta Paediatr* 1994, 83:935–940.

5. McGill HC Jr: Persistent problems in the pathogenesis of atherosclerosis. *Arteriosclerosis* 1984, 4:443–451.

Childhood Risk Factors Predict Adult Cardiovascular Risk and Strategies for Prevention: The Bogalusa Heart Study

6. Kannel WB, McGee D, Gordon T: A general cardiovascular risk profile: The Framingham Study. *Am J Cardiol* 1976, 38:46–51.

7. Gidding SS, Bao W, Srinivasan SR, Berenson GS: Effects of secular trends in obesity on coronary risk factors in children. The Bogalusa Heart Study. *J Pediatr* 1995, 127:868–874.

8. Freedman DS, Srinivasan SR, Valdez RA, *et al.*: Secular increases in relative weight and adiposity among children over two decades: The Bogalusa Heart Study. *Pediatrics* 1997, 99:420–426.

9. Mohdad AH, Serdula MK, Dietz WH, *et al.*: The spread of the obesity epidemic in the United States, 1991–1998. *JAMA* 1999, 282:1519–1522.

10. Nicklas TA, Demory-Luce D, Yang S-J, *et al.*: Children's food consumption patterns have changed over two decades (1973–1994): the Bogalusa Heart Study. *J Am Diet Assoc* 2004, 104:1127–1140.

11. Dietz WH: Critical periods in childhood for the development of obesity. *Am J Clin Nutr* 1994, 59:955–959.

12. Yoo S, Nicklas T, Baranowski T, *et al.*: Comparison of dietary intakes associated with metabolic syndrome risk factors in young adults: The Bogalusa Heart Study. *Am J Clin Nutr* 2004, 80:841–848.

13. Srinivasan SR, Bao W, Wattigney WA, Berenson GS: Adolescent overweight is associated with adult overweight and related multiple cardiovascular risk factors. The Bogalusa Heart Study. *Metabolism* 1996, 45:235–240.

14. Freedman DS, Khan LK, Dietz WH, *et al.*: Relationship of childhood obesity to coronary heart risk disease factors in adulthood: The Bogalusa Heart Study. *Pediatrics* 2001, 108:712–718.

15. Bao W, Threefoot S, Srinivasa SR, Berenson GS: Essential hypertension predicted by tracking of elevated blood pressure from childhood to adulthood: The Bogalusa Heart Study. *Am J Hypertens* 1995, 8:657–665.

16. Bao W, Srinivasan SR, Wattigney WA, Berenson GS: Persistence of multiple cardiovascular risk clustering related to syndrome X from childhood to young adulthood: The Bogalusa Heart Study. *Arch Intern Med* 1997, 154:1842–1847.

17. Reaven GM: Banting lecture 1988: role of insulin resistance in human disease. *Diabetes* 1988, 37:1595–1607.

18. DeFronzo RA, Ferrannini E: Insulin resistance: a multifaceted syndrome responsible for NIDM, obesity, hypertension, dyslipidemia, and atherosclerosis cardiovascular disease. *Diabetes Care* 1991, 14:173–194.

19. Srinivasan SR, Myers L, Berenson GS: Predictability of childhood adiposity and insulin for developing insulin resistance syndrome (syndrome X) in young adulthood: The Bogalusa Heart Study. *Diabetes* 2005, 51:204–209.

20. Srinivasan SR, Myers L, Berenson GS: Temporal association between obesity and hyperinsulinemia in children, adolescents, and young adults: The Bogalusa Heart Study. *Metabolism* 1999, 48:928–934.

21. Berenson GS for the Bogalusa Heart Study research group: Childhood risk factors predict adult risk associated with subclinical cardiovascular disease: The Bogalusa Heart Study. *Am J Cardiol* 2002, 90:3L–7L.

22. Lauer RM, Clarke WR, Mahoney LT, Witt J: Childhood predictors for high adult blood pressure. The Muscatine Study. *Pediatr Clin North Am* 1993, 40:23–40.

23. Voors AW, Berenson GS, Dalferes ER Jr, *et al.*: Racial differences in blood pressure control. *Science* 1979, 204:1091–1094.

24. Berenson GS, Voors AW, Webber LS, *et al.*: Racial differences of parameters associated with blood pressure levels in children: The Bogalusa Heart Study. *Metabolism* 1979, 28:1218–1228.

25. Third Report of the National Cholesterol Education Program (NCEP) Expert Panel on Detection, Evaluation, and Treatment of High Blood Cholesterol in Adults (Adult Treatment Panel III) final report. *Circulation* 2002, 106:3143–3421.

26. World Health Organization: *Definition, Diagnosis and Classification of Diabetes Mellitus and its Complications: Report of a WHO Consultation.* Geneva: World Health Organization; 1999.

27. Newman WP III, Freedman DS, Voors AW, *et al.*: Relation of serum lipoprotein levels and systolic blood pressure to early atherosclerosis: The Bogalusa Heart Study. *N Engl J Med* 1986, 314:138–144.

28. Berenson GS, Srinivasan SR, Bao W, *et al.*: Association between multiple cardiovascular risk factors and atherosclerosis in children and young adults. *N Engl J Med* 1998, 338:1650–1656.

29. Pathobiological Determinants of Atherosclerosis in Youth (PDAY) Research Group: Natural history of aortic and coronary atherosclerotic lesions in youth: findings from the PDAY study. *Arteriosl Thromb* 1993, 13:1291–1298.

30. McGill HC: *The Geographic Pathology of Atherosclerosis.* Baltimore: William and Wilkins; 1968.

31. Enos WF, Beyer JC, Holmes RH: Pathogenesis of coronary disease in American soldiers killed in Korea. *JAMA* 1955, 158:912–914.

32. McNamara JJ, Molot MA, Stremple JF, Vatting RT: Coronary artery disease in combat casualties in Vietnam. *JAMA* 1971, 216:1185–1187.

33. Napoli C, Glass CK, Witztum JL, *et al.*: Influence of maternal hypercholesterolemia during pregnancy on progression of early atherosclerotic lesions in childhood: fate of early lesions in children (FELIC) study. *Lancet* 1999, 354:1234–1241.

34. Stary HC, Blankenhorn DH, Chandler AB, *et al.*: A definition of the intima of human arteries and of its atherosclerosis-prone regions. *Circulation* 1992, 85:391–405.

35. Freedman DS, Newman WP III, Tracy RE, *et al.*: Black/white differences in aortic fatty streaks in adolescence and early childhood: The Bogalusa Heart Study. *Pediatrics* 1997, 99:420–426.

36. Tracy RE, Newman WP III, Wattigney WA, *et al.*: Histologic features of atherosclerosis and hypertension from autopsies of young individuals in a defined geographic population: The Bogalusa Heart Study. *Atherosclerosis* 1995, 116:163–179.

37. Levy D, Garrison RJ, Savage DD, *et al.*: Left ventricular mass and incidence of coronary heart disease in an elderly cohort: the Framingham Heart Study. *Ann Intern Med* 1989, 110:101–107

38. Urbina EM, Gidding SS, Bao W, *et al.*: Association of fasting blood sugar level, insulin level, and obesity with left ventricular mass in healthy children and adolescents: The Bogalusa Heart Study. *Am Heart J* 1999, 138:122–127.

39. Li X, Li S, Ulusoy E, *et al.*: Childhood adiposity as a predictor of cardiac mass in adulthood: the Bogalusa Heart Study. *Circulation* 2004, 110:3488–3492.

40. Mahoney LT, Burns TL, Stanford W, *et al.*: Coronary risk factors measured in childhood and young adult life is associated with coronary artery calcification in young adults: The Muscatine Study. *J Am Coll Cardiol* 1996, 27:277–284.

41. Ku DN, Giddens DP, Zarins CK, Glagov S: Pulsatile flow and atherosclerosis in the human carotid bifurcation: positive correlation between plaque location and low and oscillating shear stress. *Arteriosclerosis* 1985, 5:293–302.

42. Fry DL: Responses of the arterial wall to certain physical factors. In *Atherogenesis: Initiating Factors: Ciba Foundation Symposium 12.* Amsterdam: Associated Scientific (Elsevier); 1973:93–125.

43. Riley WA, Freedman DS, Higgs NA, *et al.*: Decreased arterial elasticity associated with CV disease risk factors in the young: The Bogalusa Heart Study. *Arteriosclerosis* 1986, 6:378–386.

44. Urbina EM, Srinivasan SR, Kieltyka RL, *et al.*: Correlates of carotid artery stiffness in young adults: The Bogalusa Heart Study. *Atherosclerosis* 2004, 176:157–164.

45. Berenson GS, Harsha DW, Johnson CC, Nicklas TA: Teach families to be Heart Smart. *Patient Care* 1993, 135–145.

46. Johnson CC, Nicklas TA: Health Ahead: the Heart Smart family approach to prevention of cardiovascular disease. *Am J Public Health* 1995, 85:979–982.

47. Nicklas TA, Webber LA, Kem J, *et al.*: Fort Polk Heart Smart Program Part III: assessment of dietary intake of military wives. *Mil Med* 1993, 158:312–316.

48. Johnson CC, Nicklas TA, Arbeit ML, *et al.*: Cardiovascular intervention for high risk families: The Bogalusa Heart Study. *South Med J* 1991, 84:1305–1312.

49. Berenson GS, Pickoff AS: Preventive cardiology and its potential influence on the early natural history of adult heart diseases: The Bogalusa Heart Disease and the Heart Smart Program. *Am J Med Sci* 1995, 310:S133–S138.

50. Berenson GS: *Introduction of Comprehensive Health Promotion for Elementary School: The Health Ahead/ Heart Smart Program.* New York: Vintage Press; 1998:1–281.

51. Downey AM, Greenberg JS, Virgilio SJ, Berenson GS: Health promotion model for "Heart Smart:" The medical school, university and community. *Am J Health Promot* 1989, 13:31–46.

52. Downey AM, Frank GC, Webber LS, *et al.*: Implementation of "Heart Smart:" a cardiovascular school health promotion program. *J Sch Health* 1987, 57:98–104.

53. Downey AM, Cresanta JL, Berenson GS: Cardiovascular health promotion: "Heart Smart" and the changing role of the physician. *Am J Prev Med* 1989, 5:279–295.

54. Kuntzleman CT: *Instructor's Guide for Feelin' Good.* Spring Arbor: Fitness Finders; 1985.

55. Virgilio SJ: *Fitness Education for Children: A Team Approach.* Champaign, IL: Human Kinetics; 1997.

Risk Factors in the Elderly

Daniel E. Forman

The population of older adults is growing rapidly, and aging itself involves constitutive changes in the vasculature and heart that fundamentally predispose to cardiovascular disease. Consistently, incidence and prevalence of acute coronary events are high among the elderly, a growing problem as the population ages. Similarly, high incidence and prevalence of hypertension and heart failure among older adults evolve from the same substrate of vascular and myocardial senescence. Cardiovascular diseases tend to compound on themselves, with hypertension adding to the likelihood of coronary heart disease events in older adults, and hypertension and coronary heart disease contributing to likelihood of heart failure. Therefore, advancing age is a key risk factor for progressive cardiovascular disease.

Cardiac risk factors exacerbate the predispositions to cardiac disease created by aging. Hypertension, hypercholesterolemia, and smoking are among the key coronary heart disease risk factors that increase likelihood of cardiovascular instability, and all can be modified to improve cardiovascular health. Similarly, improved diabetes care, weight control, and regular exercise can significantly improve cardiovascular health profiles among the senior population. In this overview, the author will briefly describe intrinsic aging changes that predispose to cardiovascular disease, and discuss the benefits of risk factor modification to allay these patterns.

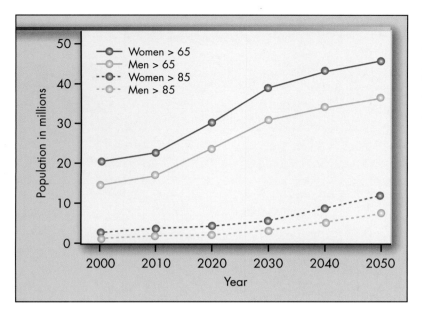

Figure 21-1.
Population projections in the United States: 2000–2050. The population of older adults is increasing rapidly. According to US Census Bureau projections, the number of individuals 65 years of age or older will increase from 34.8 million in the year 2000, to 82.0 million in 2050, an increase of 135%. Growth will be greatest among those aged 85 years and older, a subgroup expected to increase 350%. (*Data from* US Census Bureau [1].)

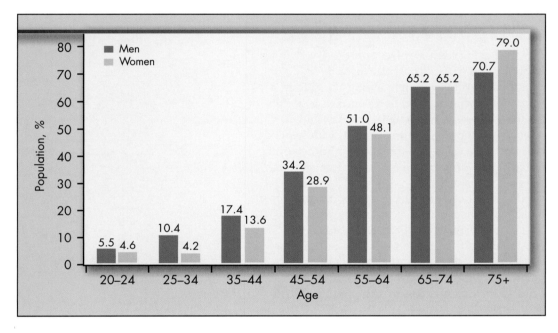

Figure 21-2.
Estimated prevalence of cardiovascular disease in Americans age 20 and older by age and gender: United States, 1988–1994. Incidence and prevalence of cardiovascular disease increase with advancing age. More than 70% of men and women over age 75 have clinically manifest cardiovascular disease. Although cardiovascular disease is more prevalent in men than in women under age 65, after age 75, prevalence is higher in women.

Coronary heart disease risk is intrinsically linked to the physiologic changes associated with typical aging, because these changes fundamentally predispose men and women to coronary heart disease pathophysiology, as well as related disease states (*eg*, hypertension, heart failure). Although aging itself is immutable, risk factor modification can allay progression of age-associated cardiovascular changes as well as their tendency to compound upon one another in worsening instability. (*Data from* National Center for Health Statistics/Centers for Disease Control [2].)

Age as a Risk Factor for Coronary Heart Disease

Age, y	Men	Women
30–39	5%	1%
40–49	11%	5%
50–59	20%	12%
60–69	29%	15%
70–74	26%	20%

Figure 21-3.
Age as a risk factor for coronary heart disease. Increasing age is the single most potent risk factor for incident cardiovascular disease. In the Framingham Heart Study, the 12-year incidence of coronary heart disease was 5% in men 30 to 39 years of age, compared with 26% in men 70 to 74 years of age. In women, the effect of age was even more remarkable, with the 12-year incidence of coronary heart disease increasing from 1% in women aged 30 to 39 to 20% in women aged 70 to 74. (*Adapted from* Wilson and Evans [3].)

Hypertension Exacerbates Age-associated Risk of Coronary Heart Disease

Age, y	Hypertension	Prevalence, %	Absolute risk, %	Relative risk	Excess risk	Population-attributable risk
45	No	90	5	—	—	—
	Yes	10	10	2.0	5%	9.1%
75	No	50	20	—	—	—
	Yes	50	30	1.5	10%	20%

Figure 21-4.

Hypertension exacerbates age-associated risk of coronary heart disease. High incidence of hypertension is linked to incidence of coronary heart disease among older adults. In part, this relates to the fact that hypertension adds to the heart's work burden as it must pump against high afterload stresses, that is, increased-demand ischemia. More fundamentally, hypertension develops from many of the same constitutive vascular changes that also underlie coronary heart disease (as will be described later in this chapter).

Given these the links between hypertension and coronary heart disease, older adults with hypertension have substantially greater likelihood of developing subsequent coronary events. This is an example of population attributable risk, a value based on the high prevalence of hypertension with aging and the relative risk for coronary heart disease associated with that risk factor. Dyslipidemia, smoking, diabetes, sedentary lifestyle, obesity, and other cardiovascular risk factors also have high attributable risks for coronary events among the elderly.

Absolute risk refers to the likelihood of an incident event occurring within a specified period of time. For example, in the Framingham Offspring Study, the 10-year absolute risk of an incident coronary event in a 45-year-old man without other major risk factors is 5%. For someone with hypertension, the absolute 10-year risk increases to 10%. The difference between these two values, that is, 5%, represents the excess risk related to hypertension, whereas the ratio 10:5 = 2.0 defines the relative risk. Among the elderly, relative risk may decrease as a function of the high prevalence of coronary heart disease even among normotensive adults, however excess risk and population attributable risk increase. (*Adapted from* Vokonas *et al.* [4] and Rich [5].)

Epidemiology of Acute Myocardial Infarction in the United States

Age, y	Population, %	Myocardial infarctions, n (%)	Myocardial infarction deaths, %
15–64	66.3	320,000 (38.6)	< 20
65–74	12.6	509,000 (61.4)	> 80
75 or older	6.1	305,000 (36.8)	~ 60

Figure 21-5.

Epidemiology of acute myocardial infarction in the United States. High incidence of cardiac events similarly relates to age-related physiologic changes and the intrinsic predisposition to coronary heart disease, especially given the mounting coronary heart disease risk factors among the elderly. In the United States, persons over 65 years of age comprise 12.6% of the population but account for over 60% of all hospitalizations for acute myocardial infarction (MI) and over 80% of all MI deaths. Moreover, the 6.1% of the population over age 75 accounts for approximately 37% of all MI hospitalizations and 60% of MI deaths. These hospital discharge data do not include "silent" infarctions, which are also common and have similarly grave prognostic implications. (*Adapted from* Center for Disease Control and Prevention [6] and Aronow [7].)

Figure 21-6.

Heart failure increasing with age. Heart failure is also a disease of aging, with heart failure prevalence skyrocketing among older adults. Framingham data show a 10-fold increase in the prevalence of heart failure among adults in their 80s (with prevalence in women greater than in men) as compared to those in their 50s. (*Adapted from* Ho *et al.* [8].)

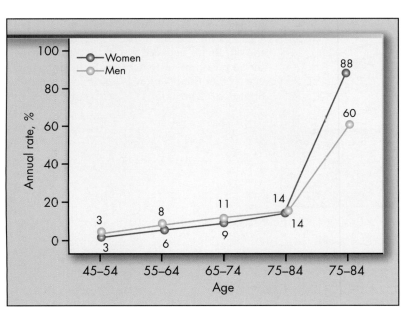

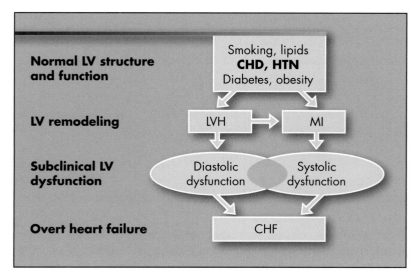

Figure 21-7.
Heart failure incidence extends from age-related hypertension, coronary heart disease (CHD), and mounting cardiovascular risks in a cycle of progressive disease. High incidence of heart failure among senior adults originates in part from the intrinsic vascular changes associated with aging, and associated vulnerabilities to antecedent CHD and hypertension (HTN). Other cardiovascular disease states (*eg*, diabetes) and behaviors (*eg*, smoking, obesity) compound these vulnerabilities. CHF—coronary heart failure; LV—left ventricle; LVH—left ventricular hypertrophy; MI—myocardial infarction. (*Adapted from* Vasan and Levy [9].)

Aspects of Aging that Predispose Elderly Individuals to Coronary Heart Disease

Increased vascular stiffness
Increased calcium, collagen, collagen cross-linking
Decreased elastin
Decreased endothelial peptide function (along the lumen)
Loss of nitric oxide
Reduced vasodilatory capacity
Loss of anti-atherosclerosis benefits

Figure 21-8.
Aspects of aging that predispose elderly to coronary heart disease. Age-associated changes in the blood vessels constitute a key vulnerability of elderly to coronary heart disease. Calcium and cross-linked collagen accumulate in vessel walls, inducing intrinsic stiffness. Elastin fibers also tend to fragment, exacerbating stiffening. Consequently, vascular impedance increases with age even among normotensive seniors, and the heart must contend 24 hours, 7 days with high afterload pressures. This age-related myocardial work burden is even greater among seniors with hypertension.

Aging also leads to diminished synthesis of vital peptides from vascular endothelium along the vessel lumen. In particular, diminished nitric oxide synthesis leads to reduced nitric oxide–mediated vasodilation, and diminished coronary flow reserve (*ie*, greater vulnerability to demand ischemia). Because nitric oxide also serves to allay atherosclerosis, diminished nitric oxide with aging leads to more coronary heart disease and coronary supply ischemia. (*Adapted from* Pugh and Wei [10] and Orlandi *et al.* [11].)

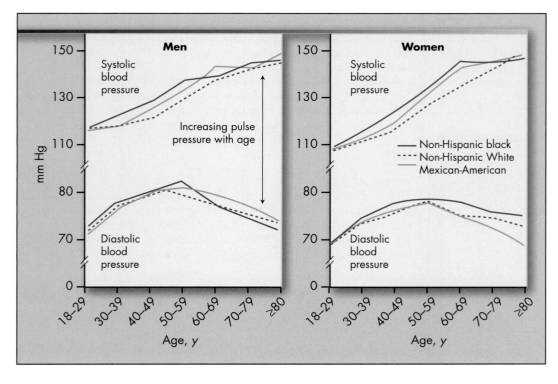

Figure 21-9.
Mean systolic and diastolic blood pressure in the United States by age, gender, and race. Because of, in large part, age-related vascular stiffening, systolic blood pressure increases progressively with advancing age in men and women, whereas diastolic blood pressure peaks and plateaus in middle age, then declines at older age. As a result, prevalence of isolated systolic hypertension increases with age, particularly in women, and may approach 30% in individuals over 80 years of age. Pulse pressure, an index for vascular stiffness calculated from the difference between systolic and diastolic blood pressures, also increases with advancing age. (*Data from* National Center for Health Statistics/Centers for Disease Control [2].)

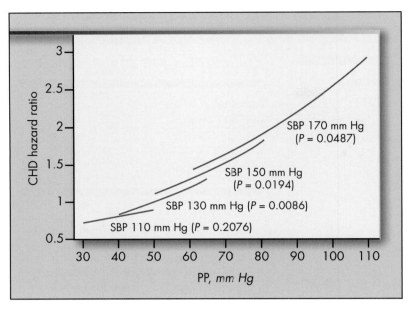

Figure 21-10.
Framingham and other studies implicate widened pulse pressure (PP) as the most powerful blood pressure parameter for assessing cardiovascular risk in the elderly. CHD—coronary heart disease; SBP—systolic blood pressure. (*Adapted from* Franklin [12].)

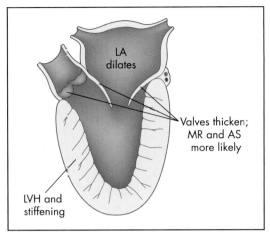

Figure 21-11.
As vasculature stiffens with age, the senescent heart pumps constantly against high afterload pressures, central pressures mount even among senior adults who are normotensive. Myocardial work demands are high, and even greater in those with coexistent hypertension and valvular disease. There is natural tendency for burdened myocytes to hypertrophy (to modify wall stresses). However, such hypertrophy is associated with higher likelihood of subendocardial ischemia, arrhythmia, and apoptosis (with associated ventricular stiffening).

Diastolic filling abnormalities are also common as filling into senescent ventricle chambers is encumbered by hypertrophy and intrinsic wall stiffening. Moreover diastolic ventricular relaxation involves energy-dependent shifts of calcium into the sarcoplasmic reticulum. These processes are hindered by supply and demand ischemia that arise from age-related coronary artery vascular changes, and typically exacerbate diastolic filling impairments that start with ventricular stiffening. (*Adapted from* Pugh and Wei [10].)

Aging Effects in Other Organ Systems That Add Cardiovascular Risk

Lungs
Kidneys
Skeletal muscle
Metabolism (thyroid, diabetes mellitus)
Infections

Figure 21-12.
Aging effects in other organ systems add to cardiovascular risk. Lung stiffening reduces vital capacity, increases V/Q mismatching, and reduces pulmonary reserve. Renal changes predispose to electrolyte disturbances as well as to volume overload and dehydration. Renal changes also affect medication metabolism, with greater susceptibility to iatrogenic medication complications. Muscle mass declines, decreasing strength, work efficiency, and worsening prognosis. Age-associated changes increase incidence of thyroid disease, diabetes, and infections, all commonly contributing to demand stresses, arrhythmias, fluid shifts, and cardiovascular instability.

Age-related Lifestyle Patterns That Compound Cardiovascular Risk

Sedentary
Diet (quantity, salt)
Serum alcohol level (ETOH)
Depression/isolation

Figure 21-13.
Age-related lifestyle patterns also compound cardiovascular risk. Baseline activity of most adults diminishes with aging, with sedentary lifestyle a notorious risk for coronary heart disease. Excessive caloric intake, particularly with fats and carbohydrates, contributes to an epidemic of obesity and associated cardiovascular instability. High blood pressure, diabetes, vascular stiffening, and left ventricular hypertrophy are among the common sequelae of overeating. Excessive salt ingestion is also common, particularly because salt is an inexpensive way to enliven foods. Unfortunately, salt exacerbates age-related vascular stiffening and hypertension, and also increases risk of fluid congestion.

Modifying Age-related Cardiovascular Risks

Modifying coronary artery disease risk factors (hypertension, lipids, smoking) allays progression to acute events or coronary heart failure
Pharmacologic options
Changing behaviors: exercise and diet (reducing glucose and obesity)

Figure 21-14.
Although aging is inescapable, age-related cardiovascular risks can be modified with therapeutic interventions including pharmacologic and behaviorial modifications.

Antihypertensive Treatment of Elderly Individuals

Trial	Patients, n	Age, y	Risk reduction			
			CVA, %	CAD, %	CHF, %	All CVD, %
Australian	582	60–69	33	18	NR	31
European Working Party on High Blood Pressure in the Elderly	840	> 60	36	20	22	29
Coope and Warrender	884	60–79	42	-3	32	24
Swedish Trial of Old Patients with Hypertension	1627	70–84	47	13	51	40
Medical Research Council	4396	65–74	25	19	NR	17
Hypertension Detection and Follow-up Program	2374	60–69	44	15	NR	16
Systolic Hypertension in the Elderly	4736	60 ≤	33	27	55	32
Systolic Hypertension in Europe	4695	60 ≤	42	26	36	31
Shanghai Trial of Slow-release Nifedipine in the Elderly	1632	60–79	57	6	68	60
Systolic Hypertension in China	2394	60 ≤	38	33	38	37

Figure 21-15.
Antihypertensive treatment in the elderly. Multiple prospective randomized trials [13–21] have evaluated efficacy of antihypertensive drug therapy in patients 60 years of age or older and consistently showed beneficial effects, with reduced strokes, coronary events, heart failure, and total cardiovascular events. A meta-analysis of data from eight trials found that treatment of isolated systolic hypertension in older patients was associated with significant reductions in all-cause mortality (13%) and cardiovascular mortality (18%). CAD—coronary artery disease; CHF—coronary heart failure; CVA—cerebrovascular accident; CVD—cardiovascular disease; NR—not reported.

Nonpharmacologic Therapies for Hypertension

Sodium restriction
Weight control
Physical activity
Alcohol moderation
Smoking cessation

Figure 21-16.
Nonpharmacologic therapy in hypertension. Nonpharmacologic therapy is an important part of antihypertensive therapy. Dietary salt restriction and weight control are important therapeutic considerations. Data from the Trial of Nonpharmacologic Intervention in the Elderly indicate that these measures facilitate blood pressure control in hypertensive patients over 60 years of age. In addition, regular physical activity, moderation in alcohol use, avoidance of tobacco products, and control of other risk factors are recommended as part of an overall strategy to maintain cardiovascular health. (*Adapted from* the Joint National Committee 7 report [22] and Whelton *et al.* [23].)

Pharmacotherapy for Hypertension in the Elderly

Medications
Diuretics, β-blockers, calcium channel blockers (dihyropyridines), angiotensin-converting enzyme inhibitors
Dosing
Start low, titrate slowly
Monitor closely for adverse effects, especially orthostatic hypotension

Figure 21-17.
Pharmacotherapy for hypertension in the elderly. If blood pressure remains uncontrolled after lifestyle modifications, then addition of a pharmacologic agent is appropriate. Recently, the Antihypertensive and Lipid-lowering Treatment to Prevent Heart Attack Trial (ALLHAT) [24] provided strong data showing that thiazides are safe and effective blood pressure–lowering therapy for older adults, although concerns regarding possibly exacerbating incontinence among an older population should be considered. The Systolic Hypertension in Europe [15] and Systolic Hypertension in China [16] trials showed that long-acting dihydropyridine calcium channel blockers are acceptable alternatives to diuretics for treatment of isolated systolic hypertension. The value of angiotensin-converting inhibitor–modifying medications to allay coronary heart disease, particularly among diabetics, will be discussed later.

Cholesterol Levels in Men and Women in the United States

Age, y	Total, mg/dL		LDL, mg/dL		HDL, mg/dL	
	Men	Women	Men	Women	Men	Women
20–34	189	185	120	110	47	56
35–44	207	195	134	117	46	54
45–54	218	217	138	132	47	57
55–64	221	237	142	145	46	56
65–74	218	234	141	147	45	56
75 or older	205	230	132	147	45	57

Figure 21-18.
Cholesterol levels in men and women in the United States. In men, population mean total cholesterol and low-density lipoprotein (LDL) cholesterol levels increase up to age 65, then gradually decline. In women, total cholesterol and LDL cholesterol levels increase rapidly after menopause and remain substantially higher than those in men after age 60. In contrast, there is little variability in high-density lipoprotein (HDL) levels as a function of age in men or women. (*Data from* National Center for Health Statistics/Centers for Disease Control [2].)

Impact of HMG-CoA Reductase Inhibitors on Major Coronary Events

Study	Placebo, %	Active, %	Relative risk	Events preferred, n
4S [24]				
< 65	26.4	18.1	0.66	83
65 or older	33.4	23.6	0.66	98
CARE [25]				
< 65	25.6	21.1	0.81	45
65 or older	28.1	19.7	0.68	84
LIPID [26]				
< 65	13.4	10.4	0.77	30
65 or older	19.7	15.5	0.79	42

Figure 21-19.
Impact of 3-hydroxy-3-methylglutaryl coenzyme A (HMG-CoA) reductase inhibitors on major coronary events. In the Scandinavian Simvastatin Survival Study (4S) [25], Cholesterol and Recurrent Events (CARE) [26], and Long-term Intervention with Pravastatin in Ischemic Disease (LIPID) [27], subjects up to the age of 75 years were enrolled in trials studying low-density lipoprotein benefits of statin medications (HMG-CoA reductase inhibitors). Absolute risk reductions of coronary events were greatest among the older subjects.

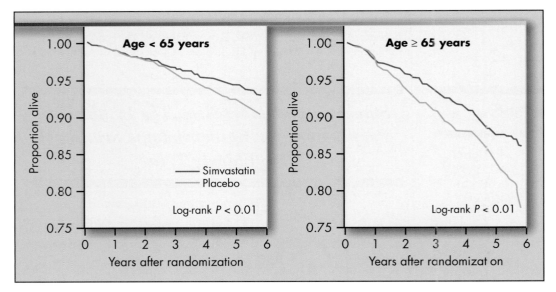

Figure 21-20.
Kaplan-Meier survival curves for all-cause mortality in patients 65 and older and 65 and younger. In the Scandinavian Simvastatin Survival Study (4S), survival benefits of statin therapy (as secondary prevention) occurred earlier in older subjects. (*Adapted from* Miettinen *et al.* [28].)

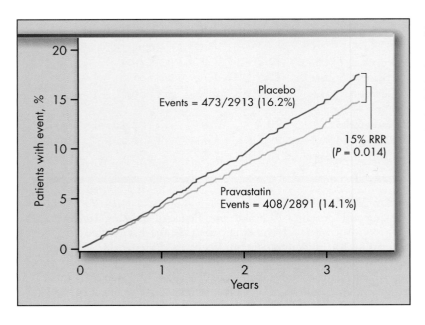

Figure 21-21.
The Pravastatin in Elderly Individuals at Risk of Vascular Disease (PROSPER) study. PROSPER was a primary and secondary prevention trial designed to specifically study efficacy of cholesterol reduction with pravastatin 40 mg among older adults. PROSPER was a randomized, controlled study of 5804 men and women aged 70 to 82 years, with a history of, or risk factors for, vascular disease. At 3.2 years, pravastatin reduced the risk of the primary endpoint (coronary death, nonfatal myocardial infarction, and fatal or nonfatal stroke) by 15%. RRR—relative risk reduction. (*Adapted from* Shepherd *et al.* [29].)

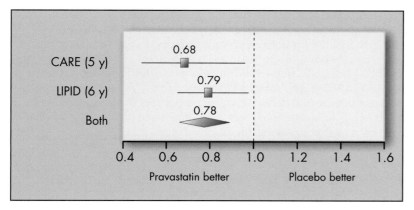

Figure 21-22.
Effects of pravastatin on fatal/nonfatal stroke in Cholesterol and Recurrent Events (CARE) [26] and Long-term Intervention with Pravastatin in Ischemic Disease (LIPID) [27] trials. Combining data from 13,173 subjects in the CARE and LIPID secondary prevention trials (as part of the Prospective Pravastatin Pooling Project [30]), monotherapy with pravastatin (40 mg/d) reduced fatal and nonfatal strokes (22% stroke reduction, *P* = 0.01, predominantly nonfatal non-hemorrhagic strokes) during the approximately 5-year follow-up.

Primary prevention
  Therapeutic lifestyle changes
  Drug therapies in high-risk patients
Secondary prevention
  Similar to younger patients
  Target low-density lipoprotein cholesterol < 100 mg/dL

Figure 21-23.
Treatment of dyslipidemia in the elderly. National Cholesterol Education Program Adult Treatment Panel III guideline [31] for the diagnosis and treatment of dyslipidemias recommends therapeutic lifestyle changes (*eg*, diet, weight loss, exercise, smoking cessation) as the initial approach to therapy in older adults without clinically manifest coronary heart disease. Pharmacotherapy therapy is advised immediately in patients at higher risk, that is, those with multiple risk factors. For those with existing coronary heart disease or diabetes mellitus, pharmacotherapy is advised immediately, with therapy oriented to reducing low-density lipoproteins less than 100 mg/dL. (*Adapted from* National Cholesterol Education Program, Expert Panel on Detection, Evaluation, and Treatment of High Blood Cholesterol in Adults [31].)

Smoking Status of Adults 1998

Age, y	Patients who never smoked, %	Patients who are former smokers, %	Patients who are current smokers, %
< 55	40.4	22.7	36.9
55–64	31.5	37.8	30.7
65–74	41.5	43.4	15.1
75–84	49.5	41.4	9.1
85 or older	64.8	30.7	4.5

Figure 21-24.
Smoking status of adults: 1998. Prevalence of smoking declines with age, in part due to smoking cessation and in part due to earlier mortality among the smoking population. In 1998, 10.4% of men and 11.2% of women 65 years of age or older were current smokers, but the proportion declined to less than 5% among persons over age 85. (*Data from* MMWR Recommendations and Reports [32].)

Smoking and Mortality: The Established Populations for Epidemiologic Studies of the Elderly Trial

	Mortality per 1000 person years			
	Men		Women	
Age, y	Rate	Relative risk	Rate	Relative risk
65–69				
Never smoked	18.5	1.0	11.7	1.0
Former smoker	28.2	1.5	9.6	0.8
Current smoker	43.5	2.3	27.8	2.4
70–74				
Never smoked	22.2	1.0	20.4	1.0
Former smoker	47.9	2.2	31.6	1.6
Current smoker	76.0	3.4	36.5	1.8
75 and older				
Never smoked	90.1	1.0	62.4	1.0
Former smoker	99.8	1.1	56.3	0.9
Current smoker	116.1	1.3	74.9	1.2

Figure 21-25.
Smoking and mortality. Although prevalence of smoking decreases with age, risks associated with smoking persist. In the Established Populations for Epidemiologic Studies of the Elderly [33], 7178 persons 65 years of age or older were studied. Current smoking was associated with a relative risk for cardiovascular death of 2.0 in men and 1.6 in women, independent of other risk factors. Adverse effect of smoking on mortality was greatest in men and women aged 65 to 74 years. Moreover, smoking was associated with a persistent survival disadvantage in seniors over 75 years. Study of 316,099 men screened in the Multiple Risk Factor Intervention Trial Research Group [34] led to similar conclusions: cigarettes per day were significant predictors of subsequent coronary heart disease death in all age groups.

Risk of Continued Smoking: The Coronary Artery Surgery Study Registry

Age, y	Relative risk of death*	Relative risk of death or myocardial infarction*
55–59	1.5	1.5
60–64	2.0	1.4
65–69	1.4	1.5
70 or older	3.3	2.9

*Compared with individuals who stopped smoking at 6-year follow-up.

Figure 21-26.
Risk of continued smoking: the Coronary Artery Surgery Study. In the Coronary Artery Surgery Study Registry [35], patients over 70 years of age with coronary heart disease who continued to smoke had a 2.9-fold greater risk of death or myocardial infarction during a 6-year follow-up period compared with patients who stopped smoking. These data suggest that smoking cessation is highly beneficial, even among adults aged older than 70 years.

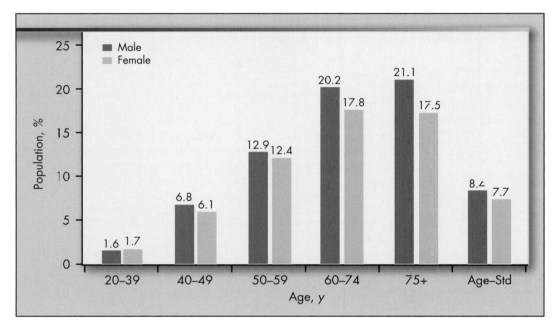

Figure 21-27.
Prevalence of diabetes in the US population. The prevalence of diabetes increases with age, approaching 20% in persons over 65 years of age, and relatively more common among men, and in African-Americans and Hispanics. In the Framingham Heart Study, relative risk for coronary heart disease in diabetic men aged over age 65 is 1.4, and it is 2.1 in diabetic women. Furthermore, coronary heart disease risk increases with the duration of diabetes. (*Adapted from* Fox *et al.* [36,37].)

Treatment Goals in Older Diabetes Patients

Optimize glucose control
Blood pressure < 130/85 mm Hg
Low-density lipoprotein cholesterol < 100 mg/dL
Smoking cessation
Body mass index < 25 mg/m^2
Regular exercise
Angiotensin-converting enzyme inhibitor

Figure 21-28.
Treatment goals in older diabetes patients. The American Diabetes Association's clinical practice recommendations do not distinguish between younger and older patients. Current recommendations stress the importance of effective glucose control and aggressively managing other cardiovascular risk factors. (*Adapted from* American Diabetes Association [38].)

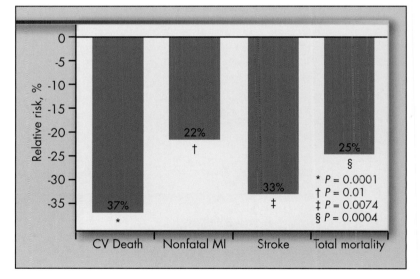

Figure 21-29.
Heart Outcomes Prevention Evaluation: effects of ramipril on cardiovascular endpoints and total mortality [38] in diabetics. Angiotensin-converting enzyme inhibition among diabetes patients is highly beneficial. The Heart Outcomes Prevention Evaluation was a prospective study of 3577 diabetes patients over the age 55 with vascular disease or at least one other cardiovascular risk factor who were randomized to ramipril 10 mg/day or placebo and observed for an average of 4.5 years. Ramipril-therapy was associated with a 26% reduction in a composite endpoint of cardiovascular death, nonfatal MI, or nonfatal stroke ($P = 0.0004$). Total mortality was reduced by 25%. (*Adapted from* [39].)

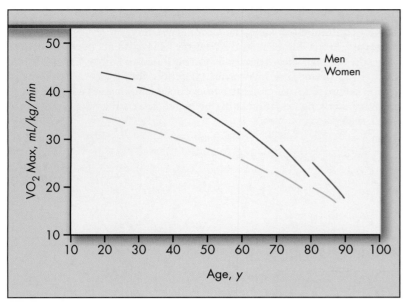

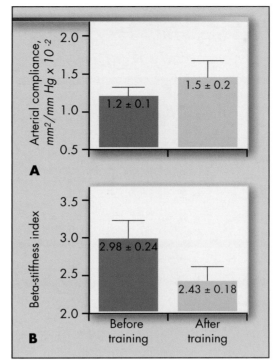

A

B

Figure 21-30.
Inactivity as a risk factor. Declining physical activity is a hallmark of typical aging [40]. Maximal aerobic capacity, typically measured as VO_2 peak, progressively falls with age, but the rate of this decline is relatively decreased among those who exercise. Whereas multiple studies demonstrate that reduced functional capacity predicts increased mortality and morbidity. Furthermore, exercise training (and relatively improved VO_2) has been demonstrated to modify these risks. Even modest exercise activity (*eg*, walking [41]) is associated with reduced mortality. (*Adapted from* [40].)

Figure 21-31.
Exercise training reduces vascular stiffness. The primary mechanism of exercise benefit for older adults is an active area of investigation as a safe, inexpensive way to help the aging population live longer and better. Tanaka *et al.* [42] showed benefits of aerobic exercise to modify vascular stiffening associated with aging. Six months of exercise training restored vascular compliance. In other words, exercise helps sustain and may even restore a more youthful physiologic profile. (*Adapted from* Tanaka *et al.* [42].)

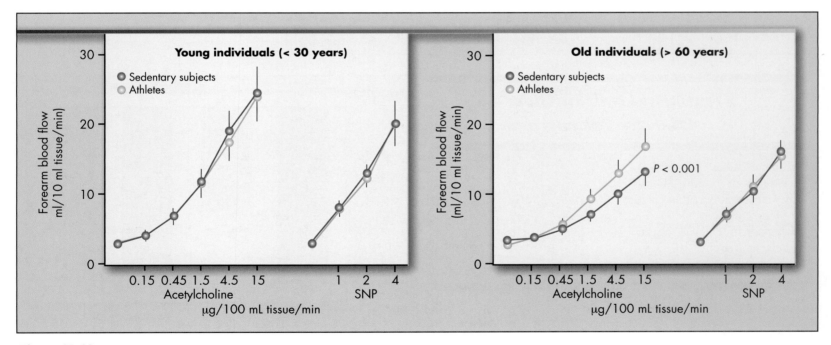

Figure 21-32.
Exercise training to improve intrinsic vasodilation. Teddei *et al.* [43] showed benefits of exercise training to improve physiologic vasodilation among elderly, through enhanced endothelial nitric oxide production. The graph compares vascular responses to acetylcholine, a stimulus of nitric oxide–mediated responses to vascular responses to nitroprusside (SNP), a nitric oxide–independent effect. Among older sedentary adults

(> 60 years), acetylcholine at 0.15, 0.45, 1.5, 4.5, and 15 µg/100 mL tissue per minute demonstrated an age-associated impairment compared to nitroprusside at 1, 2, and 4 µg/100 mL tissue per minute. However, exercise training restored nitric oxide–mediated performance. (*Adapted from* Teddei *et al.* [43]; with permission.)

Exercise Training Goals for the Elderly

Moderate activity goals include the following:
  Relatively longer sessions of moderate activity such as walking or swimming. Walking, gardening, or yard work are particularly popular moderate-intensity activities
  Or relatively shorter sessions of more vigorous activity (fast walking or stair climbing)
Those who are physically active longer or more intensely will derive greater benefits
Muscle-strengthening activities are also important for older individuals. These activities reduce the risk of falling and improve the ability to perform aerobic exercise (as well as daily tasks)

Figure 21-33.
Exercise training goals for the elderly. Exercise has broad therapeutic value in modifying overall cardiovascular risk. Reduced blood pressure, increased ischemic threshold, improved ventricular filling, improved high-density lipoprotein, improved glucose metabolism, and weight loss have all been associated with exercise training. Pulmonary and skeletal muscle benefits have been described. Exercise also reinforces other healthful behaviors including reduced smoking, improved diet, and reduced depression. Training goals are usually oriented to moderate- intensity aerobic exercises that feel appealing and comfortable. Strength training may also help build stamina and stability for an active routine.

Obesity as a Modifiable Risk Factor

Accumulating visceral fat is associated with coronary heart disease as well as with hypertension, diabetes mellitus, vascular stiffening, and left ventricular hypertrophy
Age-related skeletal muscle wasting increases the proportion of body fat and susceptibility to obesity
Weight reduction modifies these risks, but weight loss goals are confounded by concerns regarding depression or anorexia that is secondary to other diseases
Exercise is often beneficial in helping to achieve healthy weight reduction

Figure 21-34.
Obesity as a modifiable risk factor.

Subclinical Disease Markers

Carotid artery intima-media thickness
Ankle-arm index
Left ventricle systolic function
C-reactive protein

Figure 21-35.
Subclinical disease markers. In addition to targeting traditional and nontraditional risk factors, markers of subclinical cardiovascular disease provide key opportunities to recognize cardiovascular pathology in early stages and to modify progression. Such markers may be particularly important in identifying older adults most likely to benefit from risk factor modification. (*Adapted from* Psaty *et al.* [44] and Ridker *et al.* [45].)

References

1. US Census Bureau: *US Interim Projections by Age, Sex, Race, and Hispanic Origin.* Available at http://www.census.gov/ipc/www/usinterimproj.

2. National Center for Health Statistics/Centers for Disease Control: *Third National Health and Nutrition Examination Survey (NHANES III).* Available at http://www.cdc.gov.

3. Wilson PW, Evans JC: Coronary artery disease prediction. *Am J Hypertens* 1993, 6:309S–313S.

4. Vokonas PS, Kannel WB, Cupples LA: Epidemiology and risk of hypertension in the elderly: the Framingham Study. *J Hypertens Suppl* 1988, 6:S3–S9.

5. Rich MW for the Society of Geriatric Cardiology: *Cardiovascular disease in the elderly.* Module #3: Cardiovascular Risk Factors. Available at http://www.sgcard.org.

6. Centers for Disease Control and Prevention: *1999 National Hospital Discharge Survey.* Available at http://www.cdc.gov/nchs/data/series/sr_13/sr13_151.pdf.

7. Aronow WS: New coronary events at four-year follow-up in elderly patients with recognized or unrecognized myocardial infarction. *Am J Cardiol* 1989, 63:621–622.

8. Ho KK, Pinsky JL, Kannel WB, Levy D: The epidemiology of heart failure: the Framingham Study. *J Am Coll Cardiol* 1993, 22(suppl):6A–13A.

9. Vasan RS, Levy D: The role of hypertension in the pathogenesis of heart failure: a clinical mechanistic overview. *Arch Intern Med* 1996, 156:1789–1796.

10. Pugh KG, Wei JY: Clinical implications of physiological changes in the aging heart. *Drugs Aging* 2001, 18:263–276.

11. Orlandi A, Marcellini M, Spagnoli LG: Aging influences development and progression of early aortic atherosclerotic lesions in cholesterol-fed rabbits. *Arterioscler Thromb Vasc Biol* 2000, 20:1123–1136.

12. Franklin SS: Ageing and hypertension: the assessment of blood pressure indices in predicting coronary heart disease. *J Hypertens* 1999, 17(suppl):S29–S36.

13. Staessen JA, Gasowski J, Wang JG, *et al.*: Risks of untreated and treated isolated systolic hypertension in the elderly: meta-analysis of outcome trials. *Lancet* 2000, 355:865–872.

14. SHEP Cooperative Research Group: Prevention of stroke by antihypertensive drug treatment in older persons with isolated systolic hypertension: final results of the Systolic Hypertension in the Elderly Program (SHEP). *JAMA* 1991, 265:3255–3264.

15. Staessen JA, Fagard R, Thijs L, *et al.*: Randomised double-blind comparison of placebo and active treatment for older patients with isolated systolic hypertension. *Lancet* 1997, 350:757–764.

16. Liu L, Wang JG, Gong L, Liu G, for the Systolic Hypertension in China (Syst-China) Collaborative Group: Comparison of active treatment and placebo for older patients with isolated systolic hypertension. *J Hypertens* 1998, 16:1823–1829.

17. Amery A, Birkenhäger W, Brixko P, *et al.*: Mortality and morbidity results from the European Working Party on High Blood Pressure in the Elderly trial [abstract]. *Lancet* 1985, i:1349–1354.

18. Coope J, Warrender TS: Randomised trial of treatment of hypertension in elderly patients in primary care. *BMJ* 1986, 293:1145–1151.

19. Dahlöf B, Lindholm LH, Hansson L, *et al.*: Morbidity and mortality in the Swedish Trial in Old Patients with Hypertension (STOP-HTN). *Lancet* 1991, 338:1281–1285.

20. Medical Research Council Working Party: Medical Research Council trial of treatment of hypertension in older adults: principal results. *BMJ* 1992, 304:405–412.

21. Medical Research Council Working Party: Medical Research Council trial of treatment of mild hypertension: principal results. *BMJ* 1985, 291:97–104.

22. The Seventh Report of the Joint National Committee on Prevention, Detection, Evaluation, and Treatment of High Blood Pressure: the JNC 7 report. *JAMA* 2003, 289:2560–2572.

23. Whelton PK, Appel LJ, Espeland MA, *et al.*: Sodium reduction and weight loss in the treatment of hypertension in older persons: a randomized controlled trial of nonpharmacologic interventions in the elderly (TONE). TONE Collaborative Research Group. *JAMA* 1998, 279:839–846.

24. ALLHAT Officers and Coordinators for the ALLHAT Collaborative Research Group: Major outcomes in high-risk hypertensive patients randomized to angiotensin-converting enzyme inhibitor or calcium channel blocker vs diuretic: The Antihypertensive and Lipid-Lowering Treatment to Prevent Heart Attack Trial (ALLHAT). *JAMA* 2002, 288:2981–2997.

25. Scandinavian Simvastatin Survival Study Group: Randomised trial of cholesterol lowering in 4444 patients with coronary heart disease: the Scandinavian Simvastatin Survival Study (4S). *Lancet* 1994, 344:1383–1389.

26. Sacks FM, Pfeffer MA, Moyé LA, *et al.*: The effect of pravastatin on coronary events after myocardial infarction in patients with average cholesterol levels. *N Engl J Med* 1996, 335:1001–1009.

27. The Long-Term Intervention with Pravastatin in Ischaemic Disease (LIPID) Study Group: Prevention of cardiovascular events and death with pravastatin in patients with coronary heart disease and a broad range of initial cholesterol levels. *N Engl J Med* 1998, 339:1349–1357.

28. Miettinen TA, Pyorala K, Olsson AG, *et al.*: Cholesterol-lowering therapy in women and elderly patients with myocardial infarction or angina pectoris: findings from the Scandinavian Simvastatin Survival Study (4S). *Circulation* 1997, 96:4211–4218.

29. Shepherd J, Blauwh GJ, Murphy MB, *et al.*: Pravastatin in elderly individuals at risk of vascular disease (PROSPER): a randomised controlled trial. *Lancet* 2002, 360:1623-1630.

30. Byington RP, Davis BR, Plehn JF, *et al.*: Reduction of stroke events with pravastatin: the Prospective Pravastatin Pooling (PPP) Project. *Circulation* 2001, 103:387–392.

31. National Cholesterol Education Program (NCEP), Expert Panel on Detection, Evaluation, and Treatment of High Blood Cholesterol in Adults (Adult Treatment Panel III): Third Report of the National Cholesterol Education Program (NCEP) Expert Panel on Detection, Evaluation, and Treatment of High Blood Cholesterol in Adults (Adult Treatment Panel III) final report. *Circulation* 2002, 106:3143–3121.

32. Reducing Tobacco Use: a report of the Surgeon General. MMWR 2000;49:797-801

33. LaCroix AZ, Lang J, Scherr P, *et al.*: Smoking and mortality among older men and women in three communities. *N Engl J Med* 1991, 324:1619–1625.

34. Neaton JD, Wentworth D: Serum cholesterol, blood pressure, cigarette smoking, and death from coronary heart disease. Overall findings and differences by age for 316,099 white men. Multiple Risk Factor Intervention Trial Research Group. *Arch Intern Med* 1992, 152:56-64.

35. Hermanson B, Omenn GS, Kronmal RA, Gersh BJ: Beneficial six-year outcome of smoking cessation in older men and women with coronary artery disease. Results from the CASS registry. *N Engl J Med* 1988, 319:1365–1369.

36. Fox CS, Coady S, Sorlie PD, *et al.*: Trends in cardiovascular complications of diabetes. *JAMA* 2004, 292:2495–2499.

37. Fox CS, Sullivan L, D'Agostino RB Sr, Wilson PW: The significant effect of diabetes duration on coronary heart disease mortality: the Framingham Heart Study. *Diabetes Care* 2004, 27:704–708.

38. American Diabetes Association: Clinical practice recommendations 1999. *Diabetes Care* 1999, 22(suppl):S1–S114.

39. Effects of ramipril on cardiovascular and microvascular outcomes in people with diabetes mellitus: results of the HOPE study and MICRO-HOPE substudy. Heart Outcomes Prevention Evaluation Study Investigators. *Lancet* 2000, 355:253–259.

40. *Circulation* 2000, 102(suppl):II–602

41. Hakim AA, Curb JD, Petrovitch H, *et al.*: Effects of walking on coronary heart disease in elderly men: the Honolulu Heart Program. *Circulation* 1999, 100:9-13.

42. Tanaka H. Dinenno FA, Monahan KD, *et al.*: Aging, habitual exercise, and dynamic arterial compliance. *Circulation* 2000, 102:1270–1275.

43. Taddei S, Galetta F, Virdis A, *et al.*: Physical activity prevents age-related impairment in nitric oxide availability in elderly athletes. *Circulation* 2000, 101:2896–2901.

44. Psaty BM, Furberg CD, Kuller LH, *et al.*: Traditional risk factors and subclinical disease measures as predictors of first myocardial infarction in older adults: the Cardiovascular Health Study. *Arch Intern Med* 1999, 159:1339–1347.

45. Ridker PM, Rifai N, Rose L, *et al.*: Comparison of C-reactive protein and low-density lipoprotein cholesterol levels in the prediction of first cardiovascular events. *N Engl J Med* 2002, 347:1557–1565.

Coronary Risk Factors in Women

Nanette K. Wenger

Coronary heart disease is the leading cause of mortality for US women [1], responsible for almost 250,000 deaths annually. Although cardiovascular disease mortality trends for men in the US have declined from 1979 to the present, mortality trends for women have remained unchanged or may even be increasing (*see* Fig. 22-1) [1].

Coronary risk factors are highly prevalent in US women of all racial and ethnic groups. Coronary risk factors predominate and cluster in older women; the high prevalence of these risk factors and menopausal status occur concomitantly as women age. Women develop hypertension at older ages than men, with isolated systolic hypertension of particular prominence in elderly women. As well, the older woman is more likely to develop de novo diabetes. Low-density lipoprotein cholesterol levels increase after middle-age in women to exceed low-density lipoprotein levels in elderly men. Similarly, triglyceride levels increase in women of middle age and older.

Of concern regarding coronary risk factors for US women is that that their smoking rates have declined less than those of men, the prevalence of obesity in women is increasing, and almost one fourth of women report no regular physical activity. More than half of all US women older than 45 years of age have hypertension, and approximately 40% of women older than age 55 have elevated levels of serum cholesterol. Six of every 10 US women are sedentary such that physical inactivity is the most prevalent coronary risk characteristic for US women. Based on data from the National Center for Health Statistics, less than one third of all women in the United States do not have at least one major coronary risk factor [2]. This percentage decreases in older women and in socioeconomically and educationally disadvantaged women. Adverse socioeconomic circumstances predominate in elderly US women, with those 55 years of age and older almost twice as likely to be below the poverty level than comparably aged men.

Abundant data identify under-representation of women in populations screened for coronary risk factors, with risk factors in women undertreated even in the secondary prevention setting. The recently released American Heart Association Evidence-based Guidelines for Cardiovascular Disease Prevention in Women [3] are designed to encourage involvement of women and their health care providers in the identification and remediation of coronary risk factors in women.

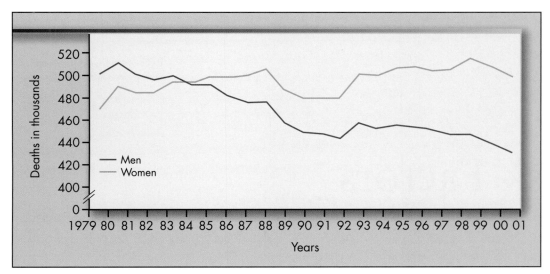

Figure 22-1.
Cardiovascular disease mortality trends for males and females in the United States, 1979 to 2001, according to the National Center for Health Statistics and the American Heart Association. (*Adapted from* American Heart Association [1]; *data from* National Center for Health Statistics/Centers for Disease Control.)

Diabetes Mellitus

Diabetes is a more powerful coronary risk factor for women than men, negating their gender-protective effect, even among premenopausal women. The relative risk for coronary death with diabetes is 2.58 for women compared with 1.85 for men [4]. This increased risk for diabetic women may reflect their more prevalent or more severe coronary risk factors. In the Nurses' Health Study, a three- to sevenfold increase in the risk of cardiovascular events was associated with diabetes and increased with the duration of the diabetes (*see* Fig. 22-2) [5].

The incidence of type 2 diabetes in a randomized trial was more effectively reduced with lifestyle modifications than with metformin, with comparable effects in women and men (*see* Fig. 22-3) [6].

Diabetes is more prevalent in black and Mexican-American women than in non-Hispanic white women (*see* Fig. 22-4) [1]. As well, the prevalence of diabetes is greatest with lowest levels of education in all races and ethnicities (*see* Fig. 22-5) [1]. Data from the Framingham Heart Study and the Framingham Offspring Study showed diabetes to be a greater predictor of subsequent coronary mortality in women than was prior established coronary heart disease; the reverse is the case for men (*see* Fig. 22-6) [7].

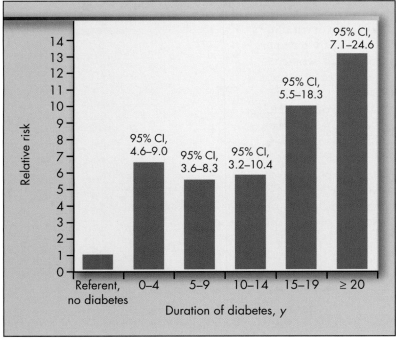

Figure 22-2.
Age-adjusted relative risks of nonfatal myocardial infarction and fatal coronary heart disease (combined in relation to duration of maturity-onset diabetes). Referent is nondiabetic women. (*Adapted from* Manson *et al.* [5].)

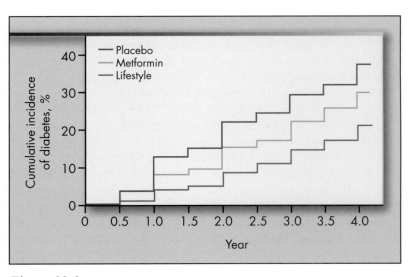

Figure 22-3.
Cumulative incidence of diabetes according to study group. The diagnosis of diabetes was based on the criteria of the American Diabetes Association. The incidence of diabetes differed significantly among the three groups (*P* < 0.001 for each comparison). (*Adapted from* Diabetes Prevention Program Research Group [6].)

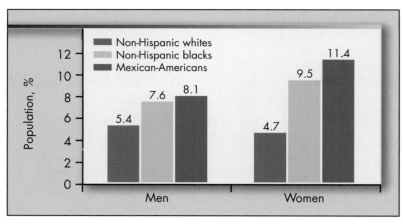

Figure 22-4.
Age-adjusted prevalence of physician-diagnosed diabetes in Americans age 20 and older by gender and race/ethnicity in the National Health and Nutrition Examination Survey III, 1988–1994. (*Adapted from* American Heart Association [1]; *data from* Harris *et al.* [7].)

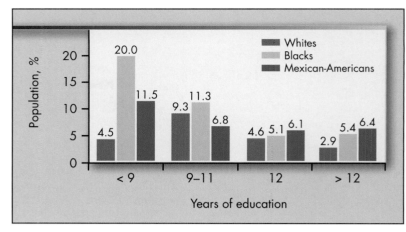

Figure 22-5.
Prevalence of non–insulin-dependent (type 2) diabetes in women aged 25 to 64 by education and race/ethnicity in the National Health and Nutrition Examination Survey III, 1988–1994. (*Adapted from* American Heart Association [1]; *data from* Winkleby *et al.* [8].)

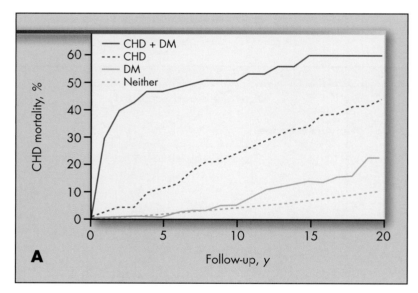

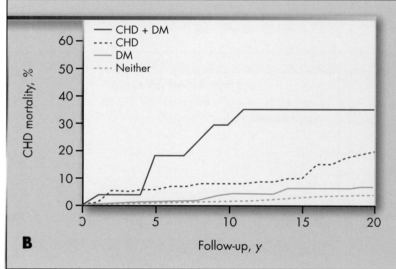

Figure 22-6.
Age-adjusted cumulative coronary heart disease (CHD) mortality by CHD and diabetes mellitus (DM) status for men (**A**) and women (**B**). (*Adapted from* Natarajan *et al.* [9].)

Hypertension

Although more men than women have hypertension before 55 years of age, the percentage of women with hypertension is slightly higher between ages 55 to 74, and far more women than men have hypertension after age 75 (*see* Fig. 22-7) [1]. Hypertension is particularly prevalent among non-Hispanic black women [1]. Within the African-American community of women, those with the highest rates of hypertension are likely to be middle-aged or older, less educated, overweight or obese, physically inactive and to have diabetes. The awareness, treatment, and control of hypertension vary substantially by race and ethnicity (*see* Fig. 22-8) [1], with levels lowest in the Mexican-American community.

Among women with cardiovascular disease in the Women's Antioxidant Cardiovascular Study, there was a strong continuous and linear association between systolic blood pressure and the risk of secondary cardiovascular events (*see* Fig. 22-9) [10].

In multiple randomized controlled trials of antihypertensive treatment, the risk for fatal and nonfatal stroke and fatal and nonfatal coronary events was significantly reduced by pharmacologic treatment and was comparable for women and for men (*see* Fig. 22-10) [11].

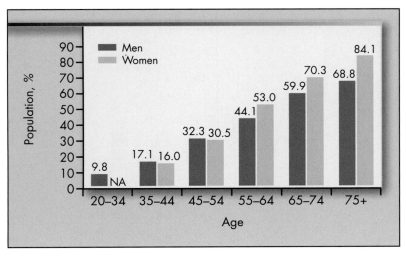

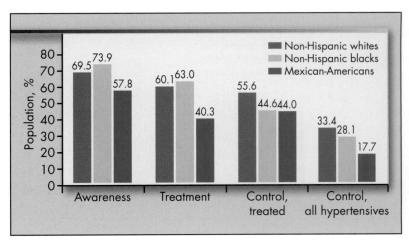

Figure 22-7.
Prevalence of high blood pressure in Americans age 20 and older by age and gender in the National Health and Nutrition Examination Survey IV, 1999–2000. Prevalence estimates for women ages 20 to 34 are not considered reliable. NA—no data available. (*Adapted from* American Heart Association [1]; *data from* National Center of Health Statistics/Centers for Disease Control.)

Figure 22-8.
Extent of awareness, treatment, and control of high blood pressure by race/ethnicity in National Health and Nutrition Examination Survey IV, 1999–2000. (*Adapted from* American Heart Association [1]; *data from* Hajjar and Kotchen [12].)

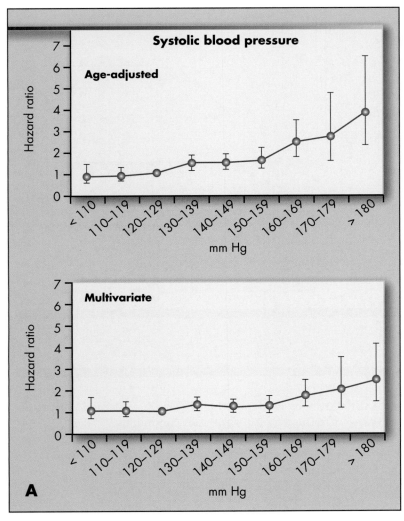

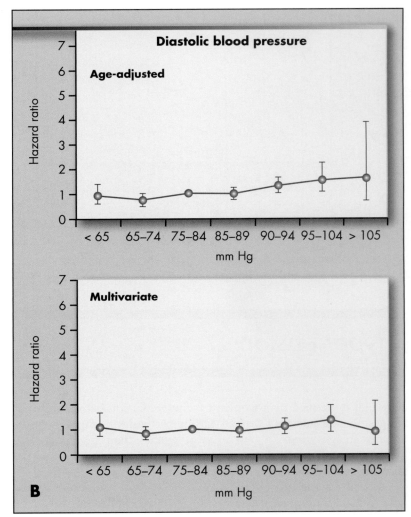

Figure 22-9.
Relative risk (95% CI) of cardiovascular disease events according to systolic ([**A**] SBP) and diastolic blood pressure ([**B**] DBP) category. Referent categories are SBP (120 to 129 mm Hg) and DBP (75 to 84 mm Hg). Relative risk is adjusted for age, randomized treatment assignments, body mass index, tobacco use, alcohol use, exercise frequency, diabetes, history of elevated cholesterol, antihypertensive therapy, prior myocardial infarction, prior stroke, and prior revascularization. (*Adapted from* Mason *et al.* [10].)

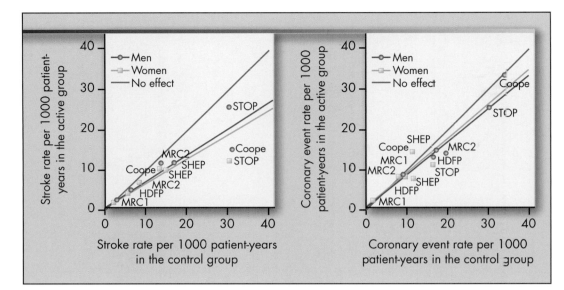

Figure 22-10.
Effect of antihypertensive treatment on absolute risk for fatal and nonfatal stroke (*left panel*) and fatal and nonfatal coronary events (*right panel*). The points show subgroups in each trial by gender; the x-axis represents risk in the control group, and the y-axis represents risk in the treatment group. The risk is given as the rate for 1000 patient-years. The two *dashed lines* represent the odds ratios in women and men. Coope—Coope and Warrender; HDFP—Hypertension Detection and Follow-up Program; MRC1—Medical Research Council trial of treatment of mild hypertension; MRC2—Medical Research Council trial of treatment of hypertension in older adults; SHEP—Systolic Hypertension in the Elderly Program; STOP—Swedish Trial in Old Patients with Hypertension. (*Adapted from* Gueyffier *et al.* [11].)

Cigarette Smoking

Cigarette smoking accounts for approximately 60% of coronary risk in middle-aged US women. US data show that the current prevalence of smoking in young women is greatest for white women; for all races and ethnicities, cigarette smoking decreases with increased levels of education (*see* Fig. 22-11) [1,13].

In the Nurses' Health Study, the number of cigarettes smoked daily was associated with the increase in risk of fatal coronary heart disease, nonfatal myocardial infarction, and angina pectoris (*see* Figs. 22-12, 22-13, and 22-14) [14]. Total mortality for former smokers in the Nurses' Health Study decreased nearly to that of never smokers within 10 to 14 years of smoking cessation (*see* Fig. 22-15) [15].

Smoking cessation lessens the risk of death after myocardial infarction in older as well as younger coronary patients [16]. The benefits of quitting were similar for women and men.

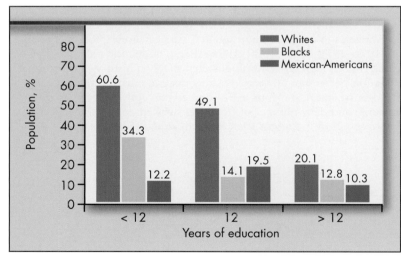

Figure 22-11.
Prevalence of current smoking for women ages 18 to 24 by education and race/ethnicity in National Health and Nutrition Examination Survey III, 1988–1994. (*Adapted from* American Heart Association [1] and Winkleby *et al.* [13].)

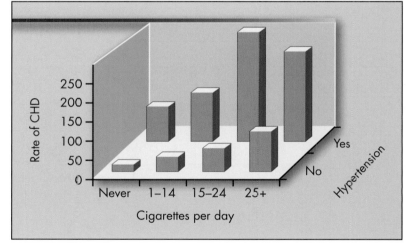

Figure 22-12.
Age-standardized rates of coronary heart disease (CHD) per 100,000 person-years among women, according to cigarette use and history of hypertension. (*Adapted from* Willett *et al.* [14].)

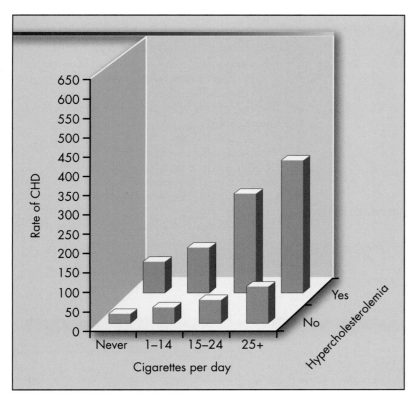

Figure 22-13.
Age-standardized rates of coronary heart disease (CHD) per 100,000 person-years among women, according to cigarette use and history of hypercholesterolemia. (*Adapted from* Willett *et al.* [14].)

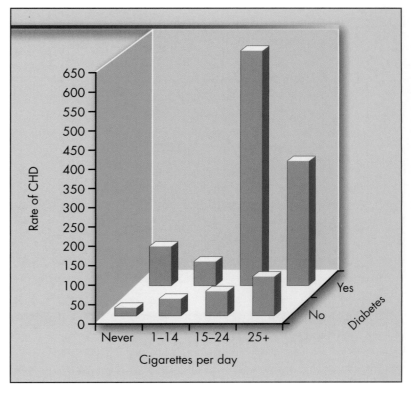

Figure 22-14.
Age-standardized rates of coronary heart disease (CHD) per 100,000 person-years among women, according to cigarette use and history of diabetes. (*Adapted from* Willett *et al.* [14].)

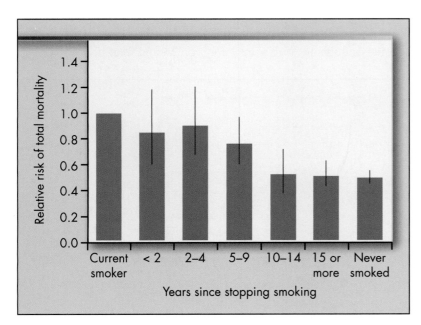

Figure 22-15.
Risk of total mortality by time since quitting. Multivariate relative risk for total mortality by time since quitting (reference category: current smokers). *Error bars* represent 95% CI. Nonfatal coronary heart disease, stroke, and cancer (except non-melanoma skin cancer) were excluded at baseline and at the beginning of each successive 2-year follow-up period. Variables in model include age in 5-year categories, follow-up period (1976–1978, 1978–1980, 1986–1988), body mass index, history of hypertension, high cholesterol, diabetes, parental history of myocardial infarction before age 60 years, postmenopausal estrogen therapy, menopausal status, previous use of oral contraceptives, age at starting smoking, and daily number of cigarettes smoked during the period before cessation. (*Adapted from* Kawachi *et al.* [15].)

Dyslipidemia

In adolescence, cholesterol levels remain highest among black women, but cholesterol levels in all women declined from 1966 to 1970 to 1988 to 1994 (*see* Fig. 22-16) [1,17].

In a systematic review of lipid data [18], higher levels of total cholesterol, low-density lipoprotein cholesterol and triglycerides, and lower levels of high-density lipoprotein cholesterol increased the risk of coronary death for women younger than 65 years of age (*see* Fig. 22-17) [19]. For older women, only low high-density lipoprotein cholesterol and increased triglycerides were associated with an increase in risk. The cardiovascular risk associated with hypertriglyceridemia is higher for women than for men (*see* Fig. 22-18) [16]. Triglyceride baseline values were primary determinants of long-term total and event-free survival after coronary artery bypass graft surgery for women but not for men (*see* Fig. 22-19) [20].

In five clinical trials of the effect of statin therapy, the overall reduction in major coronary events was similar in treated women and men, although mortality benefit was not evident for women, likely owing to the small numbers of women enrolled (*see* Fig. 22-

20) [21]. Subsequently, in the Heart Protection Study, comparable benefit of lipid lowering with statin therapy was evident for women and men [22,23]. The number of women enrolled in the Heart Protection Study was greater than the total number of women studied in clinical trials of statin therapy prior to that time.

In a systematic review of the efficacy of lipid-lowering therapy to reduce coronary heart disease risk in women [24], lipid-lowering therapy reduced coronary mortality by 26%, nonfatal myocardial infarction by 36%, and major coronary events by 21%. Statin therapy attenuated the increase in C-reactive protein during estrogen therapy in postmenopausal women (*see* Fig. 22-21) [25]. In the Heart and Estrogen/progestin Replacement Study, statin use was associated with lower rates of cardiovascular events, venous thromboembolism, and total mortality (*see* Fig. 22-22) [23].

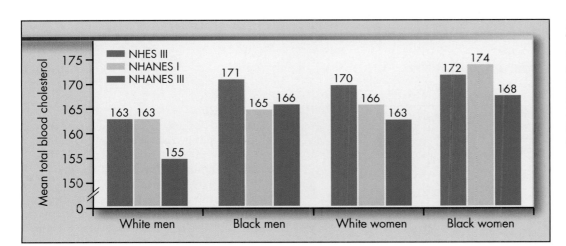

Figure 22-16.
Trends in mean total blood cholesterol among adolescents ages 12 to 17 by gender, race, and survey in National Health Examination Survey (NHES) III, National Health and Nutrition Examination Survey (NHANES) I and III, 1966–1970, 1971–1974, and 1988–1994. (*Adapted from* American Heart Association [1] and Hickman *et al.* [17].)

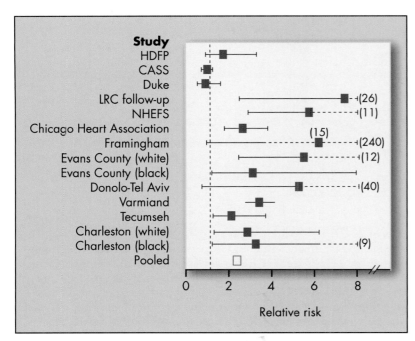

Figure 22-17.
Relative risk and 95% CI of fatal coronary heart disease associated with cholesterol levels of 6.20 mmol/L or higher compared with cholesterol levels less than 5.17 mmol/L in middle-aged women. CASS—Coronary Artery Surgery Study; HDFP—Hypertension Detection and Follow-up Program; LRC—Lipid Research Clinics; NHEFS—National Health and Nutrition Examination Survey I Epidemiologic Follow-up Study. (*Adapted from* Manolio *et al.* [18].)

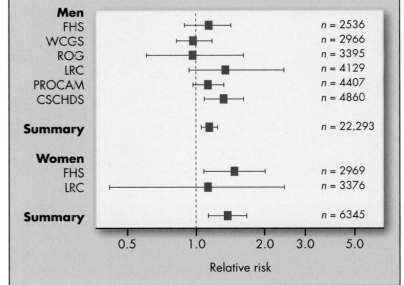

Figure 22-18.
Multivariate-adjusted relative risk (RR) estimates and 95% CI for the association between incident cardiovascular disease and a 1-mmol/L increase in triglyceride, by gender, for those studies that adjusted for high-density lipoprotein cholesterol. RR values are given on the x-axis on a natural logarithm scale. The y-axis lists each study included in the meta-analysis, ordered by sample size, and the summary RR. An RR of 1.0 (*vertical dotted line*) represents no association, and CI that do not cover 1.0 indicate RRs that are statistically significant at the $P = 0.05$ level. CSCHDS—Caerphilly and Speedwell Collaborative Heart Disease Studies; FHS—Framingham Heart Study; LRC—Lipid Research Clinics; PROCAM—Prospective Cardiovascular Munster Study; ROG—Rome Occupational Groups; WCGS—Western Collaborative Health Study. (*Adapted from* Austin *et al.* [19].)

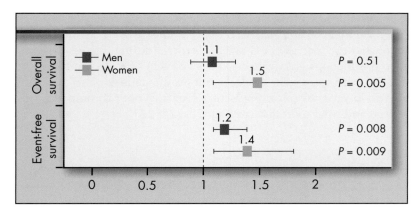

Figure 22-19.

Top (> 231 mg/dL) versus bottom (< 117 mg/dL) triglyceride quartile hazard ratios (with 95% CI) for men and women (overall and event-free survival). (*Adapted from* Sprecher *et al.* [20].)

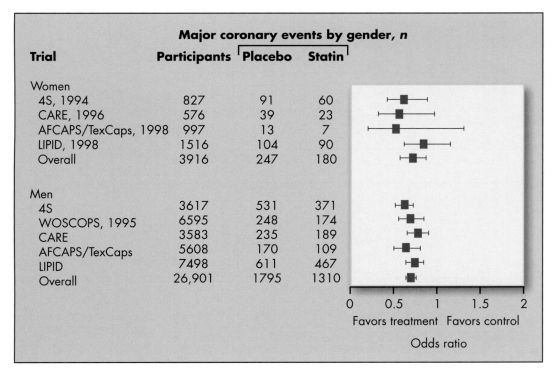

Figure 22-20.

Relative odds of major coronary events associated with statin treatment from individual trials and overall by gender and age. 4S—Scandinavian Simvastatin Survival Study; AFCAPS/TexCAPS—Air Force/Texas Coronary Atherosclerosis Prevention study; CARE— Cholesterol and Recurrent Events trial; LIPID— Long-Term Intervention with Pravastatin in Ischemic Disease trial; WOSCOPS—West of Scotland Coronary Prevention Study. (*Adapted from* LaRosa *et al.* [21].)

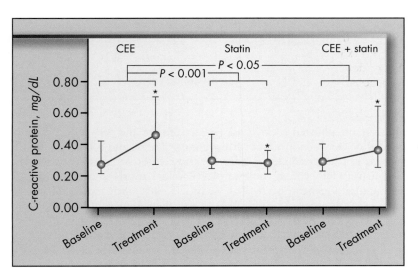

Figure 22-21.

Baseline and treatment values of C-reactive protein are shown for conjugated equine estrogens (CEEs), simvastatin (statin), and the treatments combined. Data are presented as 25th percentile, median, and 75th percentile. *Asterisks* mean $P = 0.02$ or less versus respective baseline values. Brackets with significance figures indicate post hoc comparisons between treatment periods after demonstration of significance among periods by analysis of variance ($P < 0.001$) [22–24]. (*Adapted from* Koh *et al.* [25].)

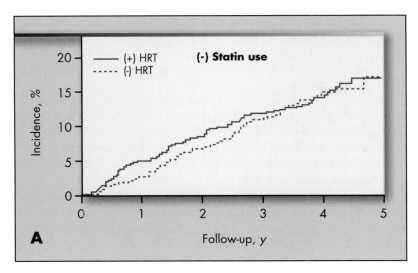

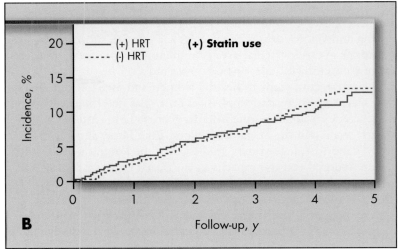

Figure 22-22.
Cumulative incidence of primary events (nonfatal myocardial infarction and coronary heart disease deaths) according to baseline use of statin therapy and treatment assignment. **A,** Hormone therapy (*solid line*) versus placebo (*dashed line*) among women not on statins at baseline.

B, Hormone therapy (*solid line*) versus placebo (*dashed line*) among baseline statin users. HRT—hormone replacement therapy. (*Adapted from* Herrington *et al.* [26].)

Obesity

The prevalence of obesity has increased substantially in women from the 1960s to the present, with obesity more common in women than in men (*see* Fig. 22-23) [1]. More than one half of African-American and one third of white women weigh 20% more than their desirable weight, with obesity increased and more severe among populations with lower educational and income levels.

In the Iowa Women's Health Study [27], an increased waist-to-hip ratio was best associated with mortality from coronary heart disease and other cardiovascular diseases.

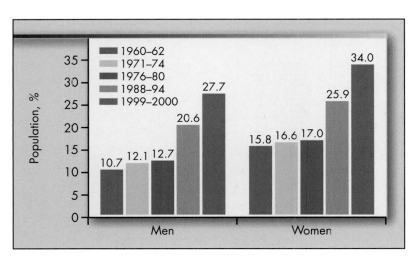

Figure 22-23.
Age-adjusted prevalence of obesity in Americans ages 20 to 74 by gender and survey in National Health Examination Survey (NHES), National Health and Nutrition Examination Survey (NHANES) I, NHANES II, NHANES III, NHANES IV, 1960–1962, 1971–1974, 1976–1980, 1988–1994, and 1999–2000. Obesity is defined as a body mass index of 30.0 or higher. (*Adapted from* American Heart Association [1]; *data from* National Center for Health Statistics/Centers for Disease Control.)

Physical Inactivity

Moderate or vigorous physical activity is lowest in non-Hispanic blacks and Mexican-American women compared with white women and is inversely related to body mass index (*see* Fig. 22-24) [1]. The leisure-time physical activity patterns among overweight adults showed that although modest numbers of women used physical activity to lose weight, a very small percentage met the physical activity guidelines.

In an older population, high-density lipoprotein cholesterol levels were higher and triglyceride levels were lower with moderate levels of exercise (although high-density lipoprotein cholesterol levels were higher in women who were users than nonusers of estrogen; *see* Fig. 22-25) [28].

Brisk walking and vigorous exercise were associated with substantial and comparable reduction in the incidence of coronary events in

Coronary Risk Factors in Women

the Nurses' Health Study (*see* Fig. 22-26) [29]. A further report from the Nurses' Health Study (*see* Fig. 22-27) [30] identified that walking and vigorous exercise were associated with substantial reductions in cardiovascular events in menopausal women, irrespective of race, ethnicity, age, or body mass index.

In a prospective study of healthy women and men, all-cause mortality was inversely related to physical fitness, as determined by maximal exercise treadmill testing in both genders [31]. Among asymptomatic women in the St. James Women Take Heart Project, the largest cohort of such women studied over the longest period of follow-up, reduced exercise capacity as measured by stress testing was an independent predictor of death (*see* Fig. 22-28) [32]. A 17% reduction in mortality rate was associated with each 1-metabolic equivalent increase in exercise capacity [32]. Among women undergoing coronary angiography for suspected myocardial ischemia in

the Women's Ischemia Syndrome Evaluation cohort study, higher self-reported physical fitness was independently associated with fewer coronary risk factors, less angiographic coronary disease, and lower risk for adverse events. Obesity was not independently associated with the outcomes (*see* Fig. 22-29) [33].

Examination of physical activity and mortality in women in the Framingham Heart Study [34] showed that active women lived longer; however, there was no association between activity levels and cardiovascular morbidity or mortality such that the beneficial effect of physical activity did not appear to be the result of a decrease in cardiovascular disease.

Efficacy of counseling for encouraging physical activity indicated important gender differences, in that women required more substantive follow-up than men to induce the behavioral changes and reversal of a sedentary lifestyle (*see* Fig. 22-30) [35].

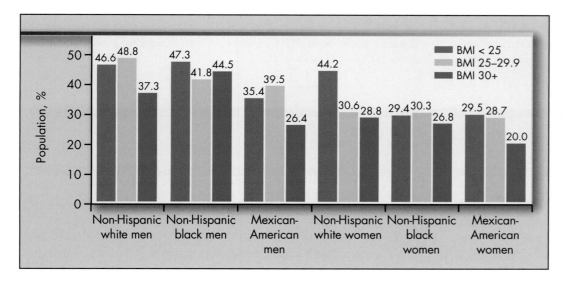

Figure 22-24.
Prevalence of moderate or vigorous physical activity in Americans age 20 and older by gender, race/ethnicity, and body mass index (BMI) in National Health and Nutrition Examination Survey III, 1988–1994. (*Adapted from* American Heart Association [1]; *data from* National Center for Health Statistics/Centers for Disease Control.)

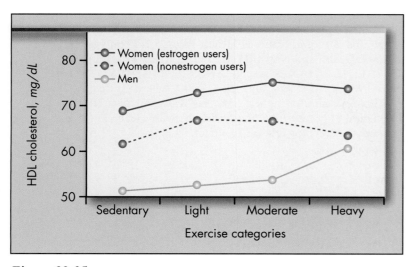

Figure 22-25.
Mean age-adjusted high-density lipoprotein (HDL) cholesterol levels by exercise category in men and women aged 50 to 89 who were not currently using cholesterol-lowering medications (Rancho Bernardo, California, 1984 to 1987). (*Adapted from* Reaven *et al.* [28].)

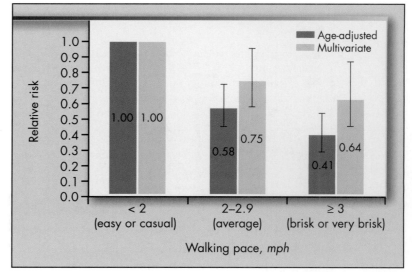

Figure 22-26.
Age-adjusted and multivariate relative risks of coronary events (nonfatal myocardial infarction or death from coronary causes) according to walking pace. mph—miles per hour. (*Adapted from* Manson *et al.* [29].)

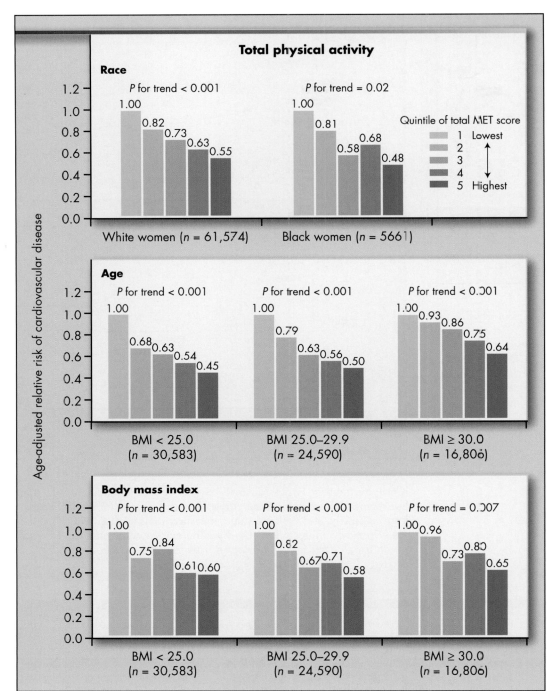

Figure 22-27.
Age-adjusted relative risks of cardiovascular disease according to quintile of total metabolic equivalent (MET) score in subgroups defined by race, age, and body mass index (BMI). The reference category is the lowest quintile of MET score. (*Adapted from* Manson *et al.* [30].)

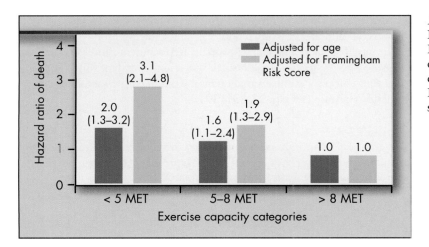

Figure 22-28.
Hazards ratios of all-cause death when adjusted for age and Framingham Risk Score for each of the exercise capacity categories (in metabolic equivalents [MET]) less than 5, 5 to 8, and greater than 8. The highest exercise capacity category (> 8 MET) was the reference category. Hazards ratios are listed within the bars; 95% CI are shown in parentheses. (*Adapted from* Gulati *et al.* [32].)

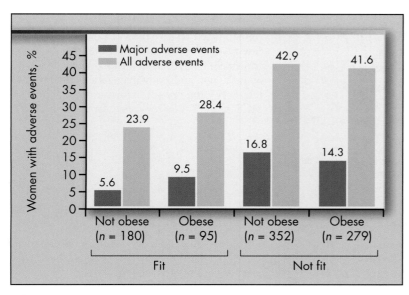

Figure 22-29.
Proportion of women with adverse events by categories of obesity and fitness. Mean (SD) follow-up time was 3.9 (1.8) years. *Not obese* was defined as body mass index less than 30.0, and *obese* was defined as body mass index of 30 or greater; *fit* was defined as a Duke Activity Status Index score 25 or greater and *not fit* as a Duke Activity Status Index score less than 25. *Asterisk* means $P = 0.002$ χ^2 test. *Dagger* means $P = 0.001$ by χ^2 test. (*Adapted from* Wessel *et al.* [33].)

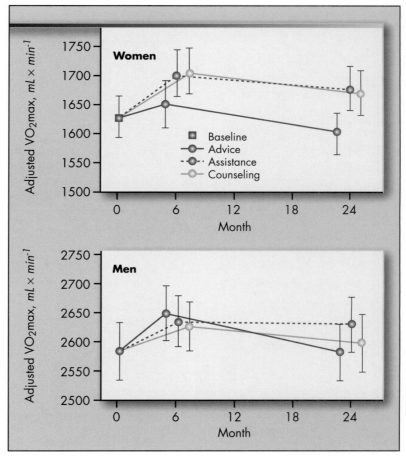

Figure 22-30.
Cardiorespiratory FitnessMaximal oxygen uptake, VO_2max in mL/min, for men and women by intervention group, adjusted for clinical center, race/ethnicity, and baseline value; measurements at months 0, 6, and 24. *Error bars* indicate 95% CI. Baseline marker represents the adjusted mean for all participants. (*Adapted from* the Writing Group for the Activity Counseling Trial Research Group [35].)

Depression/Hostility

Women are twice as likely as men to have abnormal depression scores after myocardial infarction; higher mortality rates are evident in depressed post-infarction patients, particularly those with increased ventricular ectopy (*see* Fig. 22-31) [36]. Even after controlling for established cardiovascular risk factors among menopausal women enrolled in the Women's Health Initiative, depressive symptoms significantly related to an increased risk of cardiovascular death and all-cause mortality (*see* Fig. 22-32) [37]. Despite this, interventions for depression and social isolation in a random-ized controlled clinical trial [38] failed to improve event-free survival. The current evidence-based American Heart Association Guidelines for Cardiovascular Disease Prevention in Women recommend screening for depression in high-risk women and referral for intervention [3].

In the Heart and Estrogen/progestin Replacement Study, hostility as measured by the Cook-Medley Score was an independent risk factor for recurrent coronary events in menopausal women with established coronary heart disease (*see* Fig. 22-33) [39].

Figure 22-31.
Bar graph of 18-month cardiac mortality in relation to premature ventricular contractions (PVCs) and Beck Depression Inventory (BDI) scores in the hospital after myocardial infarction. (*Adapted from* Frasure-Smith *et al.* [36].)

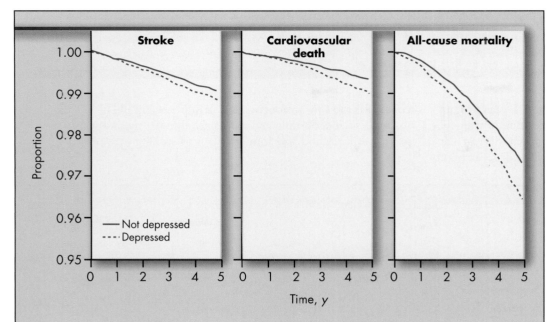

Figure 22-32.
Survival curves for those depressed and not depressed. (*Adapted from* Wassertheil-Smoller *et al.* [37].)

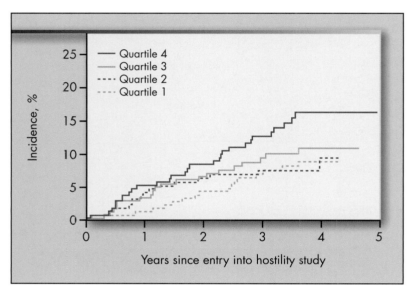

Figure 22-33.
Kaplan-Meier estimates of the cumulative incidence of coronary heart disease events (nonfatal myocardial infarction and coronary heart disease death) by hostility score quartile, Hostility Ancillary Study, Heart and Estrogen/progestin Replacement Study, United States, 1993–1998. (*Adapted from* Chaput *et al.* [39].)

Coronary Risk Factors in Women

Socioeconomic Status

Socioeconomic status differences in case fatality and 1-year prognosis after initial myocardial infarction in women and men in the Finnish Monitoring of Trends and Determinants in Cardiovascular Disease Myocardial Infarction Register Study predicted adverse outcomes for the low socioeconomic group (*see* Fig. 34) [40]. Low versus high socioeconomic groups received fewer medications with proven efficacy and had longer delays in seeking care [40].

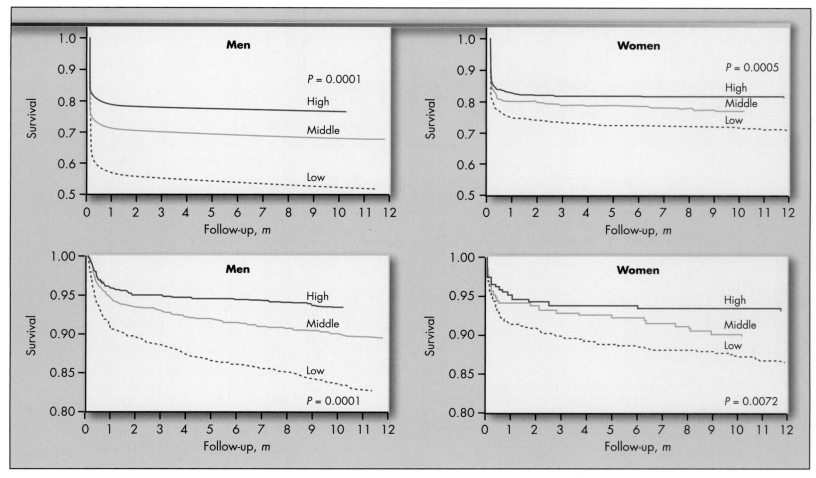

Figure 22-34.
Kaplan-Meier 1-year survival curves by income group for all patients aged 35 to 64 years with their first myocardial infarction event (*left panels*, *n* = 6485 for men and *n* = 1942 for women) and for patients who have survived more than 1 day since the beginning of symptoms of their first myocardial infarction (*right panels*, *n* = 4647 for men and *n* = 1617 for women) in the Finnish Monitoring of Trends and Determinants in Cardiovascular Disease Myocardial Infarction Register Study. The *P* values are based on log rank tests for the difference between the income groups. (*Adapted from* Salomaa *et al.* [40].)

Homocysteine

Elevated levels of serum homocysteine appear to increase coronary risk for women and for men (*see* Fig. 22-35) [41]. However, a meta-analysis of observational data suggested that elevated homocysteine at most modestly independently predicted coronary and stroke risk in a healthy population (*see* Fig. 22-36) [42]. In the American Heart Association Evidence-based Guidelines for Cardiovascular Disease Prevention in Women, therapy of elevated homocysteine levels (if measured) is recommended for high-risk women who have not undergone a revascularization procedure, with a IIb level of evidence [3].

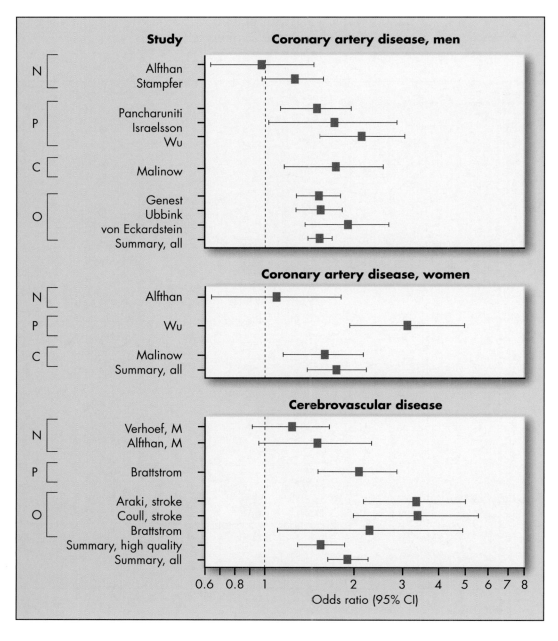

Figure 22-35.

Quantitative analysis of studies of total homocysteine (tHcy) and vascular disease presented as odds ratios (ORs) with 95% CI on a log scale based on a 5-μmol/L increase in tHcy. An OR greater than 1.0 indicates that elevated tHcy levels increase the risk for vascular disease. For each study, the OR estimate was calculated from the mean levels of total homocysteine in cases and controls by the linear discriminant function method. Unless indicated, ORs are for males (M) and females. The *Summary, All* includes all studies in each figure, and the *Summary, High Quality* includes only those studies classified as high quality. C—cross-sectional studies; N—prospective nested case-control studies; O—other case-control studies; P—population-based case-control studies. (*Adapted from* Boushey *et al.* [41].)

C-reactive Protein

Increased levels of high-sensitivity C-reactive protein were associated with a greater risk of cardiovascular events among more than 28,000 apparently healthy menopausal women in the Women's Health Study (*see* Fig. 22-36) [43]. In this prospective study, high-sensitivity C-reactive protein better predicted cardiovascular events than did levels of low-density lipoprotein cholesterol (*see* Fig. 22-37) [44], adding prognostic information to that derived from the Framingham Risk Score.

Interrelationships were examined among C-reactive protein, the metabolic syndrome, and incident cardiovascular events in an 8-year follow-up study of almost 15,000 initially healthy women in the Women's Health Study. C-reactive protein measurement added clinically important prognostic information about future vascular risk to the clinical characteristics of the metabolic syndrome: upper body obesity, hypertriglyceridemia, low high-density lipoprotein cholesterol, hypertension and abnormal glucose levels (*see* Fig. 22-38) [45]. Clinical trials of therapy to reduce levels of high-sensitivity C-reactive protein are in progress.

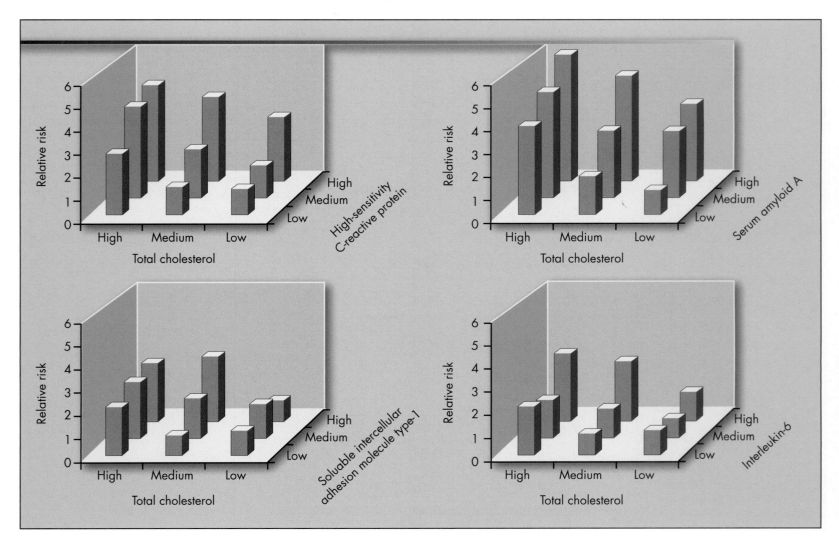

Figure 22-36.
Relative risk of cardiovascular events among apparently healthy postmenopausal women according to baseline levels of total cholesterol and markers of inflammation. Each marker of inflammation improved risk-prediction models based on lipid testing alone, an effect that was strongest for high-sensitivity C-reactive protein and serum amyloid A. (*Adapted from* Ridker *et al.* [43].)

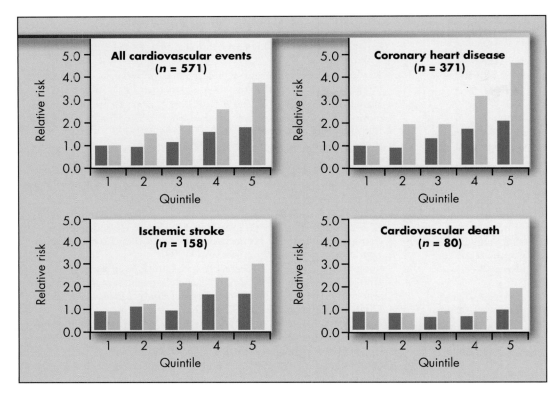

Figure 22-37.
Age-adjusted relative risk of future cardiovascular events, according to baseline C-reactive protein levels and low-density lipoprotein cholesterol levels. (*Adapted from* Ridker *et al.* [44].)

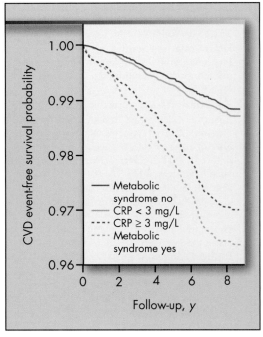

Figure 22-38.
Comparison of cardiovascular event-free survival for those with and without metabolic syndrome to those with baseline C-reactive protein (CRP) levels greater than or less than 3.0 mg/L. CVD—cardiovascular disease. (*Adapted from* Ridker *et al.* [45].)

References

1. American Heart Association: *Heart Disease and Stroke Statistics: 2004 Update*. Dallas: American Heart Association; 2003.

2. Wenger NK, Speroff L, Packard B: Cardiovascular health and disease in women. *N Engl J Med* 1993, 329:247–256.

3. Mosca L, Appel LJ, Benjamin EJ, *et al.*: Evidence-based guidelines for cardiovascular disease prevention in women. *Circulation* 2004, 109:672–692.

4. Lee WL, Cheung AM, Cape D, *et al.*: Impact of diabetes on coronary artery disease in women and men: a meta-analysis of prospective studies. *Diabetes Care* 2002, 23:962–968.

5. Manson JE, Colditz GA, Stampfer MJ, *et al.*: A prospective study of maturity-onset diabetes mellitus and risk of coronary heart disease and stroke in women. *Arch Intern Med* 1991, 151:1141–1147.

6. Diabetes Prevention Program Research Group: Reduction in the incidence of type 2 diabetes with lifestyle intervention or metformin. *N Engl J Med* 2002, 346:393–403.

7. Harris MI, Flegal KM, Cowie CC, *et al.*: Prevalence of diabetes, impaired fasting glucose, and impaired glucose tolerance in U.S. adults. The Third National Health and Nutrition Examination Survey, 1988–1994. *Diabetes Care* 1998, 21:518–524.

8. Winkleby MA, Kraemer HC, Ahn DK, Varady AN: Ethnic and socioeconomic differences in cardiovascular disease risk factors: findings for women from the Third National Health and Nutrition Examination Survey, 1988–1994. *JAMA* 1998, 280:356–362.

9. Natarajan S, Liao Y, Cao G, *et al.*: Sex differences in risk for coronary heart disease mortality associated with diabetes and established coronary heart disease. *Arch Intern Med* 2003, 163:1735–1740.

10. Mason PJ, Manson JE, Sesso HD, *et al.*: Blood pressure and risk of secondary cardiovascular events in women. The Women's Antioxidant Cardiovascular Study (WACS). *Circulation* 2004, 109:1623–1629.

11. Gueyffier F, Boutitie F, Boissel J-P, *et al.*: The INDANA Investigators. Effect of antihypertensive drug treatment on cardiovascular outcomes in women and men: a meta-analysis of individual patient data from randomized, controlled trials. *Ann Intern Med* 1997, 126:761–767.

12. Hajjar I, Kotchen TA: Trends in prevalence, awareness, treatment, and control of hypertension in the United States, 1988–2000. *JAMA* 2003, 290:199–206.

13. Winkleby MA, Robinson TN, Sundquist J, *et al.*: Ethnic variation in cardiovascular disease risk factors among children and young adults: findings from the Third National Health and Nutrition Examination Survey, 1988–1994. *JAMA* 1999, 281:1006–1013.

14. Willett WC, Green A, Stampfer MJ, *et al.*: Relative and absolute excess risks of coronary heart disease among women who smoke cigarettes. *N Engl J Med* 1987, 317:1303–1309.

15. Kawachi I, Colditz GA, Stampfer MJ, *et al.*: Smoking cessation in relation to total mortality rates in women: a prospective cohort study. *Ann Intern Med* 1993, 119:992–1000.

16. Hermanson B, Omenn GS, Kronmal RA, *et al.*, and participants in the Coronary Artery Surgery Study: Beneficial six-year outcome of smoking cessation in older men and women with coronary artery disease. Results from the CASS Registry. *N Engl J Med* 1988, 319:1365–1369.

17. Hickman TB, Briefel RR, Carroll MD, *et al.*: Distributions and trends of serum lipid levels among United States children and adolescents ages 4–19 years: data from the Third National Health and Nutrition Examination Survey. *Prev Med* 1998, 27:879–890.

18. Manolio TA, Pearson TA, Wenger NK, *et al.*: Cholesterol and heart disease in older persons and women. Review of an NHLBI Workshop. *Ann Epidemiol* 1992, 2:161–176.

19. Austin MA, Hokanson JE, Edwards KL: Hypertriglyceridemia as a cardiovascular risk factor. *Am J Cardiol* 1998, 81:7B–12B.

20. Sprecher DL, Pearce GL, Cosgrove DM, *et al.*: Relation of serum triglyceride levels to survival after coronary artery bypass grafting. *Am J Cardiol* 2000, 86:285–288.

21. LaRosa JC, He J, Vupputuri S: Effect of statins on risk of coronary disease: a meta-analysis of randomized controlled trials. *JAMA* 1999, 282:2340–2346.

22. Heart Protection Study Collaborative Group: MRC/BHF Heart Protection Study of cholesterol lowering with simvastatin in 20,536 high-risk individuals: a randomised placebo-controlled trial. *Lancet* 2002, 360:7–22.

23. *The Lancet* web site. Available at http://www.thelancet.com.

24. Agency for Healthcare Research and Quality: *Diagnosis and Treatment of Coronary Heart Disease in Women: Systematic Reviews of Evidence on Selected Topics. Evidence Report/Technology Assessment Number 81.* Bethesda, MD: US Department of Health and Human Services, Public Health Services; 2003. [AHRQ Pub. No. 03-E036.]

25. Koh KK, Schenki WH, Waclawiw MA, *et al.*: Statin attenuates increase in C-reactive protein during estrogen replacement therapy in post-menopausal women. *Circulation* 2002, 105:1531–1533.

26. Herrington DM, Vittinghoff E, Lin F, *et al.*, for the HERS Study Group: Statin therapy, cardiovascular events, and total mortality in the Heart and Estrogen/progestin Replacement Study (HERS). *Circulation* 2002, 105:2962–2967.

27. Folsom AR, Kushi LH, Anderson KE, *et al.*: Associations of general and abdominal obesity with multiple health outcomes in older women: The Iowa Women's Health Study. *Arch Intern Med* 2000, 160:2117–2128.

28. Reaven PD, McPhillips JB, Barrett-Connor EL, *et al.*: Leisure time exercise and lipid and lipoprotein levels in an older population. *JAGS* 1990, 38:847–854.

29. Manson JE, Hu FB, Rich-Edwards JW, *et al.*: A prospective study of walking as compared with vigorous exercise in the prevention of coronary heart disease in women. *N Engl J Med* 1999, 341:650–658.

30. Manson JE, Greenland P, LaCroix AZ, *et al.*: Walking compared with vigorous exercise for the prevention of cardiovascular events in women. *N Engl J Med* 2002, 347:716–725.

31. Blair SN, Kohl HW III, Paffenbarger RS Jr, *et al.*: Physical fitness and all-cause mortality: a prospective study of healthy men and women. *JAMA* 1989, 262:2395–2401.

32. Gulati M, Pandey DK, Arnsdorf MF, *et al.*: Exercise capacity and the risk of death in women. The St James Women Take Heart Project. *Circulation* 2003, 108:1554–1559.

33. Wessel TR, Arant CB, Olson MB, *et al.*: Relationship of physical fitness vs body mass index with coronary artery disease and cardiovascular events in women. *JAMA* 2004, 191:1179–1187.

34. Sherman SE, D'Agnostino RB, Cobb JL, *et al.*: Physical activity and mortality in women in the Framingham Heart Study. *Am Heart J* 1994, 128:879–884.

35. The Writing Group for the Activity Counseling Trial Research Group: Effects of physical activity counseling in primary care: The Activity Counseling Trial: a randomized controlled trial. *JAMA* 2001, 286:677–687.

36. Frasure-Smith N, Lespérance F, Talajic M: Depression and 18-month prognosis after myocardial infarction. *Circulation* 1995, 91:999–1005.

37. Wassertheil-Smoller S, Shumaker S, Ockene J, *et al.*: Depression and cardiovascular sequelae in postmenopausal women. The Women's Health Initiative (WHI). *Arch Intern Med* 2004, 164:289–298.

38. Writing Committee for the ENRICHD Investigators: Effects of treating depression and low perceived social support on clinical events after myocardial infarction. The Enhancing Recovery in Coronary Heart Disease Patients (ENRICHD) Randomized Trial. *JAMA* 2003, 289:3106–3116.

39. Chaput LA, Adams SH, Simon JA, *et al.*, for the Heart Estrogen/progestin Replacement Study (HERS) Research Group: Hostility predicts recurrent events among postmenopausal women with coronary heart disease. *Am J Epidemiol* 2002, 156:1092–1099.

40. Salomaa V, Miettinen H, Niemelä M, *et al.*: Relation of socioeconomic position to the case fatality, prognosis and treatment of myocardial infarction events; the FINMONICA MI Register Study. *J Epidemiol Community Health* 2001, 55:475–482.

41. Boushey CJ, Beresford SAA, Omenn GS, *et al.*: A quantitative assessment of plasma homocysteine as a risk factor for vascular disease. Probable benefits of increasing folic acid intakes. *JAMA* 1995, 274:1049–1057.

42. The Homocysteine Studies Collaboration: Homocysteine and risk of ischemic heart disease and stroke: a meta-analysis. *JAMA* 2002, 288:2015–2022.

43. Ridker PM, Hennekens CH, Buring JE, *et al.*: C-reactive protein and other markers of inflammation in the prediction of cardiovascular disease in women. *N Engl J Med* 2000, 342:836–843.

44. Ridker PM, Rifai N, Rose L, *et al.*: Comparison of C-reactive protein and low-density lipoprotein cholesterol levels in the prediction of first cardiovascular events. *N Engl J Med* 2002, 347:1557–1565.

45. Ridker PM, Buring JE, Cook NR, *et al.*: C-reactive protein, the metabolic syndrome, and risk of incident cardiovascular events: an 8-year follow-up of 14,719 initially healthy American women. *Circulation* 2003, 107:391–397.

Multiple Intervention Studies in Secondary Prevention

C. Tissa Kappagoda and Ezra A. Amsterdam

The traditional approach to prevention strategies for coronary artery disease (CAD) has been based on the manifestation of symptoms. Individuals with no evidence of cardiovascular disease were considered to require primary prevention measures, whereas those with documented disease required secondary prevention measures that were more intensive. The basis for this dichotomy was the data from the Lipid Research Clinics Primary Prevention Program, which identified direct relationships between serum lipids and coronary heart disease mortality in patients with and without evidence of CAD [1].

However, it has been recently recognized that this model of primary and secondary prevention is an oversimplification of a complex disease. CAD risk is a continuum in which some persons without overt disease actually may be at higher risk than those with documented disease depending on the severity of their cardiac risk factors. The concept of primary and secondary prevention was replaced by "global risk" in the recommendations of the Adult Treatment Panel of the National Cholesterol Education Program [2]. Global risk, which is determined by the basic cardiac risk factor profile, is defined as the probability of developing a myocardial infarction or fatal CAD (coronary death) during a 10-year period. Three levels of global risk were established on the basis of seven risk factors utilized in the Framingham Heart Study: age, gender, serum total cholesterol, high-density lipoprotein cholesterol concentration, systolic blood pressure, treatment of hypertension, and smoking status [3].

Although the management of lipid abnormalities is an important aspect of preventing CAD, it is only one of multiple risk factors requiring therapeutic intervention. As indicated in this chapter, other risk factors, such as hypertension and smoking, require equal attention. The increasing incidence of type 2 diabetes in the US population and the high prevalence of CAD in these patients imply that other means of treating risk factors, such as exercise training and weight management, are also essential components of multiple risk factor intervention. New, emerging risk factors such as C-reactive protein, the coronary calcium score, and homocysteine are under investigation in the assessment of risk. Their therapeutic implications have not been clearly established. This chapter overviews: 1) individual risk factors and their treatment; 2) the interaction of traditional cardiovascular risk factors; 3) major randomized trials of individual and multiple risk factor reduction; and 4) application of the results of these trials to clinical practice.

Risk category	10-year global risk	Treatment goals (LDL-C)
Low risk	< 10%	< 160 mg/dL
Intermediate risk	10%–20%	< 130 mg/dL
High risk	> 20%	< 100 mg/dL
Very high risk	> 20%	< 70 mg/dL

Figure 23-1.

Adult Treatment Panel III global risk guidelines. Recently, the Adult Treatment Panel III has extended global risk to a very broad spectrum of coronary artery disease from clearly defined very low-risk asymptomatic subjects to very high-risk individuals with a 10-year global risk greater than 20 [2]. The high-risk category includes patients with clinical forms of atherosclerotic disease (coronary artery disease, peripheral arterial disease, abdominal aortic aneurysms, and symptomatic carotid artery disease), multiple risk factors, diabetes, and the metabolic syndrome. A very high-risk category has been added that includes patients with 1) acute coronary syndrome; 2) multiple risk factors, especially diabetes mellitus; 3) severe and poorly controlled risk factors, especially cigarette smoking; and 4) multiple risk factors of the metabolic syndrome [4]. Thus, it is important to recognize that the high-risk category could include individuals who are symptomatic (overt atherosclerotic disease) *and* asymptomatic (no overt atherosclerotic disease). In terms of treatment, the general consensus is that the therapeutic target for low-density lipoprotein cholesterol (LDL-C) is inversely related to the level of risk. (*Adapted from* the Adult Treatment Panel III [2] and Grundy *et al.* [4].)

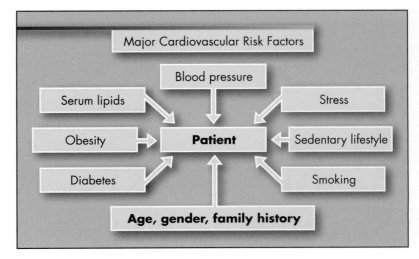

Figure 23-2.

Definition of a cardiovascular risk factor. Risk factors are conditions or characteristics that render an individual more likely to develop cardiovascular disease. They include, but are not limited to, family history, smoking, hypertension, high cholesterol, obesity, sedentary lifestyle, psychosocial factors, and diabetes mellitus. These risk factors have independent associations with the incidence of coronary artery disease. Apart from age, gender, and family history, the other factors are potentially reversible. Prospective randomized clinical trials designed to ameliorate reversible risk factors have established that directed therapy reduces the incidence of coronary artery disease. These studies provide presumptive evidence of a causative link between the reversible risk factors and coronary artery disease.

Combined Endpoints in the SHEP trial

	Active treatment (*n* = 2365)	Placebo (*n* = 2371)	Relative risk (95% CI)
Nonfatal, myocardial infarction*, or CAD[†] death	104	141	0.73 (0.57–0.94)
Fatal or nonfatal stroke, nonfatal myocardial infarction*, or CAD[†] death	199	289	0.67 (0.56–0.80)
	140	184	0.75 (0.60–0.94)
Cardiovascular disease[‡]	289	414	0.68 (0.58–0.79)

*Nonfatal myocardial infarction did not include silent myocardial infarction.

[†]CAD includes definite nonfatal and fatal myocardial infarction, sudden cardiac death, rapid cardiac death (within 24 hours), coronary artery bypass surgery, and coronary angiography.

[‡]Cardiovascular disease includes nonfatal myocardial infarction* and nonfatal and fatal stroke, transient ischemic attack, aneurysm, and endarterectomy.

Figure 23-3.

The Systolic Hypertension in the Elderly Program (SHEP). SHEP was performed to assess the ability of antihypertensive treatment to reduce the risk of fatal and nonfatal stroke in older people with isolated systolic hypertension [5]. The secondary endpoints related to cardiac disease and were defined as shown in this figure. It was a multicenter, randomized, double-blind, placebo-controlled study undertaken in 4736 men and women with a mean age of 72 years. The treatment goals were set according to the pressure at baseline. Those with a systolic pressure greater than 180 mm Hg had a target less than 160 mm Hg. In those between 160 and 179 mm Hg, the goal was a reduction of 20 mm Hg. The therapy in the treatment arm was started with chlorthalidone at a dose of 12.5 mg/d and then increased to 25 mg/d. Individuals failing

to achieve their goal were given atenolol at a dose of 25 mg/d. (Reserpine 0.05 mg/d was substituted when atenolol was contraindicated.) The average follow-up was 4.5 years. There was a significant reduction in combined endpoints.

Since completion of the SHEP study, several other placebo-controlled trials have addressed the effect of blood pressure control on the incidence of coronary artery disease (CAD). Regimens based on angiotensin-converting enzyme (ACE) inhibitors reduced the risk of CAD by 20% compared with placebo, whereas calcium antagonist–based regimens had a weaker beneficial effect [6]. (*Adapted from* SHEP Cooperative Research Group [5].)

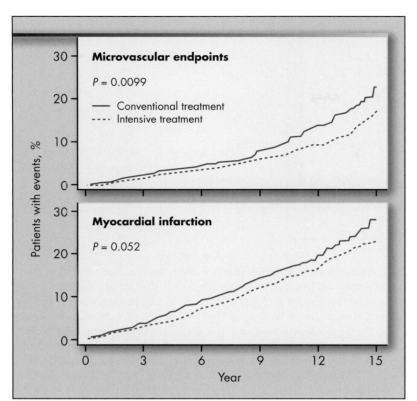

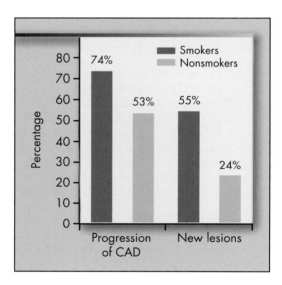

Figure 23-4.

Effect of treatment of type 2 diabetes. The United Kingdom Prospective Diabetes Study was planned to determine whether improved glycemic control of maturity-onset diabetes would diminish the morbidity and mortality of the disease. The study reported on 3867 newly diagnosed patients with type 2 diabetes (median age 54 years) followed-up for up to 15 years. Those who had a mean of two fasting plasma glucose (FPG) concentrations of 6.1 to 15.0 mmol/L after 3 months of diet treatment were randomly assigned to an intensive treatment regimen (sulphonylurea or insulin), or conventional dietary management. The endpoint in the intensive group was FPG less than 6 mmol/L (×18 for conversion to mg/dL). In the conventional group, the aim was the best achievable FPG with diet alone, with drugs being added only if there were hyperglycemic symptoms or FPG greater than 15 mol/L [7]. Intensive glycemic control minimally and insignificantly reduced macrovascular complications. However, the overall cardiovascular events were significantly decreased probably because of a reduction in microvascular complications, which included the need for retinal photocoagulation. These observations were similar to those of the Diabetes Control and Complications Trial [8]. No study has conclusively established that glycemic control alone results in a significant reduction in macrovascular complications. To assess this issue, the Veterans Administration initiated a subsequent trial to assess this issue in 2000; it has not been completed as yet [9]. (*Adapted from* UK Prospective Diabetes Study Group [7].)

Figure 23-5.

Effect of smoking cessation. Cigarette smoking has been recognized as a potent risk factor in the development of coronary artery disease (CAD) for several decades. Unlike other risk factors, there are no clinical trials that have addressed the specific issue of the effect of smoking cessation on the progression of atherosclerosis and cardiovascular events. However, several studies have addressed the effect of continued smoking on the progression of CAD with and without medical therapy. The Canadian Cardiovascular Atherosclerosis Intervention Trial [10] examined the progression of coronary atherosclerosis over 2 years in 90 smokers and 241 exsmokers and nonsmokers. Both categories were randomized to receive lovastatin for treatment of hyperlipidemia indicated by a total serum cholesterol at entry between 200 to 300 mg/dL. The degree of atherosclerosis was determined by quantitative coronary angiography. The findings are summarized in the figure. The data that were adapted from the study shows the effect of smoking on progression of CAD in the placebo group. Smokers showed significantly more progression and new lesions than nonsmokers. These differences between smokers and nonsmokers were not evident in the lovastatin-treated group (not shown). It was concluded that smoking accelerates progression of CAD and new lesion formation as assessed by serial quantitative coronary angiography. These differences were not evident in patients given lovastatin. The trial did not include CAD events. (*Adapted from* Waters *et al.* [10])

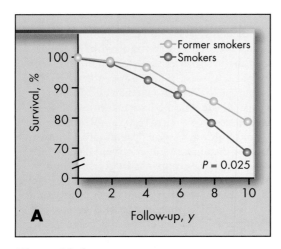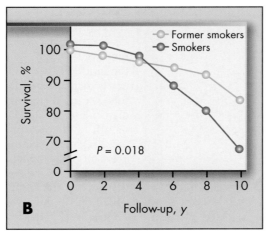

Figure 23-6.

Effect of smoking cessation: The Coronary Artery Surgery Study. The Coronary Artery Surgery Study was a prospective randomized trial of the effect of medical versus surgical treatment in symptomatic patients with angiographically proven coronary artery disease [11]. Patients were recruited from 15 sites in the United States and Canada. Seven hundred eighty patients recruited into the study were classified according to smoking behavior and followed-up for 11.2 years. The 10-year survival in 468 patients who reported no smoking during the follow-up was 82% compared with 77% in the 312 who smoked. This difference was not significant. However, the survival among those who quit at entry into the study was 80% compared with 69% who continued to smoke. Further, in those randomized to the surgical group, the 10-year survival among quitters was 84% compared with 68% in those who did

not. In the group assigned to medical management, the rates were similar in quitters and smokers. It was concluded that among patients with documented coronary artery disease undergoing coronary artery bypass surgery, continued smoking may result in decreased survival [12].

A, Ten-year survival among medical and surgical patients who were smoking at study entry. Ninety-seven patients who quit smoking within 6 months after surgery had a better survival rate after 10 years than the 187 who did not quit smoking (80% vs 69%).

B, Ten-year survival in patients randomized to surgery. Fifty-three patients who quit smoking within 6 months after surgery had a better survival rate at 10 years compared with the 86 who did not quit smoking (84% vs 68%). (*Panels A and B adapted from* Cavender *et al.* [12].)

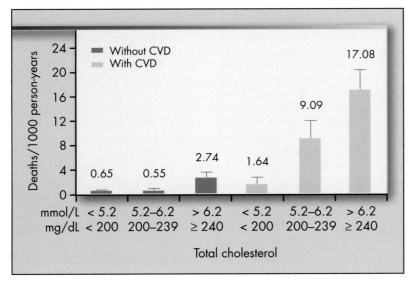

Figure 23-7.

Effect of treatment of serum lipids. Control of serum lipids is the cornerstone of preventive cardiology [2]. During the past two decades, effective cholesterol-lowering medications have become a reality, and this has altered our approach to the long-term management of patients with coronary artery disease. One of the most important investigations supporting the relationship between cardiovascular disease (CVD) and serum cholesterol levels was obtained as part of the Lipid Research

Clinics Program Prevalence Study [1], which was conducted in 10 North American populations between 1972 and 1976. After baseline serum lipid data were obtained, 2541 white males were followed-up for an average of 10.1 years. Individuals with definite diabetes and those taking lipid-lowering medications were excluded. Age-adjusted death rates for coronary heart disease increased with less favorable levels of serum lipids in people with and without prior evidence of CVD. These differences were significant even after adjustment for other risk factors (hypertension, smoking, body mass index, and physical activity). It was concluded that in men between 40 and 69 years of age, total, low- (LDL) and high-density lipoprotein (HDL) cholesterol predicted subsequent mortality. This finding was especially true for people with preexisting CVD. Individuals were considered to have CVD if there was evidence of the following: 1) a definite myocardial infarction; 2) an abnormal stress test defined by the occurrence of an arrhythmia, chest pain, hypotension, or intracardiac block in ECG; 3) specific ECG abnormalities defined by Minnesota codes; 4) angina pectoris as identified by a Rose questionnaire; or 5) miscellaneous conditions such as hospitalization for stroke, heart failure, arrhythmias, and inability to continue a graded treadmill test beyond stage 1.

In this figure, individuals without CVD are shown in the *light-shaded bars* and those with CVD are represented by *dark-shaded bars*. Risk in the highest tertile of the non-CVD group exceeds that lowest tertile in the CVD group. A similar relationship was found between serum LDL cholesterol concentration and deaths due to coronary heart disease. The serum HDL cholesterol concentration was inversely related to deaths due to coronary heart disease. (*Adapted from* Pekkanen *et al.* [1].)

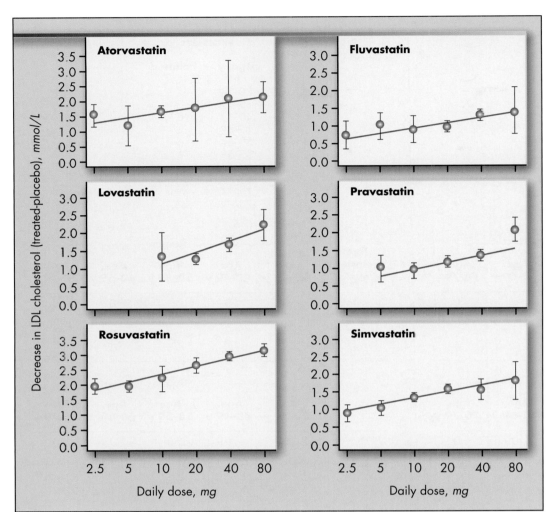

Figure 23-8.
Effect of cholesterol lowering on coronary artery disease. Multiple studies have established that 3-hydroxy-3-methylglutaryl coenzyme A reductase inhibitors not only lower serum cholesterol and serum low-density lipoprotein (LDL) concentrations significantly but also have a significant beneficial effect on the incidence of clinical events attributable to coronary atherosclerosis. The reduction in serum cholesterol is dose dependent. The figure shows the reductions in low-density lipoprotein cholesterol concentration (95% CI) in 164 trials according to 3-hydroxy-3-methylglutaryl coenzyme A reductase inhibitor and dose. The data were not standardized to pretreatment concentrations. This meta-analysis has suggested that the beneficial effects are related to cholesterol lowering per se and not linked to a particular drug. In fact, it has been suggested that the important factor is the lowering of serum cholesterol and not the means by which it is accomplished [13]. (*Adapted from* Law *et al.* [13].)

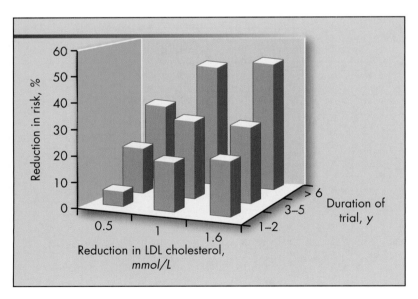

Figure 23-9.
How does cholesterol lowering translate into reduction in risk? Reducing low-density lipoprotein (LDL) cholesterol has a favorable impact on cardiovascular morbidity. Meta-analysis of 49 randomized placebo-controlled trials suggests that the outcome is related to the degree of cholesterol lowering and the duration of follow-up. The reduction in risk (%) of events attributable to ischemic heart disease refers to relative odds reduction in the 49 randomized trials grouped according to number of years in the trial at time of event and reduction in serum cholesterol concentration [13]. It is seen that in the short-term trials, risk reduction requires a larger decrease in LDL cholesterol compared with long-term trials. (*Adapted from* Law *et al.* [13].)

Men

Age, y	Points
20–34	-9
35–39	-4
40–44	0
45–49	3
50–54	6
55–59	8
60–64	10
65–69	11
70–74	12
75–79	13

Total cholesterol, mg/dL	Points				
	Age 20–39 y	Age, 40–49 y	Age 50–59 y	Age, 60–69 y	Age, 70–79 y
< 160	0	0	0	0	0
160–199	4	3	2	1	0
200–239	7	5	3	1	0
240–279	9	6	4	2	1
≥ 280	11	8	5	3	1

	Points				
	Age 20–39 y	Age, 40–49 y	Age 50–59 y	Age, 60–69 y	Age, 70–79 y
Nonsmoker	0	0	0	0	0
Smoker	8	5	3	1	1

HDL, mg/dL	Points
≥ 60	-1
50–59	0
40–49	1
> 40	2

Systolic BP, mm Hg	If Untreated	If Treated
< 120	0	0
120–129	0	1
130–139	1	2
140–159	1	2
≥ 160	2	3

Point Total	10-Year Risk, %
< 0	< 1
0	1
1	1
2	1
3	1
4	1
5	2
6	2
7	3
8	4
9	5
10	6
11	8
12	10
13	12
14	16
15	20
16	25
≥ 17	≥ 30

Women

Age, y	Points
20–34	-7
35–39	-3
40–44	0
45–49	3
50–54	6
55–59	8
60–64	10
65–69	11
70–74	12
75–79	13

Total cholesterol, mg/dL	Points				
	Age 20–39 y	Age, 40–49 y	Age 50–59 y	Age, 60–69 y	Age, 70–79 y
< 160	0	0	0	0	0
160–199	4	3	2	1	1
200–239	8	6	4	2	1
240–279	11	8	5	3	2
≥ 280	13	10	7	4	2

	Points				
	Age 20–39 y	Age, 40–49 y	Age 50–59 y	Age, 60–69 y	Age, 70–79 y
Nonsmoker	0	0	0	0	0
Smoker	9	7	4	2	1

HDL, mg/dL	Points
≥ 60	-1
50–59	0
40–49	1
> 40	2

Systolic BP, mm Hg	If Untreated	If Treated
< 120	0	0
120–129	1	3
130–139	2	4
140–159	3	5
≥ 160	4	6

Point Total	10-Year Risk, %
< 9	< 1
9	1
10	1
11	1
12	1
13	2
14	2
15	3
16	4
17	5
18	6
19	8
20	11
21	14
22	17
23	22
24	27
≥ 25	≥ 30

Figure 23-10. (*continued on next page*)

Figure 23-10. *(on previous page)*
The concept of global risk. Calculation of 10-year risk for men and women [2]. The 10-year risk for developing coronary artery disease is carried out using the Framingham risk-scoring table. The risk factors included are age, total cholesterol, high-density lipoprotein cholesterol, systolic blood pressure, treatment for hypertension, and cigarette smoking. Using the appropriate table for gender, first assign the number of points for each risk factor. Then determine the total score. The bottom part of each table permits the determination of the 10-year risk of developing coronary heart disease, that is, myocardial infarction or coronary death.

Observe that the total cholesterol was a more robust predictor of coronary heart disease in the Framingham database probably because of the magnitude of the sample. However, the low-density lipoprotein cholesterol is used as the primary treatment target based on the overall risk. Caveats: 1) The total and high-density lipoprotein cholesterol values should be the average of at least two measurements in a lipid panel. 2) The blood pressure value is that obtained at the time of examination regardless of therapy. If the patient is on antihypertensive therapy, an extra point weights the score. 3) Designation of "smoker" is based on any cigarette smoking during the previous month. (*Adapted from* the Adult Treatment Panel III [2].)

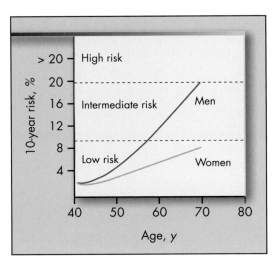

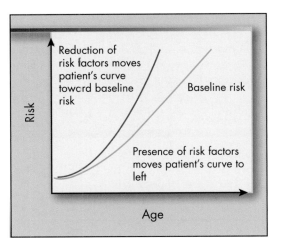

Figure 23-11.
The additive effects of multiple risk factors on the incidence of coronary artery disease. The National Cholesterol Education Panel (Adult Treatment Panel) established a working definition of cardiac risk based on the interaction of various "conventional" cardiovascular risk factors [2]. Cardiac risk was defined as the probability of experiencing a myocardial infarction or a coronary death over 10 years. A risk greater than 20% was considered high and less than 10% was considered low. Risk of 10% to 20% was considered intermediate. The concepts outlined in the report are shown graphically for men and women in this figure. Every individual has a "baseline" risk, which is dependent on age and gender. In the case of a man it increases from 4% in the fourth decade to nearly 20% at the seventh decade.

Figure 23-12.
Modification of baseline risk. In men and women, presence of additional risk factors increases the gradient of this relationship, resulting in the attainment of a high-risk status earlier in life. In women, the risk increases at a slower rate compared with men. The aim of multiple risk factor intervention is to move the risk curve to the right so that it approaches the one determined by age and gender (*ie*, the baseline curve shown in figure).

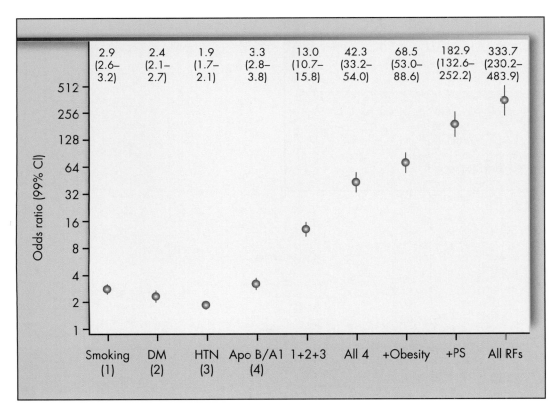

Figure 23-13.
Global risk: "the international dimension." The recently reported INTERHEART study [14] has extended the concept of global risk beyond the findings derived from the Framingham Heart Study. Much of the current views on cardiovascular risk factors have been based on findings in developed countries. The INTERHEART study was a standardized case-control study of acute myocardial infarction undertaken in 52 countries drawn from every inhabited continent. Patients enrolled included 15,152 cases and 14,820 controls. The relationship of smoking, history of hypertension (HTN) or diabetes (DM), waist/hip ratio, dietary patterns, physical activity, consumption of alcohol, apolipoproteins, and psychosocial factors to myocardial infarction were studied. It was observed that, worldwide, abnormal lipids, smoking, hypertension, diabetes, abdominal obesity, psychosocial factors (PS), low consumption of fruit and vegetables, alcohol, and lack of physical activity accounted for 90% of the risk of myocardial infarction in men and 94% in women.

The figure shows the odds ratios for individual factors and multiple risk factors. Observe the scale on the y-axis, which increases by geometric progression. RFs—risk factors. (*Adapted from* Yusuf *et al.* [14].)

Multiple Intervention Studies in Secondary Prevention

Risk factor	Definition	Most significant component
Current smokers	Smoked within the past 12 months	Smoker vs nonsmoker
Hypertension	Self-reported history	Presence or absence
Diabetes mellitus	Self-reported history	Presence or absence
Apo B/Apo A	Ratio of lipoproteins preferred to LDL because latter is affected by fasting state	Highest vs lowest quintile
Abdominal obesity	Waist/hip ratio	Highest tertile (> 0.95 for men and > 0.90 for women) vs lowest tertile (< 0.9 for men and < 0.83 for women)
Psychosocial factors	A composite score based on depression, life stress, financial stress, low locus of control, and major illness	Presence or absence of all factors
Exercise	Moderate (walking, cycling, or gardening) of vigorous exercise (jogging, swimming, soccer) > 4 hours per week	Presence or absence
Diet	Consumption of fruits and vegetables	Presence or absence

Figure 23-14.
The risk factors and protective factors identified in the INTERHEART study [14].
Apo—apoliloproteins; LDL—low-density lipoprotein.

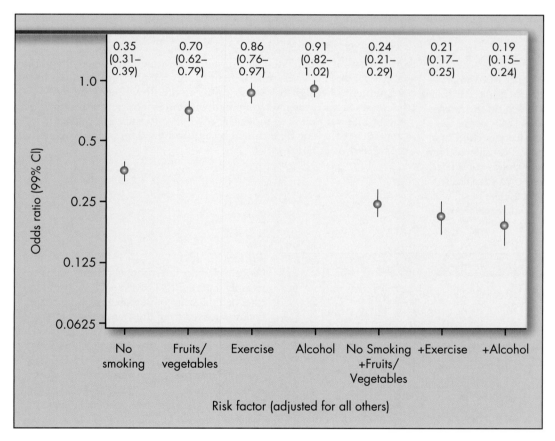

Figure 23-15.
The absence of risk factors. The INTERHEART study also reported on the effect of the absence of these factors on the relative risk of developing a myocardial infarction. Avoidance of smoking, daily consumption of fruit and vegetables, and regular physical activity significantly reduces the risk of myocardial infarction (nearly 75% reduction in risk compared with a smoker with an inappropriate lifestyle). These findings provide a basis for interventions in primary prevention. (*Adapted from* Yusuf *et al.* [14].)

Main Endpoints Used in Multiple Intervention Clinical Trials

"Hard" events
  Myocardial infarction
  Stroke
  Cardiac death
Other cardiovascular events
  Unstable angina
  Arrhythmias
  Heart failure
  Percutaneous coronary intervention
  Coronary artery bypass surgery
Angiographic evidence of regression of coronary atherosclerosis
Noninvasive imaging evidence of improved myocardial perfusion

Figure 23-16.
Multiple risk factor intervention involves the normalization of the reversible risk factors described in Figure 23-1. In practice the process involves the management of 1) serum lipids, 2) blood pressure, 3) diet, 4) weight, 5) exercise training, and 6) psychosocial stress. Such an intervention requires a multidisciplinary approach to patient care involving physicians, nurses, clinical psychologists (or other behaviorists), dieticians, and exercise physiologists. Various psychologic factors, such as depression, anxiety, and social isolation, have been associated with the prevalence of coronary artery disease and with the outcome of treatment programs. Because multiple risk factor interventions involve significant changes in lifestyle and compliance becomes a significant issue, the clinical psychologist has a unique role in facilitating this change. This figure summarizes the main endpoints used in multiple intervention clinical trials.

The Oslo Heart Study: Inclusion and Exclusion Criteria

Inclusion criteria
  Serum cholesterol 280–380 mg/dL
  Systolic blood pressure > 150 mm Hg
  Smoking (80%)
  Normal ECG at rest
  Absence of angina during stress test (regardless of
    ECG changes)
Exclusion criteria
  Presence of other cardiovascular diseases including history and
    symptoms of CAD
  Blood sugar > 135 mg/dL
  Cancer
  Psychopathologic disease
  Physically disabling conditions
  Alcoholism

Figure 23-17.
The Oslo Heart Study: a primary prevention trial. One of the first multiple risk factor intervention trials was the Oslo study, which was undertaken in normotensive men aged 40 to 49 years [15]. By current National Cholesterol Education Program III criteria these patients would be considered to be at high risk of developing coronary artery disease (CAD). In addition, it is very likely that many of these patients would also be considered to have the metabolic syndrome (high-density lipoprotein < 40 mg/dL, hypertension, triglycerides > 150 mg/dL) by current criteria. The subjects were randomized into an intervention group and a control group, which had usual care. The aim of the study was to determine whether lowering high levels of blood lipids by dietary changes and the cessation of smoking, if maintained for many years, would lead to a reduction in the incidence of first events attributable to CAD.

Dietary Interventions from the Oslo Study

	Intervention group	Control group	AHA
Protein, *% calorie/d*	18.8	15.5	12–18
Carbohydrates, *% calorie/d*	52	38.8	55
Total fat, *% calorie/d*	27.9	44.1	30
Saturated fat, *% calorie/d*	8.2	18.3	10
Cholesterol intake, *mg/d*	289	527	200
Crude fiber, *g/d*	8.3	6.5	25

Figure 23-18.
The dietary intervention in the Oslo study. The interventions in the Oslo study were limited to dietary advice and counseling to stop smoking. The dietary advice was directed at reducing saturated fat and increasing fiber intake. In patients with hypertriglyceridemia, additional counseling was provided related to reducing caloric intake, alcohol intake, and sugar consumption. Wives of the patients in the intervention group were involved as support persons in the study. This figure shows the main dietary changes resulting from the intervention. Observe the similarity between the dietary recommendation of the American Heart Association (AHA) and the diet in the intervention group with respect to the daily total fat, saturated fat, and cholesterol intakes [16]. (*Adapted from* Hjermann *et al.* [16] amd Krauss *et al.* [17].)

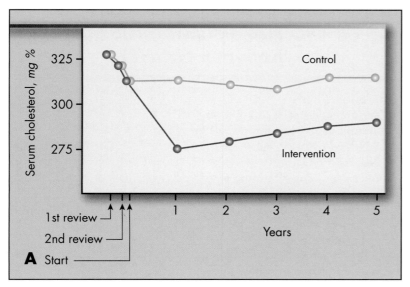

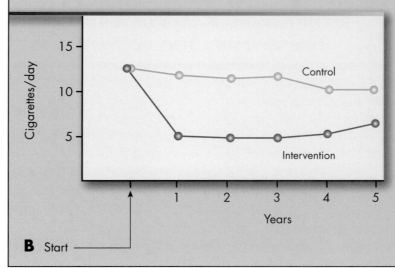

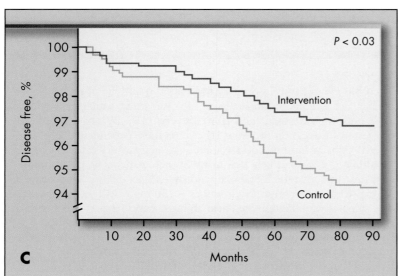

Figure 23-19.

Results of the Oslo Heart Study. The individuals in the intervention group had reductions in serum cholesterol of 13%, a 20% reduction in serum triglycerides, and a 45% reduction in overall cigarette smoking (cigarettes per man). However, only 25% in the intervention group gave up smoking compared with 17% in the control group. At the end of the study, the incidence of sudden death and myocardial infarction (fatal and nonfatal) was 47% lower in the intervention group ($P = 0.028$, two-tailed log rank test).

A, Changes in serum cholesterol. *1st review* and *2nd review* refers to two preliminary examinations before formal start of study. **B**, Changes in cigarette consumption. **C**, Outcome in Oslo Heart Study. (*Panels A and B adapted from* Leren *et al.* [15]; *panel C adapted from* Hjermann *et al.* [16].)

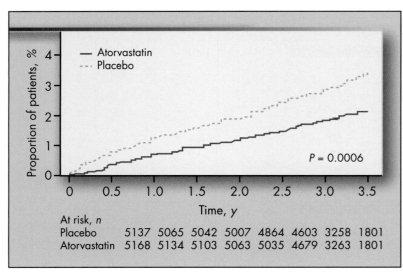

Figure 23-20.

The effect of treating high blood pressure and hyperlipidemia. The recently reported Anglo-Scandinavian Cardiac Outcomes Trial trial is an example of pharmacologic treatment of two risk factors on the combined outcome of nonfatal myocardial infarction and fatal coronary artery

disease. The risk factors treated were hypertension and hyperlipidemia [18]. Men and women were recruited into the trial and randomization was undertaken at two levels. In the first, those individuals meeting inclusion criteria for high blood pressure (systolic blood pressure 160 and 140 mm Hg or greater, and diastolic blood pressure 100 and 90 mm Hg or greater for untreated and treated hypertension, respectively) were randmonized to a β-blocker ± diuretic arm or a calcium channel blocker ± angiotensin-converting enzyme arm. Among those randomized, individuals with serum cholesterol of 6.5 mmol/L or less (×40 for mg/dL) were assigned to receive open-label lipid-lowering therapy (10%) or randomized to receive atorvastatin (10 mg/day) or placebo. At the end of follow-up (median 3.3 years), blood pressures in each treatment arm were similar (138.3/80.4 and 138.4/80.4 mm Hg). The serum cholesterol, low- and high-density lipoprotein, and triglycerides in the atorvastatin arm were 4.21, 2.32, 1.31, and 1.29 mmol/L, respectively. The corresponding values in the lipid-lowering arm were 5.21, 3.27, 1.29, and 1.49 mmol/L, respectively. There was a significant reduction in the cumulative incidence of nonfatal myocardial infarction and fatal coronary artery disease, as shown in this figure. Because all patients were effectively treated for hypertension (*ie*, there was no "true" placebo group), the study addresses the additional benefit of lipid-lowering therapy in hypertensive high-risk patients with effective blood pressure control. HR—hazard ratio. (*Adapted from* Sever *et al.* [19].)

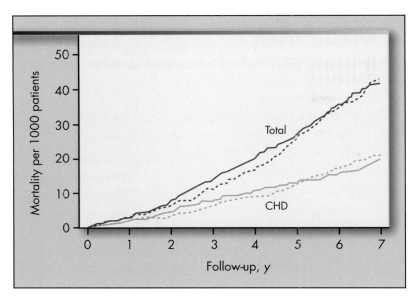

Figure 23-21.
The Multiple Risk Factor Intervention Trial (MRFIT). MRFIT was undertaken in the United States with aims similar to the Oslo Heart Study [20]. MRFIT was a randomized primary prevention trial to test the effect of a multifactor intervention on mortality from coronary heart disease. A total of 12,866 men aged 35 to 79 years were randomly assigned to a special intervention (SI) or usual care (UC) provided by community physicians. The SI consisted of stepped care for treatment for hypertension, counseling for cigarette smoking, and dietary advice to lower blood cholesterol levels. Over 7 years, the mortality in the SI group (*dotted line*) was 19.9/1000 and 19.3/1000 in the UC group (*solid line*). This difference was not statistically significant. The corresponding total mortality was 41.2 (*dotted line*) and 40.5 (*solid line*), respectively. In a second report published after 10.5 years of follow-up (*ie*, 3.5 years after the conclusion of the trial), it was suggested that the overall mortality was significantly less in the original SI group [21]. This difference was attributed to a 24% reduction in deaths related to myocardial infarction. However, there is no definite information regarding the care these patients received during the post-trial period with respect to the interventions. Over the past two decades, there have been several attempts to explain the discrepancies between the findings of MRFIT and the Oslo Heart Study. The most plausible one is that patients assigned to the UC arm in MRFIT had better than anticipated blood pressure control and rate of quitting smoking. (*Adapted from* Sever *et al.* [19].)

Stanford Coronary Risk Intervention Project Study Results [22,23]

Risk factors
  LDL cholesterol: -22%
  HDL cholesterol: +12%
  Body weight: -4%
  Exercise capacity: +20%
  Dietary fat: -24%; cholesterol intake: -40%
Endpoints
  Cardiac events (cardiac death and myocardial infarction) unchanged
  Combined endpoint of cardiac deaths, nonfatal myocardial infarction, PTCA, and CABG was significantly lower
  The rate of narrowing of the coronary arteries in the treatment group was 47% less than that in the subjects in the usual care group (change in minimal diameter: -0.024 ± 0.066 mm/y vs -0.045 ± 0.073 mm/y [P < 0.02; two-tailed test])
  Reduction in new lesion formation in the risk reduction group

Figure 23-22.
The Stanford Coronary Risk Intervention Project (SCRIP) secondary prevention trial. The SCRIP study was a multiple risk factor intervention trial undertaken in patients with documented coronary artery disease. Two hundred fifty-nine men and 41 women were recruited and randomized into usual-care or an individualized program of multiple risk reduction, which included a low-fat, low-cholesterol diet, advice regarding weight loss, exercise, and smoking cessation, as well as medications favoring improvement in lipid profiles. Interventions were provided through periodic clinic visits and by telephone calls from nurse coordinators. The endpoints were quantitative coronary angiography and cardiac events.

The study was unique for the following reasons: 1) it was undertaken in an outpatient setting with "free-living" individuals; and 2) the bulk of the intervention was carried out by nurse coordinators who contacted patients at frequent intervals throughout the 4-year study [22]. In association with favorable changes in risk factors, there were beneficial effects on combined cardiovascular events and angiographic measures of coronary lesions. CABG—coronary artery bypass graft; HDL—high-density lipoprotein; LDL—low-density lipoprotein; PTCA—percutaneous transluminal coronary angiography.

Smaller Multiple Intervention Trials

Trial	Patients, n	Follow-up, y	Intervention	Change in total-C	Change in LDL-C	Endpoint	Events
Watts *et al.* [24]	74*	3	Diet alone; Diet + cholestyra-mine; Usual care	-14.2%; -25.3%; -4%	25.3%; 35.7%; No change	Lesions improved (QCA)	Myocardial infarction and cardiac deaths significantly lower in the intervention groups
Arntzenius *et al.* [25]	39	2	Low-fat vegetarian diet	Total HDL-C ratio	Not reported	Lesions improved in patients with total-C/HDL-C ratio < 6.9 (QCA)	None reported
Niebauer *et al.* [26]	36	5	Low-diet + exercise; Usual care	-14%; +8%	-4%; +30%	Lesion progression reduced (QCA)	None reported

*Sixteen patients did not complete this study.

Figure 23-23.

Examples of small multiple intervention trials. There were three other relatively small multiple intervention trials for secondary prevention of coronary artery disease reported from European countries that supported the data shown in Figures 23-16 through 23-22. These other trials are summarized in this figure. HDL-C—high-density lipoprotein; LDL-C—low-density lipoprotein cholesterol; QCA—quantitative coronary angiography; total-C—total cholesterol.

Intensive Program of Nonpharmacologic Management of Lipids with Lifestyle Modification

Risk factors	Control group		Experimental group	
	Initial	Final	Initial	Final
Total cholesterol, *mmol/L**	6.34 ± 1.02	6.00 ± 1.55	5.88 ± 1.29	4.45 ± 1.15
LDL-C, *mmol/L*	4.32 ± 0.77	4.07 ± 1.17	3.92 ± 1.25	2.46 ± 1.55
Apo B, *mg/dL*	104 ± 21	105 ± 28	104 ± 33	81.0 ± 11.4
LDL-C/HDL-C	3.59 ± 1.37	3.33 ± 1.42	4.18 ± 1.53	2.89 ± 1.92
Weigh, *kg*	80.4 ± 22.8	81.8 ± 25	91.1 ± 15.5	81.0 ± 11.4

*×40 for conversion to mmol/L.

Figure 23-24.

Intensive program of nonpharmacologic management of lipids with lifestyle modification. In 1990, Ornish *et al.* [27] reported the findings from a small randomized trial in a group of patients with documented coronary artery disease. The experimental group participated in an intensive risk factor modification program which was more rigorous than the Stanford Coronary Risk Intervention Project study. The intervention consisted of a very low-fat vegetarian diet (10%–12% fat), exercise, support groups, and psychologic stress management. Smokers were not accepted. Lipid-lowering medications were not used and take-home meals were provided for those who wanted them. The significant changes in risk factors are shown in this figure (mean ± standard deviation).

There were no significant changes in blood pressure, triglycerides, apolipoprotein (Apo) A1 lipoproteins. These changes were accompanied by a significant improvement in lumen diameter as determined by quantitative coronary angiography. HDL-C—high-density lipoprotein cholesterol; LDL-C—low-density lipoprotein cholesterol.

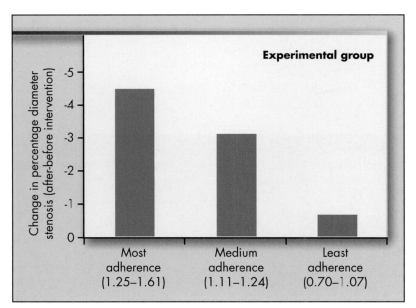

Figure 23-25.

Intensive lifestyle modification and changes in coronary artery lesions. The figure shows that in the experimental group (**A**), the degree of improvement in the coronary arteries was directly correlated with the level of participation in the program (*n* = 21). The trend was evident when the entire study population (*n* = 40) was examined as well. This was the first coronary angiographic trial that did not use lipid-lowering medications and included men and women.

However, there are certain methodologic issues that merit comment. The patients were randomized before enrollment in the study. Fifty-three patients were randomly assigned to the experimental group, and 43 to the control group. Of these, 28 and 20 subjects elected to participate in the two arms of the study protocol, respectively. A further seven patients (one in the control group and six in the experimental group) did not complete the study because of a variety of reasons. Twenty two patients in the experimental group and 19 in the control group completed the protocol, although data from one other patient were not included in the figure. Thus, it was not possible to perform an intention-to-treat analysis on the data. (*Adapted from* Ornish *et al.* [27].)

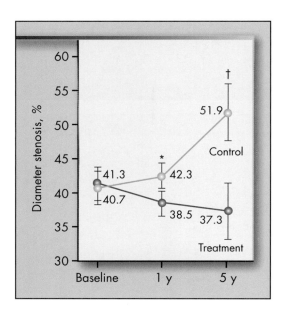

Figure 23-26.

Effect of a sustained intensive lifestyle intervention. In a second report, Ornish *et al.* [28] described the 5-year data on the controlled trial reported. The nature of the interventions was unchanged from that described previously. Twenty of 28 patients in the experimental group completed the 5-year follow-up, whereas 17 of 20 did so in the control group. There was continuing improvement in the mean diameter of the coronary arteries over the 5 years in the experimental group (1.5% at 1 year to 3.1% at 5 years). In contrast the average percent stenosis increased by 2.3% after 1 year and by 11.8% after 5 years. Twenty-five cardiac events occurred in the experimental group and 40 in the control group. All these differences were significant. The figure shows the mean percent diameter stenosis in the treatment and control groups at baseline, 1 year, and 5 years. (*Asterisk* indicates *P* < 0.02 and *dagger* indicates *P* < 0.001 by two-tailed test). As in the previous study, Ornish *et al.* [27] showed that the improvement in the angiographic appearance of the coronary arteries as determined by quantitative coronary angiography was directly related to the degree of compliance in the lifestyle modification program [28]. (*Adapted from* Ornish *et al.* [28].)

A. Study Design

Patients signed a consent form for cardiac PET scans and for intensive lifestyle treatment. Those in the moderate- and low-intensity treatment groups signed a consent form for only the PET scan

At the second PET scan, the patients were designated by blinded observers into the three categories of intensity of treatment during the period between the scans

The three categories of intensity were:

Low intensity—not on diet, not on lipid-lowering therapy and continued to smoke.

Moderate intensity—20%–30% fat diet with lipid-lowering drugs or a < 10% fat diet without lipid-lowering medications

High intensity—low-fat diet (10–20 g of fat, 60–80 g of protein per day with unlimited vegetables), exercise > 30 minutes/day 4–5 days per week, and lipid lowering, blood pressure and anti-anginal medications as needed

Patients were contacted 5 years after the second PET scan to determine the incidence of cardiac events (cardiac death, myocardial infarction, coronary artery bypass surgery, and percutaneous coronary intervention). The level of adherence to the initial treatment regimen during this second period was not reported

Figure 23-27.

A, Multiple risk factor intervention and improvement in coronary perfusion. Although the findings were undertaken against a background of no lipid-lowering medications, it is unlikely that all patients encountered in clinical practice are diet sensitive to the extent reported by Ornish *et al.* [27,28]. The study by Sdringola *et al.* [29] combined the use of lipid-lowering medications with intensive lifestyle modification. In their study, 408 consecutive patients underwent dypyridamole cardiac positron emission tomography (PET) scans at baseline and again at an average of 2.6 years. They were followed-up for a further 5 years to determine the number of cardiac events. The aim of the study was to determine if combined intensive lifestyle and pharmacologic lipid treatment reduced myocardial perfusion abnormalities and coronary events in comparison with usual care and cholesterol-lowering drugs *and whether perfusion changes predicted outcomes.*

(*continued on next page*)

	Maximal (n = 92)	Moderate (n = 142)	Poor (n = 92)	P value
Total cholesterol, mg/dL	140 ± 20	184 ± 35	226 ± 45	< 0.0001
LDL cholesterol, mg/dL	74 ± 16	111 ± 34	143 ± 44	< 0.0001
HDL cholesterol, mg/dL	49 ± 11	45 ± 15	51 ± 16	0.05
TG, mg/dL	87 ± 30	158 ± 93	169 ± 93	< 0.0001
SBP, mm Hg	126 ± 18	126 ± 17	129 ± 15	NS
DBP, mm Hg	71 ± 11	70 ± 10	73 ± 11	NS
Regular exercise, %	75	52	45	< 0.01
Weight change, lb	-5.8 ± 10	+0.2 ± 13	+3.3 ± 10	< 0.0001
Statins, %	89	64	15	< 0.0001
ACE inhibitors, %	22	18	10	NS
β-blockers	30	28	15	NS
Aspirin	76	63	73	NS

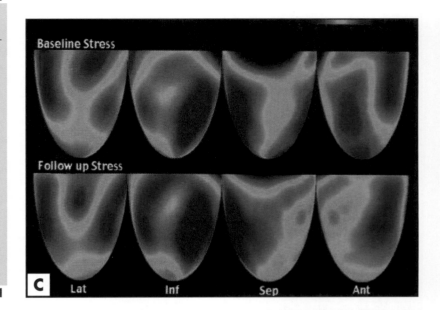

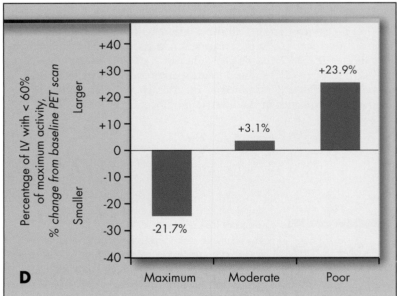

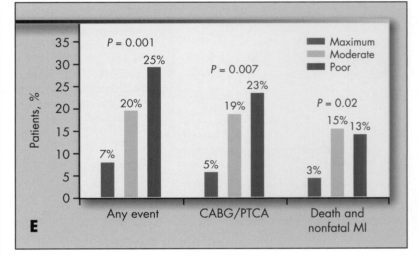

Figure 23-27. *continued*

B, Changes in coronary artery disease risk factors associated with improved myocardial perfusion. In the interval between the two PET scans there were no significant changes in cardiac events even though there were significant alterations in myocardial perfusion depending on the intensity of adherence to the program. However, the cardiovascular risk profiles were different in the three categories of patients at the time of the second PET scan. The data for the maximally adherent group were significantly different from the other two.

C, Improvement in perfusion as shown by PET. Three-dimensional topographic dipyridamole PET showing improved perfusion following treatment. *Upper row* shows baseline and *lower row* shows 2.6 year follow-up. Red depicts the highest perfusion and blue the lowest.

D, Changes in myocardial perfusion and intensity of the intervention. The changes in myocardial perfusion are correlated with the level of intensity of the lifestyle management program. The ordinate shows the "size severity" of the myocardium with less than 60% of the maximum perfusion

detected by the PET scan. Negative values indicate an improvement in perfusion. It appears that the intensive management of risk factors as depicted in *panel B* is necessary to improve myocardial perfusion abnormalities.

E, Multiple risk factor intervention, improved perfusion and prognosis. As the figure below shows, the individuals who were considered to be in the intensive lifestyle management program during the initial 2.6 years experienced a significantly lower rate of all cardiac events over the subsequent 5 years. This benefit extended to both hard events and physician-driven events such as coronary artery bypass surgery and percutaneous transluminal coronary angioplasty. ACE—angiotensin-converting enzyme; CABG—coronary artery bypass graft; DBP—diastolic blood pressure; HDL—high-density lipoprotein; LDL—low-density lipoprotein; MI—myocardial infarction; NS—not significant; PTCA—percutaneous transluminal coronary angioplasty; TG—triglycerides; SBP—systolic blood pressure. (*Panels A, B, D,* and *E adapted from* Sdringola *et al.* [29]; *panel C from* Sdringola *et al.* [29]; with permission.)

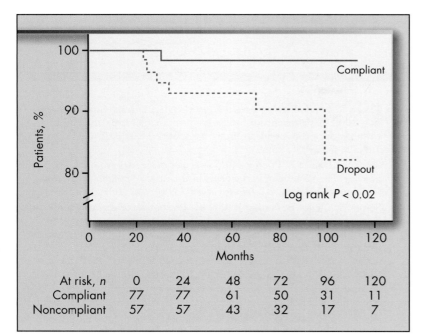

At risk, n	0	24	48	72	96	120
Compliant	77	77	61	50	31	11
Noncompliant	57	57	43	32	17	7

Figure 23-28.

Effect of a comprehensive lifestyle modification program in an outpatient setting of a tertiary care hospital. The study reported by Sdrigola et al. [29] showed that intensive lifestyle modification over a period of 2 years resulted in a better long-term prognosis for patients with angiographically documented coronary artery disease and evidence of myocardial ischemia based on PET scan. Rutledge et al. [30] studied the prognosis in a group of 134 patients who enrolled in a 2-year intensive lifestyle modification program for patients with angiographically documented coronary artery disease. The program included exercise training, dietary counseling, stress management, and therapeutic education. One hundred thirty-four patients enrolled in the program that was offered as a part of the outpatient services of a tertiary care hospital. Seventy-seven patients completed the program and 57 failed to do so. Those who completed the program improved their effort tolerance and had serum lipids and blood pressures at recommended goals. The cumulative event rate (cardiac death, myocardial infarction, and stroke) over 10 years in the patients who completed the program was 1.5%. The corresponding event rate in patients who dropped out was 18% ($P < 0.02$). It appears that patients who complete a 2-year lifestyle modification program had a better long-term prognosis.

A. Characteristics of 1821 Patients with Myocardial Infarctions Eligible to Participate in Cardiac Rehabilitation

	Nonparticipant, % (n = 812)	Participants, % (n = 1000)	P value
Hypertension	65	49	< 0.001
Current smoker	21	37	< 0.001
Hyperlipidemia	30	38	< 0.001
Family history of CAD	15	29	< 0.001
Previous history of CAD	69	63	< 0.01
Charlson index*			< 0.001
Ejection fraction	47	53	< 0.001
Body mass index	27	28	< 0.001
Diabetes	26	14	< 0.001
Medications			
Aspirin	58	75	< 0.001
β-blockers	42	66	< 0.001
ACE inhibitors	22	17	< 0.005
Statin	7	14	< 0.001

*More in nonparticipants.

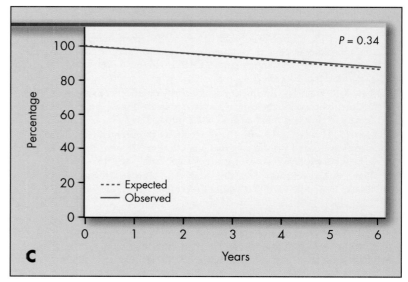

Figure 23-29.

A, The overall impact of organized cardiac rehabilitation programs in secondary prevention of coronary artery disease (CAD). In an epidemiologic study, Witt et al. [31] examined the effect on overall mortality of participation in an organized structured cardiac rehabilitation program after myocardial infarction in a single county in the United States. Participation was defined as documented attendance at the first session of a structured program that included exercise training, counseling, and education. It was observed that women and the elderly were found to be less likely to participate in the program. As this figure shows, the participants in cardiac rehabilitation programs had a worse risk profile (with the exception of diabetes) than those who did not. Further, the profile of medications was also better in the group that participated. The comorbid conditions were quantified in terms of the Charlson index [32].

B and **C**, Effect of cardiac rehabilitation on all-cause mortality. When the data were analyzed in terms of overall survival, it appeared that over 6 years, those who participated in cardiac rehabilitation had a cumulative mortality (approximately 10%) that was similar to their expected mor

tality. Compared with those who did not, they had a mortality that was considerable higher (50%). It was also observed that there was a 28% reduction in the risk of a recurrent myocardial infarction. These differences were evident even after adjusting for the deaths associated with comorbid conditions using the Charlson index [32]. ACE—angiotensin-converting enzyme. (*Panel A adapted from* Witt et al. [31]; *panels B and C adapted from* Charlson et al. [32].)

References

1. Pekkanen J, Linn S, Heiss G, *et al.*: Ten-year mortality from cardiovascular disease in relation to cholesterol level among men with and without preexisting cardiovascular disease. *N Engl J Med* 1990, 322:1700–1707.

2. Executive Summary of the Third Report of The National Cholesterol Education Program (NCEP) Expert Panel on Detection, Evaluation, And Treatment of High Blood Cholesterol In Adults (Adult Treatment Panel III). *JAMA* 2004, 285:2486–2497.

3. Wilson PWF, D'Agostino RB, Levy D, *et al.*: Prediction of coronary heart disease using risk factor categories. *Circulation* 2004, 97:1837–1847.

4. Grundy SM, Cleeman JI, Merz CN, *et al.*: Implications of recent clincial trials for the National Cholesterol Education Program Adult Treatment Panel III Guidelines. *J Am Coll Cardiol* 2004, 44:720–732.

5. SHEP Cooperative Research Group: Prevention of stroke by antihypertensive drug treatment in older persons with isolated systolic hypertension: final results of the Systolic Hypertension in the Elderly Program (SHEP). *JAMA* 1991, 265:3255–3264.

6. Blood Pressure Lowering Treatment Trialist Collaboration: Effects of different blood-pressure lowering regimens on major cardiovascular events; results of prospectively designed overviews of randomized trials. *Lancet* 2003, 362:1527–1535.

7. UK Prospective Diabetes Study (UKPDS) Group: Intensive blood-glucose control with sulphonylureas or insulin compared with conventional treatment and risk of complications in patients with type 2 diabetes (UKPDS 33). *Lancet* 1998, 352:837–853.

8. The Diabetes Control and Complications Trial Research Group: The effect of intensive treatment of diabetes on the development and progression of long-term complications in insulin-dependent diabetes mellitus. *N Engl J Med* 1993, 329:977–986.

9. Abraira C, Duckworth W, McCarren M, *et al.*: Design of the cooperative study on glycemic control and complications in diabetes mellitus type 2: Veterans Affairs Diabetes Trial. *J Diabetes Complications* 2003, 17:314–322.

10. Waters D, Lesperance J, Gladstone P, *et al.*: Effects of cigarette smoking on the angiographic evolution of coronary atherosclerosis. A Canadian Coronary Atherosclerosis Intervention Trial (CCAIT) Substudy. CCAIT Study Group. *Circulation* 1996, 94:614–621.

11. Alderman EL, Bourassa MG, Cohen LS, *et al.*: Ten-year follow-up of survival and myocardial infarction in the randomized Coronary Artery Surgery Study. *Circulation* 1990, 82:1629–1646.

12. Cavender JB, Rogers WJ, Fisher LD, *et al.*: Effect of smoking on survival and morbidity in patients randomized to medical and surgical therapy in the coronary artery surgery study (CASS): 10 year follow-up. *J Am Coll Cardiol* 1992, 20:287–294.

13. Law MR, Wald NJ, Rudnicka AR: Quantifying effects of statins on low density lipoprotein, cholesterol, ischaemic heart disease, and stroke: systematic review and meta-analysis. *BMJ* 2003, 326:1–7.

14. Yusuf S, Hawken S, Ounpuu S, *et al.*: Effect of potentially modifiable risk factors associated with myocardial infarction in 52 countries (the INTERHEART study): case-control study. *Lancet* 2004, 364:937–952.

15. Leren P, Askevold EM, Foss OP, *et al.*: The Oslo Study: cardiovascular disease in middle-aged and young Oslo men. *Acta Med Scand* 1975, 588(suppl):1–38.

16. Hjermann I, Velve Byre K, Holme I, Leren P: Effect of diet and smoking intervention on the incidence of coronary heart disease. Report from the Oslo Study Group of a randomised trial in healthy men. *Lancet* 1981, 2:1303–1310.

17. Krauss RM, Eckel RH, Howard B, *et al.*: AHA Dietary Guidelines: revision 2000: A statement for healthcare professionals from the Nutrition Committee of the American Heart Association. *Circulation* 2000, 102:2284–2299.

18. Sever PS, Dahlof B, Poulter NR, *et al.*: Rationale, design, methods, and baseline demography of participants in the Anglo-Scandinavian Cardiac Outcomes Trial. ASCOT Investigators. *J Hypertens* 2001, 19:1139–1147.

19. Sever PS, Dahlof B, Poulter NR, *et al.*: Prevention of coronary and stroke events with atorvastatin in hypertensive patients who have average or lower-than-average cholesterol concentrations in the Anglo-Scandinavian Cardiac Outcomes Trial: Lipid-Lowering Arm (ASCOT-LLA): a multicenter randomized controlled trial. *Lancet* 2003, 361:1149–1158.

20. Multiple Risk Factor Intervention Trial Research Group: Multiple risk factor intervention trial. Risk factor changes and mortality results. *JAMA* 1982, 248:1465–1477.

21. The Multiple Risk Factor Intervention Trial Research Group: Mortality rates after 10.5 years for participants in the Multiple Risk Factor Intervention Trial. Findings related to a priori hypotheses of the trial. *JAMA* 1990, 263:1795–1801.

22. Haskell WL, Alderman EL, Fair JM, *et al.*: Effects of intensive multiple risk factor reduction on coronary atherosclerosis and clinical cardiac events in men and women with coronary artery disease. The Stanford Coronary Risk Intervention Project (SCRIP). *Circulation* 1994, 89:975–990.

23. Quinn TG, Alderman EL, McMillan A, Haskell W: Development of new coronary atherosclerotic lesions during a 4-year multifactor risk reduction program: the Stanford Coronary Risk Intervention Project (SCRIP). *J Am Coll Cardiol* 1994, 24:900–908.

24. Watts GF, Lewis B, Brunt JN, *et al.*: Effects on coronary artery disease of lipid-lowering diet, or diet plus cholestyramine, in the St Thomas' Atherosclerosis Regression Study (STARS). *Lancet* 1992, 339:563–569.

25. Arntzenius AC, Kromhout D, Barth JD, *et al.*: Diet, lipoproteins, and the progression of coronary atherosclerosis. The Leiden Intervention Trial. *N Engl J Med* 1985, 312:805–811.

26. Niebauer J, Hambrecht R, Schlierf G, *et al.*: Five years of physical exercise and low fat diet: effects on progression of coronary artery disease. *J Cardiopulm Rehabil* 1995, 15:47–64.

27. Ornish D, Brown S, Scherwitz LW, *et al.*: Can lifestyle changes reverse coronary heart disease? The Lifestyle Heart Trial. *Lancet* 1990, 336:129–133.

28. Ornish D, Scherwitz LW, Billings JH, *et al.*: Intensive lifestyle changes for reversal of coronary heart disease. *JAMA* 1998, 280:2001–2007.

29. Sdringola S, Nakagawa K, Nakagawa Y, *et al.*: Combined intense lifestyle and pharmacologic lipid treatment further reduce coronary events and myocardial perfusion abnormalities compared with usual-care cholesterol-lowering drugs in coronary artery disease. *J Am Coll Cardiol* 2003, 41:263–272.

30. Rutledge JC, Hyson DA, Garduno D, *et al.*: Lifestyle modification program in management of patients with coronary artery disease: the clinical experience in a tertiary care hospital. *J Cardiopulm Rehabil* 1999, 19:226–234.

31. Witt B, Jacobsen SJ, Weston SA, *et al.*: Cardiac rehabilitation after myocardial infarction in the community. *J Am Coll Cardiol* 2004, 44:988–996.

32. Charlson ME, Pompei P, Ales KL, *et al.*: A new method of classifying prognostic comorbidity in longitudinal studies: development and validation. *J Chron Dis* 1987, 40:373–383.

Community-based Prevention in Cardiovascular Disease

David Chiriboga and Ira S. Ockene

Although it is well recognized that "an ounce of prevention is worth a pound of cure," much of the efforts in cardiovascular disease (CVD) in the past half-century have focused on the diagnostic and therapeutic aspects of the disease, with much less emphasis on prevention. Despite the significant decline in the age-adjusted coronary heart disease (CHD) mortality since the 1960s, the actual number of patients with coronary heart disease has increased dramatically, with an incidence of 1.3 million new cases per year [1]. Hospital discharges for acute myocardial infarction rose from 430,000 in 1980 [1]. This increase in total number of cases per year is related to the growth of the total US population during the period and to improvements in diagnoses and available treatments, so that smaller infarctions are detected and patients are living longer after cardiac events. Approximately 25% of the decrease in CHD mortality observed in the United States has been attributed to a decrease in the incidence of the disease, whereas the bulk of the decline (75%) has been ascribed to a reduction in death rates among patients with known CHD. Of the latter, approximately half of the decline is related to a reduction in risk factors among patients with known CHD (secondary prevention); approximately a third to a reduction in mortality from acute myocardial infarction; and the rest to specific medical and surgical treatments [1]. Given the increase in the actual number of cases, efforts in primary prevention, and specifically community-based interventions oriented toward primary prevention of the disease, are required to increase the odds of effectively controlling the CVD epidemic.

This chapter presents a series of tables and diagrams that represent a comprehensive review of community-based interventions for the prevention of CVD. The review will cover the rationale for the implementation of such programs and their efficacy, and extend to a detailed analysis of the different components of community-based preventive interventions, their strengths and limitations, and a discussion of the limited data available on cost analysis.

Rationale: The Population Versus High-risk Approach to Cardiovascular Disease Prevention

	Population approach (community-based interventions)	High-risk approach (health provider interventions)
Advantages	Timely intervention in disease progression – effective for primary prevention	Individual is motivated to make changes, because of perception of risk
	Directed at entire population	Delivered through existing health care system structure
	Seeks to affect the origins of disease in a population	High motivation of health care provider
	Aims at shifting the entire risk curve of a population	Health care provider advice has overall significant impact on behavior
	Progressive decrease in the incidence of disease	Most widely applied in secondary prevention
	Changes occurring in an entire population make it easier for an individual to change	Late in the process of disease progression
Limitations	Poor motivation of individuals, since there is a perception of "low-risk" and "little gain"	Directed mostly at high-risk, individual patients
	Poor motivation of health care providers	Does not affect the root cause of the problem
	Complex interventions	Next generation will have the same burden of disease as the last
	Limited resources for long-term interventions	Will not reach the largest subgroup affected by CVD: the highest number of clinical events occurs among individuals who are in the middle of the risk distribution
	Prevention paradox: preventive measures that greatly benefit the population as a whole may bring little benefit to individuals who are at relatively low risk [2]	
	"Blame the victim"	"Blame the victim"
		Costs associated with screening

Figure 24-1.

Rationale: the population versus high-risk approach to cardiovascular disease (CVD) prevention. A large proportion of what needs to be done in CVD prevention lies outside the domain of traditional Western medicine. Currently, lifestyle modification through behavior change in nutrition, physical activity, and smoking is considered the foundation of CVD prevention, but the impact of medical practice on behavior change is limited in terms of the timing of the intervention and the modest segment of the population over which it exerts its influence. Medical provider interventions (known also as *high-risk interventions*) tend to come late in the process of disease progression; physician- and nurse-initiated behavioral interventions are often offered as a means of secondary prevention, that is, once the relevant cardiac risk factors, or even CVD, are already established; at the same time, such interventions are directed mostly at high-risk, individual patients, as opposed to the entire population. However, population-based efforts, including community-based strategies, offer an alternative way to deliver timely and population-wide prevention interventions and seek to affect the origins of disease in a population.

Changes occurring in an entire population make it easier for an individual to change—it is easier to quit smoking when the workplace is smoke-free, and easier to observe a low saturated-fat diet when such choices are widely available in the company or school cafeteria and in restaurants. The population-based strategy does have an inherent downside, however, which Rose [3] has called the *prevention paradox*: preventive measures that greatly benefit the population as a whole may bring little benefit to individuals who are at relatively low risk. Because the gain for a given person is small, motivating that person to make lifestyle changes may be difficult. Another limitation of the population approach, which to some extent is shared by the high-risk approach, is that it may "blame the victim," that is, each individual in the society. Individuals respond to the manner in which the environment has been constructed; therefore, the results of this interaction (health or disease) also are the responsibility of the system that created the determining conditions in the first place. The behavioral approach, shared by the high-risk and the population approaches, tends to place a disproportionate portion of the blame on the individual's will power.

Impact of Population Versus High-risk Approach on Rates of Cardiovascular Disease Morbidity and Mortality

Author	Intervention level	Intervention component	Impact
Kottke *et al.* [4]	Entire population	Decrease serum cholesterol by 4%	Incidence of nonfatal MI decreased by 13%
		Decrease smoking rates by 15%	CHD mortality decreased by 18%
		Decrease diastolic blood pressure by 3%	
	Only high-risk population with all three risk factors	Decrease serum cholesterol by 34%	Incidence of nonfatal MI decreased by 6%–8%
Goldman *et al.* [5]	Entire population	Decrease smoking rates by 20%	CHD mortality decreased by 2%–9%
		Decrease diastolic blood pressure to 90 mm Hg	
	All high-risk patients with cholesterol over 250	Decrease 10 mg/dL cholesterol	Similar impact as below
		Decrease blood cholesterol to 250 mg	CHD incidence decreased by 8%–10% in men 35–54 years
			CHD incidence decreased by 1%–4% in men 55–74 years

Figure 24-2.

Impact of population versus high-risk approach on rates of cardiovascular disease morbidity and mortality. The importance of the population approach is made clear by simulations carried out by several investigators. Kottke *et al.* [4] and Goldman *et al.* [5] tested the effects of several intervention strategies on coronary heart disease (CHD) mortality rates using prediction models. More recently several other methods for risk prediction have been developed and compared [6]. Thus, it is clear that efforts targeting only high-risk segments of the overall population are inadequate to significantly reduce the population burden of disease.

If we are to improve the cardiovascular health of the nation, we must develop population approaches that build on the high-risk approach offered by the individual practitioner, while fostering changes in policy to create a favorable environment for the changes to occur. There are reports in the literature suggesting a similar level of impact of the intervention in CHD prevention when comparing a low-cost community-based approach versus a high-intensity, high-risk approach, suggesting a significant cost-benefit ratio for the population-based approach [7].

Outline of Community-based Prevention Interventions in Cardiovascular Disease

Overall goal
  Control of modifiable CVD risk factors
    Elevated serum cholesterol levels
    Smoking
    Overweight and obesity
    Sedentary lifestyle
    High blood pressure
Methods
  Lifestyle behavior modification
  Dissemination of knowledge in the community
    Prevalence of CVD
    Root causes of CVD
    Training on early recognition of symptoms of CVD

Figure 24-3.

Community-based intervention programs in cardiovascular disease (CVD). In the past few decades, increasing attention has been paid to community organizations as a means of accomplishing large-scale change for the prevention of chronic health problems [8,9,10,12–18]. In general, community interventions for CVD attempt to reduce the prevalence of risk factors associated with the disease, such as high blood pressure, elevated serum cholesterol level, smoking, overweight, and sedentary lifestyle, primarily through behavior modification, and they also disseminate information regarding the prevalence of CVD in the community, the root causes of the disease, and early recognition of symptoms of CVD. An outline of community-based CVD prevention programs is summarized in this figure. At the level of the community the lifestyle changes in diet, physical activity, and smoking that need to take place are promoted via behavior modification on the level of the individual, and also socioenvironmental (*ie*, ecologic) changes needed to support the desired lifestyle. There is also a need for dissemination of knowledge regarding the prevalence of CVD in the community, the root causes of the disease, and training in early recognition of the symptoms of CVD [19].

The American Heart Association published a comprehensive guide for CVD health at the community level [19], which describes a list of strategies, goals, and recommendations that may be implemented at the community level. Some of the suggestions within the environmental change category in this guide include:

Dietary goals of saturated fat (< 10% of calories), decreased sodium intake, grains (> six servings per day, with > three of whole grains), fruits (> two servings per day) and vegetables (> three servings per day);

Physical activity goals: Assure access to safe, appropriate, and enjoyable forms of physical activity, meeting national guidelines (30 minutes of moderate physical activity on most days of the week);

Assure a tobacco-free environment for all citizens.

The goals include the dissemination of knowledge that CVD is the leading cause of morbidity and mortality in the population, the "provision of information to all community members regarding the burden, causes and early symptoms of CVD," as well as "provision of materials and programs to motivate and teach skills for changing risk behaviors that will target multiple population subgroups" [19].

A. Program Components for Community-based Prevention in Cardiovascular Disease

Community organization
Needs assessment
Intervention planning
Implementation, monitoring, and evaluation
Program maintenance

B. Needs Assessment for Community-based Prevention in Cardiovascular Disease

Prevalence of CVD morbidity and mortality
Prevalence of cardiac risk factors
Evaluation of subpopulations
Qualitative data: knowledge, attitudes, and practices
Screening

Figure 24-4.

A, Program components. The concept of community participation and ownership is essential to community-based prevention efforts and is considered necessary for generating community support and building capacity for engaging in community activities [20]. In fact, the community organization process is considered the core of a successful program [15]. This involves identification and activation of key community leaders, stimulation of citizens and organizations to volunteer time and offer resources for cardiovascular disease (CVD) prevention, and the promotion of prevention as a community theme. Community health professionals play a vital role in providing program endorsement and stimulating the participation of community leaders. Community interventions can be applied through a variety of channels: contacting community leaders and existing formal and informal community groups (such as social, religious, ethnic, and school programs; adult education programs; and self-help programs), using the existing mass media network, and supporting community organization efforts.

B, Needs assessment. The basis for any type of community-based interventions in CVD is needs assessment. It requires careful evaluation of various aspects, including the demographic characteristics of the population and the epidemiologic profile of the residents in the community, as well as the incidence and prevalence of CVD and known cardiac risk factors. Such information, readily gathered through secondary sources such as local, state, or federal government agencies [21] (eg, State or Federal Bureau of Health Statistics, Centers for Disease Control, Behavioral Risk Factor Surveillance System), can be used for justification purposes and at the same time as baseline information. However, a comprehensive needs assessment also requires gathering information about the knowledge, attitudes, and practices of the people in the

community with regards to cardiac risk factors and CVD. Qualitative data can be obtained through secondary sources in the published literature, or through the use of qualitative research techniques, including surveys, key informant interviews, and focus groups [16,22–26]. This qualitative information can be obtained through collaborations with local community-based organizations identified through the community organization efforts. After the prevalence of CVD or cardiac risk factors has been established in a specific community, determining the knowledge, attitudes, and practices of the people in the community, with regard to CVD and cardiac risk factors, will assist in refining and tailoring the community-based intervention [27,28]. Contacting community-based organizations can lead to productive collaborations [29].

A common barrier to contacting the individuals in the community is the traditional mistrust of certain population subgroups toward academic research. To confront this issue, community-based organizations can provide a bridge to reach the population, for example, through clergy/academic partnerships [30].

Community outreach strategies can be used to provide access to screening, counseling, and referral services for CVD risk factors [31]. A specific strategy for carrying out screening through partnerships with community organizations is through religious groups. A review of the literature on this topic proposes seven key elements found to be beneficial in establishing religious group–based community health promotion programs [32]. Key elements identified by the review, based on outcomes, included the following: "partnerships, positive health values, availability of services, access to church facilities, community-focused interventions, health behavior change, and supportive social relationships" [32].

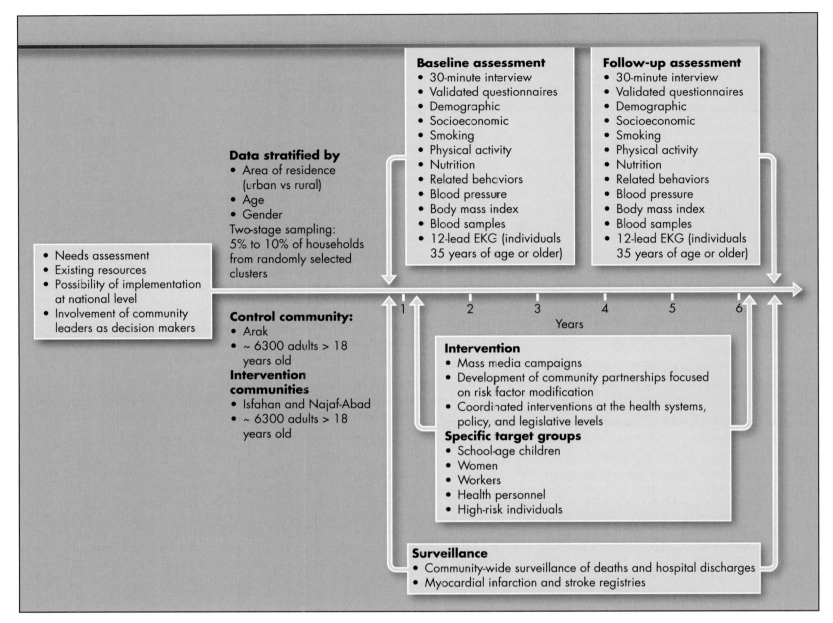

Figure 24-5.

Planning and implementation of a community-based prevention program in cardiovascular disease (CVD): a working example in Iran. As an example of the process of implementation of community-based programs for CVD prevention, and the transition from needs assessment and gathering of baseline measurements to an active program, the Isfahan Healthy Heart Program (IHHP), based in Iran [33], will be described in greater detail. The IHHP is a 6-year comprehensive, integrated, community-based program for cardiovascular disease prevention. The program focuses on CVD risk factors modification. A primary survey was administered to collect baseline data from the intervention (Isfahan and Najaf-Abad) and reference (Arak) communities. In a two-stage sampling method, the researchers randomly selected 5% to 10% of households from randomly selected clusters. A total of 12,600 adults 19 years of age and older from each of the communities were selected for the survey. Data were collected and stratified according to area of residence (urban vs rural), age, and gender. Participants also underwent a 30-minute interview to complete validated questionnaires (including demographic and socioeconomic data, as well as smoking, physical activity, nutrition, and other related behaviors). Blood pressure and

body mass index measurements were obtained as well as blood samples. A 12-lead EKG was recorded in all persons 35 years of age or older. Community-wide surveillance of deaths and hospital discharges, as well as myocardial infarction and stroke registries, were established in the intervention and control areas.

The interventions were planned based on the results of the needs assessment, the existing resources, and the possibility of implementation at the national level, with the involvement of community leaders as decision makers. The interventions also were tailored to target specific groups, including school-age children, women, workers, health personnel, and high-risk individuals. The intervention specifically included mass media campaigns, development of community partnerships focused on risk factor modification, and coordinated interventions at the health systems, policy and legislative levels.

The researchers plan to monitor samples of the intervention and control communities to assess the effect of the interventions throughout the 5-year intervention period, as well as monitor changes via epidemiologic surveillance. At the end of the intervention period, the baseline assessment will be repeated [33].

Monitoring and Evaluation of Community-based Interventions for Cardiovascular Disease

Landmark programs (1970s)
  North Karelia Project in Finland [34]
  US
    Stanford Five-City Project [35]
    Minnesota Heart Health Program [36]
    Pawtucket Heart Health Program [37,38]
Characteristics of monitoring and evaluation
  Continuing and timely
  Diffusion of results of the intervention
  Collaborations with all sectors of the community
  Maintenance of contact with national authorities
Evidence from community-based CVD prevention programs
    suggest
  High degree of generalizability,
  Cost effectiveness
  Can influence health policy
  Decrease in prevalence of risk factors
  Decrease in CVD morbidity and mortality

Figure 24-6.
Continuing and timely monitoring and evaluation of the impact of the intervention is necessary to appropriately adjust community-based interventions. Diffusion of the results of the intervention also provides the necessary evidence for policy-makers to endorse such programs.

Starting with the landmark North Karelia Project in Finland [34], in the 1970s, and continuing with similar projects in other parts in Europe [39] and the United States (*eg*, the Stanford Five-City Project [35], The Minnesota Heart Health Program [36], and the Pawtucket Heart Health Program [37,38]), the accumulated evidence from community-based interventions suggests that these programs have a high

degree of generalizability, are cost effective, and can influence health policy [40]. However, careful attention must be paid to planning, implementation, and evaluation according to clear principles and rules. Collaborations with all sectors of the community and maintenance of close contact with national authorities are critical components. Also, clearly defined guidelines, which can be adapted to local cultures, are very useful [40].

The long-term impact of successful cardiovascular disease (CVD) prevention and its influence on premature mortality is clearly evident in Finland, particularly in North Karelia. Active community-based CVD prevention began in the early 1970s in the province of North Karelia (population ~ 200,000). Toward the end of the 1970s, the program was extended to the rest of the country, based on the experience in North Karelia. Comprehensive community-based interventions aimed at changing the target risk factors and health behaviors (serum cholesterol, blood pressure, smoking, and diet) at the population level have been implemented across the country. A study comparing age-adjusted mortality rates for CVD, coronary heart disease [CHD], cerebrovascular disease, and all-cause mortality in the population aged 35 to 64 years from baseline (1969–1971) to 1995 [34] found that among men and women there was a significant reduction in deaths from CVD, CHD, and all causes in the entire country. From 1969–1971 to 1995, the age-standardized CHD mortality rate (per 100,000) decreased in North Karelia by 73% (from 672 to 185) and nationwide by 65% (from 465 to 165). The reduction in CVD mortality was of a similar magnitude. These results show that a major reduction in CVD mortality among the working-age population can take place in association with active reduction of major risk factors, with a positive impact on cancer and all-cause mortality [34].

Outcomes from other community-based interventions in Europe [41,42] and the United States [43] have demonstrated significant changes in risk behavior and clinical outcomes. A study from the United States, in rural Maine, even suggests the existence of dose-dependent reductions in cardiovascular and total mortality related to the intensity of the intervention during a two-decade long community intervention [44]. Despite the modest impact and the methodologic limitations, the prominence of the community-based prevention approach in the United States is highlighted by the creation of the Task Force on Community Preventive Services, which was established by the Centers for Disease Control and Prevention (CDC) [45].

Heart health–related behavioral and lifestyle characteristics in the "developed" world
   Physical inactivity
   Over-eating
   Engagement in self-destructive behaviors such as smoking.
"Development" is in many ways responsible for most of the chronic diseases that we face today, sharing a common pathway stemming
      from overweight and obesity
Physical activity: morbidly sedentary way of life
   From automobiles to washing machines to remote controls
   A small portion of Americans (~ 25% of all adults) participate in regular physical activity
   Physical activity appears to be even lower among women, minority populations, the elderly and the less educated
Industry's development and economic growth has provided widespread access to:
   Tobacco
   Unprecedented array of modified food items
      Processing techniques
      Addition of sugar, salt and fats, making foods more addictive, usually higher in calories
      Foods require minimum amount of time and effort for preparation and utilization
      Fast-food restaurants
      Consumption of soft drinks
      Increase in portion size

Figure 24-7.
The ecologic model. The combination of a comprehensive, individual (high-risk) intervention with population-based strategies directed at change in the social environment, as well as policy and legislative intervention, is known as the ecologic model [8]. From the preventive health perspective, the current way of life in the "developed" world is characterized by physical inactivity, overeating, and engaging in self-destructive behaviors, such as smoking. Development has been responsible for many achievements benefiting the population—it has saved the modern world from most of the infectious diseases that affected our ancestors for millennia, primarily through the widespread availability of safe drinking water, sewage systems, and improved housing. However, development is also in many ways responsible for most of the chronic diseases that we face today [46]. From automobiles to washing machines to remote controls, technology has "developed" us into a morbidly sedentary way of life. Industry's growth, based on the population's consumption patterns, has fashioned many unessential needs. We now have widespread access to cigarettes and other tobacco products and to an unprecedented array of food items, many of which have been modified by processing techniques and by the inclusion of ingredients such as sugar, salt, and fat, making these foods more attractive, usually higher in calories, and requiring the minimum amount of time and effort for preparation and utilization. The end result is an unfortunate combination of habits: a sedentary lifestyle, excess food intake, and engagement in harmful behaviors such as smoking [46]. Given our current way of life, the challenge confronting us is how we, as a society, can develop healthier lifestyle habits. The answer probably requires an approach combining behavioral change with environmental and policy regulations, namely an ecologic approach [8]. Most of the initiatives to date have centered on behavioral change geared to modifying individual undesirable habitual patterns (smoking, diet, and physical activity) [47]. However, a number of reports have recently appeared in the literature highlighting the importance of environmental changes supported by policy regulations as a means of enhancing and facilitating behavioral change [48–50]. Despite the significant reduction in fat consumption in the United States in the past few decades, which may be, in part, related to the decrease in incidence of coronary heart disease in past two decades, the obesity epidemic continues to increase [51,52] among adults and children [53,54]. One of the proposed explanations for this phenomenon is a decrease in physical activity levels [55]. Body weight is a function of caloric intake and energy expenditure. Among factors significantly increasing caloric intake on a population basis are consumption of soft drinks and sugar [55–58] and an increase in portion size [59].

On the energy expenditure side of the equation, exercise in all its forms should be promoted. The current decrease in physical activity is primarily related to our modern way of life, with its dependence on labor-saving technology [60]. A small proportion of Americans (~ 25% of all adults) participate in regular physical activity [48,61], and a study evaluating cross-sectional data from the National Health Interview Survey concluded that there is a significant decline of physical activity with age [51]. The two major activities among active older adults were walking and gardening [62]. Physical activity appears to be lower among women, minority populations, the elderly, and the less educated [63].

The Ecologic Model: Environmental, Policy, and Legislative Components

Environmental policy and legislative components
  Regulatory agencies and Congress
    Smoking
      Increased taxation on cigarettes
      Banning of smoking in public places
      Use of tobacco settlement monies for prevention efforts
      Support of media campaigns against smoking by public agencies such as the
        National Cancer Institute
    Diet: the US food supply
      Regulated by a series of laws
        Department of Health and Human Services
        Department of Agriculture
      FDA regulations
        Nutrition labeling
          Regulations requiring standardized nutrition labeling
          Illegality of using any health claim or nutrient content claim in food labeling
            unless the FDA has approved the claim in advance
          Effective way to spread knowledge
          Limitations
            Basic concepts regarding healthful dietary choices are not clear
            Enforcement al the local level
            Inaccuracy of nutrient composition
  Physical activity levels
    Urban planning and zoning regulations
      Restricting downtown centers to foot or bicycle traffic
      Making stairways more attractive and convenient
      Developing and improving greenways
      Creating exercise-friendly zoning regulations
      Developing community exercise facilities
        Parks
        Swimming pools
        Bike-paths
    Encouraging local and state health departments to collaborate with parks, education
      and transportation departments to facilitate physical activity
    Designing tax rebates programs for businesses offering physical activity programs
    Health insurance
      Decreasing health insurance premiums for people engaged in regular physical
        activities
      Health-center fee rebates

Figure 24-8.

Components of the ecologic model. Smoking, diet, and physical activity have increasingly become a source of concern at the national level, with regulatory agencies and the US Congress progressively more involved in suggesting or enacting rules and regulations that respond to public concern. For smoking, such approaches have included increased taxation on cigarettes, the banning of smoking in public places, the use of tobacco settlement monies for prevention efforts [64], and the support of media campaigns against smoking by public agencies such as the National Cancer Institute. The US Department of Health and Human Services has funded programs to develop interventions to improve diet and physical activity, and currently overweight and obesity. The recent Internal Revenue Service ruling considering obesity to be a disease highlights the importance of the prob-

lem and, as a policy decision, may have an impact on the entire population [65].

The US food supply is regulated by a series of laws administered by the Department of Health and Human Services and the Department of Agriculture. The Food and Drug Administration's (FDA) requirements concerning the provision of basic, standard-format nutrition information ("nutrition labeling") on food products have changed dramatically over the past 50 years. The new FDA regulations that became effective in 1994 require standardized nutrition labeling on most food products carried in interstate commerce [66]. Under the new FDA regulations, it is illegal to use any health claim or nutrient content claim in food labeling unless the FDA has approved the claim in advance.

Food labeling is an especially important and interesting interface between policy and preventive medicine. Dietary choices are complex and, compared with cigarette smoking, the consumer needs a great deal of information to make intelligent choices. The awareness of the nutritional content of foods influences people's choices [67–70]. The use of labels seems to be an effective way to spread knowledge. At the same time, studies show that the general public is currently overloaded with nutritional information and that many basic concepts regarding healthful dietary choices are not clear [71]. There are also problems in the implementation of labeling guidelines with regard to enforcement al the local level and accuracy of nutrient composition [46,72].

The emphasis of community-based cardiovascular disease prevention programs should be directed toward reaching and maintaining a healthy body weight [73]. The food service industry could support efforts geared to control obesity by offering "petite" portions (as opposed to "super-sized") as a menu option, and by focusing on improving flavor and nutritional composition instead of increasing size [45].

Environmental and policy approaches to cardiovascular disease prevention through physical activity [48,49] include the following suggestions: restricting downtown centers to foot or bicycle traffic; making stairways more attractive and convenient; encouraging local and state health departments to collaborate with parks, education and transportation departments to facilitate physical activity; developing and improving greenways; creating exercise-friendly zoning regulations; developing community exercise facilities such as parks, swimming pools, and bike-paths; designing tax rebates programs for businesses that offer physical activity programs, decreasing health insurance premiums for people engaged in regular physical activities; and implementing health-center fee rebates [46].

Location for Community-based Prevention in Cardiovascular Disease

Communities defined as neighborhood, town, city, and so forth

Schools

Work site

Religious organizations

Community/grass-roots
    organizations/nongovernmental
    organizations

Figure 24-9.
Most adult coronary heart disease (CHD) is attributable to risk factor–related behaviors that are often established in early childhood [75–79]. By age 12, at least one modifiable risk factor for CHD exists in 36% to 60% of children in the United States [80]. There are also reports of high prevalence of CHD risk factors among children in Europe [81]. There is a general awareness that the psychosocial environment of childhood contributes to behaviors in adult life, including those related to CHD morbidity and mortality [82]. These behavioral risks—cigarette smoking, inappropriate dietary habits, and insufficient exercise—are all difficult to modify once established. In the United States, more than 50 million children attend private and public schools, for an average of 5 to 8 hours a day, 5 days a week, for 36 weeks a year, making schools a major window of opportunity for promoting health-related behaviors among children [81,83,84].

For the most part, the model for school health services that has guided the development of school health programs in the United States includes three components: health instruction, a healthful school environment, and the provision of school health services. Health instruction includes teaching health-related knowledge, attitudes, and practices. The school environment relates to the actual physical setting, as well as to an awareness of its influence on the attitude and behavior of students. School health services include medical examinations, screening programs, communicable disease control, and correction of remediable problems. This model has been used to tailor CHD interventions as well as interventions for other acute and chronic diseases in the school setting [46].

Before 1980, the goal of most school health education programs was to transmit information with the hope that increased knowledge would lead students to adopt positive health behaviors [75]. However, there is substantial evidence that such an approach is ineffective. A modified approach has evolved that places less emphasis on knowledge acquisition and more on skills development, social influences, and behavioral competencies, with the goal of intervening before risk behaviors become established [86].

Finally, regarding interventions in the work site, the number of health promotion programs in the work site has increased in recent years, with most of the programs aimed at individual behavior change [85]. Earlier results from the first National Survey of Worksite Health Promotion Activities found that 65.5% of responding work sites had one or more types of health promotion activities [86]. Work site preventive health programs typically include, in decreasing order of frequency, smoking cessation, health risk assessment, back care regimens, stress management, exercise and fitness programs, accident prevention, nutrition education, high blood pressure treatment, and weight control. The frequency of these activities is directly related to the size of the work site and varies by industry type [85,87].

The work site provides a vehicle for helping people reduce risk through changes in the work organization and environment. CHD risks may be reduced by eliminating or reducing exposures to hazardous substances such as cigarette smoke or by altering work conditions that are associated with increased disease incidence, such as the stressful work combination of high demand and low control [88–90]. Over three quarters (76%) of US civilian, noninstitutionalized men age 20 and over are currently employed; the corresponding figure for women is 60.8% [91]. Even a small intervention effect in this large segment of the population has the potential to change health behaviors so as to result in substantial changes in CHD event rates [3,92]. At the same time, interventions in this group can be an important window into the usefulness of work site policy/regulation and for implementation of environmental changes that would, in turn, foster changes in individual behavior. Increasingly, businesses themselves are taking an active role in this process, as they perceive prevention as a way of holding down health care costs related to absenteeism, insurance claims, and disability [93–100]. However, the efficacy of such efforts is limited by their availability and the degree of interest that employees show in participating in these programs. Low levels of employee participation can limit the potential health impact of otherwise effective work-based interventions [101].

Health education can also be channeled through allied health personnel, such as pharmacists, who have traditionally had a limited role in prevention; there is mounting evidence of their potential effectiveness, particularly in the areas of secondary prevention and adherence to medication regimens [102].

Effective Community-based Strategies in Cardiovascular Disease Prevention

Health education
  Content beyond traditional fact-transmission
  Specific tips on lifestyle modification
  Culturally-appropriate tailoring
  Channel specific messages for high-risk subgroups
Systematic involvement of and coordination with health care
    services
Community organization
  Community involvement from the start
  Involvement of lay opinion leaders
  Development of collaboration networks
    Local community-based initiatives, providers, grocery stores,
        schools, worksite, health authorities, and the public
    Close collaboration between community-based projects and
        health authorities
Ecologic approach
    Develop collaborations with industry and businesses
    Involvement of governmental regulatory agencies

Figure 24-10.
Effective community-based strategies. Successful strategies at the community level include health education, the systematic involvement of and coordination with health care services, and a comprehensive involvement of the community organizations, highlighting the importance of utilizing an ecologic approach. Health education and media campaigns have played a prominent role in many community-based programs. Although the impact of media campaigns by themselves has been limited, such campaigns are useful and necessary components in the comprehensive package [40]. However, in certain communities, because of concurrent secular trends, which may dilute the impact of the mass media campaign, the content may need to go beyond the traditional fact-transmission,

and include more detailed information about specific tips for lifestyle modification. Intensity of the media campaign is also a key aspect, as is the design of culturally appropriate and channel-specific messages to reach certain subgroups of the population.

Health service interventions may not have as much visibility as major media campaigns; however, the systematic involvement of and coordination with primary health care centers can become a critical component of community-based interventions. This may be particularly true when the intervention deals with biologic risk factors such as hypertension or elevated blood cholesterol [40].

Community organization means involvement and collaboration with various sectors of the community. This has been the particular strength of the North Karelia Project, in which the involvement of many nongovernmental organizations was considered to be a key component. The North Karelia Project also demonstrated the potential of involving lay opinion leaders, a concept that has been successfully applied on many occasions in developing countries [40,103].

It is difficult for community-based interventions in small communities to include collaboration with industry and businesses, but this policy may be very cost-effective in large interventions or those at the national level. The experience of a community-based prevention program in cardiovascular disease in Mauritius [104], in which the project managed to have the industry collaborate in the substitution of saturated fatty acids in cooking oil, is a good example of the population-wide impact of such a measure. The dramatic and important reduction of blood cholesterol levels in Finland was the result of collaboration with the food industry, through the widespread availability of lower fat food product options, which was also supported by governmental policy decisions [105]. In fact, the response of the industry and governmental regulatory agencies may be in part responsible for the secular trends [51] in certain cardiac risk factors in the United States.

Comprehensive community-based cardiovascular disease prevention projects tend to have a stronger impact. For example, a successful intervention in Norsjo, Sweden [106] created collaborations among local community-based initiatives, providers, grocery stores, schools, municipal authorities, and the public to develop a national model for community intervention. Close collaboration between the community-based projects and national health authorities has been important in sustaining the activity and for addressing policy implications at the national level [40].

Limitations and Challenges of Community-based Interventions in Cardiovascular Disease Prevention

Methodologic issues
Limitations of the intervention itself
Poorly defined theoretical framework
Challenges to community participation
  Inclusion of the community in problem definition
  Differences in goals between the community members and
      researchers
  Poor capacity for establishing community ownership of the
      intervention
Challenges in coalition building

Figure 24-11.
Limitations and challenges of community-based interventions. Although significant progress has been achieved in community-based prevention, much remains to be understood about the process of change at the population level [8,107]. Preventing cardiovascular disease through community interventions makes theoretic sense but has been difficult to demonstrate. Despite a strong design and conceptual foundation, the major community-based cardiovascular disease prevention programs conducted in the 1980s in the United States resulted in limited population-level change in health behaviors and heath status outcomes [8]. However, the overall results of these interventions suggest that there is great potential for community-based prevention interventions in cardiovascular disease.

A critical review and analysis of community-based health promotion projects, primarily those in the United States, by Merzel and D'Afflitti [8] provides insights regarding the limitations and difficulties in the implementation of such programs, with reference to community-based prevention interventions, emphasizing the particular challenges in dealing with chronic conditions such as cardiovascular disease, in which the population perception of imminent risk may be low. Among the potential reasons for the modest impact of such programs in the US, the authors highlight several aspects including methodologic issues, the influence of secular trends, the magnitude of effects, limitations of the intervention itself, limitations in the theoretic basis, and several challenges to community participation.

Methodologic Limitations and Challenges of Community-based Interventions in Cardiovascular Disease Prevention

Absence of a clearly defined theoretic framework
Use of quasi-experimental designs
Difficulty finding comparable communities to include in RCTs
High turnover of people within a community limit value of serial surveys
Contamination effect in control communities
Low statistical power
Magnitude of effects
  Modest effects in the order of 5%–10%
  Related to low intensity of interventions
Complex statistical analyses related to nested nature of sampling
Influence of secular trends dilutes impact

Figure 24-12.
Methodologic limitations and challenges of community-based interventions. The absence of a clearly defined theoretic framework for community-based prevention interventions has hindered the development and evaluation of such projects [8]. Most of the community-based interventions in cardiovascular disease have used quasi-experimental designs, as opposed to more rigorous scientific methods, generally because of budgetary and feasibility constraints. One of the limitations of randomized controlled trials, recognized early on in the history of implementation of community-based prevention, is the inherent difficulty of obtaining comparable baseline characteristics in the communities involved [12]. This problem is compounded further in communities with high turnover rates in the population. However, high dropout rates in the community cohort and difficulties with comparisons of serial survey results limit the ability to evaluate the impact of the intervention, because subsequent surveys may include a significant proportion of individuals who have not been exposed to the intervention [8]. In this age of rapid communication, information can disseminate quickly and interfere with classic intervention/evaluation control designs through contamination, particularly if the intervention and control communities are geographically close to one another. Therefore, alternative experimental designs for assessing the effectiveness of long-term intervention programs need to be considered. These should not rely solely on the use of reference populations but should balance the measurement of outcome with an assessment of the process of change in communities [108]. At the same time, there are limitations of community-based interventions for cardiovascular disease related to low statistical power to detect differences in the effects of the intervention and the nested nature of the individual observations, which make the statistical analysis far more complex. Koepsell *et al.* [109] suggest that at least 10 communities per arm would be needed to address some of the issues regarding statistical power; however, the feasibility of carrying out such large studies comes into question [8].

The influence of secular trends on the general population has been sited by many reports as one of the main reasons to explain the lack of statistically significant differences in effects between the intervention and the control communities [8]. Secular trends in this context refer to trends in the general population regarding cardiac risk factor–related behaviors. For example, Merzel and D'Afflitti [8] reported that during the late 1970s and 1980s, while community interventions were implementing activities designed to reduce at-risk behaviors, a general shift also was occurring in US society with favorable changes regarding attitudes toward those same behaviors. Reports from the Minnesota Heart Health Program illustrate this phenomenon [110]. One of the factors that could explain the difficulty in outperforming secular trends is the limited ecologic component, or failure to have an impact in the social environment through environmental and political/legislative interventions [111]. Furthermore, the magnitude of the effect of community-based prevention interventions in cardiovascular disease has proved to be more modest than expected (< 5%–10% [112]), based on a comparison with high-risk interventions. Therefore, this divergence probably contributes to a lack of statistical power to determine statistically significant differences. The low intensity of the intervention at the level of the entire population also may contribute to the lower-than-expected impact [8].

Limitations and Challenges of the Intervention Itself in Community-based Interventions for Cardiovascular Disease

Short- to mid-term interventions
  Limited by grant-based model
Most interventions have been of low intensity
Failure to reach high-risk subgroups in the population
Limited ecologic components in studies

Figure 24-13.
Limitations and challenges of the intervention itself. Regarding the intervention itself, there are a few pitfalls to consider. Some of the specific weaknesses in the delivery of the intervention include shorter-length interventions in the United States [113] (compared with successful trials in Europe), and that community-based interventions in the United States have been reported to reach a maximum of approximately 60% of the population within a particular community [8], with special difficulty encountered in reaching population subgroups with higher prevalence of risk factors, because of limitations in the development of specifically tailored interventions [113,114]. Populations of low socioeconomic status or differing cultural backgrounds may require specific approaches that differ from those applicable to the general population [113,116]. The New York State Healthy Heart Program studied a population of approximately 200,000 people, predominantly Hispanic and of low socioeconomic status, living in northern Manhattan in New York City [115]. Potential barriers to diffusion of the community-based disease prevention model in disadvantaged inner city communities were identified, including issues of scale and complexity, adaptation of the model to a "community" without geopolitical boundaries or infrastructure, linguistic and cultural diversity, competing problems, and sustainability of the program in a poor community. Strategies used to address obstacles to model adoption included legitimizing the program, building program infrastructure, setting realistic expectations, focusing on one risk factor at a time, defining target population segments, and emphasizing a small number of communication channels.

Challenges to Community Participation in Community-based Interventions for Cardiovascular Disease Prevention

Inclusion of the community in problem definition
Differences in goals between the community members and
  researchers
Poor capacity for establishing community ownership of the
  intervention
Challenges in coalition building:
  Development of broad-based community support
  Community capacity building and program maintenance
  Institutionalization of the interventions

Cost Implications of Community-based Cardiovascular Disease Prevention Interventions

A cost-effective population approach
  Use of inexpensive intervention
  Implementation on a mass scale
  Maintenance of intervention over a long period of time
An illustration of economic benefits
  North Karelia Project [34]
    During 20 year (1972–1992) period the age-adjusted CVD
      rates had decreased significantly
    Decrease in annual costs in all Finland has been approximate-
      ly US $100 million for persons over 64 years old and US
      $600 million for those from 35 to 64 years of age [120]
Decrease in CHD morbidity and mortality may result in
      long-term increase in the nation's net health care costs
  Shift of health-related costs to a number of other diseases that
    affect people living to an older age—mainly cancer
As a society, sensible to explore the alternatives using health
    prediction models [121,25]
Even large community projects have used resources that are very
    small compared with the huge health services costs for
    CVD treatment
Urgent need for cost-benefit analyses for community-based
    CVD prevention efforts

Figure 24-14.
Challenges to community participation. Community participation is a complex process and requires careful attention to each individual component. Failure to include the community in defining the problem and differences in goals between the community members and researchers [114] can lead to a mismatch, which could significantly reduce the likelihood of establishing community ownership of the intervention [117]. However, it is common for outside agencies to control the resources through a grant-based approach [117,118], which promotes competition for limited resources and exerts pressures on the community and the researchers, becoming another factor that limits the maintenance over time of community-based prevention interventions.

It is worth considering that in many community interventions, an initial favorable effect in groups that already have a given risk factor for coronary heart disease seems to abate with time, despite the increased level of awareness of the community as a whole. It may be that for people at risk, community interventions are useful to initiate change but that this "high-risk" subgroup may ultimately need a more intensive intervention, or a sustained—that is, over time—lower level intervention, so as to maintain the desired behavior and to prevent a "rebound effect." At the same time, the rest of the population (the majority) may slowly assimilate the information and work toward behavior modification. The diffusion of innovations learning theory [119] could explain some of the differences in adoption of new behaviors between "early" and "late" adopters.

Regarding community participation, Merzel and D'Afflitti [8] highlight the critical importance of the process of coalition building and the challenges and pitfalls at each stage. Coalition building should start with inclusion of the community in definition of the problem [113], then continue with careful attention to the development of a broad-based community support that will facilitate the process of capacity building and eventually will lead to institutionalization of the interventions [8].

Figure 24-15.
Cost implications of community-based interventions. A cost-effective population approach calls for inexpensive measures that can be implemented on a mass scale and maintained over a long period of time. An illustration of the overall economic consequences of successful heart health interventions comes from the North Karelia Project [34]. This project assessed the overall cardiovascular disease (CVD)–related costs in North Karelia and in the whole of Finland in 1972 (at the beginning of the intervention) and again in 1992. During this period, the age-adjusted CVD rates had decreased significantly [34]. Kiiskisen [120] calculated that the decrease in annual costs in all Finland has been approximately US $100 million for persons over 64 years of age, and US $600 million for those from 35 to 64 years of age. The estimated proportional reduction was greater in North Karelia than in all Finland. This could translate into savings of US $35 million in 1992 alone [40,120].

The primary modifiable behavioral risk factors for coronary heart disease (CHD) are smoking, diet, and physical activity. A number of reports have attempted to predict the change in morbidity and mortality associated with relatively small changes in these factors on a population level [6,122–126]. However, these improvements in health may result in a long-term increase in the nation's net health-care costs related to the shift of health-related costs to a number of other diseases that affect people living to an older age. Therefore, it is prudent to explore the alternatives using health prediction models, and as a society make conscious decisions as to the appropriate approach [121,122].

A clear observation is that even the large community projects have used resources that have been very small compared with the huge health services costs for CVD treatment. The data on costs reported by many of the community projects support this conclusion [40]. However, there is a clear need for further cost-benefit analyses for community-based CVD prevention efforts [46].

References

1. Goldman L: The decline in coronary heart disease: determining the paternity of success. *Am J Med* 2004, 117:274–276.

2. Rose G: Sick individuals and sick populations. *Int J Epidemiol* 1985, 14:32–38.

3. Rose G: Strategy of prevention: lessons from cardiovascular disease. *BMJ (Clin Res Ed)* 1981, 282:1847–1851.

4. Kottke TE, Gatewood LC, Wu SC, Park HA: Preventing heart disease: is treating the high risk sufficient? *J Clin Epidemiol* 1988, 41:1083–1093.

5. Goldman L, Weinstein MC, Williams LW: Relative impact of targeted versus populationwide cholesterol interventions on the incidence of coronary heart disease. Projections of the Coronary Heart Disease Policy Model. *Circulation* 1989, 80:254–260.

6. Durrington PN, Prais H: Methods for the prediction of coronary heart disease risk. *Heart* 2001, 85:489–490.

7. Rossouw JE, Jooste PL, Chalton DO, *et al.*: Community-based intervention: the Coronary Risk Factor Study (CORIS). *Int J Epidemiol* 1993, 22:428–438.

8. Merzel C, D'Afflitti J: Reconsidering community-based health promotion: promise, performance, and potential. *Am J Public Health* 2003, 93:557–574.

9. Blackburn H: Research and demonstration projects in community cardiovascular disease prevention. *J Public Health Policy* 1983, 4:398–421.

10. Elder JP, Schmid TL, Dower P, Hedlund S: Community heart health programs: components, rationale, and strategies for effective interventions. *J Public Health Policy* 1993, 14:463–479.

11. Blackburn H: Epidemiological basis of a community strategy for the prevention of cardiopulmonary diseases. *Ann Epidemiol* 1997, 7(suppl):S8–S13.

12. Farquhar JW: The community-based model of life style intervention trials. *Am J Epidemiol* 1978, 108: 103–111.

13. Jeffery RW: Community programs for obesity prevention: the Minnesota Heart Health Program. *Obes Res* 1995, 3(suppl):283S–288S.

14. Jeffery RW, Gray CW, French SA, *et al.*: Evaluation of weight reduction in a community intervention for cardiovascular disease risk: changes in body mass index in the Minnesota Heart Health Program. *Int J Obes Relat Metab Disord* 1995, 19:30–39.

15. Mittelmark MB, Hunt MK, Heath GW, Schmid TL: Realistic outcomes: lessons from community-based research and demonstration programs for the prevention of cardiovascular diseases. *J Public Health Policy* 1993, 14:437–462.

16. Neal WA, Demerath E, Gonzales E, *et al.*: Coronary Artery Risk Detection in Appalachian Communities (CARDIAC): preliminary findings. *W V Med J* 2001, 97:102–105.

17. Shea S, Basch CE: A review of five major community-based cardiovascular disease prevention programs. Part II: intervention strategies, evaluation methods, and results. *Am J Health Promot* 1990, 4:279–287.

18. Sowden A, Arblaster L: Community interventions for preventing smoking in young people. *Cochrane Database Syst Rev* 2000, 2.

19. Pearson TA, Bazzarre TL, Daniels SR, *et al.*: American Heart Association guide for improving cardiovascular health at the community level: a statement for public health practitioners, healthcare providers, and health policy makers from the American Heart Association Expert Panel on Population and Prevention Science. *Circulation* 2003, 107:645–651.

20. Goodman RM: Principles and tools for evaluating community-based prevention and health promotion programs. *J Public Health Manag Pract* 1998, 4:37–47.

21. Armstrong D, Barnett E, Casper M, Wing S: Community occupational structure, medical and economic resources, and coronary mortality among U.S. blacks and whites, 1980–1988. *Ann Epidemiol* 1998, 8:184–191.

22. Wendel VI, Durso SC, Remsburg RE: Studying coronary artery disease in the retirement community. *Nurse Pract* 2001, 26:48–55.

23. Muratova VN, Demerath EW, Spangler E, *et al.*: The relation of obesity to cardiovascular risk factors among children: the CARDIAC project. *W V Med J* 2002, 98:263–267.

24. Muratova VN, Islam SS, Demerath EW, *et al.*: Cholesterol screening among children and their parents. *Prev Med* 2001, 33:1–6.

25. Boreham C, Twisk J, Murray L, *et al.*: Fitness, fatness, and coronary heart disease risk in adolescents: the Northern Ireland Young Hearts Project. *Med Sci Sports Exerc* 2001, 33:270–274.

26. Farooqi A, Nagra D, Edgar T, Khunti K: Attitudes to lifestyle risk factors for coronary heart disease amongst South Asians in Leicester: a focus group study. *Fam Pract* 2000, 17:293–297.

27. Narevic E, Schoenberg NE: Lay explanations for Kentucky's "Coronary Valley". *J Community Health* 2002, 27:53–62.

28. Vale A: Heart disease and young adults: is prevention important? *J Community Health Nurs* 2000, 17:225–233.

29. Bone LR, Hill MN, Stallings R, *et al.*: Community health survey in an urban African-American neighborhood: distribution and correlates of elevated blood pressure. *Ethn Dis* 2000, 10:87–95.

30. Becker DM, Tuggle MB, Prentice MF: Building a gateway to promote cardiovascular health research in African American communities: lessons and findings from the field. *Am J Med Sci* 2001, 322:276–281.

31. Kirk-Gardner R, Steven D: Hearts for Life: a community program on heart health promotion. *Can J Cardiovasc Nurs* 2003, 13:5–10.

32. Peterson J, Atwood JR, Yates B: Key elements for church-based health promotion programs: outcome-based literature review. *Public Health Nurs* 2002, 19:401–411.

33. Sarraf-Zadegan N, Sadri G, Malek Afzali H, *et al.*: Isfahan Healthy Heart Programme: a comprehensive integrated community-based programme for cardiovascular disease prevention and control. Design, methods and initial experience. *Acta Cardiol* 2003, 58:309–320.

34. Puska P, Vartiainen E, Tuomilehto J, *et al.*: Changes in premature deaths in Finland: successful long-term prevention of cardiovascular diseases. *Bull World Health Organ* 1998, 76:419–425.

35. Farquhar JW, Fortmann SP, Maccoby N, *et al.*: The Stanford Five-City Project: design and methods. *Am J Epidemiol* 1985, 122:323–334.

36. Perry C, Klepp KI, Sillers C: Community-wide strategies for cardiovascular health: The Minnesota Heart Health Program youth program. *Health Educ Res* 1989, 4:87–101.

37. Hunt MK, Lefebvre RC, Hixson ML, *et al.*: Pawtucket Heart Health Program point-of-purchase nutrition education program in supermarkets. *Am J Public Health* 1990, 80:730–732.

38. Eaton CB, Lapane KL, Garber CE, *et al.*: Effects of a community-based intervention on physical activity: the Pawtucket Heart Health Program. *Am J Public Health* 1999, 89:1741–1744.

39. Comprehensive cardiovascular community control programmes in Europe. *EURO Rep Stud* 1988, 106:1–91.

40. Nissinen A, Berrios X, Puska P: Community-based noncommunicable disease interventions: lessons from developed countries for developing ones. *Bull World Health Organ* 2001, 79:963–970.

41. Weinehall L, Hellsten G, Boman K, *et al.*: Can a sustainable community intervention reduce the health gap? 10-year evaluation of a Swedish community intervention program for the prevention of cardiovascular disease. *Scand J Public Health Suppl* 2001, 56:59–68.

42. Hoffmeister H, Mensink GB, Stolzenberg H, *et al.*: Reduction of coronary heart disease risk factors in the German cardiovascular prevention study. *Prev Med* 1996, 25:135–145.

43. Weinehall L, Lewis C, Nafziger AN, *et al.*: Different outcomes for different interventions with different focus!—A cross-country comparison of community interventions in rural Swedish and US populations. *Scand J Public Health Suppl* 2001, 56:46–58.

44. Record NB, Harris DE, Record SS, *et al.*: Mortality impact of an integrated community cardiovascular health program. *Am J Prev Med* 2000, 19:30–38.

45. Gold MR, McCoy KI, Teutsch SM, Haddix AC: Assessing outcomes in population health: moving the field forward. *Am J Prev Med* 1997, 13:3–5.

46. Chiriboga D, Ockene I: Prevention strategies: from the office to the community and beyond. In *Clinical Trials in Heart Disease: A Companion to Braunwald's Heart Disease.* Edited by Gaziano J. Philadelphia: Elsevier-Saunders; 2004.

47. Wilson MG: Cholesterol reduction in the workplace and in community settings. *J Community Health* 1991, 16:49–65.

48. King AC, Jeffery RW, Fridinger F, *et al.*: Environmental and policy approaches to cardiovascular disease prevention through physical activity: issues and opportunities. *Health Educ Q* 1995, 22:499–511.

49. Schmid TL, Pratt M, Howze E: Policy as intervention: environmental and policy approaches to the prevention of cardiovascular disease. *Am J Public Health* 1995, 85:1207–1211.

50. Glasgow RE, McKay HG, Piette JD, Reynolds KD: The RE-AIM framework for evaluating interventions: what can it tell us about approaches to chronic illness management? *Patient Educ Couns* 2001, 44:119–127.

51. Caspersen CJ, Pereira MA, Curran KM: Changes in physical activity patterns in the United States, by sex and cross-sectional age. *Med Sci Sports Exerc* 2000, 32:1601–1609.

52. Flegal KM, Carroll MD, Kuczmarski RJ, Johnson CL: Overweight and obesity in the United States: prevalence and trends, 1960–1994. *Int J Obes Relat Metab Disord* 1998, 22:39–47.

53. Fulton JE, McGuire MT, Caspersen CJ, Dietz WH: Interventions for weight loss and weight gain prevention among youth: current issues. *Sports Med* 2001, 31:153–165.

54. Flegal KM, Troiano RP: Changes in the distribution of body mass index of adults and children in the US population. *Int J Obes Relat Metab Disord* 2000, 24:807–818.

55. Nestle M, Jacobson MF: Halting the obesity epidemic: a public health policy approach. *Public Health Rep* 2000, 115:12–24.

56. Johnson RK, Frary C: Choose beverages and foods to moderate your intake of sugars: the 2000 dietary guidelines for Americans. What's all the fuss about? *J Nutr* 2001, 131:2766S–2771S.

57. Bodenheimer T: A public health approach to cholesterol. Confronting the 'TV-auto- supermarket society'. *West J Med* 1991, 154:344–348.

58. Jacobson MF, Brownell KD: Small taxes on soft drinks and snack foods to promote health. *Am J Public Health* 2000, 90:854–857.

59. Young LR, Nestle M: The contribution of expanding portion sizes to the US obesity epidemic. *Am J Public Health* 2002, 92:246–249.

60. Goran MI, Treuth MS: Energy expenditure, physical activity, and obesity in children. *Pediatr Clin North Am* 2001, 48:931–953.

61. US Centers for Disease Control and Prevention: Increasing physical activity: a report on recommendations of the Task Force on Community Preventive Services. *MMWR* 2001, 50:RR18.

62. Yusuf HR, Croft JB, Giles WH, *et al.*: Leisure-time physical activity among older adults, United States 1990. *Arch Intern Med* 1996, 156:1321–1326.

63. US Centers for Disease Control and Prevention: Prevalence of sedentary lifestyle: behavioral risk factor surveillance system, United States 1991. *MMWR* 1993, 42:576.

64. Kessler DA, Myers ML: Beyond the tobacco settlement. *N Engl J Med* 2001, 345:535–537.

65. McCaffree J: The new IRS weight-loss deduction: what it means to dietetics professionals. *J Am Diet Assoc* 2002, 102:632–633.

66. McNamara S: The brave new world of FDA nutrition regulation: some thoughts about current trends and long-term effects. *Crit Rev Food Sci Nutr* 1994, 34:215–221.

67. Shide DJ, Rolls BJ: Information about the fat content of preloads influences energy intake in healthy women. *J Am Diet Assoc* 1995, 95:993–998.

68. Daillant-Spinner B, Issanchou S: Influence of label and location of testing on acceptability of cream cheese varying in fat content. *Appetite* 1995, 24:101–105.

69. Aaron JI, Mela DJ, Evans RE: The influences of attitudes, beliefs and label information on perceptions of reduced-fat spread. *Appetite* 1994, 22:25–37.

70. Tuorila H, Cardello AV, Lesher LL: Antecedents and consequences of expectations related to fat-free and regular-fat foods. *Appetite* 1994, 23:247–263.

71. Goldberg JP: Nutrition and health communication: the message and the media over half a century. *Nutr Rev* 1992, 50:71–77.

72. Allison DB, Heshka S, Sepulveda D, Heymsfield SB: Counting calories: caveat emptor. *JAMA* 1993, 270:1454–1456.

73. Willett WC: *Eat, Drink, and Be Healthy.* New York: Simon & Schuster Source; 2004.

74. Marcus BH, Owen N, Forsyth LH, *et al.*: Physical activity interventions using mass media, print media, and information technology. *Am J Prev Med* 1998, 15:362–378.

75. Eriksen M: School intervention. In *Prevention of Coronary Heart Disease.* Edited by Ockene IS. Boston: Little-Brown; 1992.

76. Hunter SM, Bao W, Berenson GS: Understanding the development of behavior risk factors for cardiovascular disease in youth: the Bogalusa Heart Study. *Am J Med Sci* 1995, 310(suppl):S114–S118.

77. Gidding SS, Bao W, Srinivasan SR, Berenson GS: Effects of secular trends in obesity on coronary risk factors in children: the Bogalusa Heart Study. *J Pediatr* 1995, 127:868–874.

78. Ockene IS, Ockene JK: Barriers to lifestyle change, and the need to develop an integrated approach to prevention. *Cardiol Clin* 1996, 14:159–169.

79. Berenson GS: Prevention of heart disease beginning in childhood through comprehensive school health: the Heart Smart Program. *Prev Med* 1993, 22:507–512.

80. Williams CL, Carter BJ, Wynder EL: Prevalence of selected cardiovascular and cancer risk factors in a pediatric population: the "Know Your Body" project, New York. *Prev Med* 1981, 10:235–250.

81. Schwandt P, Geiss HC, Ritter MM, *et al.*: The prevention education program (PEP). A prospective study of the efficacy of family-oriented life style modification in the reduction of cardiovascular risk and disease: design and baseline data. *J Clin Epidemiol* 1999, 52:791–800.

82. Perry CL, Stone EJ, Parcel GS, *et al.*: School-based cardiovascular health promotion: the child and adolescent trial for cardiovascular health (CATCH). *J Sch Health* 1990, 60:406–413.

83. Frank G: Primary prevention in the school arena: a dietary approach. *Health Values* 1983, 7:14–21.

84. Iverson DC, Kolbe LJ: Evolution of the national disease prevention and health promotion strategy: establishing a role for the schools. *J Sch Health* 1983, 53:294–302.

85. Sorensen G, Himmelstein J: Worksite intervention. In *Prevention of Coronary Heart Disease.* Edited by Ockene IS. Boston: Little-Brown; 1992.

86. Fielding JE, Piserchia PV: Frequency of worksite health promotion activities. *Am J Public Health* 1989, 79:16–20.

87. Fisher B, Golaszewski T, Barr D: Measuring worksite resources for employee heart health. *Am J Health Promot* 1999, 13:325–332.

88. Karasek RA, Theorell TG, Schwartz J, *et al.*: Job, psychological factors and coronary heart disease. Swedish prospective findings and US prevalence findings using a new occupational inference method. *Adv Cardiol* 1982, 29:62–67.

89. Karasek RA, Theorell T, Schwartz JE, *et al.*: Job characteristics in relation to the prevalence of myocardial infarction in the US Health Examination Survey (HES) and the Health and Nutrition Examination Survey (HANES). *Am J Public Health* 1988, 78:910–918.

90. Theriault G: Cardiovascular disorders. In *Occupational Health: Recognizing and Preventing Work-Related Disease.* Edited by Levy BS. Boston: Little-Brown; 1988.

91. Bureau of Labor Statistics: *Report on Employment Situation.* Washington, DC: US Department of Labor; 2002.

92. Terborg J: The organization as a context for health promotion. In *Social Psychology and Health: The Clargmont Symposium on Applied Social Psychology.* Newbury Park: Sage Press; 1988.

93. Warner KE, Wickizer TM, Wolfe RA, *et al.*: Economic implications of workplace health promotion programs: review of the literature. *J Occup Med* 1988, 30:106–112.

94. Sloan R, Gruman JC, Allegrante JP: *Investing in Employee Health: A Guide to Effective Health Promotion in the Workplace.* San Francisco: Josey-Bass; 1987.

95. Angotti CM, Levine MS: Review of 5 years of a combined dietary and physical fitness intervention for control of serum cholesterol. *J Am Diet Assoc* 1994, 94:634–638; quiz 639–640.

96. Blake SM, Caspersen CJ, Finnegan J, *et al.*: The shape up challenge: a community-based worksite exercise competition. *Am J Health Promot* 1996, 11:23–34.

97. Braeckman L, De Bacquer D, Maes L, De Backer G: Effects of a low-intensity worksite-based nutrition intervention. *Occup Med (Lond)* 1999, 49:549–555.

98. Shipley RH, Orleans CT, Wilbur CS, *et al.*: Effect of the Johnson & Johnson Live for Life program on employee smoking. *Prev Med* 1988, 17:25–34.

99. Max W: The financial impact of smoking on health-related costs: a review of the literature. *Am J Health Promot* 2001, 15:321–331.

100. Bertera RL: The effects of behavioral risks on absenteeism and health-care costs in the workplace. *J Occup Med* 1991, 33:1119–1124.

101. Linnan LA, Sorensen G, Colditz G, *et al.*: Using theory to understand the multiple determinants of low participation in worksite health promotion programs. *Health Educ Behav* 2001, 28:591–607.

102. Blenkinsopp A, Anderson C, Armstrong M: Systematic review of the effectiveness of community pharmacy-based interventions to reduce risk behaviours and risk factors for coronary heart disease. *J Public Health Med* 2003, 25:144–153.

103. Puska P, Koskela K, McAlister A, *et al.*: Use of lay opinion leaders to promote diffusion of health innovations in a community programme: lessons learned from the North Karelia project. *Bull World Health Organ* 1986, 64:437–446.

104. Uusitalo U, Feskens EJ, Tuomilehto J, *et al.*: Fall in total cholesterol concentration over five years in association with changes in fatty acid composition of cooking oil in Mauritius: cross sectional survey. *BMJ* 1996, 313:1044–1046.

105. Puska P: Nutrition and mortality: the Finnish experience. *Acta Cardiol* 2000, 55:213–220.

106. Weinehall L, Hellsten G, Boman K, Hallmans G: Prevention of cardiovascular disease in Sweden: the Norsjo community intervention program—motives, methods and intervention components. *Scand J Public Health Suppl* 2001, 56:13–20.

107. Fortmann SP, Flora JA, Winkleby MA, *et al.*: Community intervention trials: reflections on the Stanford Five-City Project Experience. *Am J Epidemiol* 1995, 142:576–586.

108. Nutbeam D, Smith C, Murphy S, Catford J: Maintaining evaluation designs in long term community based health promotion programs: Heartbeat Wales case study. *J Epidemiol Community Health* 1993, 47:127–33.

109. Koepsell TD, Wagner EH, Cheadle AC, *et al.*: Selected methodological issues in evaluating community-based health promotion and disease prevention programs. *Annu Rev Public Health* 1992, 13:31–57.

110. Luepker RV, Murray DM, Jacobs DR Jr, *et al.*: Community education for cardiovascular disease prevention: risk factor changes in the Minnesota Heart Health Program. *Am J Public Health* 1994, 84:1383–1393.

111. Richard L, Potvin L, Kishchuk N, *et al.*: Assessment of the integration of the ecological approach in health promotion programs. *Am J Health Promot* 1996, 10:318–328.

112. Fishbein M: Great expectations, or do we ask too much from community-level interventions? *Am J Public Health* 1996, 86:1075–1076.

113. Freudenberg N, Silver D, Carmona JM, *et al.*: Health promotion in the city: a structured review of the literature on interventions to prevent heart disease, substance abuse, violence and HIV infection in US metropolitan areas, 1980–1995. *J Urban Health* 2000, 77:443–457.

114. Goodman RM, Wheeler FC, Lee PR: Evaluation of the Heart To Heart Project: lessons from a community-based chronic disease prevention project. *Am J Health Promot* 1995, 9:443–455.

115. Shea S, Basch CE, Lantigua R, Wechsler H: The Washington Heights-Inwood Healthy Heart Program: a third generation community-based cardiovascular disease prevention program in a disadvantaged urban setting. *Prev Med* 1992, 21:203–217.

116. Fardy PS, Azzollini A, Magel JR, *et al.*: Gender and ethnic differences in health behaviors and risk factors for coronary disease among urban teenagers: the PATH program. *J Gend Specif Med* 2000, 3:59–68.

117. Cheadle A, Beery W, Wagner E, *et al.*: Conference report: community-based health promotion—state of the art and recommendations for the future. *Am J Prev Med* 1997, 13:240–243.

118. Goodman RM, Wandersman A, Chinman M, *et al.*: An ecological assessment of community-based interventions for prevention and health promotion: approaches to measuring community coalitions. *Am J Community Psychol* 1996, 24:33–61.

119. Rogers EM: Lessons for guidelines from the diffusion of innovations. *Jt Comm J Qual Improv* 1995, 21:324–328.

120. Kiiskisen U: The costs of cardiovascular diseases. In *The North Karelia Project: 20 Year Results and Experiences*. Edited by Vartiainen E. Helsinki: The National Public Health Institute; 1996:255–270.

121. Cowen ME, Bannister M, Shellenberger R, Tilden R: A guide for planning community-oriented health care: the health sector resource allocation model. *Med Care* 1996, 34:264–279.

122. Douglas MJ, Conway L, Gorman D, *et al.*: Developing principles for health impact assessment. *J Public Health Med* 2001, 23:148–154.

123. Haq IU, Ramsay LE, Jackson PR, Wallis EJ: Prediction of coronary risk for primary prevention of coronary heart disease: a comparison of methods. *QJM* 1999, 92:379–385.

124. Menotti A, Lanti M, Puddu PE, *et al.*: First risk functions for prediction of coronary and cardiovascular disease incidence in the Gubbio Population Study. *Ital Heart J* 2000, 1:394–399.

125. Jones AF, Walker J, Jewkes C, *et al.*: Comparative accuracy of cardiovascular risk prediction methods in primary care patients. *Heart* 2001, 85:37–43.

126. Torremocha F, Hadjadj S, Carrie F, *et al.*: Prediction of major coronary events by coronary risk profile and silent myocardial ischaemia: prospective follow-up study of primary prevention in 72 diabetic patients. *Diabetes Metab* 2001, 27:49–57.

Community-based Prevention in Cardiovascular Disease

Primary Prevention of First Stroke

Tobias Kurth and Carlos S. Kase

Annually, 15 million people worldwide suffer a stroke; 5 million of these are fatal, and an equal number are left permanently disabled and in need of assistance for activities of daily living [1]. In the United States alone, approximately 700,000 people have a stroke each year, of which approximately 23% are fatal and 500,000 are first stroke events. The estimated direct and indirect cost for stroke treatment and care in the United States exceeds $50 billion per year, and the costs are rising [2]. Stroke mortality has declined since the beginning of the past century. However, the rate of decline has slowed over the past three decades. Stroke is a heterogeneous disorder that can be divided into two major subtypes: ischemic (which includes several subtypes) and hemorrhagic (which includes intracerebral and subarachnoid hemorrhages). In the United States the vast majority of strokes (85%) are ischemic in nature and approximately 15% are hemorrhagic, of which approximately two thirds are intracerebral and one third are subarachnoid in location [3]. With respect to primary prevention and treatment, ischemic and hemorrhagic strokes should be distinguished. It is beyond the scope of this chapter to differentiate all risk factors for ischemic stroke subclasses as well as between the two types of hemorrhagic strokes. Despite advances in acute treatment for ischemic stroke [4] few patients are eligible or receive treatment [5,6]. Furthermore, treatment options for hemorrhagic strokes are limited. Thus, primary prevention remains an important factor in reducing the burden of this disease [7–9].

The evidence for risk factors comes from a variety of sources. In situations in which an effective treatment exists (*eg*, antihypertensive treatment to reduce the risk of stroke from hypertension), placebo-controlled randomized trials contribute to the evidence, whereas with regard to most modifiable and behavioral risk factors, the data have been derived from observational epidemiologic studies [10,11]. Because the numbers of incident hemorrhagic strokes are much smaller than those of ischemic strokes, the association between some risk factors and hemorrhagic stroke is less clear. For ischemic stroke, there is good evidence from randomized clinical trials that treatment of hypertension [12], hyperlipidemia [13], atrial fibrillation [14], asymptomatic carotid stenosis [15], and subgroups of patients with myocardial infarction [16] is beneficial with respect to decreasing stroke occurrence [10]. With regard to modifiable risk factors, observational studies over the past decades established associations between smoking [17], exercise [18], alcohol consumption [19], obesity [20,21], as well as dietary factors [22] and the risk of stroke, mostly ischemic stroke. Nonmodifiable risk factors for stroke include older age, male gender, nonwhite race, congestive heart failure, prevalent transient ischemic attack, and a positive family history of stroke [23].

The most important measures for reducing the risk of stroke are awareness of risk factors; a healthy lifestyle (including tobacco abstention, moderate alcohol consumption, regular exercise, lean body weight, and a balanced diet); treatment of hypertension, hyperlipidemia, and antithrombotic therapy after myocardial infarction or in high-risk patients.

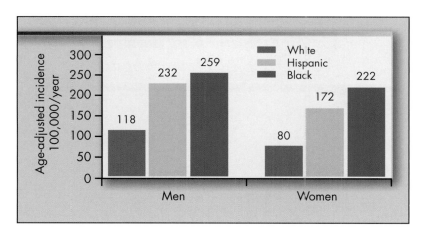

Figure 25-1.

Incident rate of first stroke according to gender and race/ethnicity. These data are from a New York City population-based study [24]. Stroke incidence was greater in men than in women. The average annual age-adjusted stroke incidence rate at age 20 years or older, per 100,000 individuals, was 223 for blacks, 196 for Hispanics, and 93 for whites. Blacks had a 2.4-fold and Hispanics a twofold increase in stroke incidence compared with whites. In this study, cerebral infarct accounted for 77% of all strokes, intracerebral hemorrhage for 17%, and subarachnoid hemorrhage for 6%. These data from the Northern Manhattan Stroke Study suggest that part of the reported excess stroke mortality among blacks in the United States may be a reflection of racial/ethnic differences in stroke incidence.

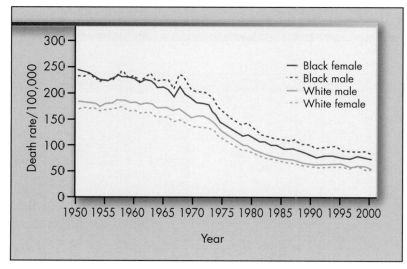

Figure 25-2.

The steep increase in the risk of stroke with increasing age. As seen in the previous figure (*see* Fig. 25-1), black men and women have the highest incidence rate of stroke and a somewhat steeper increase with advancing age. Before the age of 45, stroke risk is very low. (*Adapted from* American Heart Association [2].)

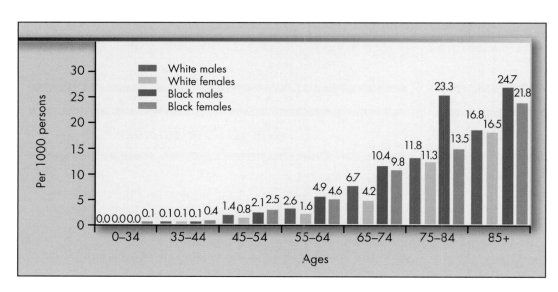

Figure 25-3.

Age-adjusted death rate from stroke by race and gender from between 1995 and 2000. There is a steep decline in the age-adjusted death rate from stroke in the United States that started in the beginning of the past century and may be explained by improved care but also may be related to changes in lifestyle factors [11,25]. The steep decline from the 1970s to the end of the 1980s subsequently slowed-down, which may be related to the detection of less severe stroke cases due to improved brain imaging techniques [26]. (*Data from* the National Heart, Lung, and Blood Institute [27].)

Figures 25-4.

A–E, Risk factors for stroke in categories of nonmodifiable (genetic predisposition, age, gender, or race) or modifiable (metabolic factors, factors associated with vascular structural damage, nonstroke cardiovascular events, and behavioral factors).

(*continued on next page*)

B. Nonmodifiable Risk Factors: Ischemic and Hemorrhagic

Age
  Most powerful independent risk factor for stroke
  After age 55, the risk doubles every decade
Gender
  Men have slight increased risk for ischemic stroke
  Women have increased risk for hemorrhagic stroke
Ethnicity
  Increased stroke risk for African-Americans, some Hispanic-Americans, and Asian populations
Heredity or family history
  Increased risk if a first-degree blood relative has had coronary heart disease or stroke before age 55 (for a male relative) or 65 years (for a female relative)

C. Modifiable Risk Factors: Ischemic and Hemorrhagic

Ischemic	Hemorrhagic
Behavioral	Behavioral
Smoking	Smoking
Low exercise level	Alcohol abuse
Rare or heavy alcohol consumption	Metabolic
Unhealthy diet	Hypertension
Metabolic	Diabetes
Hypertension	
Diabetes	
Overweight/obesity	
High cholesterol among high-risk patients	

D. Cardiovascular Disease Risk Factors

Atrial fibrillation
Coronary heart disease
Myocardial infarction
  With ventricular dysfunction
Carotid stenosis
Prior transient ischemic attack or stroke
Postmenopausal hormone use

Figures 25-4. continued

E. Novel Risk Factors

Excess homocysteine in blood
  High levels may be associated with increased risk of ischemic stroke
  Association with hemorrhagic stroke (?)
Inflammation
  Several inflammatory markers, such as C-reactive protein, are associated with increased risk of ischemic stroke
Abnormal blood coagulation
  Elevated blood levels of fibrinogen and other markers of blood clotting increase the risk of ischemic stroke

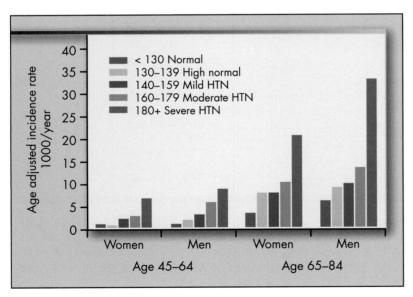

Figure 25-5.
Stroke incidence by systolic blood pressure: Framingham Study [28]. After the nonmodifiable risk factor of age, hypertension (HTN) is the strongest predictor for ischemic and hemorrhagic stroke. This figure shows the incidence rate of total stroke according to age and gender. Increasing systolic blood pressure is associated with an increased risk of stroke in the young and older population although the association is stronger among individuals age 65 years and older. (*Adapted from* Wolf [28].)

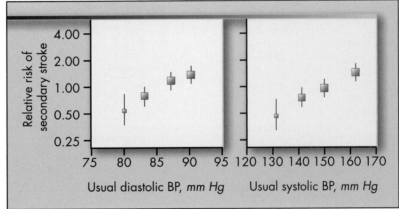

Figure 25-6.
There is a continuous relationship between blood pressure (BP) levels and recurrent stroke risk. This figure shows the association between diastolic and systolic BP and risk of recurrent stroke [29]. These data indicate that among patients with a history of transient cerebral ischemia or minor ischemic strokes, there are steep, direct, and continuous relationships between usual level of systolic and diastolic BP and the subsequent risk of stroke. From these analyses, it was estimated that a prolonged decline of about 12 mm Hg in usual systolic BP and 5 mm Hg in usual diastolic BP would be expected to reduce the risk of recurrent stroke by approximately one third. (*Adapted from* Rodgers *et al.* [29].)

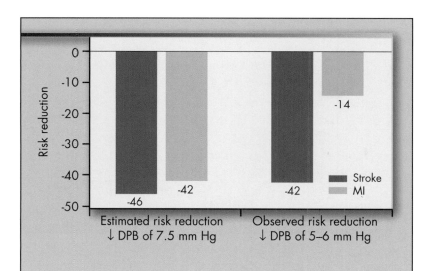

Figure 25-7.
Meta-analytic estimated and observed risk reduction associated with reduction in diastolic blood pressure (DBP). Randomized placebo-controlled trials have shown that lowering blood pressure among hypertensive individuals is effective in the primary prevention of ischemic and hemorrhagic stroke. The risk reduction varies between 35% and 45% [23]. The benefit of antihypertensive treatment is also apparent in the elderly (> 80 years) [30].

The figure shows the risk reduction on stroke in comparison with myocardial infarction comparing the evidence from randomized trials [31] and observational studies [12]. It is apparent that the risk reduction for stroke is more consistent across the randomized trials and observational studies than for myocardial infarction. (*Adapted from* Collins *et al.* [12] and MacMahon *et al.* [31].)

Smoking as a Risk Factor for Cardiovascular Disease

Event	Never smoker	Former smoker	Current smoker	Cigarettes smoked per day: current smokers, $n^{\S}$			
				1–14	15–24	25–34	35 or more
Total stroke*							
Cases, n	126	114	208	40	92	38	35
RR[†]	1.00	1.34 (1.04–1.73)	2.58 (2.08–3.19)	1.79 (1.26–2.54)	2.84 (2.19–3.67)	2.70 (1.91–3.84)	1.23 (2.99–6.00)
RR[‡]	1.00	1.35 (0.98–1.85)	2.73 (2.18–3.41)	2.02 (1.29–3.14)	3.34 (2.38–4.70)	3.08 (1.94–4.87)	4.48 (2.78–7.23)
Subarachnoid hemorrhage*							
Cases, n	19	25	64	13	21	17	11
RR[†]	1.00	2.01 (1.12–3.61)	4.96 (3.13–7.87)	3.68 (1.91–7.11)	4.05 (2.30–7.14)	7.31 (4.15–12.85)	8.28 (4.45–15.42)
RR[‡]	1.00	2.26 (1.16–4.42)	4.85 (2.90–8.11)	4.28 (1.88–9.77)	4.02 (1.90–8.54)	7.95 (3.50–18.07)	10.22 (4.03–25.94)
Ischemic stroke*							
Cases, n	85	70	120	23	58	19	18
RR[†]	1.00	1.20 (0.88–1.65)	2.25 (1.72–2.95)	1.54 (0.98–2.44)	2.69 (1.95–3.72)	2.06 (1.27–3.36)	3.43 (2.13–5.51)
RR[‡]	1.00	1.27 (0.85–1.89)	2.53 (1.91–3.35)	1.83 (1.04–3.23)	3.57 (2.36–5.42)	2.73 (1.49–5.03)	3.97 (2.09–7.53)
Cerebral hemorrhage*							
Cases, n	19	16	18	4	10	4[¶]	
RR[†]	1.00	1.27 (0.66–2.44)	1.46 (0.77–2.78)	1.18 (0.40–3.46)	2.01 (0.94–4.28)	1.18 (0.41–3.46)	
RR[‡]	1.00	1.24 (0.64–2.42)	1.24 (0.64–2.42)	1.68 (0.34–5.28)	2.53 (0.71–6.05)	1.41 (0.39–5.05)	

*95% CI are in parentheses.
[†]Age-adjusted relative risk.
[‡]Adjusted for age in 5-year intervals, follow-up period (1976–1978, 1978–1980, 1980–1982, 1982–1984, 1984–1986, or 1986–1988), hypertension history, diabetes, high cholesterol levels, body mass index, use of oral contraceptives, postmenopausal estrogen therapy, and age started smoking.
[§]Number of cigarettes smoked per day were unknown in four cases, including two cases of subarachnoid hemorrhage and two cases of ischemic stroke.
[¶]The last two columns combined because of small numbers.

Figure 25-8.
Smoking is a well-established risk factor for ischemic stroke [17,32], as well as for subarachnoid hemorrhage [33,34]. Only recently has smoking been linked with incident intracerebral hemorrhage [35,36]. The risk of stroke from smoking is dose-related, and there is good evidence that smoking cessation can reduce the risk [17]. This figure shows the associated risk of total stroke as well as stroke subtypes according to the numbers of cigarettes smoked. The data are from the Nurses' Health Study, which only included women [17]. The magnitude of association is similar in men [32,36]. RR—relative risk. (*Adapted from* Kawachi *et al.* [17].)

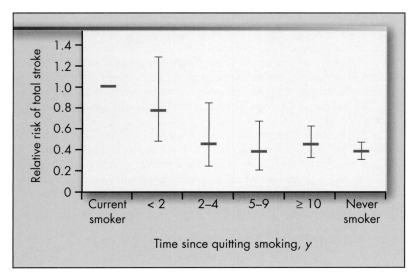

Figure 25-9.

Time from quitting smoking and risk of stroke. The figure illustrates the risk reduction associated with time from smoking cessation [17]. The data are from the Nurses' Health Study, and current smokers are used as the reference group. For less than 2 years after cessation, the age-adjusted relative risk (RR) among former smokers compared with continuing smokers was 0.78, that is, a reduction in risk by 22% compared with continuing smokers. Nevertheless, this level of risk among former smokers was still about double that among never smokers. Between 2 and 4 years after cessation, the RR among former smokers was 0.46 (95% CI, 0.25–0.85), indicating that almost 90% of the full potential benefit of cessation had occurred, as the RR for never smokers compared with continuing smokers was 0.39 (95% CI, 0.31–0.48).This figure indicates convincingly that smoking cessation leads to a reduction in the risk of stroke. Already after approximately 4 years after stopping smoking, the risk of stroke reaches the level of never smokers. Because the finding was independent of age, the data support the concept that it is never too late to quit smoking. (*Adapted from* Kawachi *et al.* [17].)

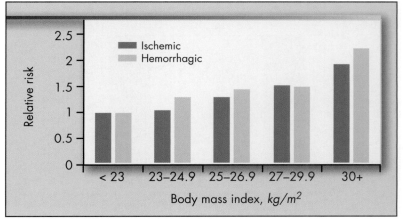

Figure 25-10.

Body mass index and stroke risk in men. Overweight and obesity have been consistently associated with increased risk of ischemic stroke [20,21,37–40]. In contrast, the association between obesity and hemorrhagic stroke remains unclear. Several studies showed an increased risk of hemorrhagic stroke among the lean [21,39,41]. Other studies, however, found no association [37,38,42] or even found an increased risk with increasing body mass index [20]. Because obesity is associated with increased risk of developing hypertension [43] and diabetes [44], which are strong stroke risk factors, obesity should be regarded as one of the major targets in stroke prevention. This figure shows the association between body mass index and risk of ischemic, as well as hemorrhagic, stroke in the Physicians' Health Study [20]. The relative risks are adjusted for age, smoking status, alcohol consumption, exercise, history of angina, parental history of myocardial infarction at an age younger than 60 years, as well as randomized aspirin and beta-carotene assignment. There was a significant linear trend across categories for ischemic ($P < 0.01$) and hemorrhagic stroke ($P = 0.05$). After additional adjustment for history of hypertension, diabetes, and elevated cholesterol, each one-unit increase of body mass index was associated with a statistically significant 4% increase in the risk of ischemic stroke and a 6% increase in the risk of hemorrhagic stroke. (*Adapted from* Kurth *et al.* [20].)

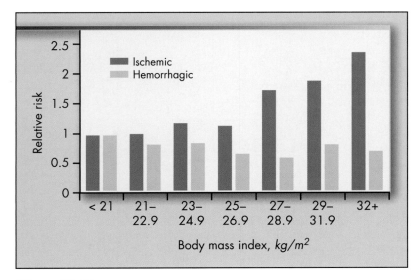

Figure 25-11.

Body mass index and stroke risk in women. The association between body mass index and ischemic stroke is similar in women [21]. However, as shown in this figure, the association between increasing body mass index and hemorrhagic stroke is not evident in women: the highest relative risk for hemorrhagic stroke was seen among women in the lean body mass index category and the relative risk decreased with increasing body mass index. (*Adapted from* Rexrode *et al.* [21].)

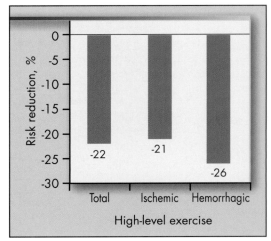

Figure 25-12.

Risk reduction of high-level leisure time physical activity on stroke occurrence. Physical activity is inconsistently associated with risk of stroke. Findings from a recent meta-analysis of observational studies [18] showed that moderately intense physical activity compared with inactivity had a protective effect on total stroke for occupational (relative risk [RR] = 0.64; 95% CI, 0.48–0.87) and leisure-time physical activity (RR = 0.85; 95% CI, 0.78–0.93). High-level occupational physical activity protected against ischemic stroke compared with moderate occupational physical activity (RR = 0.77; 95% CI, 0.60–0.98) and inactive occupational levels (RR = 0.57; 95% CI, 0.43–0.77). High-level compared with low-level leisure time physical activity protected against total stroke (RR = 0.78; 95% CI, 0.71–0.85), hemorrhagic stroke (RR = 0.74; 95% CI, 0.57–0.96), and ischemic stroke (RR = 0.79; 95% CI, 0.69–0.91). The figure shows the relative risk reduction of high-level leisure time physical activity for total, ischemic, and hemorrhagic stroke. (*Adapted from* Wendel-Voss *et al.* [18].)

Atlas of Cardiovascular Risk Factors

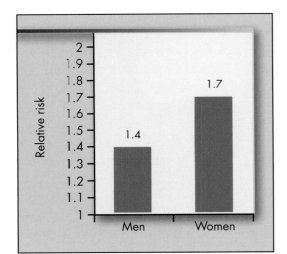

Figure 25-13.
Stroke risk and diabetes: Framingham Study. Patients with diabetes are at increased risk for stroke [45]. As the figure shows, the risks seem somewhat higher in women compared with men. In contrast to coronary heart disease, results from randomized trials did not provide evidence that better glucose control results in a substantial risk reduction of stroke [23]. (*Adapted from* Wolf [45].)

Relative Risk of Subtypes of Stroke According to Alcohol Consumption*: Results from the Physicians' Health Study

Alcohol consumption	Ischemic stroke			Hemorrhagic stroke		
	Cases, *n*	Relative risk (95% CI)	*P*	Cases, *n*	Relative risk (95% CI)	*P*
< One drink/week	168	1.00	0.10†	26	1.00	0.67†
One drink/week	54	0.73 (0.52–1.00)		13	1.17 (0.58–2.40)	
Two to four drinks/week	91	0.74 (0.56–0.98)		14	0.70 (0.33–1.46)	
Five or six drinks/week	68	0.81 (0.59–1.12)		11	1.00 (0.46–2.23)	
One or more drink/day	176	0.79 (0.62–1.00)		24	0.90 (0.48–1.69)	

*Values are adjusted for age (y), randomized treatment assignment (aspirin; beta-carotene [yes/no]), systolic blood pressure, smoking (four categories), history of diabetes (yes/no), current treatment for hypertension, body mass index (quartiles), and exercise (four categories). Men who consumed less than one drink per week were the reference category.
†*P* values = linear trend across all categories of alcohol consumption.

Figure 25-14.
Relative risk of subtypes of stroke according to alcohol consumption: results from the Physicians' Health Study. This figure shows results from a large prospective cohort study of 21,870 male physicians, aged 40 to 84 years old, in whom risk of stroke was analyzed in relationship to alcohol consumption [46]. At baseline, the participants reported that they had no history of stroke, transient ischemic attack, or myocardial infarction, and were free of cancer. Alcohol intake was self-reported at baseline and ranged from none or almost none to two or more drinks per day. After an average of 12.2 years of follow-up, 679 strokes were reported and confirmed. Compared with participants who had less than one drink per week, those who drank at least one drink per week had a reduced overall risk of stroke (relative risk, 0.79; 95% CI, 0.66–0.94) and a reduced risk of ischemic stroke. There was no statistically significant association between alcohol consumption and hemorrhagic stroke in this study. The analysis was controlled for major risk factors for stroke. (*Adapted from* Berger *et al.* [46].)

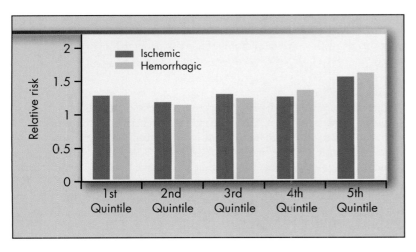

Figure 25-15.
Western diet and risk of stroke: results from the Nurses' Health Study. This figure shows the association between a Western diet defined by higher intakes of red and processed meats, refined grains, and sweets and desserts, and risk of ischemic as well as hemorrhagic stroke [22]. During 14 years of follow-up, 791 incidents of stroke were identified, including 476 ischemic and 189 hemorrhagic strokes; the remaining 126 cases were of undetermined mechanism. The risk estimates are adjusted for age, smoking status, body mass index, menopausal status, aspirin use, energy intake, alcohol intake, and hours of moderate and vigorous physical activity. The *P* trend was significant for ischemic stroke (*P* = 0.02) and marginally significant for hemorrhagic stroke (*P* = 0.098). The study also evaluated the association between a diet pattern characterized by higher intakes of fruits, vegetables, legumes, fish, and whole grains and risk of stroke. The relative risks comparing extreme quintiles were 0.78 (95% CI, 0.61–1.01) for total stroke and 0.74 (95% CI, 0.54–1.02) for ischemic stroke. Overall the data suggest that a Western dietary pattern may increase stroke risk, whereas a diet rich in fruits, vegetables, whole grain, and fish may protect against stroke. (*Adapted from* Fung *et al.* [22].)

Primary Prevention of First Stroke

Type/severity of stroke and prior cardiovascular disease	Simvastatin-allocated (10,269), n (%)	Placebo-allocated (10,267), n (%)	Stroke rate ratio (95% CI)	Heterogeneity P value
(1) Type of stroke				
Ischemic				
Cerebrovascular disease	100 (6.1%)	122 (7.5%)		
No prior cerebrovascular	190 (2.2%)	287 (3.3%)		P = 0.2
Subtotal: ischemic	**290 (8.2%)**	**409 (4.0%)**	0.70 (0.60–0.81) P < 0.0001	
Hemorrhagic				
Cerebrovascular disease	21 (1.3%)	11 (0.7%)		
No prior cerebrovascular	30 (0.3%)	42 (0.5%)		P = 0.03
Subtotal: hemorrhagic	**51 (0.5%)**	**53 (0.5%)**	0.95 (0.65–1.40) P = 0.8	
(2) Severity of stroke				
Severe/fatal				
Cerebrovascular disease	56 (3.4%)	58 (3.5%)		
No prior cerebrovascular	82 (1.0%)	112 (1.3%)		P = 0.3
Subtotal: severe/fatal	**138 (1.3%)**	**170 (1.7%)**	0.81 (0.64–1.01) P = 0.06	
Mild/moderate				
Cerebrovascular disease	95 (5.8%)	94 (5.7%)		
No prior cerebrovascular	163 (1.9%)	271 (3.1%)		P = 0.003
Subtotal: mild/moderate	**258 (2.5%)**	**365 (3.6%)**	0.70 (0.60–0.82) P < 0.0001	
All patients	**444 (4.3%)**	**585 (5.7%)**	0.75 (0.66–0.85) P < 0.0001	

0.4 0.6 0.8 1.0 1.2 1.4

Simvastatin better   Placebo better

Figure 25-16.

Randomized trials among high-risk patients for cardiovascular events have proven that lipid-lowering drugs significantly reduce the risk of ischemic stroke [13,47]. In contrast to this and the well-established association between cholesterol and increased risk of coronary heart disease, only few studies have suggested that elevated total cholesterol and low-density lipoprotein cholesterol is associated with increased risk of ischemic stroke. With regard to hemorrhagic stroke, several studies have suggested an inverse association between serum cholesterol and hemorrhagic stroke. However, lowering serum cholesterols with simvastatin did not yield excess risk of hemorrhagic stroke [13].

The figure summarizes the results of a large randomized placebo controlled clinical trial of 40 mg simvastatin daily or matching placebo among 3280 adults with prevalent cerebrovascular disease, and an additional 17,256 with other occlusive arterial disease or diabetes [13]. This figure shows the effects of simvastatin allocation on type and severity of stroke in participants subdivided by prior cerebrovascular disease. For stroke type, the analyses are of the numbers of participants having a first ischemic or a first hemorrhagic stroke (with 11 having both stroke types), whereas those having only strokes that could not be classified were not included. There was an overall 30% reduction in the risk of ischemic stroke (P < 0.0001) and no indication that simvastatin increases the risk of hemorrhagic stroke. The effect of simvastatin on stroke severity was of similar magnitude. This study shows that lipid lowering therapy with simvastatin among high-risk patients is beneficial with regard to stroke occurrence. (*Adapted from* Collins *et al.* [13].)

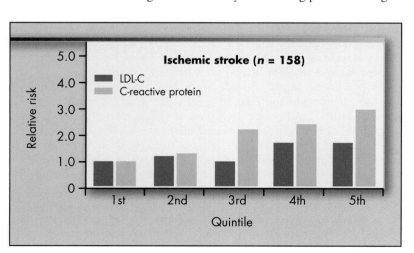

Figure 25-17.

C-reactive protein, low-density lipoprotein, and risk of ischemic stroke. Recently, markers of inflammation, such as C-reactive protein, have been associated with increased risk of ischemic but not hemorrhagic stroke. In a large prospective cohort study of 27,939 apparently healthy women, Ridker *et al.* [48] showed that C-reactive protein and low-density lipoprotein cholesterol (LDL-C) were associated with risk of ischemic stroke. This figure shows the age-adjusted relative risk of future cardiovascular events, according to baseline C-reactive protein levels and LDL-C levels. (*Adapted from* Ridker *et al.* [48].)

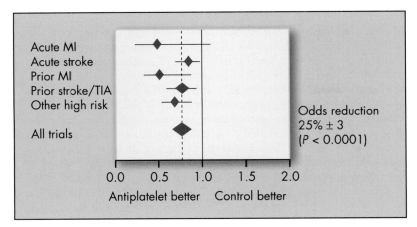

Figure 25-18.

Antithrombotic Trialists' Collaboration: reduction in risk of nonfatal recurrent stroke. Aspirin has been shown to significantly reduce the risk of non-fatal ischemic stroke among patients at high risk of occlusive arterial disease, and has been associated with a small excess risk of hemorrhagic stroke of about 0.3 per 1000 [49]. The pooled estimate for aspirin in preventing acute ischemic stroke was not as strong as for acute myocardial infarction (MI).

In primary prevention, a recent meta-analysis included the five published primary prevention trials of aspirin, which randomized over 55,000 apparently healthy individuals [50]. Overall, aspirin was associated with a statistically significant reduction of 32% in the risk of first MI and a 15% reduction in the risk of all important vascular events. Conversely, there were no significant effects on nonfatal stroke or vascular death. With respect to hemorrhagic stroke, although based on small numbers of events, aspirin use was associated with a possible 56% increase, which was of borderline statistical significance [50]. TIA—transient ischemic stroke. (*Adapted from* Antithrombotic Trialists' Collaboration [49].)

Estimates of Benefit and Harm Per 1000 Individuals Given Aspirin for 5 Years: US Preventive Services Task Force

Benefit and harm	Baseline risk for CHD over 5 years		
	1%	**3%**	**5%**
Total mortality	No effect	No effect	No effect
CHD events	1–4 avoided	4–12 avoided	6–20 avoided
Hemorrhagic stroke	0–2 caused	0–2 caused	0–2 caused
Major GI bleeding	2–4 caused	2–4 caused	2–4 caused

Figure 25-19.

Estimates of benefit and harm per 1000 individuals given aspirin for 5 years: US Preventive Services Task Force. This figure summarizes the balance of benefits and risk of treatment with aspirin based on Framingham risk for coronary heart disease. There is currently no evaluation of benefits and risk stratified by stroke risk. CHD—coronary heart disease; GI—gastrointestinal. (*Adapted from* US Preventive Services Task Force [51].)

Figure 25-20.

Asymptomatic Carotid Atherosclerosis Study. For patients with asymptomatic carotid stenosis, the optimal treatment strategy is unclear. Results from a systematic review of five randomized trials comparing medical treatment with carotid endarterectomy (CEA) among patients with a stenosis of more than 50% found that the risk of stroke was increased in the perioperative period. However, the combined endpoint of stroke or death was reduced [23]. This figure shows the results from the Asymptomatic Carotid Atherosclerosis Study [52], in which subjects with asymptomatic internal carotid artery stenosis of 60% or more were randomized to CEA or best medical treatment, while control of vascular risk factors was applied to both groups. The CEA group had a significant reduction of stroke risk (relative risk reduction = 53%, *P* = 0.004) when follow-up was projected to 5 years. (*Adapted from* Executive Committee for the Asymptomatic Carotid Atherosclerosis Study [52].)

Patients with ≥ 60% stenosis by ultrasound
Mean age: 67/Median follow-up: 2.7 years

Medical treatment (n = 834) | Surgery (CEA) (n = 825)

Perioperative stroke/death — 2.3%

Ipsilateral stroke — 2.2%/y | 1%/y

Relative risk reduction: 53% - *P* = 0.0004

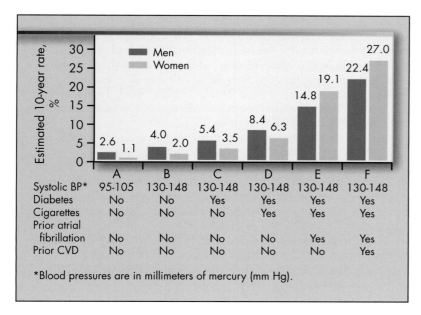

Figure 25-21.

Risk prediction model. For primary prevention, only one risk prediction model has been published. This tool has been developed by the Framingham investigators and is based on 472 cerebrovascular events (total strokes and transient ischemic attacks) in a cohort of 2372 men and 3362 women between the ages of 55 and 84 years. This risk profile for stroke uses a point system to weight each risk factor and its level of presence in a linear function to predict an event for any period from 1 to 10 years [53,54]. The risk factors included in this algorithm are age, systolic blood pressure (BP), use of antihypertensive therapy, diabetes mellitus, cigarette smoking, prior cardiovascular disease ([CVD] coronary heart disease, cardiac failure, or intermittent claudication), atrial fibrillation, and left ventricular hypertrophy. That other risk factors for stroke (such as obesity) have not been included does not diminish their importance but only indicates that they do not add substantially to the prediction. This figure shows the estimated 10-year stroke risk in 55-year-old adults according to levels of various risk factors based on the Framingham Heart Study stroke risk prediction score [2,53,54]. For men and women, the risk of overall stroke increases with increasing numbers of risk factors (systolic blood pressure, diabetes, cigarettes, prior atrial fibrillation, and prior CVD). (*Adapted from* Wolf *et al.* [53].)

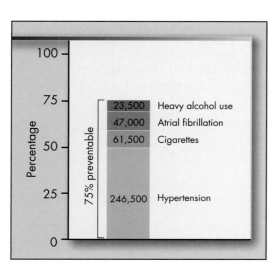

Figure 25-22.

Number of first strokes prevented in the United States. This figure summarizes the estimated preventable numbers of stroke per year in the United States [55]. The numbers of strokes prevented for specific stroke risk factors have been estimated by using the population-attributable risk estimates for hypertension, cigarette smoking, atrial fibrillation, and heavy alcohol consumption. The projected numbers of strokes that could be prevented are substantial and highest after control of hypertension and cigarette smoking cessation. The figure emphasizes the value of modifying behavioral stroke risk factors, treating hypertension, or a combination of these approaches. (*Adapted from* Gorelick [55].)

References

1. World Health Organization: *Atlas of Heart Disease and Stroke. Part 3: The Burden.* Edited by Mackay J, Mensah G. Geneva: World Health Organization; 2004.

2. American Heart Association: *Heart Disease and Stroke Statistics: 2004 Update.* Dallas: American Heart Association; 2004.

3. Mohr JP, Caplan LR, Melski JW, *et al.*: The Harvard Cooperative Stroke Registry: a prospective registry. *Neurology* 1978, 28:754–762.

4. Hacke W, Donnan G, Fieschi C, *et al.*: Association of outcome with early stroke treatment: pooled analysis of ATLANTIS, ECASS, and NINDS rt-PA stroke trials. *Lancet* 2004, 363:768–774.

5. Heuschmann PU, Berger K, Misselwitz B, *et al.*: Frequency of thrombolytic therapy in patients with acute ischemic stroke and the risk of in-hospital mortality: the German Stroke Registers Study Group. *Stroke* 2003, 34:1106–1113.

6. Heuschmann PU, Kolominsky-Rabas PL, Misselwitz B, *et al.*: Predictors of in-hospital mortality and attributable risks of death after ischemic stroke: the German Stroke Registers Study Group. *Arch Intern Med* 2004, 164:1761–1768.

7. Gorelick PB, Sacco RL, Smith DB, *et al.*: Prevention of a first stroke: a review of guidelines and a multidisciplinary consensus statement from the National Stroke Association. *JAMA* 1999, 281:1112–1120.

8. Hankey GJ, Warlow CP: Treatment and secondary prevention of stroke: evidence, costs, and effects on individuals and populations. *Lancet* 1999, 354:1457–1463.

9. Hankey GJ: Stroke: how large a public health problem, and how can the neurologist help? *Arch Neurol* 1999, 56:748–754.

10. Holloway RG, Benesch C, Rush SR: Stroke prevention: narrowing the evidence-practice gap. *Neurology* 2000, 54:1899–1906.

11. Bronner LL, Kanter DS, Manson JE: Primary prevention of stroke. *N Engl J Med* 1995, 333:1392–1400.

12. Collins R, Peto R, MacMahon S, *et al.*: Blood pressure, stroke, and coronary heart disease. Part 2: short-term reductions in blood pressure: overview of randomised drug trials in their epidemiological context. *Lancet* 1990, 335:827–838.

13. Collins R, Armitage J, Parish S, *et al.*: Effects of cholesterol-lowering with simvastatin on stroke and other major vascular events in 20536 people with cerebrovascular disease or other high-risk conditions. *Lancet* 2004, 363:757–767.

14. Report of the Quality Standards Subcommittee of the American Academy of Neurology: Practice parameter: Stroke prevention in patients with non-valvular atrial fibrillation. *Neurology* 1998, 51:671–673.

15. Executive Committee for the Asymptomatic Carotid Atherosclerosis Study: Endarterectomy for asymptomatic carotid artery stenosis. *JAMA* 1995, 273:1421–1428.

16. Loh E, Sutton MS, Wun CC, *et al.*: Ventricular dysfunction and the risk of stroke after myocardial infarction. *N Engl J Med* 1997, 336:251–257.

17. Kawachi I, Colditz GA, Stampfer MJ, *et al.*: Smoking cessation and decreased risk of stroke in women. *JAMA* 1993, 269:232–236.

18. Wendel-Voss GC, Schuit AJ, Feskens EJ, *et al.*: Physical activity and stroke: a meta-analysis of observational data. *Int J Epidemiol* 2004, 33:787–798.

19. Reynolds K, Lewis B, Nolen JD, *et al.*: Alcohol consumption and risk of stroke: a meta-analysis. *JAMA* 2003, 289:579–588.

20. Kurth T, Gaziano JM, Berger K, *et al.*: Body mass index and the risk of stroke in men. *Arch Intern Med* 2002, 162:2557–2562.

21. Rexrode KM, Hennekens CH, Willett WC, *et al.*: A prospective study of body mass index, weight change, and risk of stroke in women. *JAMA* 1997, 277:1539–1545.

22. Fung TT, Stampfer MJ, Manson JE, *et al.*: Prospective study of major dietary patterns and stroke risk in women. *Stroke* 2004, 35:2014–2019.

23. Straus SE, Majumdar SR, McAlister FA: New evidence for stroke prevention: scientific review. *JAMA* 2002, 288:1388–1395.

24. Sacco RL, Boden-Albala B, Gan R, *et al.*: Stroke incidence among white, black, and Hispanic residents of an urban community: the Northern Manhattan Stroke Study. *Am J Epidemiol* 1998, 147:259–268.

25. Reed DM: The paradox of high risk of stroke in populations with low risk of coronary heart disease. *Am J Epidemiol* 1990, 131:579–588.

26. Cooper R, Sempos C, Hsieh SC, Kovar MG: Slowdown in the decline of stroke mortality in the United States, 1978–1986. *Stroke* 1990, 21:1274–1279.

27. National Heart, Lung, and Blood Institute: *Morbidity and Mortality: 2004 Chart Book on Cardiovascular, Lung, and Blood Diseases*. Bethesda: National Heart, Lung, and Blood Institute; 2004.

28. Wolf PA: Cerebrovascular risk. In *Hypertension Primer: The Essentials of High Blood Pressure*, edn 3. Edited by Izzo JL, Black HR. Philadelphia: Lippincott, Williams & Wilkins; 2003:239–243.

29. Rodgers A, MacMahon S, Gamble G, *et al.*: Blood pressure and risk of stroke in patients with cerebrovascular disease. The United Kingdom Transient Ischaemic Attack Collaborative Group. *BMJ* 1996, 313:147.

30. Gueyffier F, Bulpitt C, Boissel JP, *et al.*: Antihypertensive drugs in very old people: a subgroup meta-analysis of randomised controlled trials. INDANA Group. *Lancet* 1999, 353:793–796.

31. MacMahon S, Peto R, Cutler J, *et al.*: Blood pressure, stroke, and coronary heart disease. Part 1: prolonged differences in blood pressure: prospective observational studies corrected for the regression dilution bias. *Lancet* 1990, 335:765–774.

32. Robbins AS, Manson JE, Lee IM, *et al.*: Cigarette smoking and stroke in a cohort of US male physicians. *Ann Intern Med* 1994, 120:458–462.

33. Juvela S: Prevalence of risk factors in spontaneous intracerebral hemorrhage and aneurysmal subarachnoid hemorrhage. *Arch Neurol* 1996, 53:734–740.

34. Juvela S: Risk factors for multiple intracranial aneurysms. *Stroke* 2000, 31:392–397.

35. Kurth T, Kase CS, Berger K, *et al.*: Smoking and risk of hemorrhagic stroke in women. *Stroke* 2003, 34:2792–2795.

36. Kurth T, Kase CS, Berger K, *et al.*: Smoking and the risk of hemorrhagic stroke in men. *Stroke* 2003, 34:1151–1155.

37. Abbott RD, Behrens GR, Sharp DS, *et al.*: Body mass index and thromboembolic stroke in nonsmoking men in older middle age. The Honolulu Heart Program. *Stroke* 1994, 25:2370–2376.

38. Jood K, Jern C, Wilhelmsen L, Rosengren A: Body mass index in mid-life is associated with a first stroke in men: a prospective population study over 28 years. *Stroke* 2004, 35:2764–2769.

39. Song YM, Sung J, Davey Smith G, Ebrahim S: Body mass index and ischemic and hemorrhagic stroke: a prospective study in Korean men. *Stroke* 2004, 35:831–836.

40. Suk SH, Sacco RL, Boden-Albala B, *et al.*: Abdominal obesity and risk of ischemic stroke: the Northern Manhattan Stroke Study. *Stroke* 2003, 34:1586–1592.

41. Thrift AG, McNeil JJ, Forbes A, Donnan GA: Risk factors for cerebral hemorrhage in the era of well-controlled hypertension. Melbourne Risk Factor Study (MERFS) Group. *Stroke* 1996, 27:2020–2025.

42. Rodriguez BL, D'Agostino R, Abbott RD, *et al.*: Risk of hospitalized stroke in men enrolled in the Honolulu Heart Program and the Framingham Study: A comparison of incidence and risk factor effects. *Stroke* 2002, 33:230–236.

43. Hu G, Barengo NC, Tuomilehto J, *et al.*: Relationship of physical activity and body mass index to the risk of hypertension: a prospective study in Finland. *Hypertension* 2004, 43:25–30.

44. Weinstein AR, Sesso HD, Lee IM, *et al.*: Relationship of physical activity vs body mass index with type 2 diabetes in women. *JAMA* 2004, 292:1188–1194.

45. Wolf PA: An overview of the epidemiology of stroke. *Stroke* 1990, 21:II4–II6.

46. Berger K, Ajani UA, Kase CS, *et al.*: Light-to-moderate alcohol consumption and risk of stroke among US male physicians *N Engl J Med* 1999, 341:1557–1564.

47. Hess DC, Demchuk AM, Brass LM, Yatsu FM: HMG-CoA reductase inhibitors (statins): a promising approach to stroke prevention. *Neurology* 2000, 54:790–796.

48. Ridker PM, Rifai N, Rose L, *et al.*: Comparison of C-reactive protein and low-density lipoprotein cholesterol levels in the prediction of first cardiovascular events. *N Engl J Med* 2002, 347:1557–1565.

49. Antithrombotic Trialists' Collaboration: Collaborative meta-analysis of randomised trials of antiplatelet therapy for prevention of death, myocardial infarction, and stroke in high risk patients. *BMJ* 2002, 324:71–86.

50. Eidelman RS, Hebert PR, Weisman SM, Hennekens CH: An update on aspirin in the primary prevention of cardiovascular disease. *Arch Intern Med* 2003, 163:2006–2010.

51. US Preventive Services Task Force: Aspirin for the primary prevention of cardiovascular events: recommendation and rationale. *Ann Intern Med* 2002, 136:157–160.

52. Executive Committee for the Asymptomatic Carotid Atherosclerosis Study: Endarterectomy for asymptomatic carotid artery stenosis. *JAMA* 1995, 273:1421–1428.

53. Wolf PA, D'Agostino RB, Belanger AJ, Kannel WB: Probability of stroke: a risk profile from the Framingham Study. *Stroke* 1991, 22:312–318.

54. D'Agostino RB, Wolf PA, Belanger AJ, Kannel WB: Stroke risk profile: adjustment for antihypertensive medication. The Framingham Study. *Stroke* 1994, 25:40–43.

55. Gorelick PB: Stroke prevention: an opportunity for efficient utilization of health care resources during the coming decade. *Stroke* 1994, 25:220–224.

Cost Effectiveness of Prevention

Paul A. Heidenreich and Harlan M. Krumholz

As new treatments are identified that can prevent or delay the onset of cardiovascular disease, society must weigh their costs and benefits. Given that health care funds are limited we must carefully choose where to use health care resources. For example, should we promote identification and treatment of hypercholesterolemia or increase our capability of revascularization for patients with coronary disease? Although it may seem intuitive that prevention will improve outcome and save money, the latter is rarely the case. This is primarily related to two factors. First, we cannot reliably predict who will and will not get heart disease. Thus, we will treat a lot of patients to prevent disease in a few. Second, we are paying today to prevent an outcome that is unlikely to occur for many months or years. This is important because just as a resource in the future is worth less (in net present value) than the same resource today, improving health in the future is less urgent than improving health today. Therefore, the cost and benefit of prevention must be evaluated and compared with a strategy of waiting for disease to develop. If prevention is found to be a good value, then the cost effectiveness of screening to identify candidates for preventive treatment should be evaluated.

Cost effectiveness analyses help decide between different preventive strategies and screening programs, and they help target future research and technology development by revealing the key factors in decision making. Although these analyses cannot alone determine which preventive strategies should be implemented, they are an important part of developing an efficient and equitable health policy. In this chapter, we review the cost effectiveness of different preventive treatments and screening strategies to identify patients for those treatments. All costs have been converted to 2003 US dollars.

We find that smoking cessation and exercise are highly cost effective (< 20,000 per life year gained) primary prevention strategies. Treatment of hypertension, intensive glycemic control for diabetes, and statins in high-risk patients also provide a benefit for a cost near or below $50,000 per life year gained. Screening for hypertension (age 40 and higher), diabetes (age 50), and asymptomatic left ventricular dysfunction (age 60 for men) appears to be cost effective (< $50,000 per life year gained), whereas screening for asymptomatic carotid stenosis is not economically attractive. Intracardiac defibrillators may be cost effective in certain populations.

$$\text{Cost per benefit} = \frac{(\text{Cost of strategy A} - \text{cost of strategy B})}{(\text{Benefit of strategy A} - \text{benefit of strategy B})}$$

Benefit units: life years, quality adjusted life years, or events avoided

Figure 26-1.

Definition of cost effectiveness. Cost effectiveness is defined as the difference in cost per unit of difference in benefit. The lower the ratio the more economically attractive is the strategy. One strategy is always understood in the context of alternative strategies. The ratio is conveying the incremental difference in cost per unit benefit in comparison with another approach. The preferred units for benefit are life-years or quality adjusted life-years (sometimes referred to as *cost-utility*) because they allow for comparisons of strategies across different diseases [1]. A cost per prevented event (eg, myocardial infarction) has little meaning unless the subsequent cost and outcome associated with the event are known. Most new interventions (treatments or diagnostic tests) will increase cost and outcome. Cost effectiveness ratios are not always relevant. For interventions that decrease costs and improve outcomes, there is no cost effectiveness ratio. This strategy is referred to as dominant. In addition to the best estimate of the cost effectiveness ratio (base case) a sensitivity analysis, in which important assumptions are tested by varying the model inputs and determining the impact on the results, is usually performed.

Components of Cost

Direct costs
  Hospitalization
  Outpatient procedures
  Medications
  Laboratory
  Provider visits
  Time costs
Indirect costs
  Lost wages/productivity

Figure 26-2.

Components of cost. Costs can be divided into direct costs of medical care and indirect costs because of lost productivity [2]. For many chronic cardiac diseases, hospitalizations are the main source of cost. In addition to the cost of care, there may be many other costs that are indirectly related to a given condition. If a patient suffers a complication, then family members may need to spend time away from their work, hire aids, and equip the patient's home with new equipment. These indirect costs are not directly part of the medical care, but are related to the consequences of the medical care. Indirect costs are often more difficult to measure than direct costs and are commonly not included in cost effectiveness analyses. If they are included, then interventions to prevent illnesses that affect working adults (eg, statin therapy for coronary disease) may be relatively more attractive because they have a greater impact on indirect costs than interventions that prevent illnesses of the elderly (eg, angiotensin-converting enzyme inhibitors to prevent systolic heart failure).

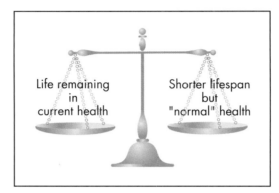

Figure 26-3.

Incorporation of quality of life. A common way to measure quality of life is to use the time-tradeoff method, which asks the patient to speculate about how they would balance length of life for quality of life [3]. For example, one may ask how many years of life a person would give up in their current health state in order to live in perfect health. This information is used to quantify their perception of the quality of their current health. If someone with a major stroke (expected survival 5 years) is willing to give up 2 years of their life expectancy to return to normal functioning, then their quality of life value (utility) is (5-2)/5 or 0.6. One year of life for this patient equals 0.6 quality adjusted life-years. Other utility assessment methods incorporate risk (standard gamble) or just ask the patient to give a value between 0 and 100 (analog scale).

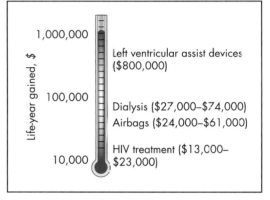

Figure 26-4.

Benchmarks for cost effectiveness. There is no precise threshold beyond which a particular strategy is not considered to have a favorable cost effectiveness ratio. Strategies with lower ratios are considered to be more economically attractive than strategies with higher ratios. However, some general guidelines have been adopted in the literature. In this figure, several accepted interventions are shown along with their respective costs per life-year (or quality-adjusted life-year) gained. Dialysis costs less than $100,000 per life-year gained, a common upper limit for cost effectiveness [4]. Antiretroviral therapy for patients with HIV infection [5] and use of automobile airbags [6] cost less than $30,000 per life-year gained. Recently the Food and Drug Administration approved the use of left ventricular assist devices as destination therapy. Their criteria do not consider cost effectiveness, which is close to one million per life-year gained [7].

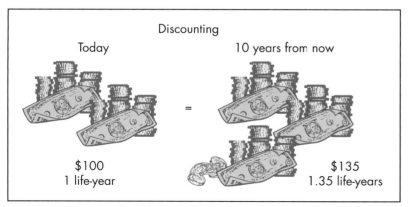

Figure 26-5.

Discounting and the effect on the cost effectiveness of prevention. The benefits of prevention often occur many years after initiation of therapy. Costs and benefits in the future are not valued as much as costs and benefits in the present. For example, a treatment that produces a benefit in 1 year is preferred to one that produces the same benefit in 5 to 10 years. The comparison of preventive strategies requires that the late benefits and costs be converted to their value in today's dollars (the net present value). Conversion to net present value is done by discounting future costs and health benefits. A discount rate of 3% per year is commonly used [2].

Cost Effectiveness of Prevention

Treatment Versus Screening Cost Effectiveness

Treatment
  Cost $4000
  Gain in survival 1 year
  Cost effectiveness = $4000 per life-year gained
Screening
  Cost $50 per person
  Prevalence of condition = 1%
    $5000 to identify one patient eligible for treatment
  Cost effectiveness ($5000 + $4000) = $9000 per life-year gained

Figure 26-6.
Cost effectiveness of screening versus treatment. Cost effectiveness
analysis of preventive strategies often focus on screening strategies. The
premise of a screening program is that there is an intervention that can
modify outcomes of a fraction of the individuals who are screened. The
cost of screening includes the cost of identifying patients and the subsequent cost of their treatment. It is possible that treating patients can be
cost effective, while identifying candidates for treatment (screening) can
make the strategy much less economically attractive. This figure illustrates how the cost of identifying patients ($5000) to be treated must
be added to the cost of treatment ($4000) to get the total cost of
implementing prevention. The prevalence of disease in the population
to be screened is often more important than the cost of the screening
test in determining the cost-effectiveness of screening [8].

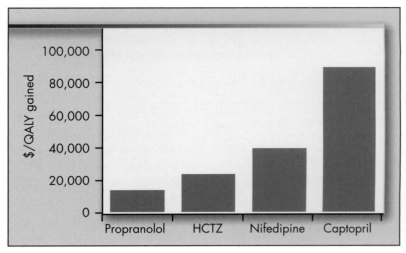

Figures 26-7.
Hypertension treatment. This figure shows an example of evaluating
the cost effectiveness of hypertension treatment. In this economic
analysis from 1990 using the Coronary Heart Disease Policy Model,
the treatment of 35- to 60-year-old patients with β-blockers or thiazides is more economically attractive than treatment with calcium
antagonists or angiotensin-converting enzyme inhibitors [9]. The cost
of medications is the variable responsible for the difference in cost
effectiveness between medications because the treatment effect is similar. HTCZ—hydrochlorothiazide; QALY—quality-adjusted life-year.

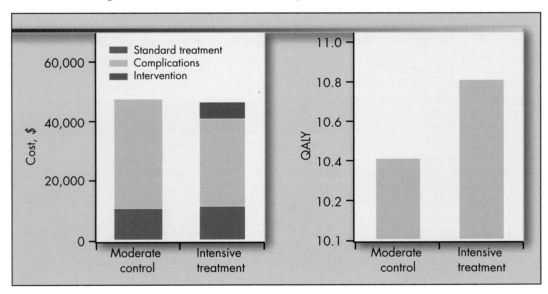

Figures 26-8.
Intensive hypertension treatment in diabetes
patients. Patients with diabetes are at high risk
for cardiovascular disease and thus are most
likely to benefit from risk factor treatment. A
study by the Centers for Disease Control Cost
Effectiveness Study Group found that when
compared with moderate hypertensive control,
intensive hypertensive control decreased costs
and improved outcomes (dominant strategy)
for patients with diabetes [10]. This finding
contrasts with Figure 26-7, in which hypertension treatment was cost effective but not cost
saving for the general population. QALY—
quality-adjusted life-year.

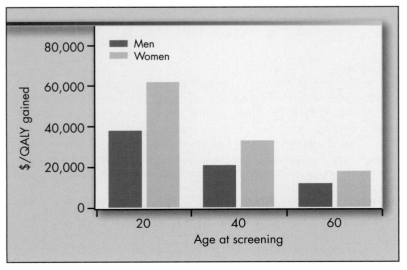

Figure 26-9.
Hypertension screening. The cost effectiveness of screening depends
importantly on the underlying prevalence of the condition in the population and the underlying risk associated with the condition. This relationship is illustrated by the impact of age and gender on the cost effectiveness ratio for hypertension screening [11]. Screening at younger
ages provides less benefit for a given dollar spent because treatment will
be provided for many years when the risk of cardiac events is low.
Similarly, screening women is less cost effective than screening men
because the cost is the same but the number of events prevented will be
less for women. QALY—quality-adjusted life-year.

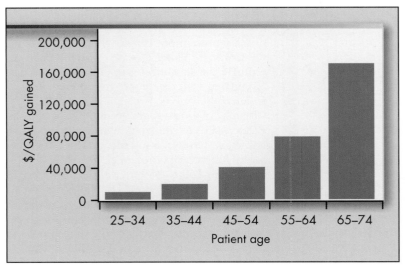

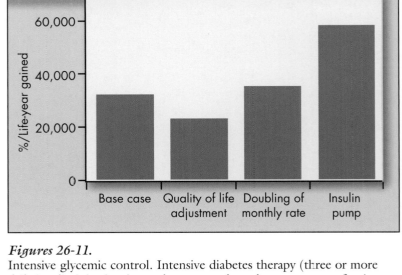

Figures 26-10.

Intensive glycemic control. Studies suggest that intensive glycemic control is effective in reducing the risk of complications [10]. A model based on the United Kingdom Prospective Diabetes Study results found that intensive glycemic control, defined as treatment with a sulfonylurea or insulin to reduce fasting glucose to less than 108 mg/dL is economically attractive for younger patients [10]. Older than age 65, intensive glycemic control is expensive per quality-adjusted life-year (QALY) gained. The cost effectiveness of intensive glycemic control for those ages 75 to 84 ($445,000/QALY gained) and those 85 and older ($2.3 million/QALY gained) suggests that it is not economically attractive in the elderly. Although the cost increase with intensive treatment was not large (near $4000) for those age 85 and older the benefit was minimal (0.6 quality adjusted life-days).

Figures 26-11.

Intensive glycemic control. Intensive diabetes therapy (three or more daily insulin injections) was shown to reduce the occurrence of retinopathy, microalbuminuria, nephropathy, and neuropathy in the Diabetes Control and Complication Trial [12]. A cost effectiveness analysis from this trial found that intensive treatment costs less than $30,000 per life-year gained (base case) [12]. In most sensitivity analyses, the authors examined the impact of a higher mortality rate, adjustment for quality of life, and the widespread use of insulin pumps on the cost effectiveness ratio. They found that including a scenario in which the mortality hazard for each patient was double, the cost per life-year gained remained less than $50,000. Adjustment for quality of life (denominator quality-adjusted life-years [QALY]) resulted in a more favorable ratio of cost effectiveness because quality of life was improved by intensive insulin treatment. Use of an insulin pump (an expensive but potentially more effective method to deliver insulin) increased costs, but the cost effectiveness remained less than $60,000 per life-year gained.

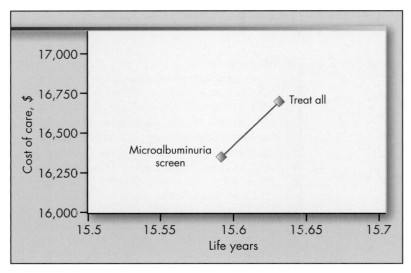

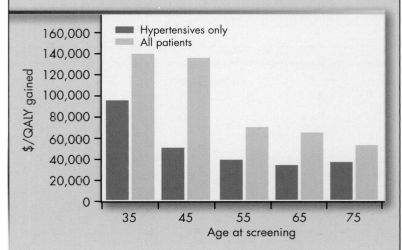

Figures 26-12.

Angiotensin-converting enzyme (ACE) inhibitors for diabetes. Patients with diabetes and microalbuminuria are known to benefit from treatment with ACE inhibitors. A cost effectiveness analysis compared screening diabetics for microalbuminuria with treating all with ACE inhibitors [13]. Treating all patients increased cost and improved outcome. The slope of the line represents the incremental cost effectiveness ratio, in this case, $8200 per life-year gained. These findings suggest that treating all patients with ACE inhibitors may be preferred to a strategy of screening first for microalbuminuria.

Figure 26-13.

Diabetes screening. Given the benefits of diabetes treatment, it seems reasonable to identify those with undiagnosed diabetes. The cost effectiveness of screening for type 2 diabetes mellitus was recently evaluated. A strategy of limiting screening to patients with hypertension was economically attractive for patients 45 and older (ratio near $50,000 per quality-adjusted life-year [QALY] gained) [14]. A strategy of screening all patients was cost effective in older patients.

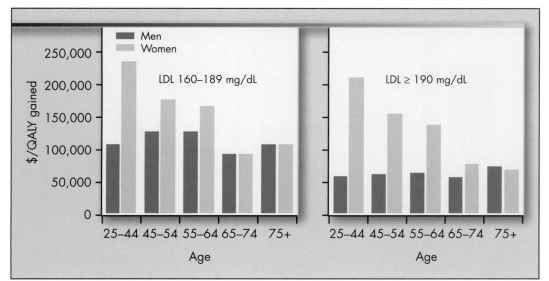

Figures 26-14.

Cost effectiveness of cholesterol treatment: primary prevention. Prosser *et al.* [15] used the Coronary Heart Disease Policy Model to estimate the cost effectiveness of statin use (compared with diet alone) for different patient populations. For high-risk populations (diastolic blood pressure 95 mm Hg or greater, current smoking, high-density lipoprotein cholesterol < 35 mg/dL), statin treatment for low-density lipoprotein (LDL) cholesterol levels from 160 to 189 mg/dL was less economically attractive. For LDL cholesterol levels greater than 190 mg/dL, statin treatment was near $50,000 per life-year gained for all men and women older than age 65. Statins were assumed to reduce LDL cholesterol by 27% based on a meta-analysis of published studies [15]. QALY—quality-adjusted life-year.

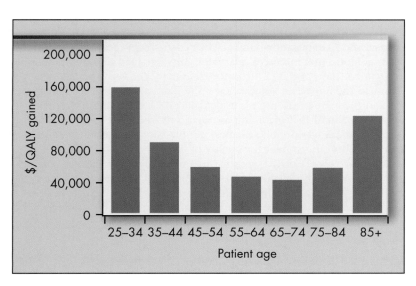

Figures 26-15.

Cost effectiveness of cholesterol treatment in patients with diabetes. The United Kingdom Prospective Diabetes Study estimated that treatment of elevated cholesterol in patients with diabetes will be cost effective for patients older than 45 and younger than 85 years (near $50,000/quality-adjusted life-year [QALY] gained) [10]. Patients were assumed to have baseline total cholesterol of at least 200 mg/dL with a reduction of 31% with pravastatin treatment ($1400 per year) as observed in the West of Scotland Coronary Prevention Study [16]. Although cholesterol reduction treatment is effective in older patients, there is limited absolute improvement in survival for a given reduction in low-density lipoprotein cholesterol compared with younger age groups. In general, treatment will be most cost effective in those populations with the most to gain in terms of life-expectancy or quality of life (*ie*, those that are younger but at high risk for disease).

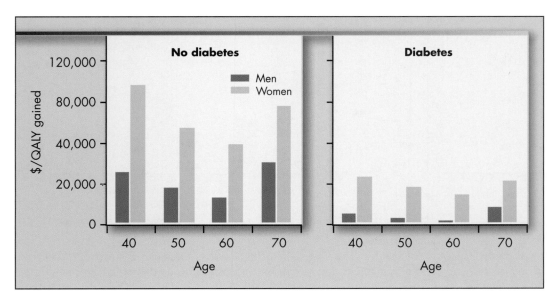

Figures 26-16.

Cost effectiveness of cholesterol treatment in patients with diabetes. Another model (Cardiovascular Life Expectancy Model) used relative effectiveness of simvastatin therapy from the Scandinavian Simvastatin Survival Study (4S) [17] to compare the cost effectiveness of primary prevention with statin treatment for patients with diabetes to statin treatment for those without diabetes [18].

Although the relative benefit of simvastatin was comparable between those with and without diabetes, the absolute benefit was much greater for patients with diabetes. Treatment with simvastatin was clearly economically attractive for all groups except women without diabetes, where it ranged from $60,000 to $100,000 per life year gained. QALY—quality-adjusted life-year.

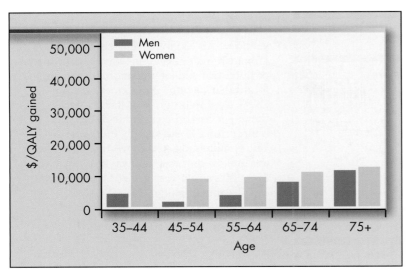

Figures 26-17.

Cost effectiveness of cholesterol treatment: secondary prevention. Data from the Coronary Heart Disease Policy Model indicates that secondary prevention is clearly economically attractive for all patients with the possible exception of women under age 45 [15]. The benefit from statins was obtained from the Scandinavian Simvastatin Survival Study (31% reduction in low-density lipoprotein cholesterol) [17].

	Difference with simvastatin	
	Men	**Women**
Cost of care	$2574	$2767
Cost of morbidity	$-824	$-832
Net cost	$1750	$1935
Life expectancy, y	0.28	0.16
Cost per life-year gained	$6200	$12,057

Figure 26-18.

Simvastatin for secondary prevention. Data on hospitalization from the Scandinavian Simvastatin Survival Study [17] were used to estimate the cost effectiveness of simvastatin for secondary prevention [17,19]. The cost of subsequent morbidity (eg, reduction in acute myocardial infarction) is reduced with statin therapy, but this only accounts for 25% of the cost of treatment. Data presented are for 59-year-old patients with a mean cholesterol level of 291 mg/dL. The cost effectiveness of secondary prevention with statin therapy was very attractive (at or below $12,000 per life-year gained).

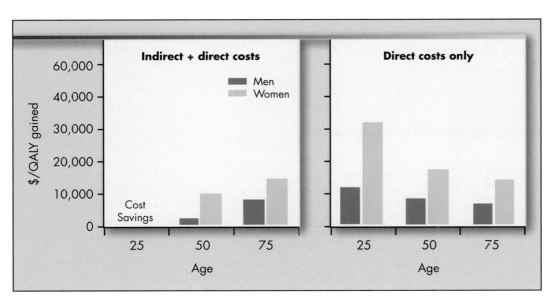

Figure 26-19.

The effect of secondary prevention on indirect cost of care. Indirect costs, such as loss of wages because of illness, can have a substantial impact on the cost effectiveness ratio. Most analyses have not included these costs because of the difficulty in measuring them and a concern over double counting if quality of life estimates incorporate time lost from work. A cost effectiveness analysis from the Scandinavian Simvastatin Survival Study [19] evaluated indirect and direct costs [19]. For young patients, the indirect costs are large and make statin therapy a dominant strategy (cost savings and life-prolonging). For the elderly, there are negligible indirect costs. Thus, an analysis of direct costs captures the important differences in cost between strategies in this age group.

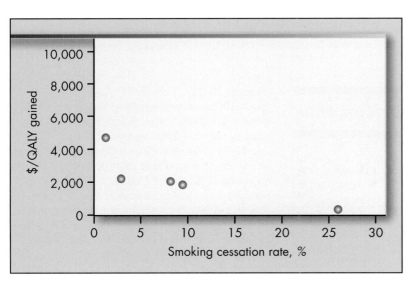

Figure 26-20.

Cost effectiveness of counseling for smoking cessation: multiple cost effectiveness analyses have found smoking cessation counseling to be one of the most economically attractive interventions for the prevention of cardiovascular disease [20–23]. These data show a clear linear relationship between effectiveness and cost effectiveness. Even when counseling led to a relatively low rate of smoking cessation (0.8%), the cost per life year gained was still less than $5000. QALY—quality-adjusted life-year.

Smoking Cessation Intervention

Strategy	Treatment cost	12-month quit rate, %	Cost per lifetime quitter	Incremental cost per life-year gained
Counseling	$65	9	$1198	—
Counseling + NRT	$189	14.7	$2153	$3672
Counseling + buproprion SR	$189	17.9	$1769	$2345
Counseling + NRT + buproprion SR	$316	21.8	$2412	$3267

Figures 26-21.
Cost effectiveness of smoking cessation interventions. An economic analysis from the United Kingdom that included a meta-analysis of published smoking cessation programs found that nicotine replacement therapy (NRT) and buproprion sustained-release (SR) therapy increased costs similarly, and that buproprion SR was slightly more effective. The combination of the two treatments led to the highest quit rate and was cost effective (< $50,000 per life-year gained) compared with each treatment alone [24].

Cost Effectiveness of Exercise

Study	Population	Intervention	Comparator	Cost effectiveness
Hatziandreu 1988	Men age 35	Unsupervised exercise (running/ jogging)	No exercise	$15,900/QALY
Munro 1997	Women and men over age 65	Supervised exercise twice per week	No exercise	$550/LY
Lowensteyn 2000	US population	Unsupervised exercise	No exercise	$13,400/LY

Figures 26-22.
Cost effectiveness of exercise programs. Several analyses of exercise for preventing heart disease have found supervised and unsupervised exercise to be economically attractive when compared with no exercise [25–27]. Exercise remained cost effective (< $20,000 per quality-adjusted life-year [QALY] gained) compared with no exercise after including the value of time lost because of exercise [25]. LY—life-year.

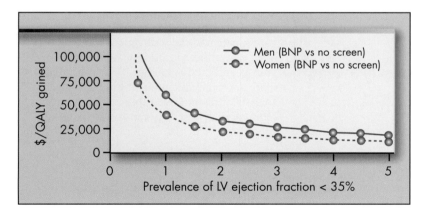

Figure 26-23.
Cost effectiveness of screening for asymptomatic left ventricular (LV) dysfunction. In a cost effectiveness analysis of screening for patients with asymptomatic LV dysfunction, Heidenreich *et al.* [8] found that screening for B-type natriuretic peptide (BNP) and confirming positive results with echocardiography was economically attractive (< $50,000 per quality-adjusted life-year [QALY] gained) compared with no screening if the prevalence of ejection fraction less than 35% was at least 1%. Men over the age of 60, those with diabetes, and those with stable angina are likely to have at least a 1% prevalence of low ejection fraction [8]. If more than 10% of the target population has an ejection fraction less than 35% then screening all with echocardiography increases outcome at a cost less than $50,000/QALY gained.

Treatment of Asymptomatic Left Ventricular Dysfunction

Population	Benefit with ACE inhibitors (QALYs)	Benefit with ACE inhibitors and β-blockers (QALYs)	Cost effectiveness (ACE inhibitors vs no treatment)
60-year-old men	0.56	0.66	< $10,000/QALY gained
60-year-old women	0.59	0.78	< $10,000/QALY gained

Figure 26-24.
Cost effectiveness of treating asymptomatic left ventricular dysfunction. A lifetime model that tracked patients from asymptomatic left ventricular systolic dysfunction through heart failure to death found that treatment with angiotensin-converting enzyme (ACE) inhibitors would improve outcome at a cost less near $5000 per quality-adjusted life-year (QALY) gained [8]. The benefit of ACE inhibitors was based on data from the Studies of Left Ventricular Dysfunction Prevention trial. A nongeneric cost of enalapril was used. Adding β-blockers (nongeneric) further improved the cost effectiveness ratio.

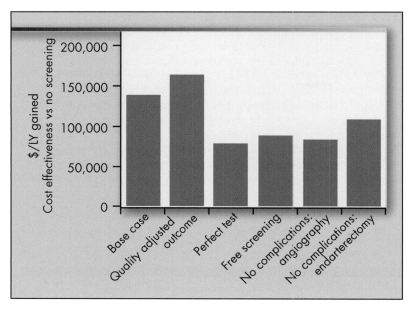

Figure 26-25.
Cost effectiveness of screening for asymptomatic carotid artery stenosis. Using data from the Asymptomatic Carotid Atherosclerosis Study, Lee *et al.* [28] evaluated the cost effectiveness of screening with Doppler ultrasonography. Screening was not recommended based on the high cost (> $100,000 per life-year [LY] gained). If the price of the test or the test characteristics could be improved, then the cost effectiveness may be reasonable. Perfect test = 100% sensitivity and specificity. (*Adapted from* Lee *et al.* [28].)

Stroke Prevention in Atrial Fibrillation

Patient population treatment	Cost	QALY	Incremental cost/QALY
Low risk (1.6%/y)			
No therapy	$7400	6.51	Reference
Aspirin	$6300	6.69	Aspirin dominates "no therapy"
Warfarin	$10,600	6.70	$434,000 (warfarin vs aspirin)
Medium risk (3.6%/y)			
No therapy	$13,400	6.23	Reference
Aspirin	$11,400	6.46	Aspirin dominates "no therapy"
Warfarin	$12,800	6.60	$9400 (warfarin vs aspirin)
High risk (5.3%/y)			
No therapy	$17,900	6.01	Reference
Aspirin	$15,500	6.27	Warfarin dominates
Warfarin	$14,700	6.51	"No therapy" and aspirin

Figures 26-26.
Cost effectiveness of treating atrial fibrillation to prevent stroke. Gage *et al.* [29] evaluated the cost effectiveness of warfarin and aspirin therapies for 60- to 69-year-old patients with nonvalvular atrial fibrillation. In all cases, aspirin was preferred to no treatment because it improved outcome and decreased cost. For patients at high risk of stroke (two or more risk factors, 5.3% stroke rate per year), warfarin dominated aspirin (better outcome and less cost). For patients at medium risk (one risk factor, 3.6% stroke rate per year), warfarin increased outcome at a cost of $9400 per quality-adjusted life-year (QALY) gained. For low-risk patients (no risk factors, 1.6% stroke rate per year), warfarin still improved outcome slightly, but the cost was high (> $400,000 per QALY). Based on these findings, aspirin is the economically attractive choice for low-risk patients and warfarin is appropriate for medium- and high-risk patients. (*Adapted from* Gage *et al.* [29].)

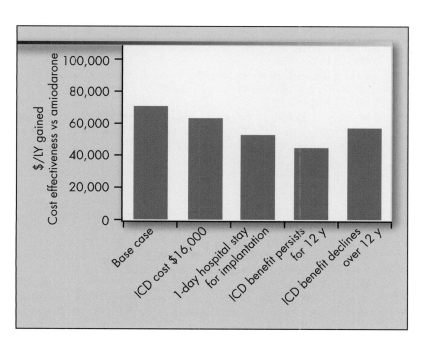

Figure 26-27.
Cost effectiveness of intracardiac defibrillators (ICDs). ICDs are known to be effective in reducing sudden death in those at risk for ventricular arrhythmias, but their expense ($20,000–$30,000) has led to efforts to determine if the benefit can be localized to certain patient subgroups. In the Canadian Implantable Defibrillator Study, the cost effectiveness of ICDs in preventing sudden death was found to be highly dependent on the number of risk factors [30]. Patients with two or more of the following risk factors were considered to be high risk: age at least 70; ejection fraction 35% or less; and New York Heart Association Class III. In patients with zero or one risk factor, the cost effectiveness of ICDs compared with amiodarone treatment was $988,700 compared with $70,400 if there were two or more risk factors. Aside from the number of risk factors, the cost effectiveness of ICDs was robust to variation in other assumptions. LY—life-year. (*Adapted from* Sheldon *et al.* [30].)

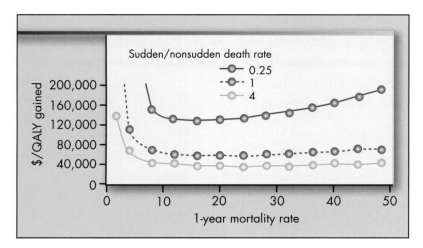

Figure 26-28.

Cost effectiveness of intracardiac defibrillators (ICDs): sudden versus nonsudden death risk. ICDs are known to be effective in reducing the rate of sudden death, but the economic value of these devices is less clear. A study by Owens *et al.* [31] evaluated the impact of the ratio of sudden to nonsudden cardiac death rate on the cost effectiveness of ICDs (vs amiodarone therapy). The cost effectiveness demonstrates a U-shaped relationship where those patients at the highest risk and those at minimal risk are not good candidates for the devices. The ratio of sudden to nonsudden death is also important. If this ratio is less than 0.25, the cost effectiveness ratio remains above $120,000 per quality-adjusted life-year (QALY) gained (economically unattractive). (*Adapted from* Owens *et al.* [31].)

References

1. Weinstein MC, Siegel JE, Gold MR, *et al.*: Recommendations of the Panel on Cost-effectiveness in Health and Medicine. *JAMA* 1996, 276:1253–1258.

2. Gold M, Siegel J, Russel L, Weinstein M: *Cost Effectiveness in Health and Medicine*. New York: Oxford University Press; 1996.

3. Fryback DG, Dasbach EJ, Klein R, *et al.*: The Beaver Dam Health Outcomes Study: initial catalog of health-state quality factors. *Med Decis Making* 1993, 13:89–102.

4. Goeree R, Manalich J, Grootendorst P, *et al.*: Cost analysis of dialysis treatments for end-stage renal disease (ESRD). *Clin Invest Med* 1995; 18:455–464.

5. Freedberg KA, Losina E, Weinstein MC, *et al.*: The cost effectiveness of combination antiretroviral therapy for HIV disease. *N Engl J Med* 2001, 344:824–831.

6. Graham JD, Thompson KM, Goldie SJ, *et al.*: The cost-effectiveness of air bags by seating position. *JAMA* 1997, 278:1418–1425.

7. Association BCBS: Left ventricular assist devices as destination therapy for endstage heart failure. Technology Evaluation Center: *Assessment Program* 2002, 17:1–13.

8. Heidenreich PA, Gubens MA, Fonarow GC, *et al.*: Cost-effectiveness of screening with B-type natriuretic peptide to identify patients with reduced left ventricular ejection fraction. *J Am Coll Cardiol* 2004, 43:1019–1026.

9. Edelson JT, Weinstein MC, Tosteson AN, *et al.*: Long-term cost-effectiveness of various initial monotherapies for mild to moderate hypertension. *JAMA* 1990, 263:407–413.

10. Cost-effectiveness of intensive glycemic control, intensified hypertension control, and serum cholesterol level reduction for type 2 diabetes. *JAMA* 2002, 287:2542–2551.

11. Littenberg B, Garber AM, Sox HC Jr: Screening for hypertension. *Ann Intern Med* 1990, 112:192–202.

12. Lifetime benefits and costs of intensive therapy as practiced in the diabetes control and complications trial. The Diabetes Control and Complications Trial Research Group. *JAMA* 1996, 276:1409–1415.

13. Golan L, Birkmeyer JD, Welch HG: The cost-effectiveness of treating all patients with type 2 diabetes with angiotensin-converting enzyme inhibitors. *Ann Intern Med* 1999, 131:660–667.

14. Hoerger TJ, Harris R, Hicks KA, *et al.*: Screening for type 2 diabetes mellitus: a cost-effectiveness analysis. *Ann Intern Med* 2004; 140:689–699.

15. Prosser LA, Stinnett AA, Goldman PA, *et al.*: Cost-effectiveness of cholesterol-lowering therapies according to selected patient characteristics. *Ann Intern Med* 2000, 132:769–779.

16. Shepherd J, Cobbe SM, Ford I, *et al.*: Prevention of coronary heart disease with pravastatin in men with hypercholesterolemia. West of Scotland Coronary Prevention Study Group. *N Engl J Med* 1995, 333:1301–1307.

17. Randomised trial of cholesterol lowering in 4444 patients with coronary heart disease: the Scandinavian Simvastatin Survival Study (4S). *Lancet* 1994, 344:1383–1389.

18. Grover SA, Coupal L, Zowall H, Dorais M: Cost-effectiveness of treating hyperlipidemia in the presence of diabetes: who should be treated? *Circulation* 2000, 102:722–777.

19. Johannesson M, Jonsson B, Kjekshus J, *et al.*: Cost effectiveness of simvastatin treatment to lower cholesterol levels in patients with coronary heart disease. Scandinavian Simvastatin Survival Study Group. *N Engl J Med* 1997, 336:332–336.

20. Meenan RT, Stevens VJ, Hornbrook MC, *et al.*: Cost-effectiveness of a hospital-based smoking cessation intervention. *Med Care* 1998, 36:670–678.

21. Krumholz HM, Cohen BJ, Tsevat J, *et al.*: Cost-effectiveness of a smoking cessation program after myocardial infarction. *J Am Coll Cardiol* 1993, 22:1697–702.

22. Cromwell J, Bartosch WJ, Fiore MC, *et al.*: Cost-effectiveness of the clinical practice recommendations in the AHCPR guideline for smoking cessation Agency for Health Care Policy and Research. *JAMA* 1997, 278:1759–1766.

23. Cummings SR, Rubin SM, Oster G: The cost-effectiveness of counseling smokers to quit. *JAMA* 1989, 261:75–79.

24. Woolacott NF, Jones L, Forbes CA, *et al.*: The clinical effectiveness and cost-effectiveness of bupropion and nicotine replacement therapy for smoking cessation: a systematic review and economic evaluation. *Health Technol Assess* 2002, 6:1–245.

25. Hatziandreu EI, Koplan JP, Weinstein MC, *et al.*: A cost-effectiveness analysis of exercise as a health promotion activity. *Am J Public Health* 1988, 78:1417–1421.

26. Munro J, Brazier J, Davey R, Nicholl J: Physical activity for the over-65s: could it be a cost-effective exercise for the NHS? *J Public Health Med* 1997, 19:397–402.

27. Lowensteyn I, Coupal L, Zowall H, Grover SA: The cost-effectiveness of exercise training for the primary and secondary prevention of cardiovascular disease. *J Cardiopulm Rehabil* 2000, 20:147–155.

28. Lee TT, Solomon NA, Heidenreich PA, *et al.*: Cost-effectiveness of screening for carotid stenosis in asymptomatic persons. *Ann Intern Med* 1997, 126:337–346.

29. Gage BF, Cardinalli AB, Albers GW, Owens DK: Cost-effectiveness of warfarin and aspirin for prophylaxis of stroke in patients with nonvalvular atrial fibrillation. *JAMA* 1995, 274:1839–1845.

30. Sheldon R, O'Brien BJ, Blackhouse G, *et al.*: Effect of clinical risk stratification on cost-effectiveness of the implantable cardioverter-defibrillator: the Canadian implantable defibrillator study. *Circulation* 2001, 104:1622–1666.

31. Owens DK, Sanders GD, Heidenreich PA, *et al.*: Effect of risk stratification on cost-effectiveness of the implantable cardioverter defibrillator. *Am Heart J* 2002, 144:440–448.

Summary of Recommendations

J. Michael Gaziano

Our ever-increasing knowledge about the pathogenesis of atherosclerosis has enhanced our understanding of the interrelationship between risk factors and heart disease. In previous chapters of this Atlas, we have defined what constitutes a major risk factor for cardiovascular disease. For each risk factor, we have provided detailed information on its prevalence, the strength of its association with risk of coronary heart disease (CHD). In addition, when available, the authors provided information regarding the benefits of intervention and guidelines for assessment and management. Because many risk factors contribute to CHD risk, for most people, successful disease prevention or amelioration requires that we simultaneously address a number of factors. In this chapter, these data are organized and presented an integrated, logical strategy that physicians and other health care providers can easily implement to assess a patients' overall risk of CHD and then implement a strategy for reducing that risk.

In prevention programs, prioritizing risk factors is key, and a number of schemes have been devised for cardiovascular disease prevention. For example, the American College of Cardiology's (ACC) Bethesda Conference [1] and the World Health Organization [2] have each developed classification schemes that consist of four categories. The ACC and the World Health Organization incorporate the concept of modifiable versus nonmodifiable risk factors, although the ACC scheme does not use those terms. I have devised a slightly different approach to organizing risk factors. First, I divide them into two broad categories, those that are useful for predicting risk—risk predictors—and those that are targets for risk reduction—risk modifiers. Some, of course, cigarette smoking and blood pressure, for example, will fall into both categories.

An important concept in developing a risk-reduction strategy understands an individuals' overall or absolute risk of developing a CHD event in the future. This is helpful in evaluating the value of a potential intervention at an individual level and determining how aggressive we should be at intervening on that risk factor. Fewer high-risk individuals require treatment to save one life or prevent one CHD event in comparison to those at lower risk. This justifies a more aggressive and more costly treatment plan for those with known cardiovascular disease our multiple risk factors. For low-risk individuals, interventions must be safe and low cost.

When predicting risk, a "perfect" risk factor is one that is prevalent in the population and that can be easily, safely, and inexpensively measured. Age and gender are examples of nonmodifiable risk factors that meet these criteria; similarly, blood pressure and smoking status are examples of modifiable factors that are easy to assess. Because many risk predictors are correlated, the point of diminishing returns is reached quickly. So although it's possible to assess many factors, in most cases, when conducting an initial screen, a handful of easily measured risk factors are sufficient to determine one's overall risk of CHD. Measuring and evaluating numerous additional risk factors will provide very little, if any, incremental information helpful in managing the patient.

One of the most basic but relevant facts to gather is whether an individual has known cardiovascular disease. It's the first question in an algorithm that I have created for clinicians to help them classify and manage patients. If the answer is yes, the patient is high risk and we should proceed with an aggressive risk factor modification plan. If the answer is no, another question needs to be answered: Does the patient have symptoms suggestive of coronary artery disease/cardiovascular disease? If the answer is yes, the patient will have to be evaluated for potentially high short-term risk with appropriate diagnostic testing. If the answer to this questions is also no, he or she should be evaluated for overall 10-year risk of experiencing a cardiac event using a simple risk prediction tool such as the well known Framingham Risk Score or another similar tool. In this way, the algorithm lays out a detailed method for categorizing patients according to their overall risk.

Following this algorithm, once the risk score is calculated, you may consider a secondary screen for those patients whose overall risk score leaves you with some remaining uncertainty about how aggressive to be with certain risk factor interventions. These patients are unlikely to be those with very high or very low scores, but rather those with intermediate scores that create some uncertainty about treatment aggressiveness for blood pressure or lipid abnormalities. Possible options include an exercise tolerance test, electron beam CT to determine calcium score, or measurement of high-sensitivity C-reactive protein, a marker of inflammation. Each of these tests appears to add prognostic information to the

Framingham Risk Score. Another key factor is whether the patient is diabetic. The algorithm incorporates all of this diagnostic information to classify patients into one of three categories: high-, intermediate-, or low-risk of a cardiac event within 10 years.

After determining the long-term risk, the clinician can implement the risk-reduction strategy that best suits a particular patient. I have prioritized these strategies into three classes based on the strength of the association, the evidence of benefit of the intervention, and on cost efficacy. Class 1 interventions are those where cause and effect is well documented and the benefits of intervention are clear and often based on data from large trials. Class 2 interventions are likely to reduce CHD risk, but randomized trial data are lacking or limited, whereas Class 3 interventions address other factors that do not have a proven causal relationship with heart disease but one is suspected or where there is uncertainty about the utility of intervention.

Class 1 interventions include smoking cessation, management of hypertension and dyslipidemia, and consideration of certain prophylactic medications in appropriate patients. Class 2 interventions include exercise and weight management programs and counseling, management of diabetes and specific dietary recommendations. Class 3 interventions include many novel but as yet unproven potential interventions, such as various dietary supplements. An awareness of interventions in the third category is essential because patients will inquire about how useful some of these are, and it is important for the provider to be able to put these in perspective with the more established risk reduction strategies in Class 1 and 2.

Steps in Disease Prevention

Measure the burden of disease in the population
Understand disease mechanisms
Identify risk factors
Establish intervention strategies
Risk and cost/benefit analyses
Establish guidelines
Implement guidelines

Figure 27-1.
Steps in disease prevention. In Chapter 3 of this Atlas, the author discusses the steps in a successful prevention strategy. In other chapters, the characteristics of the individual risk factors are discussed and, where appropriate, use of interventions are summarized. In this chapter, the author will focus on the final step in this process, implementation of a complete approach to prevention at the individual patient level. Guidelines have been established for a number of individual risk factors, including the detection and treatment of hypertension and dyslipidemia. In this chapter, the author will try to organize these guidelines and present an integrated approach to prevention that considers the major risk factors.

Development of Prevention Programs

Lower overall burden of risk factors in the entire population through population-wide public health measures, such as detection and surveillance strategies, public education campaigns, and the institution of low-cost, population-wide preventive interventions
Through screening, identify and target higher-risk subgroups of the population who stand to benefit the most from moderate, cost effective prevention interventions, such as treatment of hypertension and high cholesterol
Allocate resources to acute and chronic higher-cost treatments and secondary preventions for those with clinically manifest disease

Figure 27-2.
Our understanding of the pathophysiology of atherosclerosis and its risk factors has permitted us to develop prevention programs at two levels. A population-wide approach lowers the burden of coronary heart disease by reducing the prevalence of major risk factors through widely disseminated public health messages. Examples include national programs to promote smoking cessation and regular exercise. In this chapter, the focus is on the individual, laying out a prevention program begins with an assessment of overall risk and then targeting specific reduction strategies tailored to the particular profile of each patient.

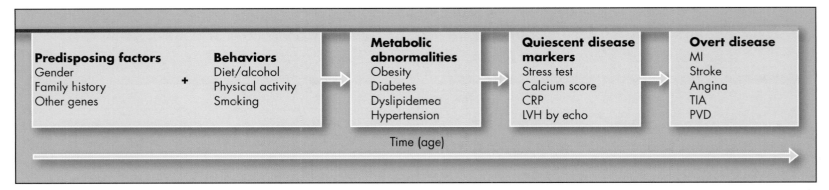

Predisposing factors		**Behaviors**	**Metabolic abnormalities**	**Quiescent disease markers**	**Overt disease**
Gender		Diet/alcohol	Obesity	Stress test	MI
Family history	+	Physical activity	Diabetes	Calcium score	Stroke
Other genes		Smoking	Dyslipidemea	CRP	Angina
			Hypertension	LVH by echo	TIA
					PVD

Time (age)

Figure 27-3.

Progression of atherosclerosis. Our knowledge of the pathogenesis of atherosclerotic disease has led us to many risk factors for disease. Risk factors can be derived from inherited characteristics, such as gender and family history. Various other behaviors such as smoking, a Western-style diet, consumption of alcohol, and level of physical activity are easily identifiable risk factors. We can measure metabolic abnormalities that are a consequence of inherited predispositions and environmental factors. These include obesity, diabetes, dyslipidemia, and hypertension. Risk can also be predicted as a measure of an underlying disease state.

Although there are many potential methods of detecting quiescent disease, this figure lists a few that are widely available and can be considered under certain circumstances to improve overall risk assessment. Finally, having had an event or known coronary artery disease is clearly a risk factor for subsequent disease. From each aspect of this progression, a systematic approach to thinking about risk factors can be developed. CRP—C-reactive protein; LVH—left ventricular hypertrophy; MI—myocardial infarction; PVD—peripheral vascular disease; TIA—transient ischemic attack.

Requirements for a Good Screening Test

Disease or its risk factor should be common
Consequences of undetected disease should be serious
Screening test should be inexpensive
Test should be easy to administer
Test must be safe
Information gained from the test must be worth the cost, and the benefits need to far exceed any risk
Test results should lead to interventions that reduce risk

Figure 27-4.

Requirements for a good screening test. There are two general approaches to screening: 1) early disease detection so that early treatment can alter the course of the disease; and 2) early detection of disease risk factors that can lead to interventions to prevent or delay disease onset. The first approach is used in cancer screening to detect disease at an early stage. With cardiovascular disease, we generally do not screen asymptomatic individuals in order to detect quiescent disease; rather we screen for risk factors and implement interventions to address the factors that are modifiable. Among the hundreds of potential risk factors, relatively few have characteristics that make them suitable as a screening test that is practical for the general population.

Risk Factors from the World Health Organization

Major modifiable risk factors
  High blood pressure
  Abnormal blood lipids
  Tobacco use
  Physical inactivity
  Obesity
  Unhealthy diets
  Diabetes mellitus
Other modifiable risk factors
  Low socioeconomic status
  Mental ill health
  Psychosocial stress
  Alcohol use
  Use of certain medications
  Lipoprotein(a)
  Left ventricular hypertrophy
Nonmodifiable risk factors
  Advancing age
  Hereditary or family history
  Gender
  Ethnicity or race
"Novel" risk factors
  Excess homocysteine in blood
  Inflammation
  Abnormal blood coagulation

Figure 27-5.

Risk factors can be classified in a number of ways. In its new *Atlas of Heart Disease and Stroke*, the World Health Organization uses a four-tiered system to categorize risk factors. Noting that more than 300 risk factors have been associated with coronary heart disease and stroke, the report identifies three criteria that define a major established risk factor: a high prevalence in many populations; a significant independent impact on the risk of coronary heart disease or stroke; and when treated and controlled, risk is reduced. Approximately 75% of cardiovascular disease can be attributed to conventional risk factors, according to the report. (*Adapted from* Mackay and Mensah [2].)

Summary of Recommendations

Risk Factors with Cardiovascular Disease: Evidence Supporting the Association, the Usefulness of Measuring Them, and Their Responsiveness to Intervention

	Evidence for association with CVD			Response to	
Risk factor	Epidemiologic	Clinical trials	Clinical measurement useful?	Nonpharmacologic therapy	Pharmacologic therapy
Category 1 (risk factor interventions that lower CVD risk)					
Cigarette smoking	+++	++	+++	+++	++
LDL-C	+++	+++	+++	+++	+++
High-fat/high-cholesterol diet	+++	++	++	++	-
Hypertension	+++	+++ (stroke)	+++	+	+++
LVH	+++	+	++	-	++
Category 2 (risk factor interventions likely to lower CVD risk)					
Diabetes mellitus	+++	+	+++	++	+++
Physical inactivity	+++	++	++	++	-
HDL-C	+++	+	+++	++	+
Triglycerides; small, dense LDL	++	++	+++	++	+++
Obesity	+++	-	+++	++	+
Postmenopausal status (for women)	+++	-	+++	-	+++
Category 3 (factors associated with increased CVD risk that may lower risk if modified)					
Psychosocial factors	++	+	+++	+	-
Lipoprotein(a)	+	-	+	-	+
Homocysteine	++	-	+	++	++
Oxidative stress	+	-	-	+	++
No alcohol consumption	+++	-	++	++	-
Category 4 (factors association with increased CVD risk that cannot be modified)					
Age	+++	-	+++	-	-
Gender (male)	+++	-	+++	-	-
Low socioeconomic status	+++	-	++	-	-
Family history of early onset CVD	+++	-	+++	-	-

Figure 27-6.

A practical, systematic approach is called for when implementing preventive strategies. The American College of Cardiology's Bethesda Conference placed risk factors into four categories based on the likelihood that modification of the factor will result in lower risk. The four categories are 1) factors for which interventions have been proved to reduce risk; 2) factors for which interventions are likely to lower the incidence of events; 3) factors clearly associated with coronary heart disease risk that, if modified, may lower the incidence of coronary events; and 4) factors associated with coronary heart disease risk that cannot be modified or, if modified, are not likely to decrease risk. However, adapting this useful scheme to clinical practice requires consideration of cost efficacy. +—weak; ++—moderately strong; +++—very strong, consistent evidence; -—poor or nonexistent evidence; CVD—cardiovascular disease; HDL—high-density lipoprotein; HDL-C—HDL cholesterol; LDL-C—low-density lipoprotein cholesterol; LVH—left ventricular hypertrophy. (*Adapted from* Pearson *et al.* [1].)

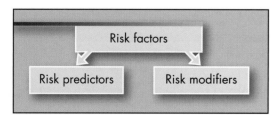

Figure 27-7.

Building on the classification schemes provided by World Health Organization and American College of Cardiology/American Heart Association, the author devised a slightly different approach, which organizes risk factors for two purposes. The first is to predict the chance of a future coronary heart disease event. The second is to identify targets for risk reduction. Some risk factors, such as smoking, are a simple predictor of risk and a target for intervention. If they can be easily and inexpensively measured, they are useful in predicting risk. Therefore, an expensive screening technique such as electron-beam computed tomography to obtain a calcium score is not practical for mass screening. Tools that are used to predict risk, which I term *risk predictors*, are presented first. This will be followed by a discussion of strategies to reduce risk, or *risk modifiers*. Included in the latter category are aspirin and other affordable preventive medications that have been added to the list of interventions because of their proven ability to lower the risk of future events.

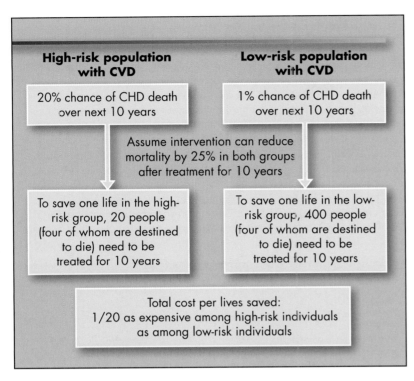

High-risk population with CVD

20% chance of CHD death over next 10 years

Assume intervention can reduce mortality by 25% in both groups after treatment for 10 years

To save one life in the high-risk group, 20 people (four of whom are destined to die) need to be treated for 10 years

Low-risk population with CVD

1% chance of CHD death over next 10 years

To save one life in the low-risk group, 400 people (four of whom are destined to die) need to be treated for 10 years

Total cost per lives saved: 1/20 as expensive among high-risk individuals as among low-risk individuals

Figure 27-8.
Why do we need to predict risk? Determining absolute risk is helpful in measuring the cost efficacy of any intervention. Because absolute risk is higher among those with known disease than among those at lower risk, fewer high-risk individuals require treatment to save one life or prevent one event, even if relative risk reductions are identical in both groups. Consequently, the National Cholesterol Education Program Adult Treatment Panel III and the Seventh Joint National Committee on Prevention, Detection, Evaluation, and Treatment of High Blood Pressure now use some assessment of absolute risk to gauge the intensity of intervention [3,4]. The American Diabetes Association also recommends a tiered approach based on absolute risk [5].

As illustrated here, if high-risk individuals can be successfully identified, the number needed to treat will be much lower, resulting in a significant cost savings. If an intervention is assumed to lower the relative risk of coronary heart disease (CHD) in high- and low-risk populations equally, then how many high-risk and low-risk patients will be needed to treat to save one life? For a high-risk patient with a 20% chance of a CHD death over the next 10 years, one needs to treat only 20 patients for 10 years. Among those 20, one of four who were destined to die (20% chance) will survive (25% risk reduction). However, one needs to treat 400 low-risk patients to save one life. Again, among these 400, one of four who were destined to die (20% chance) will survive (25% risk reduction). Thus, the cost of saving a life in the low-risk group is 20 times that in the high-risk group. This clearly illustrates the utility of understanding the risk of a given patient as a guide to using interventions. The cutpoints in current guidelines often take this into account. CVD—cardiovascular disease.

Overall Risk Assessment Tools

Framingham Risk Score
European Society of Cardiology risk tables
PROCAM risk score

Figure 27-9.
Overall risk assessment tools. As mentioned previously, the first step to developing a prevention program for a given patient is to assess his or her overall risk. There are several tools available for assessing overall risk. Each of these tools uses several easily measurable risk factors and generates an estimate of longer-term risk. The Framingham Risk Score uses gender, smoking, age, blood pressure, total and high-density lipoprotein level to estimate 10-year coronary heart disease risk.

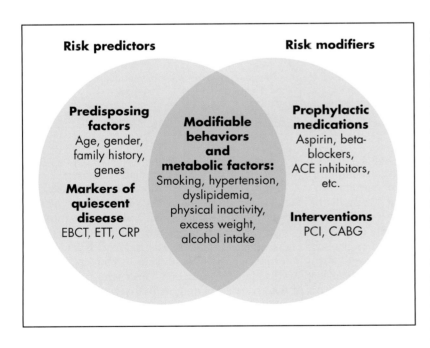

Risk predictors

Predisposing factors
Age, gender, family history, genes
Markers of quiescent disease
EBCT, ETT, CRP

Modifiable behaviors and metabolic factors:
Smoking, hypertension, dyslipidemia, physical inactivity, excess weight, alcohol intake

Risk modifiers

Prophylactic medications
Aspirin, beta-blockers, ACE inhibitors, etc.

Interventions
PCI, CABG

Figure 27-10.
The factors that predict risk can be divided into three categories: predisposing factors, modifiable behaviors and metabolic factors, and markers of quiescent disease. The factors that reduce risk can also be divided into three basic categories: modifiable behaviors and metabolic factors, prophylactic medications, and aggressive interventions. Although useful, these categories are somewhat arbitrary, and, at times, it may be difficult to classify a factor in a distinct category. For example, is hypertension a metabolic risk factor that results in part from the influence of risk-modifying behaviors, such as an atherosclerotic diet or physical inactivity, or is it a marker of endothelial dysfunction and atherosclerosis? Similarly, an inflammatory state as measured by high-sensitivity C-reactive protein (CRP) could be considered as a metabolic intermediate, such as high cholesterol, or may be a marker of ongoing atherosclerosis. Useful factors that predict risk are those that are easily obtained and easily measured and are prevalent enough in the population to warrant screening. Risk assessment should include nonmodifiable factors, such as age, gender, and family history of premature coronary disease, as well as modifiable factors, such as smoking, hypertension, dyslipidemia, excess weight, and physical inactivity. As we will see, many of these factors coexist. So, when building a prediction model such as the Framingham Risk Score, once we have half a dozen or so factors, our model will not be greatly enhanced by the inclusion of more factors. One piece of additional information that can be very useful in predicting future disease is whether the patient has known disease. ACE—angiotensin-converting enzyme; CABG—coronary artery bypass graft; EBCT—electron-beam computed tomography; ETT—exercise tolerance test; PCI—percutaneous coronary intervention.

Functional tools
  Exercise Tolerance Test
  Exercise Tolerance Test with imaging
Anatomic imaging
  Electron-beam CT or multi-detector CT
  LVH on echocardiogram
Biochemical markers
  C-reactive protein

Figure 27-11.
Possible secondary screening tools. Once the initial screen has been completed using a score such as the Framingham Risk Score or counting risk factors, we can consider a secondary screen for those patients whose profile creates some indecision concerning the aggressiveness of the intervention. For those who are deemed very low risk, a secondary screening test will likely not change the aggressiveness with which cholesterol is lowered, for example. Similarly, a very high-risk individual's recommendations will likely not be changed because of a negative secondary screening test. Among the potential secondary screening tests are a laboratory test, such as that for high-sensitivity C-reactive protein, a functional test, such as an exercise tolerance test, a calcium score measured by electron beam CT, or even an echocardiogram to detect left ventricular hypertrophy (LHV). When considering these criteria for a good screening test, C-reactive protein has many of those characteristics.

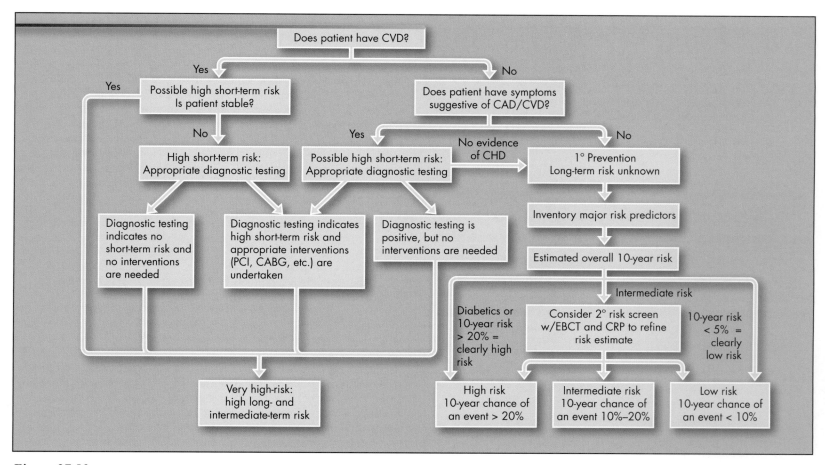

Figure 27-12.
Cardiovascular disease (CVD) risk assessment algorithm. This figure shows a scheme that can be used by clinicians to classify their patients' long-term risk of a coronary heart disease event using a few simple questions and simple office measures, such as blood pressure.

First, the clinician needs to make a distinction about high short-term risk. Patients who are unstable, and therefore have high short-term risk, need immediate referral for appropriate diagnostic testing and interventions as warranted. Once stabilized, these patients' long-term risk can be assessed. The first branch point is "Does the patient have known CVD?" and, if so, "Is it stable?" Known CVD includes prior coronary heart disease, stroke, bypass surgery, percutaneous coronary intervention (PCI), angina, or peripheral vascular disease. If the patient is stable, no further classification is necessary. This person is already at very high long-term risk and warrants the most aggressive risk factor modification. If there is an indication of instability, this patient needs to be referred for appropriate diagnostic testing (exercise tolerance testing, catheterization, and so forth) and intervention as necessary to return the patient to a stable state.

For the patient without known CVD, it is important to determine if he or she has symptoms suggestive of CVD, such as chest pain when walking up stairs. That patient also needs referral for short-term risk assessment and intervention as needed. If this testing is negative, that will return us to primary

prevention and risk assessment. If diagnosed with CVD, after appropriate intervention, this patient will be placed in the very high-risk group.

For those without CVD or symptoms, we need to first inventory major risk prediction factors, and then assess total long-term risk. For those with diabetes, long-term risk is clearly high, and they can automatically be put in the high-risk category. For those without diabetes but with a very high Framingham Risk Score that indicates greater than 20% chance of a major coronary heart disease event in 10 years, they too should be placed in this high-risk category. Those who have fewer than two risk factors or who have a Framingham 10-year risk score of less than 5% can be placed in the low-risk category.

For individuals who have intermediate risk after initial screening, particularly if they are on the cusp between high risk and intermediate risk, consider a secondary screen such as measuring C-reactive protein (CRP), an exercise tolerance test, or possibly a calcium score by electron-beam CT (EBCT). The result of this secondary test will refine the risk assessment and permit classification into one of three categories. This classification of overall risk will be used to develop a program to lower that risk. The overall level of risk is used in some guidelines to help with the decision to intervene and with the intensity of the intervention. CABG—coronary artery bypass graft; CAD—coronary artery disease; CHD—coronary heart disease.

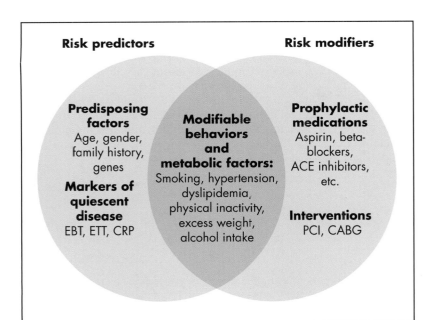

Risk predictors		Risk modifiers
Predisposing factors Age, gender, family history, genes **Markers of quiescent disease** EBT, ETT, CRP	**Modifiable behaviors and metabolic factors:** Smoking, hypertension, dyslipidemia, physical inactivity, excess weight, alcohol intake	**Prophylactic medications** Aspirin, beta-blockers, ACE inhibitors, etc. **Interventions** PCI, CABG

Figure 27-13.
Focusing on the risk modifiers, factors that are known to, or are likely to, lower risk are listed in this figure. These include modifiable behaviors and metabolic factors, such as smoking, hypertension, and alcohol intake, and prophylactic medications, such as aspirin and β-blockers, for appropriate patients. Percutaneous coronary intervention (PCI), coronary artery bypass graft (CABG), and other cardiac procedures are generally reserved for those at high near-term risk and are not generally considered as preventive strategies [6–8]. ACE—angiotensin-converting enzyme; CRP—C-reactive protein; EBT—electron-beam tomography; ETT—exercise tolerance test; PCI—percutaneous coronary intervention.

Risk Reduction Strategies

Class 1
Basic research and human observational studies indicate a clear causal relationship; intervention data (typically from randomized trials) demonstrate the magnitude of the benefit and risk; interventions are cost effective
Smoking cessation
Blood pressure management
Lipid management
Management of prophylactic medication, such as aspirin, β-blockers, and angiotensin-converting enzyme inhibitors, in selected patients
Class 2
Basic research and human observational studies indicate a clear causal relationship; intervention data from large-scale trials are limited; lack of adequate intervention data precludes determination of cost effectiveness
Weight maintenance/reduction
Physical activity
Specific dietary interventions
Control of diabetes
Class 3
Basic research and human observational studies demonstrate associations, but independent nature of a causal relationship is not yet clear; interventions are not yet available or have not been adequately tested
Interventions for psychologic factors
Other dietary modifications

Figure 27-14.
Once each individual has been classified according to his or her long-term risk, one can implement those risk-reduction strategies that make sense. Risk-reduction strategies can be prioritized into three classes, based on the strength of the association, the evidence of benefit of the intervention, and also on cost efficacy. Class 1 comprises interventions for smoking, hypertension, and other risks in which the cause and effect is well documented and the benefits of intervention are clear. For blood pressure and lipid management, the decision to treat with medications should be based on the patient's overall risk as described herewith. Class 2 interventions target obesity, diabetes, and other risks that appear to have a causal relationship with coronary heart disease and for which the data suggest that intervention will probably reduce risk, but studies regarding the benefits, risks, and costs of intervention are limited. Class 3 interventions address those risk factors for which an independent causal relationship with heart disease is suspected but as yet unproven or in which the utility of the intervention is unclear. These unproven interventions include some dietary factors, such as certain supplements, and psychosocial factors, such as having a type A personality.

The factors in Class 1 and 2 are the primary focus of our intervention efforts. However, it is very useful to be aware of some of the novel interventions in the third category because patients may read about these in the paper and have questions regarding their usefulness.

Risk Reduction Program

1. Smoking status
2. Blood pressure
3. Lipid levels
4. Prophylactic medication
5. Exercise history
6. Body weight/body mass index
7. Diabetes control history
8. Targeted dietary assessment, including alcohol

Figure 27-15.
Risk reduction program. After categorizing patients by their overall risk of future events, it is necessary to do an assessment of the Class 1 and 2 risk modifiers and to make recommendations for each in accordance with current guidelines. Fortunately, many of these have already been assessed for risk prediction. A brief history of diet and exercise is necessary to develop a plan for risk reduction. A discussion of trends in weight and realistic weight goals is also helpful. Continued monitoring and reinforcement and modification of the plan over the long term should yield substantial risk reduction for our patients.

Prevention Program

1. Assess CVD status and major risk predictors
2. Estimate overall risk using the algorithm (*see* Fig. 27-11)
3. Develop a risk reduction program using Class I and II interventions for modifiable risk factors
4. Empower the individual to track their own process
5. Monitor, reinforce, and modify the program periodically

Figure 27-16.
Prevention program. This figure summarizes the basic elements of a prevention program. This approach can be implemented by most providers with the high likelihood of success in achieving substantial risk reduction for our patients.

References

1. Pearson TA, McBride PE, Miller NH, *et al.*: Twenty-seventh Bethesda Conference: matching the intensity of risk factor management with the hazard for coronary disease events. Task Force 8. Organization of preventive cardiology service. *J Am Coll Cardiol* 1996, 27:1039–1047.

2. Mackay J, Mensah, GA: *The Atlas of Heart Disease and Stroke.* Washington, DC: World Health Organization; 2004.

3. Third Report of the National Cholesterol Education Program (NCEP) Expert Panel on Detection, Evaluation, and Treatment of High Blood Cholesterol in Adults (Adult Treatment Panel III) final report. *Circulation* 2002, 106:3143–3421.

4. Chobanian AV, Bakris GL, Black HE, *et al.*: The Seventh Report of the Joint National Committee on Prevention, Detection, Evaluation, and Treatment of High Blood Pressure: The JNC-7 Report. *JAMA* 2003, 289:2560–2572.

5. Haffner SM: Management of dyslipidemia in adults with diabetes. *Diabetes Care* 2003, 26(suppl):S83–S86.

6. Kannel, WB, Dawber TR, Kagan A, *et al.*: Factors of risk in the development of coronary heart disease—six year follow-up experience: The Framingham Study. *Ann Intern Med* 1961, 55:33–50.

7. Wilson PW, D'Agostino RB, Levy D, *et al.*: Prediction of coronary heart disease using risk factor categories. *Circulation* 1998, 97:1837–1847.

8. Orford JL, Sesso HD, Stedman M, *et al.*: A comparison of the Framingham and European Society of Cardiology coronary heart disease risk prediction models in the normative aging study. *Am Heart J* 2002, 144:95–100.